20 058 265 88

AF606288

Cancer Immunotherapy at the Crossroads

CURRENT CLINICAL ONCOLOGY

Maurie Markman, MD, **SERIES EDITOR**

Cancer Immunotherapy at the Crossroads: *How Tumors Evade Immunity and What Can Be Done,* edited by *JAMES H. FINKE AND RONALD M. BUKOWSKI,* 2004

Treatment of Acute Leukemias: *New Directions for Clinical Research,* edited by *CHING-HON PUI,* 2003

Allogeneic Stem Cell Transplantation: *Clinical Research and Practice,* edited by *MARY J. LAUGHLIN AND HILLARD M. LAZARUN,* 2003

Chronic Leukemias and Lymphomas: *Biology, Pathophysiology, and Clinical Management,* edited by *GARY J. SCHILLER,* 2003

Colorectal Cancer: *Multimodality Management,* edited by *LEONARD SALTZ,* 2002

Breast Cancer: *A Guide to Detection and Multidisciplinary Therapy,* edited by *MICHAEL H. TOROSIAN,* 2002

Melanoma: *Biologically Targeted Therapeutics,* edited by *ERNEST C. BORDEN,* 2002

Cancer of the Lung: *From Molecular Biology to Treatment Guidelines,* edited by *ALAN B. WEITBERG,* 2001

Renal Cell Carcinoma: *Molecular Biology, Immunology, and Clinical Management,* edited by *RONALD M. BUKOWSKI AND ANDREW NOVICK,* 2000

Current Controversies in Bone Marrow Transplantation, edited by *BRIAN J. BOLWELL,* 2000

Regional Chemotherapy: *Clinical Research and Practice,* edtied by *MAURIE MARKMAN,* 2000

Intraoperative Irradiation: *Techniques and Results,* edited by *L. L. GUNDERSON, C. G. WILLETT, L. B. HARRISON, AND F. A. CALVO,* 1999

Cancer Immunotherapy at the Crossroads

How Tumors Evade Immunity and What Can Be Done

Edited by

James H. Finke, PhD

and

Ronald M. Bukowski, MD

Cleveland Clinic Foundation,
Cleveland, OH

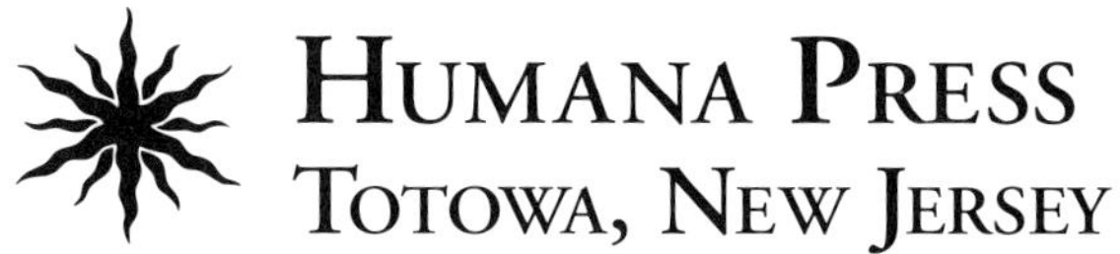

999 Riverview Drive, Suite 208
Totowa, New Jersey 07512
www.humanapress.com

For additional copies, pricing for bulk purchases, and/or information about other Humana titles, contact Humana at the above address or at any of the following numbers: Tel.: 973-256-1699; Fax: 973-256-8341, E-mail: humana@humanapr.com; or visit our Website: humanapress.com

Production Editor: Mark J. Breaugh.

Cover Illustration: Association of abnormalities in HLA class I antigen expression with tumor-cell differentiation. See Fig. 3 on p. 8.

Cover design by Patricia F. Cleary.

This publication is printed on acid-free paper. ∞
ANSI Z39.48-1984 (American National Standards Institute) Permanence of Paper for Printed Library Materials.

Printed in the United States of America. 10 9 8 7 6 5 4 3 2 1

E-ISBN: 1-59259-743-2

Library of Congress Cataloging-in-Publication Data

Cancer immunotherapy at the crossroads : how tumors evade immunity and what can be done / edited by James H. Finke and Ronald M. Bukowski.
p. ; cm. -- (Current clinical oncology)
Includes bibliographical references and index.
ISBN 1-58829-183-9 (alk. paper)
1. Cancer--Immunological aspects. 2. Cancer--Immunotherapy.
[DNLM: 1. Neoplasms--therapy. 2. Antibody Formation. 3. Immunity, Cellular. 4. Immunotherapy--methods. 5. Neoplasms--immunology. 6. T-Lymphocytes--immunology. QZ 266 C2145 2003] I. Finke, James H., 1944- II. Bukowski, Ronald M. III. Current clinical oncology (Totowa, N.J.)
RC268.3.C346 2003
616.99'4079--dc21

2003014354

Dedication

This book is dedicated to my wife (Jeane) and to my parents (Lillian and Bill Finke) for their never-ending support and encouragement.

Preface

The immune system plays a critical role in controlling and eliminating infectious organisms, including many pathogenic bacteria and viruses. More controversial has been the debate pertaining to whether the immune system can effectively control tumor growth and metastases. However, many studies suggest that appropriate activation of the immune system can lead to tumor regressions in experimental animal models. Thus, there is significant interest in harnessing the immune system for the treatment of tumors. The main focus of immunotherapy has been on T lymphocytes, since they have been shown to be the major effector cells in various animal tumor models. Removal of T cells typically eliminates the antitumor activity of most therapeutic approaches, while conversely, the adoptive transfer of tumor-reactive T cells mediates regression of malignant lesions. Furthermore, in several histologically distinct types of human tumors, the degree of T-cell infiltrate demonstrated a positive correlation with patient survival, suggesting a role for these cells in controlling malignant growth.

Significant progress has been made in the past several decades in our understanding of the host immune response to tumors. This has included: (1) identification of antigens expressed on human tumors as well as epitopes from these proteins that can serve as targets for the $CD4^+$ and $CD8^+$ T-cell populations; (2) defining and characterizing antigen presenting cells (e.g., dendritic cells), and the co-stimulatory requirements for effective peptide presentation; (3) identifying the role various cytokines play in regulating cellular and humoral immune responses; and (4) understanding the intracellular signaling pathways that control T and APC differentiation, effector functional and survival. There have also been important advances in our ability to monitor antitumor immune responses in tumor-bearing hosts. This has included the use of major histocompatibility complex (MHC)-tetramers to detect antigen-specific T cells in the blood and tumor, as well as the development of techniques to measure cytokine expression by subsets of T cells (ELISPOT, flow cytometry-based intracellular staining, and real-time PCR). These insights are leading to new approaches in immunotherapy, and to more precise ways of assessing the impact that such therapy has on antitumor effector T cells.

Prior clinical trials employing cytokines (IL-2 and IL-12) and interferons alone, or in different combinations, have demonstrated antitumor activity in select sets of patients. Overall, the response rate in patients with advanced disease has been in the 10–20% range. More recent clinical studies using various vaccine strategies (peptides, peptide-pulsed dendritic cells, etc.) have demonstrated an ability to increase the frequency of tumor reactive T cells in the blood and in tumors. However, in the majority of these trials, the modest antitumor activity observed was not commensurate with the augmented number of effector cells. Although these studies suggest that boosting T cell-mediated antitumor immunity has some clinical activity, it currently is beneficial only to a minority of patients. It seems plausible that the effectiveness of immunotherapy will continue to improve as we develop more effective means of enhancing the appropriate effector cells through our better understanding of the tumor immune response at both the cellular and molecular levels. There is growing evidence, however, that tumors can evade the immune system by multiple mechanisms, each potentially representing a significant barrier to immunotherapy. Thus, understanding these processes may be critical to implementing new and more effective forms of immunotherapy.

It has been well documented that the tumor environment can have a negative impact on the development of an effective antitumor immune response. This concept is illustrated by the fact that a significant number of T cells infiltrating human tumors are functionally impaired in their ability to proliferate and mediate important effector functions. Furthermore, impaired immune function, including unresponsiveness to recall antigens, has been noted in peripheral blood T cells, suggesting that systemic effects can occur in cancer patients. There is also evidence to suggest that the antigen-specific T-cell response to some tumor antigens is impaired.

Part I of *Cancer Immunotherapy at the Crossroads: How Tumors Evade Immunity and What Can Be Done* outlines the basic mechanisms that may be operative in cancer patients that contribute to the poor development of antitumor immune responses. Tumors may escape detection by immune cells owing to defective MHC expression and/or antigen processing by the tumor, or because the tumors fail to migrate or interact with T cells at secondary lymphoid organs. Tumors may also evade the immune system by directly or indirectly modulating the normal activation and signaling cascades of immune cells. Indeed, tumors can alter the differentiation and function of dendritic cells, resulting in ineffective antigen presentation, and hence causing T-cell unresponsiveness or anergy. Thus, the tumor environment can impair both CD4+ helper and CD8+ effector T-cell responses. Also discussed within these chapters is the involvement of immunosuppressive products produced either by the tumor or the immune cells themselves, which are likely responsible for some of the immune dysfunction observed in both the antigen-presenting cells and T cells. It is also becoming clear that the tumor environment may alter the sensitivity of T cells and dendritic cells to programmed cell death, or apoptosis. This may occur as a natural response to antigen, leading to activation-induced cell death, or by the elaboration of tumor products that directly sensitize or induce apoptosis in immune cells.

Several chapters address mechanisms of optimizing antigen presentation and the delivery of T cells to tumor sites as well as ways to promote their survival. These modifications appear to enhance T-cell effector function and may render tumors less capable of immune evasion. Also discussed is the notion that malignant cells utilize some of the same immune escape mechanisms employed by various pathogens, suggesting that lessons learned from the study of infectious diseases may benefit the understanding of immune dysfunction in cancer. Although the majority of mechanisms examined in these pages focus on the tumor-induced dysfunction of immune cells, also included is a chapter appraising molecular alterations within the tumor cells themselves that afford resistance to apoptosis. These modifications enhance not only the resistance of tumors to immune-mediated attack, but also may significantly reduce their susceptibility to radiation and chemotherapy.

Additional chapters address immune dysfunction and evasion mechanisms in histologically diverse human tumors. These chapters highlight both the immunosuppressive tactics common to multiple tumor types, and the unique evasive mechanisms employed by biologically and histologically distinct tumors.

In Part II, the clinical relevance of immune evasion is reviewed. The functional and signaling defects in T cells and antigen-presenting cells and their relation to impaired antitumor immune responses and to poor clinical outcome are discussed. These investigations also ask whether measurably impaired signaling and effector function in T cells may one day serve as biomarkers for patient prognosis. These types of analysis are clearly important and suggest that defects in T cell signaling and immune function impact on clinical outcome, however, more studies are needed to address this issue.

The future development of effective immunotherapeutic protocols for treating cancer will incorporate strategies that can abrogate the mechanisms by which tumors evade the immune system in different histologic types of tumors. It is thus relevant to study and understand these evasion mechanisms in order to devise ways to prevent and/or circumvent their capacity to enhance progressive tumor growth.

James H. Finke, PhD
Ronald M. Bukowski, MD

Contents

Contributors

LEVENT BALKIR, MD, PhD • *Department of Pathology, University of Pittsburgh School of Medicine and the University of Pittsburgh Cancer Institute, Pittsburgh, PA*

RAJ K. BATRA, MD • *Division of Pulmonary and Critical Care Medicine, David Geffen School of Medicine at UCLA, Los Angeles, CA*

WILLIAM H. BROOKS, MD • *Department of Microbiology, Immunology, and Molecular Genetics, University of Kentucky Medical Center, Lexington, KY*

RONALD M. BUKOWSKI, MD • *Experimental Therapeutics Program, Taussig Cancer Center, Cleveland Clinic Foundation, Cleveland, OH*

PAUL CAIRNS, PhD • *Departments of Surgical Oncology and Pathology, Fox Chase Cancer Center, Philadelphia, PA*

MICHAEL CAMPOLI, BS • *Department of Immunology, Roswell Park Cancer Institute, Buffalo, NY*

CRISTIAN A. CARVALLO, MD • *Urologic Oncology Branch, National Cancer Institute, Bethesda, MD*

CHIEN-CHUNG CHANG, MS • *Department of Immunology, Roswell Park Cancer Institute, Buffalo, NY*

GURKAMAL S. CHATTA, MD • *Department of Medicine, University of Pittsburgh School of Medicine and the University of Pittsburgh Cancer Institute, Pittsburgh, PA*

LIEPING CHEN, MD, PhD • *Department of Immunology, Mayo Clinic, Rochester, MN*

RICHARD W. CHILDS, MD • *National Heart, Lung, and Blood Institute, National Institutes of Health, Bethesda, MD*

PETER A. COHEN, MD • *Center for Surgery Research, Cleveland Clinic Foundation, Cleveland, OH*

CYNTHIA COMBS, BS • *Department of Immunology, Lerner Research Institute, Cleveland Clinic Foundation, Cleveland, OH*

PELAYO CORREA, MD • *Department of Pathology, Stanley S. Scott Cancer Center, Louisiana State University Health Sciences Center, New Orleans, LA*

ITHAAR H. DERWEESH, MD • *Department of Immunology, Lerner Research Institute, Glickman Urological Institute, Cleveland Clinic Foundation, Cleveland, OH*

ARJAN DIEPSTRA, MD • *Department of Pathology and Laboratory Medicine, University Medical Center Groningen, Groningen, The Netherlands*

STEVEN M. DUBINETT, MD • *UCLA Lung Cancer Research Program, Division of Pulmonary and Critical Care Medicine, David Geffen School of Medicine at UCLA, Los Angeles, CA*

NICKOLAI DULIN, PhD • *Department of Medicine, The University of Chicago, Chicago, IL*

LUCINDA H. ELLIOTT, PhD • *Department of Biology, Shippensburg University, Shippensburg, PA*

PAUL ELSON, ScD • *Department of Biostatistics, Taussig Cancer Center, Cleveland Clinic Foundation, Cleveland, OH*

DEAN E. EVANS, PhD • *Earle A. Chiles Research Institute, Robert W. Franz Cancer Research Center, Providence Portland Medical Center, Portland, OR*

SOLDANO FERRONE, MD, PhD • *Department of Immunology, Roswell Park Cancer Institute, Buffalo, NY*

JAMES H. FINKE, PhD • *Department of Immunology, Lerner Research Institute, Cleveland Clinic Foundation, Cleveland, OH*

BRIAN R. GASTMAN, MD • *Department of Plastic Surgery, University of Pittsburgh School of Medicine, Pittsburgh, PA*

ERIC M. HORWITZ, MD • *Department of Radiation Oncology, Fox Chase Cancer Center, Philadelphia, PA*

MIN HUANG, MD • *Division of Pulmonary and Critical Care Medicine, David Geffen School of Medicine at UCLA, Los Angeles, CA*

ARTHUR A. HURWITZ, PhD • *Department of Microbiology and Immunology, SUNY Upstate Medical University, Syracuse, NY*

VLADIMIR KOLENKO, MD, PhD • *Department of Surgical Oncology, Fox Chase Cancer Center, Philadelphia, PA*

STEPHAN LADISCH, MD • *Center for Cancer and Immunology Research, Children's Research Institute, Children's National Medical Center; George Washington University School of Medicine, Washington, DC*

EDMUND C. LATTIME, PhD • *Departments of Surgery and Molecular Genetics, Microbiology & Immunology, UMDNJ-Robert Wood Johnson Medical School and The Cancer Institute of New Jersey, New Brunswick, NJ*

EWERTON M. MAGGIO, MD, PhD • *Department of Pathology and Laboratory Medicine, University Medical Center Groningen, The Netherlands*

JENNY T. MAO, MD • *Division of Pulmonary and Critical Care Medicine, David Geffen School of Medicine at UCLA, Los Angeles, CA*

FRANCESCO M. MARINCOLA, MD • *Immunogenetics Section, Department of Transfusion Medicine, Clinical Center, National Institutes of Health, Bethesda, MD*

LUIS MOLTO, MD, PhD • *Servicio de Immunologia, Hospital Clinico San Carlos, Madrid, Spain*

CHRISTINA MOON, BS • *Lerner Research Institute, Department of Immunology, Cleveland Clinic Foundation, Cleveland, OH*
LORRI A. MORFORD, PhD • *Department of Microbiology, Immunology and Molecular Genetics, University of Kentucky Medical Center, Lexington, KY*
AUGUSTO C. OCHOA, MD • *Tumor Immunology Program, Stanley S. Scott Cancer Center, Department of Pediatrics, Louisiana State University Health Sciences Center, New Orleans, LA*
THOMAS OLENCKI, DO • *Experimental Therapeutics Program, Taussig Cancer Center, Cleveland Clinic Foundation, Cleveland, OH*
LORI PEREZ • *Department of Pathology, University of Pittsburgh School of Medicine and the University of Pittsburgh Cancer Institute, Pittsburgh, PA*
GREGORY E. PLAUTZ, MD • *Center for Surgery Research, Cleveland Clinic Foundation, Cleveland, OH*
ALAN POLLACK, MD, PhD • *Department Radiation Oncology, Fox Chase Cancer Center, Philadelphia, PA*
SIBRAND POPPEMA, MD, PhD • *Department of Pathology and Laboratory Medicine, University Medical Center Groningen, The Netherlands*
HANNAH RABINOWICH, PhD • *Department of Pathology, University of Pittsburgh School of Medicine and the University of Pittsburgh Cancer Institute, Pittsburgh, PA*
PATRICIA RAYMAN, MS • *Department of Immunology, Lerner Research Institute, Cleveland Clinic Foundation, Cleveland, OH*
DANIEL RE, MD • *Molecular Tumor Biology and Tumor Immunology Laboratory, Department of Internal Medicine I, University Cologne, Cologne, Germany*
PAULO C. RODRIGUEZ, MSc • *Tumor Immunology Program, Stanley S. Scott Cancer Center, Louisiana State University Health Sciences Center, New Orleans, LA*
THOMAS L. ROSZMAN, PhD • *Department of Microbiology, Immunology and Molecular Genetics, University of Kentucky Medical Center, Lexington, KY*
JOACHIM L. SCHULTZE, MD • *Molecular Tumor Biology and Tumor Immunology Laboratory, Department of Internal Medicine I, University Cologne, Cologne, Germany*
SHERVEN SHARMA, PhD • *Division of Pulmonary and Critical Care Medicine, David Geffen School of Medicine at UCLA, Los Angeles, CA*
SUYU SHU, PhD, *Center for Surgery Research, Cleveland Clinic Foundation, Cleveland, OH*
GALINA V. SHURIN, PhD • *Department of Pathology, University of Pittsburgh School of Medicine and the University of Pittsburgh Cancer Institute, Pittsburgh, PA*

MICHAEL R. SHURIN, MD, PhD • *Department of Pathology and Immunology, University of Pittsburgh School of Medicine and the University of Pittsburgh Cancer Institute, Pittsburgh, PA*

WALTER J. STORKUS, PhD • *Department of Surgery, University of Pittsburgh School of Medicine and the University of Pittsburgh Cancer Institute, Pittsburgh, PA*

KOJI TAMADA, MD • *Department of Immunology, Mayo Clinic, Rochester, MN*

CHARLES TANNENBAUM, PhD • *Department of Immunology, Lerner Research Institute, Cleveland Clinic Foundation, Cleveland, OH*

TOMOHIDE TATSUMI, MD, PhD • *Department of Surgery, University of Pittsburgh School of Medicine and the University of Pittsburgh Cancer Institute, Pittsburgh, PA*

IRINA L. TOURKOVA, PhD • *Department of Pathology, University of Pittsburgh School of Medicine and the University of Pittsburgh Cancer Institute, Pittsburgh, PA*

ROBERT G. UZZO, MD • *Division of Urology, Department of Surgical Oncology, Fox Chase Cancer Center, Philadelphia, PA*

ANKE VAN DEN BERG, PhD • *Department of Pathology and Laboratory Medicine, University Medical Center Groningen, Groningen, The Netherlands*

MICHAEL VON BERGWELT-BAILDON, MD, PhD • *Molecular Tumor Biology and Tumor Immunology Laboratory, Department of Internal Medicine I, University Cologne, Cologne, Germany*

ENA WANG, MD • *Immunogenetics Section, Department of Transfusion Medicine, Clinical Center, National Institutes of Health, Bethesda, MD*

XIN-HUI WANG, MD, PhD • *Department of Immunology, Roswell Park Cancer Institute, Buffalo, NY*

ANDREW D. WEINBERG, PhD • *Earle A. Chiles Research Institute, Robert W. Franz Cancer Research Center, Providence Portland Medical Center, Portland, OR*

AMY WESA, PhD • *Department of Surgery, University of Pittsburgh School of Medicine and the University of Pittsburgh Cancer Institute, Pittsburgh, PA*

THERESA L. WHITESIDE, PhD • *Departments of Pathology, Immunology, and Otolaryngology, University of Pittsburgh School of Medicine and the University of Pittsburgh Cancer Institute, Pittsburgh, PA*

JÜRGEN WOLF, MD • *Molecular Tumor Biology and Tumor Immunology Laboratory, Department of Internal Medicine I, University Cologne, Cologne, Germany*

ARVIN S. YANG, PhD • *Departments of Surgery and Molecular Genetics, Microbiology and Immunology, UMDNJ-Robert Wood Johnson Medical School and The Cancer Institute of New Jersey, New Brunswick, NJ*

ZOYA R. YURKOVETSKY, PhD • *Department of Molecular Genetics and Biochemistry, University of Pittsburgh School of Medicine and the University of Pittsburgh Cancer Institute, Pittsburgh, PA*

JOVANNY ZABALETA, MSc • *Tumor Immunology Program, Stanley S. Scott Cancer Center, Louisiana State University Health Sciences Center, New Orleans, LA*

THOMAS ZANDER, MD • *Molecular Tumor Biology and Tumor Immunology Laboratory, Department of Internal Medicine I, University Cologne, Cologne, Germany*

ARNOLD H. ZEA, PhD • *Department of Microbiology, Stanley S. Scott Cancer Center, Louisiana State University Health Sciences Center, New Orleans, LA*

I Basic Mechanisms of Immune Evasion

1 HLA Class I Antigen-Processing Machinery and HLA Class I Antigen-Derived Peptide-Complex Defects in Tumor-Cell Escape

Michael Campoli, BS,
Chien-Chung Chang, MS,
Xin-Hui Wang, MD, PhD,
and Soldano Ferrone, MD, PhD

CONTENTS

1. INTRODUCTION

The rationale behind the use of T-cell-based immunotherapy for the treatment of solid tumors relies on the convincing evidence in animal model systems *(1)* and more recently in patients with cutaneous melanoma *(2,3)* that major histocompatibility complex (MHC) class I antigen-restricted, tumor-associated antigen (TAA)-specific cytotoxic T lymphocytes (CTLs) control tumor growth. Taking advantage of the many TAA identified in malignant cells *(4–6)* and of the multiple strategies to enhance an immune response *(7–11)*, a

From: *Current Clinical Oncology: Cancer Immunotherapy at the Crossroads: How Tumors Evade Immunity and What Can Be Done*
Edited by: J. H. Finke and R. M. Bukowski © Humana Press Inc., Totowa, NJ

number of clinical trials designed to induce CTL-mediated immune responses in patients with malignant disease have been implemented *(12)*. Contrary to the expectations, clinical response rates have only been observed in a limited number of patients (10–30%) *(12)*. With the exception of the results reported by Boon and colleagues *(13,14)*, the general evidence has been that results of immunomonitoring assays in patients with active specific immunotherapy have poor, if any, predictive value *(12)* and that lack of clinical response and/or recurrence of disease occur frequently, despite induction and/or persistence of TAA-specific immune responses *(12)*. Considering the genetic instability of tumor cells *(15)*, this discrepancy is likely to reflect the ability of malignant cells to escape from immune recognition and destruction. Therefore, one of the major challenges facing tumor immunologists is the characterization of the molecular mechanisms by which tumor cells evade immune recognition and destruction and the development of strategies to counteract these escape mechanisms.

Through the efforts of many investigators, a number of escape mechanisms have been identified and characterized, as evidenced by recent reviews on this topic *(16–18)*. We have primarily focused our investigations on the analysis of defects in the expression and/or function of HLA class I antigens in malignant cells, because of the critical role these antigens play in the presentation of TAA-derived peptides to TAA-specific CTLs *(19)*, as well as their ability to modulate the interactions of natural killer (NK) cells *(20)* and T-cell subpopulations *(21,22)* with target cells (Fig. 1). In this chapter, we first summarize the available information about abnormalities in HLA class I antigen expression in malignant cells, the underlying molecular defects, and their potential clinical significance. Then, we address the question of whether the evaluation of HLA class I antigen expression by tumor cells represents a reliable measure of the actual level of HLA class I antigen-TAA-derived peptide complexes on the

---

Fig. 1. *(see facing page)* Generation and interaction of HLA class I antigen-peptide complexes with T cells and NK cells. Intracellular protein antigens, which are mostly endogenous, are marked for ubiquitination within the cytosol, and are subsequently degraded into peptides by the proteasome. Peptides are then transported into the ER through TAP. Nascent, HLA class I antigen heavy chains are synthesized in the ER, and these associate with the chaperone immunoglobulin heavy-chain binding protein (BiP), a universal ER chaperone involved in the translation and insertion of proteins into the ER. Following insertion into the ER, the HLA class I heavy-chain associates with the chaperone calnexin and the thiol-dependent reductase E*Rp57*. Calnexin dissociation is followed by HLA class I heavy-chain association with $\beta_2 m$, tapasin, and the chaperone calreticulin. Calnexin, calreticulin, and ER*p57* play a role in folding of the HLA class I heavy chain. Tapasin brings the HLA class I heavy-chain $\beta_2 m$, chaperone complex into association with TAP, and plays a role in both quantitative and qualitative peptide selection. The trimeric HLA class I-β_2m-peptide complex is then transported to the plasma membrane, where it plays a major role in the interactions between target cells and (*a*) activation of peptide-specific CTL through TCR; (*b*) inhibition of T-cell subpopulations through inhibitory receptors KIR or (*c*) CD94/NKG2A *(21,22)*; (*d*) inhibition of NK cell-mediated killing through KIR *(20)*.

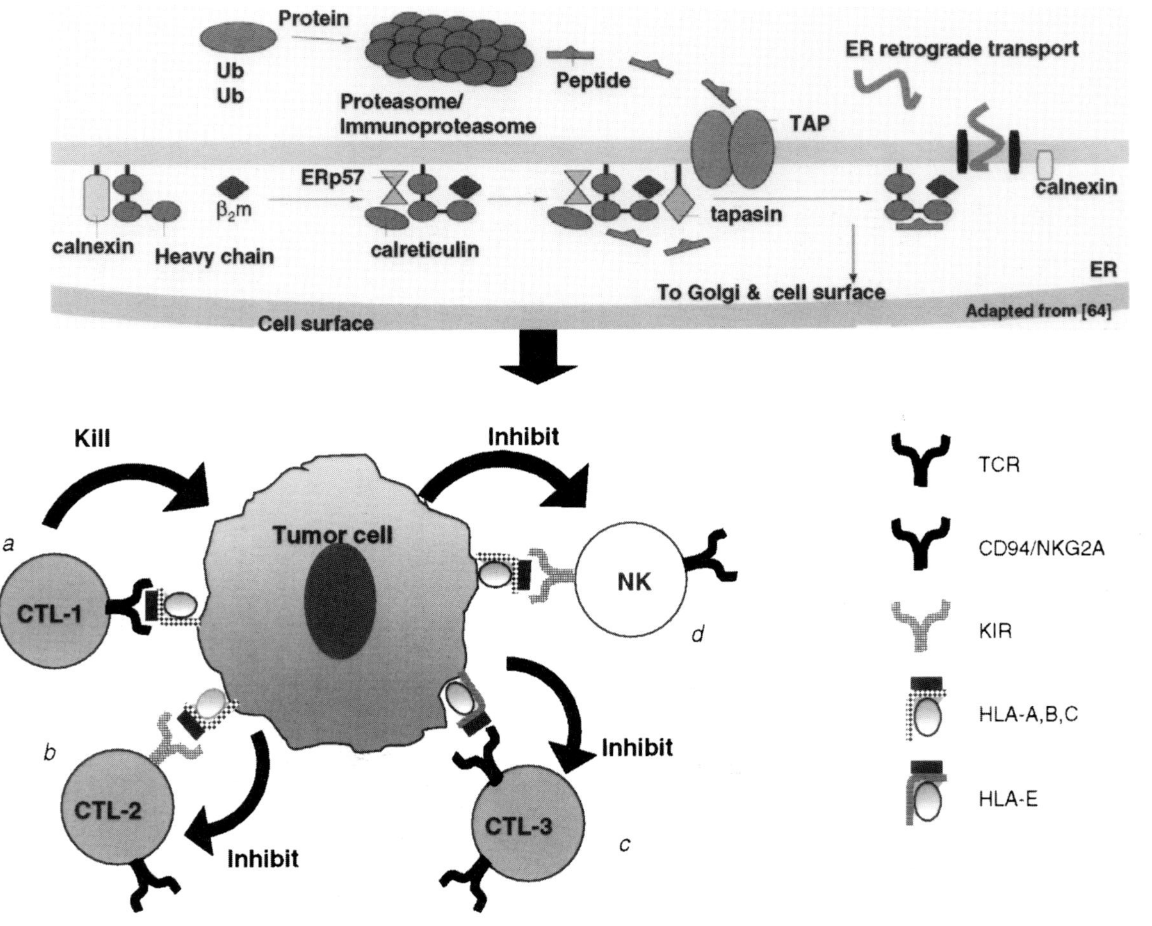

Protein
Ub
Ub
Proteasome/
Immunoproteasome
Peptide
TAP
ER retrograde transport
calnexin
Heavy chain
β_2m
ERp57
calreticulin
tapasin
calnexin
ER
To Golgi & cell surface
Cell surface
Adapted from [64]
Kill
Inhibit
Tumor cell
a
CTL-1
NK
d
b
CTL-2
Inhibit
CTL-3
Inhibit
c
TCR
CD94/NKG2A
KIR
HLA-A,B,C
HLA-E

surface of tumor cells. Finally, we discuss strategies used to develop probes to measure HLA class I antigen-TAA-derived peptide complex expression on the surface of tumor cells and the questions that have not remain to be addressed in order to develop, from the available probes, reagents useful to select and monitor patients to be treated with T-cell-based immunotherapy.

2. HLA CLASS I ANTIGEN DEFECTS IN MALIGNANT LESIONS

2.1. Detection and Frequency of Abnormalities

The analysis of cell lines in long-term culture, through a combination of binding and immunochemical assays, has identified distinct defects in the expression of HLA class I antigens in tumor cells *(23)*. These include i) total loss of the gene products of HLA-A, B, and C loci; ii) total downregulation of all HLA class I antigens expressed by a cell; iii) total loss of the HLA class I antigens encoded in one haplotype; iv) selective downregulation of the gene products of one HLA class I locus; v) selective loss of one HLA class I allospecificity; and vi) a combination of the previously mentioned defects (Fig. 2). These defects do not represent artifacts of in vitro cell culture, since they have also been identified in surgically removed tumors by immunohistochemical staining with monoclonal antibodies (MAbs). A large number of lesions removed from patients with different types of tumors have been analyzed over the years *(16,23)*. Most of the studies have utilized frozen tissue sections as substrates in immunohistochemical staining because the determinants recognized by the large majority of the available anti-HLA class I antigen MAbs are lost during the fixation procedure. More recently, MAbs that detect monomorphic determinants of HLA class I antigens in formalin-fixed, paraffin-embedded tissues have been identified (*16*; Fig. 3). These reagents have enabled the use of formalin-fixed, paraffin-embedded tissues to analyze HLA class I antigen expression in surgically removed tumors, thus facilitating the use of archived clinical samples in retrospective studies. It is hoped that the availability of this methodological improvement will facilitate the participation of pathologists in the analysis of HLA class I antigen expression in malignant tumors, since formalin-fixed, paraffin-embedded tissues represent the substrate of choice in immunohistochemical reactions in departments of pathology. Nevertheless, it should be emphasized that frozen tissue sections have not yet been used as substrates in order to characterize HLA class I allospecificity expression, since the polymorphic determinants that identify each allospecificity are conformational in nature and are lost during the fixation of tissues with formalin and their embedding with paraffin.

The immunohistochemical technique has proven to be very valuable in the analysis of HLA class I antigen expression in surgically removed tumors, yet it suffers from three limitations. First, the evaluation of results is subjective.

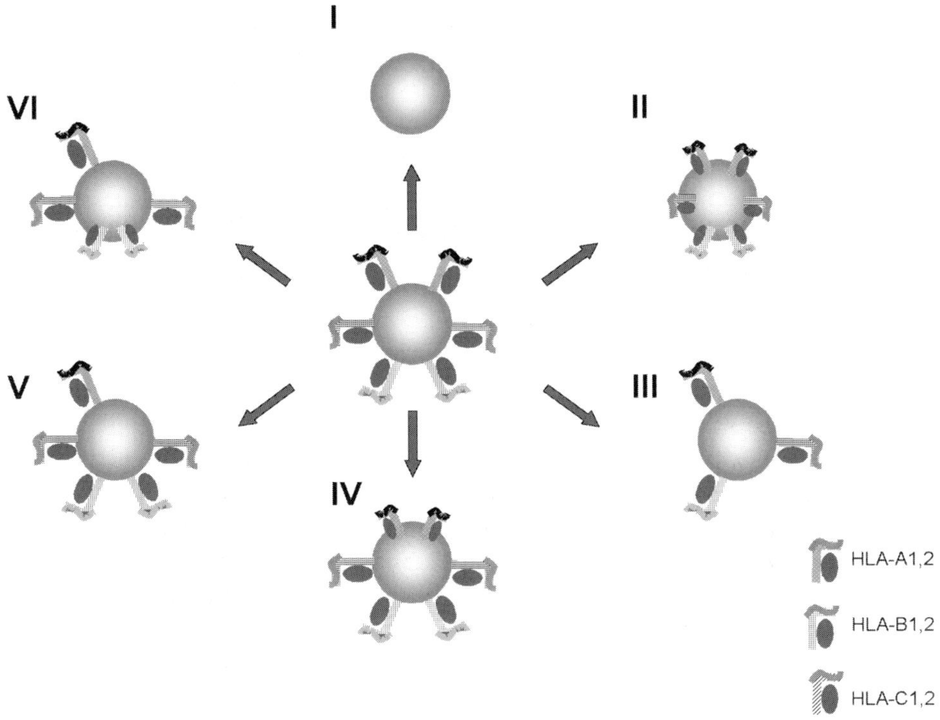

Fig. 2. Defective HLA class I phenotypes identified in malignant cells. The phenotypes identified in tumor cells include: (I) total loss of the gene products of the HLA-A, B and C loci; (II) total downregulation of all HLA class I antigens expressed by a cell; (III) total loss of all HLA class I antigens encoded in one haplotype; (IV) selective downregulation of the gene products of one HLA class I locus; (V) selective loss of one HLA class I allospecificity; or (VI) complex phenotype resulting from a combination of two or more of the described phenotypes.

This limitation is likely to be overcome in the near future by the development of equipment for computer-based reading of immunohistochemical staining. Second, the differentiation between total HLA class I antigen loss and marked downregulation is difficult to evaluate because of the technical limitations. Finally, it is not known whether the lack of staining of tumor cells by anti-HLA class I antigen MAbs in immunohistochemical reactions is a reliable predictor of tumor-cell resistance to TAA-specific CTL-mediated lysis, since no study has compared the sensitivity of antibody-based and CTL-based assays to detect HLA class I antigens on the cell membrane. Furthermore, HLA class I antigen expression does not represent the only requirement for TAA-specific CTL recognition of tumor cells, since—as discussed later—the level of HLA class I antigen expression may not correlate with that of HLA class I antigen-TAA-derived peptide complex expression on tumor cells.

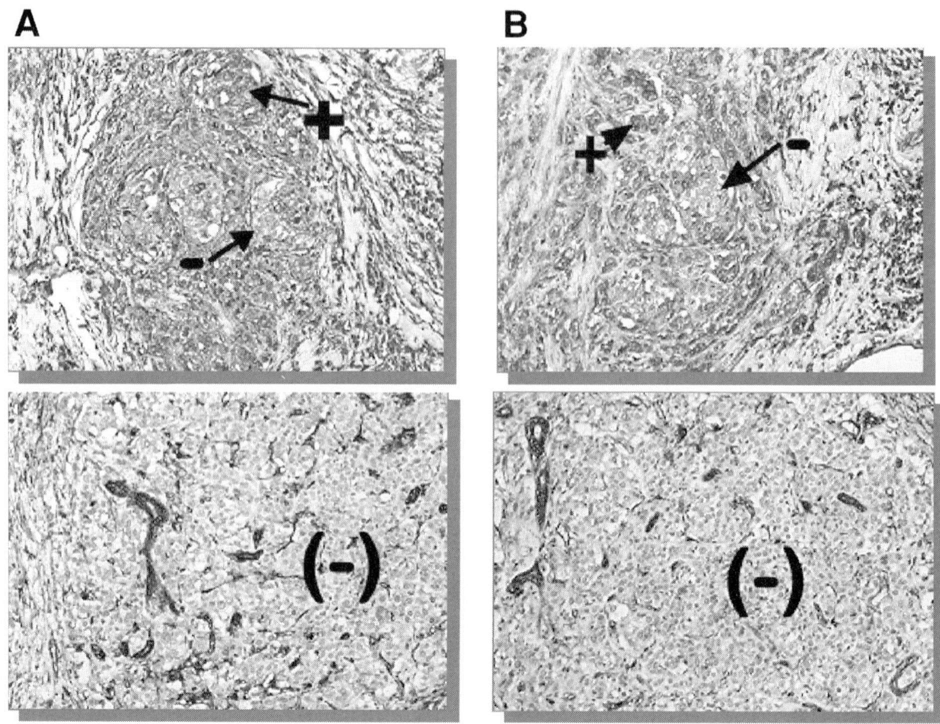

Fig. 3. Association of abnormalities in HLA class I antigen expression with tumor-cell differentiation. Serial formalin-fixed, paraffin-embeded sections of a breast carcinoma lesion were stained with **(A)** anti-HLA class I heavy-chain MAb HC-10 and **(B)** anti-$\beta_2 m$ MAb L368 in the immunohistochemical reaction. Heterogeneous (+/–) HLA class I antigen and $\beta_2 m$ expression was detected in lesions with a differentiated phenotype, and negative (–) HLA class I antigen and $\beta_2 m$ expression were found in lesions with a undifferentiated phenotype.

Convincing evidence in the literature indicates that malignant transformation of cells is associated with HLA class I antigen defects, although with different frequencies in various malignancies (Fig. 4). Data regarding the frequency of HLA class I antigen abnormalities in malignant lesions should be interpreted with caution, since not all the defective HLA class I antigen phenotypes identified in tumor-cell lines, such as selective loss of a HLA class I allospecificity, can be easily evaluated in malignant lesions. The reason for this limitation is that either MAbs with the appropriate specificity are unavailable or unsuitable for use in immunohistochemical staining. To the best of our knowledge, the only known exceptions to the general rule of HLA class I antigen loss or downregulation in malignant lesions are liver carcinoma *(24–26)* and leukemia *(27)*. In the latter, defects in HLA class I antigen expression in malignant cells have only occasionally been identified. This finding may reflect the time interval between the onset of the disease and the diagnosis, which is likely to be shorter than that usually found in solid tumors. However, the higher frequency of HLA class I antigen abnormalities in sporadic diffuse large-cell lymphoma than in immunodeficient and transplant-related lymphomas *(28)* argues against lack of an immune response to leukemic cells and of immune-selective pressure in patients with leukemia. Several studies have suggested that lack of immune-selective pressure plays a major role in the generation of malignant cell populations with HLA class I antigen abnormalities *(29–31)*. It is also unlikely that genetic and/or epigenetic changes in the gene(s) involved in HLA class I antigen expression are rare in leukemic cells, since these types of abnormalities are often found in leukemic cells *(32)*. In the liver, normal hepatocytes, which do not express or express very low levels of HLA class I antigens *(24)*, acquire the expression of these antigens during malignant transformation. This finding is likely to reflect an upregulation of these antigens by cytokines secreted by immune cells that infiltrate malignant lesions *(24)*.

2.2. Molecular Abnormalities Underlying Abnormal HLA Class I Antigen Phenotypes in Malignant Cells

Distinct molecular mechanisms have been found to be the basis of abnormalities in HLA class I antigen expression in malignant cells. The frequency of complete HLA class I antigen loss has been found to be between about 15% in primary cutaneous melanoma lesions and 50% in primary prostate carcinoma lesions (*16*; Fig. 4). These differences are likely to reflect the time between onset of tumor and diagnosis, since a long interval gives tumor cells more chances to mutate in the genes involved in HLA class I antigen expression and allows mutated cells to overgrow cells without abnormalities in their HLA class I phenotype in the presence of T-cell selective pressure. Complete HLA class I antigen loss is caused by defects in β_2-microglobulin ($\beta_2 m$), which is required for the formation of the HLA class I heavy-chain-β_2m-peptide complex and its transport to the cell membrane *(17)*. The frequency of this phenotype varies significantly between different malignancies, with breast carcinoma and prostate carcinoma demonstrating the highest frequency, and renal cell carcinoma (RCC) and cutaneous melanoma demonstrating the lowest frequency *(16)*. It should also be noted that there are conflicting reports in the literature regarding the frequency of this phenotype in head and neck squamous cell carcinoma (HNSCC) *(33,34)*. The reasons for these differences are unknown. Since two copies of the $\beta_2 m$ gene are present in each cell and only one copy is sufficient for HLA class I antigen expression, complete HLA class I antigen loss is caused by the combination of two events. One involves loss of one copy of the $\beta_2 m$ gene because of total or partial loss of chromosome 15, which carries the $\beta_2 m$ gene in humans *(35)*. The other event involves mutations in the remaining copy of the $\beta_2 m$ gene, which inhibit its transcription in a few cases and its transla-

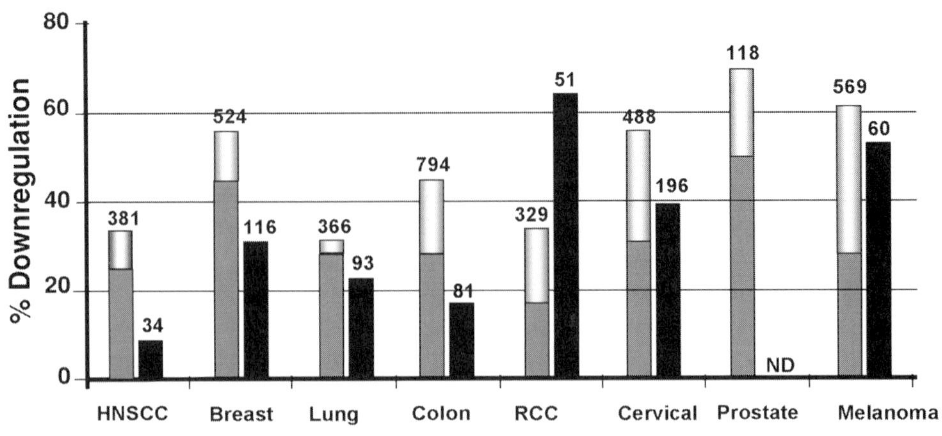

Fig. 4. Frequency of HLA class I antigen and TAP1 downregulation in malignant lesions of different embryological origin. The most common types of solid tumors for which more than 300 or 30 lesions have been analyzed for HLA class I antigen or TAP1 expression, respectively, are shown. (▒) Indicates total HLA class I antigen downregulation; (▯) indicates selective HLA class I allospecificity loss; and (■) indicates TAP1 downregulation. Figures indicate the number of lesions analyzed. ND: not determined. Data has been adapted from refs. *16,23,34,35,37,41,43,50–54,66,77–85,88,89.*

tion in most cases *(17,36–39)*. It is unknown which of these two events occurs first in malignant cells. This information will probably become available in the near future, since the analysis of tumor cells for loss of heterozygosity (LOH), which is currently widely applied to characterize malignant cells, will determine the frequency of loss of one copy of the β_2m gene in malignant cells that express HLA class I antigens.

Selective HLA class I antigen loss is caused by loss of the gene(s) encoding the lost HLA class I heavy chain(s), or by mutations that inhibit their transcription or translation. This phenotype has a higher frequency in cervical carcinoma, prostate carcinoma, and cutaneous melanoma than in HNSCC, breast carcinoma, lung carcinoma, RCC, and colon carcinoma *(16,37,40)*. The reason(s) for these differences is (are) unknown. Selective HLA class I allospecificity losses are not detected by staining of malignant cells with MAbs to monomorphic determinants of HLA class I antigens *(41,42)*. Therefore, it is expected that the frequency of this phenotype in malignant cells is higher than that described in the literature, since the expression of some HLA class I allospecificities in malignant lesions has not been evaluated because of the lack of appropriate probes. Furthermore, the methodology to detect selective HLA class I allospecificity loss, which does not require antibodies to HLA class I allospecificities *(43)*, is not suitable to test large numbers of tissue samples.

In most malignancies, the frequency of selective HLA class I antigen losses is higher than that of total HLA class I antigen losses *(16)*. This difference is likely to reflect the distinct mechanisms underlying these two phenotypes. Although two mutational events are required for total HLA class I antigen loss, only one is sufficient for selective HLA class I allospecificity loss in cells that are heterozygous for the lost allele. The mechanisms underlying selective HLA class I antigen loss include LOH of chromosome 6, which carries the HLA class I heavy-chain genes in humans *(44)*, or sequence mutations in the HLA class I heavy-chain gene. As in the case of the β_2m gene, the mutations found in HLA class I heavy chains range from large deletions to single-base deletions *(42,45–48)*. These mutations appear to occur randomly; however, LOH in the short arm of chromosome 6 appears to represent the most frequent mechanism contributing to selective HLA haplotype loss in human tumors *(49)*. Notably, selective HLA class I allospecificity loss provides a mechanism for the unexpectedly poor clinical course of the disease in some patients despite a high level of HLA class I antigen expression, as measured by staining of tumor cells with MAbs to monomorphic determinants *(16)*. In these patients, malignant cells may have acquired resistance to CTL-mediated lysis because of the selective loss of the HLA class I restricting element.

Various mechanisms have been found to cause total HLA class I antigen downregulation in different malignancies. Hypermethylation of the HLA-A, B, and C gene-promoter regions appears to represent the major mechanism of total HLA class I antigen downregulation in esophageal squamous cell carcinomas and esophageal carcinomas *(50)*. In other malignancies, total HLA class I antigen downregulation in malignant cells appears to be caused by downregulation or losses of one or multiple antigen-processing-machinery components *(16,51–53)*. The latter play a crucial role in the assembly of functional HLA class I antigen-peptide complexes and in their expression on the cell membrane (Fig. 1). Defects in antigen-processing-machinery components may affect the generation of peptides from antigens, their transport into the endoplasmic reticulum (ER), their loading on HLA class I antigens, and/or the repertoire of peptides presented by HLA class I antigens. It is noteworthy that in the majority of cases, antigen-processing-machinery component loss or downregulation can be corrected by treating cells with cytokines—e.g., IFN-γ—indicating that these abnormalities are caused by regulatory and not structural defects *(16,52)*. This mechanism may explain why the frequency of downregulation of one or multiple antigen-processing-machinery components in malignant lesions is high, despite the codominant expression of the two genes encoding each antigen-processing-machinery component. An alternative—although not exclusive—mechanism is represented by the downregulation, by IL-10, of antigen-processing-machinery components, which leads to reduced HLA class I antigen cell-surface expression *(54)*. This finding may be of clinical relevance, since a large number of human tumors secrete IL-10 *(55)*. The clinical implication of theses findings is that administration of IFN-γ and/or anti-IL-10 antibodies may enhance the efficacy of active specific immunotherapy in patients with HLA class I antigen downregulation caused by defects in the antigen-processing machinery.

To date, the information in the literature about antigen-processing-machinery component expression in various types of malignancies is sparse. To the best of our knowledge, only a few components have been analyzed, and only in a limited number of malignancies. Furthermore, there is no data concerning the quantitative levels of antigen-processing-machinery component expression in malignant cells. The lack of available information reflects the limited availability or absence of antibodies and methodology to quantitate antigen-processing-machinery components. These limitations have been overcome by the recent development of antibodies *(56)* and methodology *(57)*, which can provide quantitative information about the expression of intracellular components. Representative examples are shown in Fig. 5. Because of these limitations, most studies have utilized reverse transcription-polymerase chain reaction (RT-PCR) analysis in order to evaluate antigen-processing-machinery component expression in human tumor-cell lines *(16,52)*. Although these studies are conclusive when mRNA is not detected, they provide no information about the level and/or function of the proteins expressed when mRNA is expressed. Thus, the results of these studies should be interpreted with caution.

The generation of HLA class I antigen-TAA-derived peptide complexes begins with the cleavage of intracellular proteins into peptides by the 26S proteasome (Fig. 6). The 26S proteasome consists of four staggered heptameric rings, two outer rings composed of distinct α subunits, and two inner rings comprised of distinct β subunits, collectively known as the 20S proteasome *(58)*. The β1(delta), β2(Z) and β5 (MB1) subunits possess distinct N-terminal nucleophile hydrolase activities *(58)*. However, the 20S proteasome cannot degrade proteins unless it is complexed with the adenosine triphosphate (ATP)-dependent 19S cap, creating the 26S proteasome *(58)*. The 19S cap plays a role in the recognition and translocation of potential proteasome substrates *(58)*. The activity of the proteasome can be modulated by IFN-γ, which induces the expression of the proteasome activator 28 (PA28), also known as the 11S cap, and the exchange of the three constitutive active sites β1, β2, and β5 with the immunosubunits LMP2, LMP10 (MECL-1), and LMP7, respectively, creating the immunoproteasome (*58*; Fig. 6). PA28 and immunosubunit (LMP) expression favors the generation of antigenic peptides demonstrating increased binding affinity for HLA class I antigens and enhances the recognition of target cells

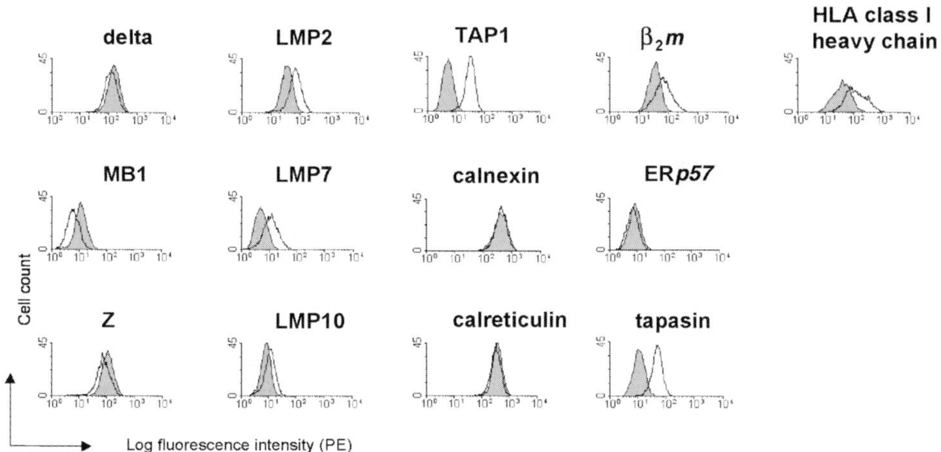

Fig. 5. Quantitative analysis of antigen-processing-machinery component expression in human uveal melanoma cells Om431. Cultured human uveal melanoma cells Om431 were analyzed for proteasome subunits delta, MB1, and Z, immunoproteasome subunits LMP2, LMP7, and LMP10, and TAP1, calnexin, calreticulin, ER*p57*, tapasin, HLA class I antigen and β_2m expression by intracytoplasmic flow cytometry with anti-delta MAb SY-5, anti-MB1 MAb SJJ-3, anti-Z MAb NB-1, anti-LMP2 MAb SY-1, anti-LMP7 MAb SY-3, anti-LMP10 MAb TO-6, anti-TAP1 MAb TO-1, anti-calnexin MAb TO-5, anti-calreticulin MAb TO-11, anti-ER*p57* MAb TO-2, anti-tapasin MAb TO-3, anti-HLA class I heavy-chain MAb HC-10, and anti-β_2m MAb L368 both prior to ( ) and following ( ) in vitro incubation of cells with IFN-γ.

by antigen-specific CTL *(58)*. However, it should be noted that some peptides, primarily those of self-origin, are not processed by the immunoproteasome *(59)*, and expression of these immunosubunits is not essential for overall antigen presentation *(58)*. It is generally assumed that immunosubunit expression is not constitutive within a cell, but induced upon exposure to cytokines such as IFN-γ, thereby increasing the number of peptides capable of binding HLA class I antigens. However, at variance with this notion, basal expression of the immunosubunits LMP2, LMP7, and LMP10 has been observed in normal cells of different histology, both in mice and in humans *(58,60,61)*. Currently, there is no information as to what constitutes normal or abnormal expression profiles of the proteasome subunits in cells, since to the best of our knowledge no study has quantitated the level of antigen-processing machinery component expression in normal cells of different embryological origin. Therefore, one must exercise caution in interpreting studies that analyze antigen-processing-machinery component expression in malignant cells, since the phenotype of the normal counterparts is unknown in many cases.

Thus far, a limited number of tumor-cell lines and human surgically removed lesions of distinct histology have been analyzed for LMP2 and LMP7 expression. When compared to normal cells, the level of LMP2 and LMP7 expression

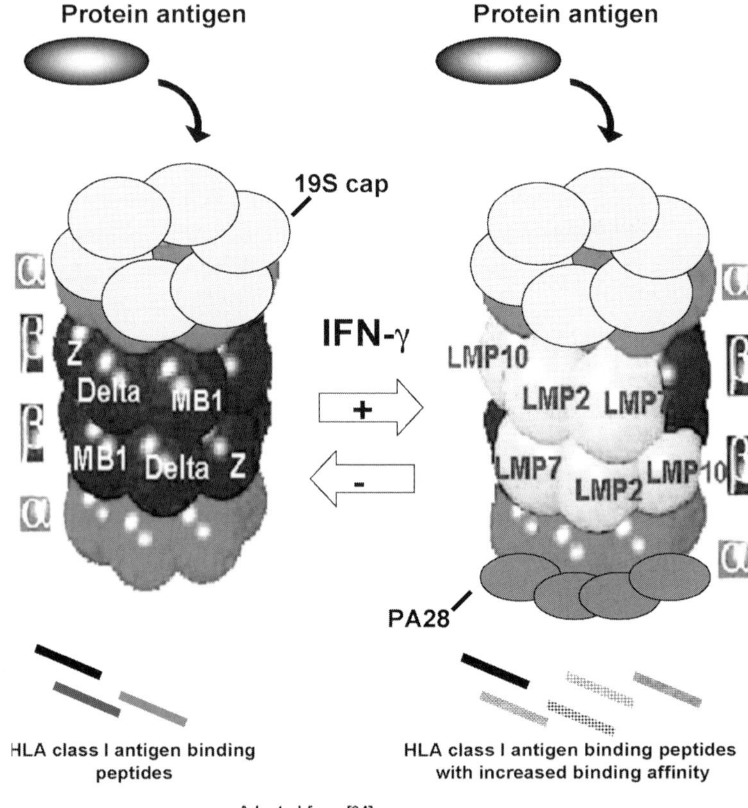

Fig. 6. Generation of high-affinity HLA class I antigen-binding peptides by the immunoproteasome. The 26S proteasome consists of four staggered heptameric rings–two outer rings comprised of distinct α subunits and two inner rings comprised of distinct β subunits, and the ATP-dependent 19S cap. The 19S cap plays a role in the recognition and translocation of potential proteasome substrates. The activity of the proteasome can be modulated by IFN-γ, which induces the expression of the proteasome activator 28 (PA28), also known as the 11S cap, and the exchange of the three constitutive active sites β1, β2, and β5 with the immunosubunits LMP2, LMP10 (MECL-1), and LMP7, respectively. Changes in both subunit composition and regulator status of the proteasome heighten the ability of the proteasome to generate peptides in terms of both quality and quantity, and are believed to be responsible for the generation of peptides with increased HLA class I antigen-binding affinity.

observed in Epstein-Barr virus (EBV)-associated Burkitt's lymphoma (BL), breast carcinoma, and RCC is impaired, whereas in several colon carcinoma cell lines only LMP2 expression appears to be downregulated *(16,51,53)*. In cutaneous melanoma, the level of LMP7 expression is downregulated, whereas that of LMP2 is elevated when compared to melanocytes in culture, which constitutively express LMP7 but not LMP2 *(16)*. Notably, these changes are not restricted to malignant transformation of melanocytes because they have also been found in nevi *(16)*. LMP10 expression has only been analyzed at the mRNA level in 39 human tumor-cell lines of different origin including breast carcinoma, small-cell lung carcinoma (SCLC), cervical carcinoma, colon carcinoma, pancreatic carcinoma, neuroblastoma, and cutaneous melanoma *(16,52,62,63)*. These studies have demonstrated LMP10 mRNA downregulation in breast carcinoma, SCLC, cervical carcinoma, neuroblastoma, and cutaneous melanoma cell lines. This deficit, which is frequently associated with antigen-processing-machinery component downregulation, is probably caused by abnormalities in regulatory mechanisms, since it could be corrected by administration of IFN-γ. The significance of impaired LMP2, LMP7, and LMP10 expression in malignant cells remains unclear because of the limitations listed here. However, the role these catalytic subunits play in the generation of TAA-derived peptides suggests that these variations may lead to alterations in the repertoire of peptides presented on HLA class I antigens by malignant cells.

Once peptides have been generated by the proteasome and further processed by cytosolic and/or ER proteases *(58)*, they are translocated into the ER by the dimeric ATP-dependent transporter associated with antigen processing (TAP1/2), which plays a role in both quantitative and qualitative peptide selection *(58)*. Among the antigen-processing-machinery components, TAP1 has been most extensively investigated. TAP1 downregulation or loss has been found in breast carcinoma, SCLC, cervical carcinoma, RCC, and cutaneous melanoma *(64,65)*. The frequency ranges from 10 to 84% in different tumor types. A few studies have investigated TAP2 expression in malignant cells, and the frequency of TAP2 downregulation usually correlates with that of TAP1 *(16)*. It is important to note that impaired TAP1 mRNA expression is usually observed in parallel with LMP2 downregulation, probably because both genes share a bi-directional promoter. Therefore, their expression may be under the control of common regulatory elements *(66)*. As mentioned previously, in some instances, TAP downregulation can be corrected by treatment with cytokines such as IFN-γ and TNF-α, and is accompanied by an increase in HLA class I antigen expression. The increase in HLA class I antigen expression following induction of TAP1 expression is correlated with an increased susceptibility to TAA-specific CTL lysis, in most but not all cases *(67–69)*. In addition, it is expected that the frequency of TAP downregulation is higher than that of total HLA class I antigen losses, because of the distinct mechanisms underlying these two phenotypes. Although two mutational events are required for total HLA class I antigen loss, TAP downregulation appears to be primarily caused by abnormalities in regulatory mechanisms. In only two cases, mutations in the *Tap1* gene have been observed. These mutations have led to altered function of the TAP1 protein itself or a lack of protein translation. An amino acid substitution was identified at position 659 (R659Q) near the ATP-binding site of *Tap1* in a human SCLC cell line *(70)*. Although this mutant TAP1 protein is expressed, it is defective in its ability to bind peptides. As a result, these cells are deficient in antigen presentation to CTL, a function that can be restored after transfection of a functional *Tap1* allele. In addition, sequence analyses of *Tap1* were isolated from the melanoma cell line buf1280, which demonstrates deficient HLA class I antigen surface expression, identified a bp deletion at position 1489 near the ATP-binding domain of *Tap1*, causing a frameshift *(71)*. This frameshift results in the early introduction of a stop codon at position 1489, leading to the lack of TAP1 and TAP2 expression. This cell line is deficient in peptide binding and transport, and is resistant to CTL-mediated lysis. These abnormalities can be corrected following transfection of cells with the wild-type *Tap1* gene, and can result in an increase in susceptibility to TAA-specific CTL.

When peptides have been translocated into the ER, subunits of HLA class I antigens—e.g., the polymorphic heavy chain and the monomorphic β_2m, which have been assembled into HLA class I antigen-β_2m dimers through the aid of multiple ER chaperones *(58)*—are brought into association with TAP through interaction with tapasin. Tapasin plays a role in both quantitative and qualitative peptide selection *(58)*. Abnormalities in tapasin expression can lead to reduced HLA class I antigen expression, alterations in the repertoire of peptides presented by HLA class I antigens and resistance of malignant cells to CTL *(58)*. Heterogeneous and reduced levels of tapasin mRNA/protein has been observed in HNSCC, SCLC, hepatoma, RCC, colon carcinoma, pancreatic carcinoma, neuroblastoma, and cutaneous melanoma cell lines (*72,73*; Fig. 7). In the majority of cases, in vitro incubation of cells with cytokines such as IFN-α, IFN-γ, TNF-α, and IL-4 has resulted in tapasin transcriptional upregulation *(72,73)*. However, in the melanoma cell line COPA159, we have identified a single-base deletion at position 684 in exon 3 of the *tapasin* gene, resulting in a reading frameshift of the mRNA with a subsequent introduction of a premature stop codon at positions 698–700. This cell line demonstrates reduced HLA class I antigen expression, which can be restored upon transfection with the wild-type *tapasin* allele (Chang et al., unpublished data). More recently, taking advantage of newly developed methodology suitable to quantitate the expression of intracellular components *(57)* and of MAbs with the appropriate characteristics *(56)*, the level of tapasin protein expression in cell lines has been quantitated (Fig. 8). These studies have shown that the level of tapasin expressed in cell lines is significantly associated with that of HLA class I antigen expression. To a limited extent, tapasin expression has been investigated in surgically removed malignant lesions. In these studies, tapasin has been found to be downregulated in both RCC and HNSCC lesions *(66,74,75)*. In the latter malignancy, this downregulation is associated with a poor prognosis *(75)*. If this is a cause-and-effect relationship, it is likely to reflect the reduced susceptibility of tumor

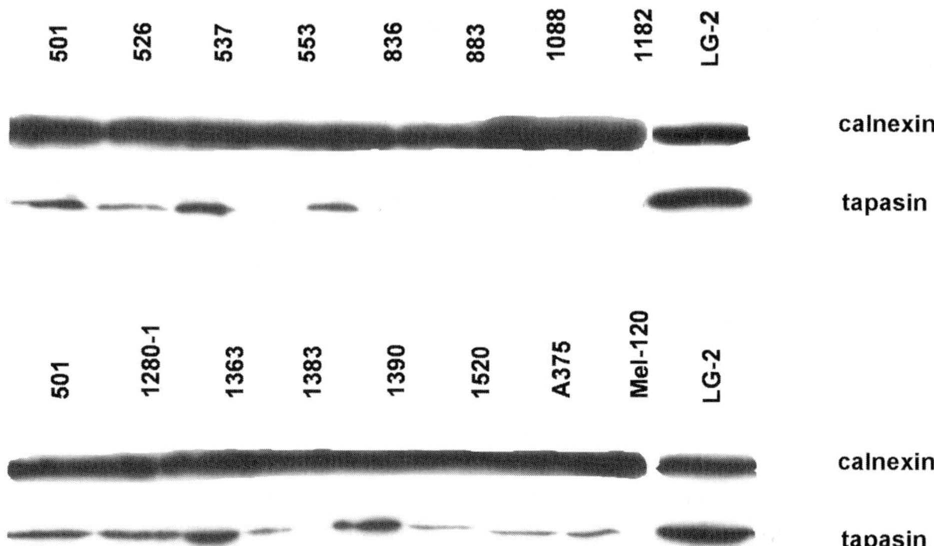

Fig. 7. Heterogeneous levels of tapasin expression in cultured human cutaneous melanoma cells. Cultured human cutaneous melanoma cells 501, 526, 537, 553, 836, 883, 1088, 1182, 1280-1, 1363, 1383, 1390, 1520, A375, and Mel-120 were analyzed for calnexin and tapasin expression by Western blot analysis with anti-calnexin MAb TO-5 and anti-tapasin MAb TO-3. The human lymphoid cell line LG-2 and the human melanoma cell line 501 were used as positive controls.

cells to CTL-mediated lysis because of HLA class I antigen downregulation and alterations in the HLA class I antigen peptide repertoire in cells with reduced tapasin expression.

2.3. Clinical Significance of HLA Class I Antigen Defects

Abnormalities in HLA class I antigen expression appear to have clinical significance, since they are associated with histopathological characteristics of the lesions and/or with clinical parameters in several malignant diseases. In general, the frequency of HLA class I antigen defects in metastatic lesions is higher than that in primary and premalignant lesions *(16)*. Furthermore, the frequency of HLA class I antigen abnormalities is significantly associated with poor histological differentiation, abnormal DNA content, and advanced clinical stage (tumor grading), each suggestive of more aggressive tumors, in primary laryngeal and hypopharyngeal carcinoma, SCLC, squamous cell carcinoma of the lung, cervical carcinoma, RCC, colon carcinoma, and cutaneous melanoma *(16,76–79)*. In prostate carcinoma, no association has been found between HLA class I antigen abnormalities and Gleason morphological grade *(80)*; however, an inverse relationship is observed between the level of HLA class I

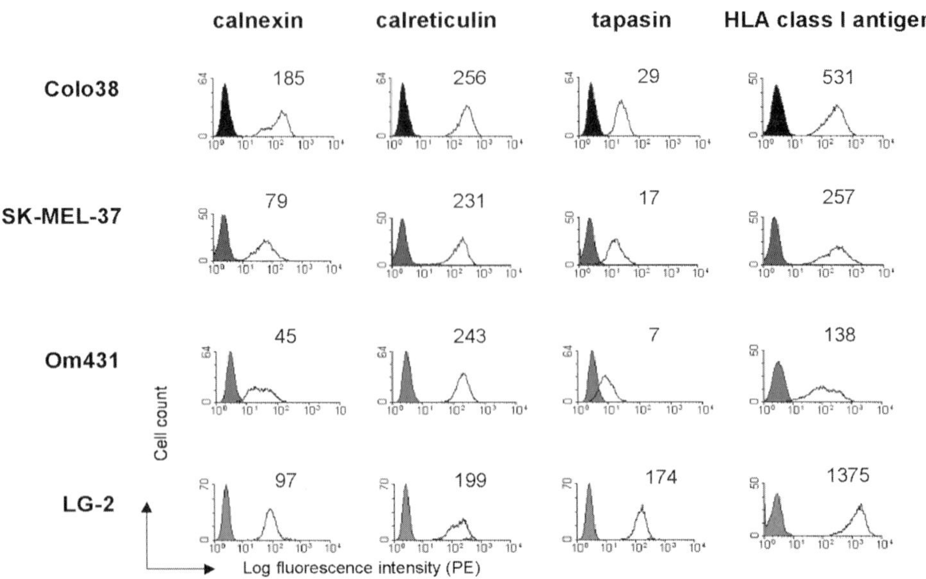

Fig. 8. Association of tapasin and HLA class I antigen levels in long-term culture melanoma cells. Cultured human cutaneous melanoma cells Colo38 and SK-MEL-37 and cultured human uveal melanoma cells Om431 were analyzed for calnexin, calreticulin, tapasin, and HLA class I antigen expression by intracytoplasmic flow cytometry with anti-calnexin MAb TO-5, anti-calreticulin MAb TO-11, anti-tapasin MAb TO-3, and anti-HLA class I heavy-chain MAb HC-10. The human lymphoid cell line LG-2 was used as a positive control.

antigen expression and degree of tumor differentiation *(81)*. It is also noteworthy that HLA-A and A2-allele loss is associated with the presence and number of tumor-positive lymph nodes in cervical carcinoma *(16)*, and total HLA class I antigen loss is associated with regional lymph-node metastases and the development of new primary aerodigestive tract cancers in HNSCC *(82)*. Moreover, the frequency of TAP1 downregulation is significantly higher in metastases than in primary lesions in breast carcinoma, cervical carcinoma, and cutaneous melanoma *(16)*. In addition, TAP1 downregulation in primary cutaneous melanoma lesions is significantly associated with the development of metastases *(83)*. Possible explanations for the association of HLA class I antigen abnormalities with later-stage and less-differentiated tumors, as well as the association of HLA class I antigen abnormalities and TAP1 downregulation with the development of metastatic lesions include immune selection of tumor cells with an abnormal HLA class I antigen phenotype and/or accumulation of mutations by tumor cells.

The findings we have summarized suggest that in the presence of T-cell selective pressure, malignant cells—which exhibit HLA class I antigen

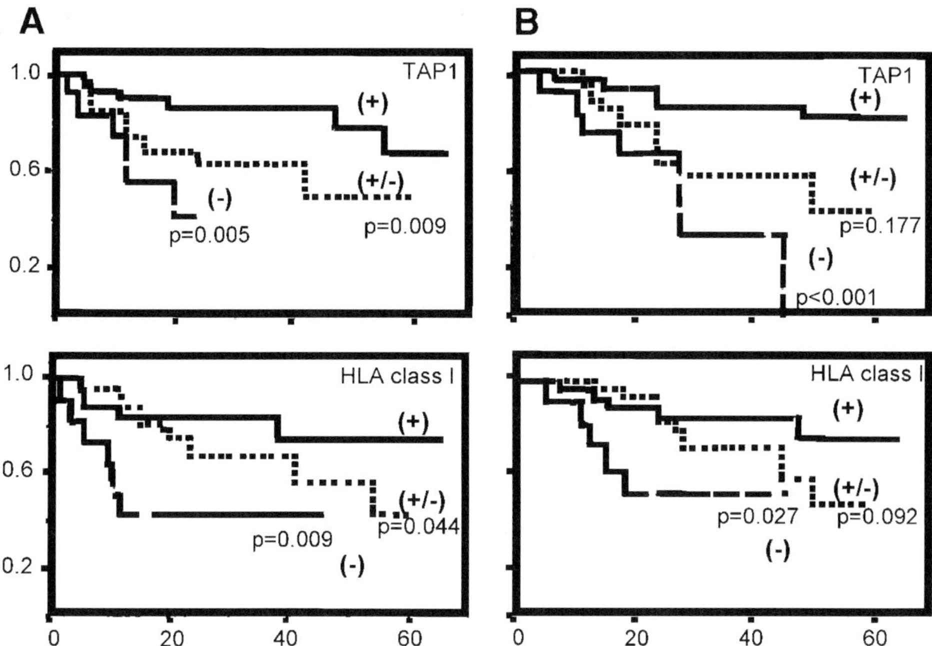

Fig. 9. Association between TAP1 and HLA class I antigen downregulation with survival in breast cancer and cutaneous melanoma patients. Reduced survival is seen in patients with **(A)** breast carcinoma and **(B)** cutaneous melanoma whose lesions demonstrate TAP1 and HLA class I antigen downregulation. (+), (+/–) and (–) denote ≥75%, 25–75% and ≤25% of cells, respectively, which stain for TAP1 and HLA class I antigen expression.

defects—overgrow cells without abnormalities in their HLA class I phenotype and progress to advanced tumor grades. This theory is supported by the association of HLA class I antigen downregulation with a reduction in disease-free interval and survival in HNSCC, breast carcinoma, SCLC, bladder carcinoma, cervical carcinoma, and cutaneous melanoma (*16,76,82,84–86*; Fig. 9). In prostate carcinoma, when the degree of tumor differentiation is considered, the disease-free interval and survival of patients with prostate carcinoma—whose lesions demonstrate HLA class I antigen abnormalities—is shorter than those of patients whose lesions have a similar degree of tumor differentiation and do not demonstrate detectable HLA class I antigen abnormalities *(81)*. These clinical findings have been suggested to reflect resistance of malignant cells to lysis by CTL through lack of TAA-derived peptides presented properly in the context of a HLA class I allospecificity. This mechanism can also explain the association of TAP1 downregulation with tumor grading, tumor staging, and reduction in patients' survival in breast carcinoma, SCLC, cervical cancer, and cutaneous melanoma (*16;* Fig. 9). Interestingly, TAP1 expression has been suggested to represent an independent prognostic marker for patients with cutaneous melanoma, since its downregulation in primary lesions has been found to correlate with metastasis development and a prognosis that is better than the traditional prognostic marker—e.g., tumor thickness *(82)*. If these findings are confirmed, the analysis of TAP1 expression in primary cutaneous melanoma lesions may represent a useful molecular marker in order to evaluate the prognosis for melanoma patients. Whether this conclusion also applies to other types of malignancies has not been determined.

It is important to note that HLA class I antigen loss or downregulation is not associated with poor clinical prognosis in every disease. For example, in uveal melanoma, HLA class I antigen downregulation is associated with a decrease in metastases and improved survival *(87)*. These findings have been attributed to the hematogeneous route of metastasis formation and its control by NK cells. This is corroborated by the high HLA class I antigen expression found in uveal melanoma metastases, which may result from the reduced susceptibility of tumor cells with high HLA class I antigen expression to NK cell-mediated lysis *(87)*. In colon carcinoma, there are conflicting reports in the literature *(79,88)*, since the correlation of HLA-A downregulation with lower tumor stage and longer disease-free survival has only been found by one group of investigators *(88)*. Whether these findings reflect differences in characteristics of the patient population or the methods of analysis is unknown.

No association has been found between HLA class I antigen abnormalities and the histological type, degree of differentiation, or clinical stage of the disease in pulmonary adenocarcinoma, squamous cell carcinoma of the uterine cervix, and cutaneous squamous cell carcinoma *(16,89,90)*. Moreover, no association has been found between HLA class I antigen abnormalities and disease-free interval and survival in both non-small-cell lung cancer (NSCLC) and large-cell or large-cell immunoblastic (B-cell or T-cell) lymphomas *(16,91,92)*. These findings may be attributed to the lack of a T-cell-mediated immune response in patients with these malignancies, the inability of a T-cell-mediated immune response to control the growth of these tumors, and/or the effect of other confounding variables. However, the identification of tumor-specific CTL, which have been expanded from tumor-infiltrating lymphocytes (TIL) of non-Hodgkin's lymphoma (NHL) and NSCLC, argues against the lack of a T-cell-mediated immune response in patients with NHL and NSCLC *(93,94)*. On the other hand, these findings may reflect differences in characteristics of the patient population, the methods of analysis, and/or the system used to score HLA class I antigen expression. In this regard, an international classification system has been established for the evaluation of HLA class I antigen expression in malignant lesions *(95)*. It is hoped that this will facilitate the standardization of the analysis of HLA class I antigen expression in malignant lesions.

3. HLA CLASS I ALLOSPECIFICITY-TAA-DERIVED PEPTIDE COMPLEXES ON TUMOR CELLS

As already discussed, a crucial role in the interactions between HLA class I antigen-restricted, TAA-specific CTLs and tumor cells is played by HLA class I antigen-TAA-derived peptide complexes. Therefore, it is important to ask whether the level of a HLA class I allospecificity on the cell membrane can be used as a measure of the respective HLA class I allospecificity-peptide complex. In other words, does the level of a HLA class I allospecificity on the cell membrane correlate closely with that of the complexes generated by its association with peptides derived from antigens? When all HLA class I antigens or the HLA class I allospecificity presenting a peptide have been lost, the HLA class I allospecificity-peptide complex of interest is not expressed. However, whether the expression of a HLA class I allospecificity excludes defects in the presentation of an actual HLA class I allospecificity-TAA-derived peptide complex on the surface of malignant cells is unknown. Furthermore, it has not been determined whether all HLA class I antigen-TAA-derived peptide complexes are homogenously downregulated when HLA class I antigens or the presenting HLA class I allospecificity are downregulated. We believe that this is unlikely, since several lines of evidence argue against this possibility and suggest that the level of a HLA class I allospecificity does not correlate with the level of HLA class I antigen-peptide complexes on the cell membrane in many experimental conditions.

First, the detection of antigen-processing-machinery components and HLA class I antigens in tissues with immunohistochemical assays does not exclude the possibility that they are nonfunctional or malfunctional because of mutations and/or changes in their conformation. Second, if one makes the assumption that all HLA class I antigens and antigen-processing-machinery components that are expressed are functional, monitoring malignant lesions for HLA class I antigen and antigen-processing-machinery component expression at the protein level does not provide an accurate interpretation of the repertoire of peptides presented by HLA class I antigens on tumor cells, since the variables that control this phenomenon have not been fully characterized. In this regard, two lines of evidence indicate that conversion of the standard proteasome to the immunoproteasome, which is induced by IFN-γ, significantly affects the presentation of peptides derived from two melanoma-associated antigens (MAA). Melanoma cells with no detectable defects in HLA class I antigens, antigen-processing machinery components, and the MAA MART1 are not recognized by HLA-A2-restricted, MART1-specific CTLs following in vitro incubation with IFN-γ, since LMP2 and LMP7 expression in the immunoproteasome inhibits presentation of the MART1-derived peptide to CTL *(96)*.

Conversely, loss of the capacity to upregulate both LMP immunosubunit and PA28 expression in response to in vitro incubation with IFN-γ is associated with the loss of the ability to present a TRP-2-derived peptide, which requires expression of PA28, a component of the immunoproteasome *(97)*. As a result, melanoma cells with this defect are resistant to HLA-A2-restricted, TRP2-specific CTL following exposure to IFN-γ. These findings imply that during the course of an active immune response against malignant cells, the presentation of specific TAA-derived peptides may be gained or lost, resulting in the switch from susceptibility to resistance of malignant cells to TAA-specific CTL. Moreover, recent evidence demonstrates that individual organs display different expression profiles of the multiple proteasome subunits in mice *(61)*. Therefore, these data suggest that tumors that express the same TAA but have originated from different tissues may have a completely different repertoire of peptides presented by HLA class I antigens because of the differential organ-specific potential to produce T-cell epitopes.

Finally, defects in the expression and/or function of several antigen-processing machinery components in malignant cells may have a significant influence on the repertoire of peptides presented by HLA class I antigens. As mentioned previously, several types of malignancies display abnormalities in LMP2 and/or LMP7 expression. Although these abnormalities do not have profound effects on the total level of HLA class I antigen expression *(58)*, it is unclear how these abnormalities influence the generation of TAA-derived peptides. Clearly, the critical role of the proteasome in the generation of TAA-derived peptides suggests that these variations may have dramatic effects on the actual repertoire of TAA-derived peptides presented on HLA class I antigens by malignant cells. TAP and tapasin downregulation may also have a major influence on the repertoire of peptides presented on the cell membrane. TAP downregulation results in a reduction in the level of HLA class I antigen expression by reducing the number of peptides transported into the ER. However, it is also likely to affect the range of peptides presented, since TAP is primarily responsible for the qualitative selection of peptides to be transported into the ER *(58)*, and TAP downregulation may increase the presentation of TAP-independent HLA class I antigen-binding peptides *(58)*. Similar effects are also likely to be caused by defects in tapasin expression. Tapasin brings the HLA class I heavy-chain, β_2m, chaperone complex into association with TAP, and plays a key role in both quantitative and qualitative peptide selection. Tapasin downregulation results in a reduction in the level of HLA class I antigen expression, and is likely to affect the peptides presented on HLA class I antigens by malignant cells. Recent evidence suggests that in the absence of tapasin, the peptides presented on HLA class I antigens can be significantly altered, resulting in the presentation of suboptimal major histocompatibility complex (MHC) class I-bound peptides *(58)*.

	Pan HLA class I antigen staining	Restricting HLA class I allospecificity expression	HLA class I allospecificity -TAA complex expression	CTL lysis
A	+	+	+	+
B	+	+	–	–
C	+	–	–	–

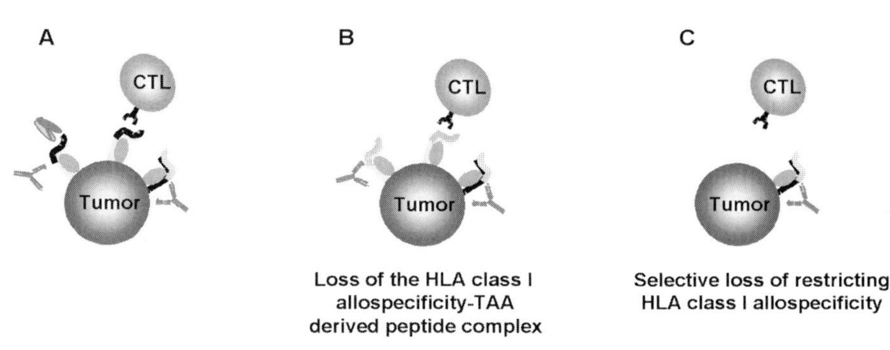

Fig. 10. Possible mechanisms that prevent a relationship between TAA-specific CTL response and clinical response in patients without detectable HLA class I antigen defects in their malignant lesions, as determined by immunohistochemical reaction. **(A)** HLA class I allospecificity-TAA-derived peptide-complex expression is required for HLA class I antigen-restricted, TAA-specific CTL recognition and lysis of tumor cells; **(B)** Downregulation or loss of the HLA class I allospecificity-TAA-derived peptide complex recognized by TAA-specific CTL despite the lack of significant changes in HLA class I antigen expression provides malignant cells with a mechanism of resistance to TAA-specific CTL; **(C)** Selective loss of the restricting HLA class I allospecificity despite of the lack of significant changes in expression of other HLA class I allospecificities provides malignant cells with a mechanism of resistance to TAA-specific CTL.

The data we have summarized, as well as the subtle variations frequently observed in the level of antigen-processing-machinery component expression during the progression of a malignant lesion, highlight the need to monitor HLA class I antigen-TAA-derived peptide-complex expression on tumor cells (Fig. 10). In recent years, probes that are capable of directly monitoring the level of MHC antigen-peptide complexes on cells are being prepared. In mice, mouse MAbs that recognize a determinant expressed on mouse MHC class I antigens, H-2K^b and H-2D^d, complexed with a peptide derived from ovalbumin *(98)* or the HIV envelope protein gp160 *(99)*, respectively, and on mouse MHC class II antigens I-A^k, complexed with peptide derived from hen egg lysozyme *(100)* have been described. Analysis of the known three-dimensional structure of the

H-$2D^d$-gp160 complex and the amino acid sequence of the Mab that is specific for the MHC class I antigen-HIV envelope protein gp160 peptide complex, suggest that this MAb binds in an orientation similar to that of the corresponding TCR. Furthermore, a single-chain immunoglobulin variable region fragment (scFv) that recognizes a determinant expressed on mouse MHC class I antigen K^k-influenza virus-derived peptide complexes has been isolated from a phage display antibody library constructed from a mouse immunized with the respective MHC class I antigen-peptide complex *(101)*. In humans, mouse MAbs that recognize determinants expressed by HLA-DR antigen-mylein basic protein-derived peptide complexes *(102)* and HLA class II antigen-invariant chain-derived peptide complexes *(103)* have been described. To the best of our knowledge, no mouse MAb that is specific for human MHC class I antigen-peptide complexes has been described. Whether this reflects the lack of immunogenicity of HLA class I antigen-peptide complexes in mice because of their overshadowing by more immunodominant epitopes is not known. More recently, Chames et al. have isolated human Fab fragments, which recognize the HLA-A1-MAGE1, HLA-A2-gp100, and HLA-A2-telomerase catalytic subunit-derived peptide complexes *(104–106)* by panning with the respective HLA class I antigen-peptide complex. These Fab fragments are capable of detecting endogenously derived HLA class I antigen-peptide complexes on the surface of cells in vitro. In addition, these Fab fragments are functional in vivo, since T cells transduced with cell-surface-anchored HLA class I antigen-TAA peptide complex-specific Fab fragments are able to eradicate tumor cells in a tumor-bearing animal model *(107)*. We have focused our efforts on the isolation of probes that recognize HLA-A2-$MART1_{27-35}$-derived peptide complexes, since this peptide has been and is extensively used as an immunogen in patients with melanoma *(12)*. Like Chames et al., we are utilizing a phage display antibody library to isolate probes that are specific for HLA class I allospecificity-TAA-derived peptide complexes over the production of mouse MAbs since: i) the isolation of scFv fragments does not depend on the immunogenicity of the complex; and ii) the range of antibody specificities present in the scFv library is much broader than that found in a panel of hybridomas generated from an immunized mouse. The steps required in order to isolate a HLA class I antigen-TAA peptide complex-specific scFv are schematically shown in Fig. 11. They include incubation of the phage library with recombinant HLA class I antigen-TAA peptide complexes, separation of phage-bound HLA class I antigen-TAA peptide complexes, and elution of bound phage from the peptide complex. This process is repeated several times in order to enrich for HLA class I antigen-TAA peptide complex-specific binding phage. Using this strategy, we have isolated scFv fragments that recognize determinants expressed on the HLA-A*0201-$MART1_{27-35}$ peptide complex. These scFv fragments are capable of recognizing the recombinant HLA-A*0201-$MART1_{27-35}$ derived

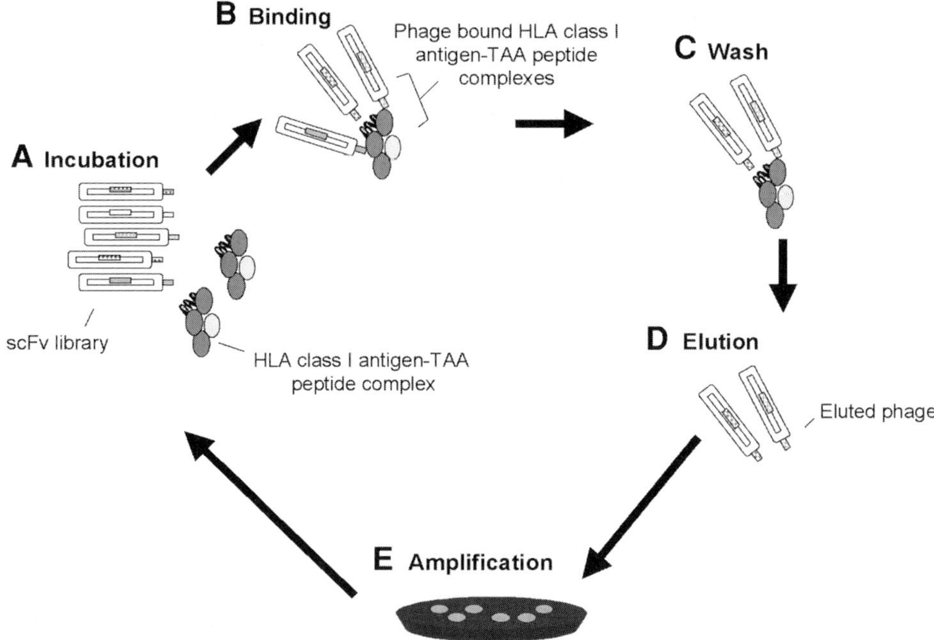

Fig. 11. Isolation of HLA class I antigen-TAA-derived peptide-complex specific scFv fragments. The steps involved in the isolation of HLA class I antigen-TAA-derived peptide-complex-specific scFv fragments are as follows: (A) incubation of the scFv phage display antibody library with recombinant HLA class I antigen-TAA-derived peptide complexes; **(B)** separation of phage-bound HLA class I antigen-TAA-derived peptide complexes; **(C)** washing of phage-bound HLA class I antigen-TAA-derived peptide complexes in order to eliminate nonspecific binding phage; **(D)** elution of phage bound to HLA class I antigen-TAA-derived peptide complexes via acid treatment; **(E)** amplification of eluted phage. This process is repeated several times in order to enrich for phage-displayed scFv fragments that bind with high affinity to HLA class I antigen-TAA-derived peptide complexes.

peptide complex, as well as MART1$_{27-35}$ peptide-pulsed T2 cells and HLA-A*0201 (+), MART1 (+) cells (Campoli et al., unpublished data) (Fig. 12).

4. CONCLUSION

In the past, studies have focused on the development of active specific T cell-based immunotherapeutic strategies for the treatment of malignant disease *(12)*. The significant progress in our understanding of the molecular steps leading to an immune response and the development of MHC class I antigen tetramers *(108)* has facilitated our ability to implement these immunotherapeutic strategies and to monitor TAA-specific CTL immune responses. However, the current challenge facing tumor immunologists is the need to understand why a TAA-specific CTL immune response, which can be detected

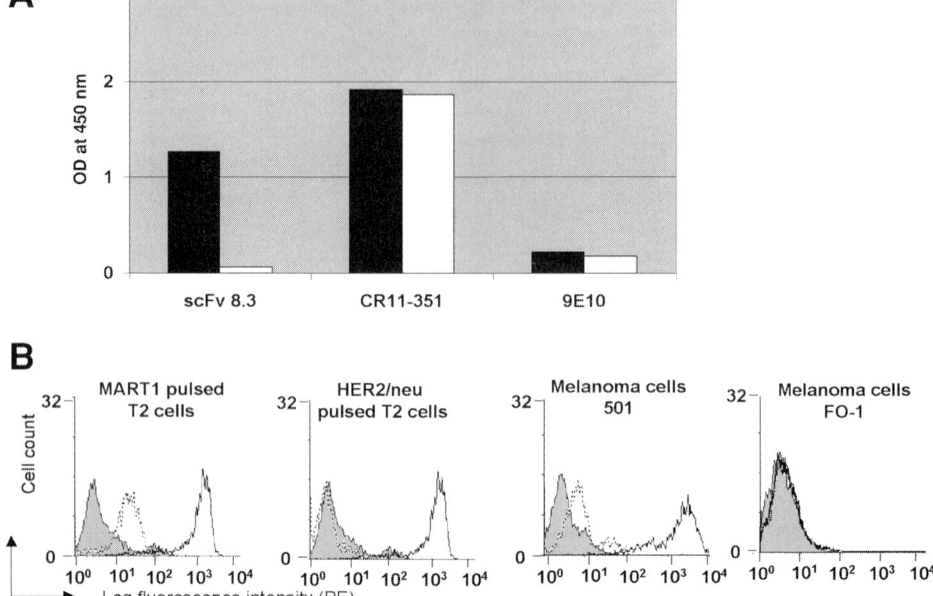

Fig. 12. Reactivity of anti-HLA-A*0201-MART1$_{27-35}$ peptide complex scFv 8.3 with recombinant HLA-A*0201-MART1$_{27-35}$ peptide complexes, MART1$_{27-35}$ peptide-pulsed T2 cells and HLA-A*0201 (+), MART1(+) human melanoma cells 501. **(A)** scFv 8.3 bound to HLA-A*0201-MART1$_{27-35}$ peptide complexes (■), but not to HLA-A*0201-HIVgag peptide complexes (□) in enzyme-linked immunosorbent assay (ELISA). The anti-HLA-A2, A24, A28 MAb CR11-351 and anti-c-*myc* MAb 9E10 were used as positive and negative controls, respectively. **(B)** scFv 8.3 stained MART1$_{27-35}$ peptide-pulsed T2 cells and HLA-A*0201 (+), MART1(+) cultured human melanoma cells 501 in flow cytometry (□). HER2/neu peptide-pulsed T2 cells, HLA-A*0201(–), MART1(–) cultured human melanoma cells FO-1, anti-HLA A2, A24, A28 mAb CR11-351 (□) and anti-*c-myc* MAb 9E10 (■) were used as controls.

in a variable percentage of immunized patients, is not matched by a clinical response in the majority of immunized patients *(12)*. A number of escape mechanisms have been identified and characterized *(16–19)*. Although no definitive proof has been demonstrated, the identification of HLA class I antigen loss variants in recurrent metastatic lesions in patients who had experienced clinical responses following T-cell-based immunotherapy *(29,30)* suggests that total HLA class I antigen loss, as well as selective HLA class I antigen loss, may play an important role in tumor-cell escape from TAA-specific CTL lysis. However, the association between HLA class I antigen defects—as determined by staining formalin-fixed, paraffin-embedded malignant lesions with MAbs to monomorphic determinants—and clinical parameters of disease is statistically significant but not absolute. This may reflect the variety of escape mechanisms utilized by tumor cells to evade immune recognition and destruction. They include selective loss of the restricting HLA class I allospecificity and/or downregulation or loss of the HLA class I allospecificity-TAA-derived peptide complex. The latter may not be identified by measuring the level of the corresponding HLA class I allospecificity. Furthermore, the level of restricting HLA class I allospecificity expression may not correlate with that of the level of HLA class I allospecificity-peptide complexes on the surface of tumor cells. Subtle changes in the expression of these complexes on tumor cells may have dramatic effects on the outcome of T-cell-based immunotherapy, since many TAA that are candidates for immunotherapy are derived from self-antigens, and low-avidity, self-reactive T cells may require a higher threshold density than non-self antigens for activation *(109,110)*. This fact indicates that subtle variations in the level of antigen-processing-machinery components may lead to the lack of presentation of HLA class I antigen-TAA peptide complexes at sufficient density on tumor cells for recognition by TAA-specific CTL. Therefore, we believe that that strategies must be developed to isolate probes capable of monitoring specific HLA class I antigen-TAA-derived peptide complex expression on the surface of tumor cells, since the expression of these complexes is essential in the interactions between TAA-specific CTL and target cells. As these probes become available, we can determine whether the actual levels of HLA class I antigen-TAA-derived peptide-complex expression correlate with the sensitivity of tumor cells to TAA-specific CTL lysis. However, before these reagents can be used effectively, several questions must still be addressed. Is the sensitivity of binding of the currently available probes comparable with the sensitivity of binding of CTL? If the currently available probes are not capable of recognizing the minimum number of complexes that are sufficient for CTL activation, can their affinity be enhanced? Notably, through a combination of light-chain shuffling, targeted mutagenesis, and in vitro selection, Chames et al. demonstrated an 18-fold improvement in affinity for an HLA-A1-MAGE1-specific Fab fragment *(104)*. If the affinity of the current probes cannot be enhanced, can we develop strategies to enhance the immunogenicity of HLA class I antigen-TAA-derived peptide complexes in order to generate mouse MAbs specific for these complexes? If these probes are capable of monitoring HLA class I antigen-TAA peptide complex expression at the appropriate levels required for CTL recognition and lysis, can the level of their binding be a predictable indicator of tumor susceptibility to CTL-mediated lysis? In addition, can these probes be used to stain surgically removed lesions, and especially formalin-fixed malignant lesions? If so, does the level of HLA class I allospecificity-TAA peptide complex expression in malignant lesions correlate with clinical parameters of the disease? Finally, can we develop, from the available probes, reagents that will improve the selection and monitoring of patients to be treated with T-cell-based immunotherapy?

ACKNOWLEDGMENTS

This work was supported by PHS grants RO1 CA67108, P30 CA16056, and T32 CA85183, awarded by the National Cancer Institute, DHHS.

REFERENCES

1. Restifo NP, Wunderlich JR (1996b) Principles of tumor immunity: biology of cellular immune responses. In: *Biologic Therapy of Cancer* (DeVita VT, Hellman S, Rosenderg SA, eds.), JB Lippincott Co., Philadelphia, PA, pp. 3–21.
2. Dudley ME, Wunderlich JR, Robbins PF, Yang JC, Hwu P, Schwartzentruber DJ, et al. Cancer regression and autoimmunity in patients after clonal repopulation with antitumor lymphocytes. *Science* 2002;298:850–854.
3. Yee C, Thompson JA, Byrd D, Riddell SR, Roche P, Celis E, et al. Adoptive T cell therapy using antigen-specific CD8+ T cell clones for the treatment of patients with metastatic melanoma: in vivo persistence, migration, and antitumor effect of transferred T cells. *Proc Natl Acad Sci USA* 2002;99:16,168–16,173.
4. Rosenberg SA. Cancer vaccines based on the identification of genes encoding cancer regression antigens. *Immunol Today* 1997;18:175–182.
5. Stevanovic S. Identification of tumour-associated T-cell epitopes for vaccine development. *Nat Rev Cancer* 2002;2:514–520.
6. Dermime S, Armstrong A, Hawkins RE, Stern PL. Cancer vaccines and immunotherapy. Br Med Bull 2002;62:149–162.
7. Naftzger C, Takechi Y, Kohda H, Hara I, Vivjayasaradhi S, Houghton AN. Immune response to a differentiation antigen induced by altered antigen: a study of tumor rejection and autoimmunity. *Proc Natl Acad Sci USA* 1996;93:14,809–14,814.
8. Nestle FO, Alijagic S, Gilliet M, Sun Y, Grabbe S, Dummer R, et al. Vaccination of melanoma patients with peptide- or tumor lysate-pulsed dendritic cells. *Nat Med* 1998;4:328–332.
9. Rosenberg SA, Yang JC, Schwartzentruber DJ, Hwu P, Marincola FM, Topalian SL, et al. Immunologic and therapeutic evaluation of a synthetic peptide vaccine for the treatment of patients with metastatic melanoma. *Nat Med* 1998;4:321–327.
10. Egen JG, Kuhns MS, Allison JP. CTLA-4: new insights into its biological function and use in tumor immunotherapy. *Nat Immunol* 2002;3:611–618.
11. Toso JF, Gill VJ, Hwu P, Marincola FM, Restifo NP, Schwartzentruber DJ, et al. Phase I study of the intravenous administration of attenuated Salmonella typhimurium to patients with metastatic melanoma. *J Clin Oncol* 2002;20:142–152.
12. Parmiani G, Castelli C, Dalerba P, Mortarini R, Rivoltini L, Marincola FM, et al. Cancer immunotherapy with peptide-based vaccines: what have we achieved? Where are we going? *J Natl Cancer Inst* 2002;94:805–818.
13. Marchand M, Weynants P, Rankin E, Arienti F, Belli F, Parmiani G, et al. Tumor regression responses in melanoma patients treated with a peptide encoded by gene MAGE-3. *Int J Cancer* 1995;63:883–885.
14. Marchand M, van Baren N, Weynants P, Brichard V, Dreno B, Tessier MH, et al. Tumor regressions observed in patients with metastatic melanoma treated with an antigenic peptide encoded by gene MAGE-3 and presented by HLA-A1. *Int J Cancer* 1999;80:219–230.
15. Onyango P. Genomics and cancer. *Curr Opin Oncol* 2002;14:79–85.
16. Marincola FM, Jaffee EM, Hicklin DJ, Ferrone S. Escape of human solid tumors from T-cell recognition: molecular mechanisms and functional significance. *Adv Immunol* 2000;74:181–273.

17. Ferrone S (guest ed.). Tumour immune escape. *Semin Cancer Biol* 2002;12.
18. Khong HT, Restifo NP. Natural selection of tumor variants in the generation of "tumor escape" phenotypes. *Nat Immunol* 2002;3:999–1005.
19. Romero P, Valmori D, Pittet MJ, Zippelius A, Rimoldi D, Levy F, et al. Antigenicity and immunogenicity of Melan-A/MART-1 derived peptides as targets for tumor reactive CTL in human melanoma. *Immunol Rev* 2002;188:81–96.
20. Moretta L, Bottino C, Pende D, Mingari MC, Biassoni R, Moretta A. Human natural killer cells: their origin, receptors and function. *Eur J Immunol* 2002;32:1205–1211.
21. Ikeda H, Lethe B, Lehmann F, van Baren N, Baurain JF, de Smet C, et al. Characterization of an antigen that is recognized on a melanoma showing partial HLA loss by CTL expressing an NK inhibitory receptor. *Immunity* 1997;6:199–208.
22. Malmberg KJ, Levitsky V, Norell H, de Matos CT, Carlsten M, Schedvins K, et al. FN-gamma protects short-term ovarian carcinoma cell lines from CTL lysis via a CD94/NKG2A-dependent mechanism. *J Clin Investig* 2002;110:1515–1523.
23. Hicklin DJ, Marincola FM, Ferrone S. HLA class I antigen downregulation in human cancers: T-cell immunotherapy revives an old story. *Mol Med Today* 1999;5:178–186.
24. Fukusato T, Gerber MA, Thung SN, Ferrone S, Schaffner F. Expression of HLA class I antigens on hepatocytes in liver disease. *Am J Pathol* 1986;123:264–270.
25. Kurokohchi K, Carrington M, Mann DL, Simonis TB, Alexander-Miller MA, Feinstone SM, et al. Expression of HLA class I molecules and the transporter associated with antigen processing in hepatocellular carcinoma. *Hepatology* 1996;23:1181–1188.
26. Bi Y, Zhang J, Hong Z, Huang J, Chen J, Wang X, et al. Association of HLA class I antigen expression in human hepatocellar carcinoma with improved prognosis. *Tissue Antigens* 2002;59 (suppl 2):105–106.
27. Wetzler M, Baer MR, Stewart SJ, Donohue K, Ford L, Stewart CC, et al. HLA class I antigen cell surface expression is preserved on acute myeloid leukemia blasts at diagnosis and at relapse. *Leukemia* 2001;15:128–133.
28. List AF, Spier CM, Miller TP, Grogan TM. Deficient tumor-infiltrating T-lymphocyte response in malignant lymphoma: relationship to HLA expression and host immunocompetence. *Leukemia* 1993;7:398–403.
29. Lehmann F, Marchand M, Hainaut P, Pouillart P, Sastre X, Ikeda H, et al. Differences in the antigens recognized by cytolytic T cells on two successive metastases of a melanoma patient are consistent with immune selection. *Eur J Immunol* 1995;25:340–347.
30. Restifo NP, Marincola FM, Kawakami Y, Taubenberger J, Yannelli JR, Rosenberg SA. Loss of functional beta 2-microglobulin in metastatic melanomas from five patients receiving immunotherapy. *J Natl Cancer Inst* 1996;88:100–108.
31. Garcia-Lora A, Algarra I, Gaforio JJ, Ruiz-Cabello F, Garrido F. Immunoselection by T lymphocytes generates repeated MHC class I-deficient metastatic tumor variants. *Int J Cancer* 2001;91:109–119.
32. Kelly LM, Gilliland DG. Genetics of myeloid leukemias. *Annu Rev Genomics Hum Genet* 2002;3:179–198.
33. Feenstra M, Rozemuller E, Duran K, Stuy I, van den Tweel J, Slootweg P, et al. Mutation in the beta 2m gene is not a frequent event in head and neck squamous cell carcinomas. *Hum Immunol* 1999;60:697–706.
34. Cabrera T, Salinero J, Fernandez MA, Garrido A, Esquivias J, Garrido F. High frequency of altered HLA class I phenotypes in laryngeal carcinomas. *Hum Immunol* 2000;61:499–506.
35. Goodfellow PN, Jones EA, Van Heyningen V, Solomon E, Bobrow M, Miggiano V, et al. The beta2-microglobulin gene is on chromosome 15 and not in the HL-A region. *Nature* 1975;254:267–269.

36. Jordanova ES, Riemersma SA, Philippo K, Schuuring E, Kluin PM. Beta2-microglobulin aberrations in diffuse large B-cell lymphoma of the testis and the central nervous system. *Int J Cancer* 2003;103:393–398.
37. McEvoy CR, Seshadri R, Morley AA, Firgaira FA. Frequency and genetic basis of MHC, beta-2-microglobulin and MEMO-1 loss of heterozygosity in sporadic breast cancer. *Tissue Antigens* 2002;60:235–243.
38. Maleno I, Lopez-Nevot MA, Cabrera T, Salinero J, Garrido F. Multiple mechanisms generate HLA class I altered phenotypes in laryngeal carcinomas: high frequency of HLA haplotype loss associated with loss of heterozygosity in chromosome region 6p21. *Cancer Immunol Immunother* 2002;51:389–396.
39. Paschen A, Mendez RM, Jimenez P, Sucker A, Ruiz-Cabello F, Song M, et al. Complete loss of HLA class I antigen expression on melanoma cells: A result of successive mutational events. *Int J Cancer* 2003;103:759–767.
40. Geertsen RC, Hofbauer GF, Yue FY, Manolio S, Burg G, Dummer R. Higher frequency of selective losses of HLA-A and -B allospecificities in metastasis than in primary melanoma lesions. *J Investig Dermatol* 1998;111:497–502.
41. Kageshita T, Wang Z, Calorini L, Yoshii A, Kimura T, Ono T, et al. Selective loss of human leukocyte class I allospecificities and staining of melanoma cells by monoclonal antibodies recognizing monomorphic determinants of class I human leukocyte antigens. *Cancer Res* 1993;53:3349–3354.
42. Wang Z, Marincola FM, Rivoltini L, Parmiani G, Ferrone S. Selective histocompatibility leukocyte antigen (HLA)-A2 loss caused by aberrant pre-mRNA splicing in 624MEL28 melanoma cells. *J Exp Med* 1999;190:205–215.
43. Luboldt HJ, Kubens BS, Rubben H, Grosse-Wilde H. Selective loss of human leukocyte antigen class I allele expression in advanced renal cell carcinoma. *Cancer Res* 1996;56:826–830.
44. Francke U, Pellegrino MA. Assignment of the major histocompatibility complex to a region of the short arm of human chromosome 6. *Proc Natl Acad Sci USA* 1977;74:1147–1151.
45. Brady CS, Bartholomew JS, Burt DJ, Duggan-Keen MF, Glenville S, Telford N, et al. Multiple mechanisms underlie HLA dysregulation in cervical cancer. *Tissue Antigens* 2000;55:401–411.
46. Koopman LA, Corver WE, van der Slik AR, Giphart MJ, Fleuren GJ. Multiple genetic alterations cause frequent and heterogeneous human histocompatibility leukocyte antigen class I loss in cervical cancer. *J Exp Med* 2000;191:961–976.
47. Jimenez P, Cabrera T, Mendez R, Esparza C, Cozar JM, Tallada M, et al. A nucleotide insertion in exon 4 is responsible for the absence of expression of an HLA-A*0301 allele in a prostate carcinoma cell line. *Immunogenetics* 2001;53:606–610.
48. Geertsen R, Boni R, Blasczyk R, Romero P, Betts D, Rimoldi D, et al. Loss of single HLA class I allospecificities in melanoma cells due to selective genomic abbreviations. *Int J Cancer* 2002;99:82–87.
49. Jimenez P, Canton J, Collado A, Cabrera T, Serrano A, Real LM, et al. Chromosome loss is the most frequent mechanism contributing to HLA haplotype loss in human tumors. *Int J Cancer* 1999;83:91–97.
50. Nie Y, Yang G, Song Y, Zhao X, So C, Liao J, et al. DNA hypermethylation is a mechanism for loss of expression of the HLA class I genes in human esophageal squamous cell carcinomas. *Carcinogenesis* 2001;22:1615–1623.
51. Murray PG, Constandinou CM, Crocker J, Young LS, Ambinder RF. Analysis of major histocompatibility complex class I, TAP expression, and LMP2 epitope sequence in Epstein-Barr virus-positive Hodgkin's disease. *Blood* 1998;92:2477–2483.
52. Ritz U, Momburg F, Pilch H, Huber C, Maeurer MJ, Seliger B. Deficient expression of components of the MHC class I antigen processing machinery in human cervical carcinoma. *Int J Oncol* 2001;19:1211–1220.

53. Miyagi T, Tatsumi T, Takehara T, Kanto T, Kuzushita N, Sugimoto Y, et al. Impaired expression of proteasome subunits and human leukocyte antigens class I in human colon cancer cells. *J Gastroenterol Hepatol* 2003;18:32–40.
54. Terrazzano G, Romano MF, Turco MC, Salzano S, Ottaiano A, Venuta S, et al. HLA class I antigen downregulation by interleukin (IL)-10 is predominantly governed by NK-kappaB in the short term and by TAP1+2 in the long term. *Tissue Antigens* 2000;55:326–332.
55. Salazar-Onfray F. Interleukin-10: a cytokine used by tumors to escape immunosurveillance. *Med Oncol* 1999;16:86–94.
56. Ogino T, Wang X, Kato S, Miyokawa N, Harabuchi Y, Ferrone S. Endoplasmic reticulum chaperone-specific monoclonal antibodies for flow cytometry and immunohistochemical staining. *Tissue Antigens* 2003;in press.
57. Ogino T, Wang X, Ferrone S. Modified flow cytometry and cell-ELSIA methodology to detect HLA clas I antigen processing machinery components in cytoplasm and endoplasmic reticulum. *J Immunol Methods* 2003;in press.
58. Yewdell J (guest ed.). Generating peptide ligands for MHC class I molecules. *Mol Immunol* 2002;39.
59. Van den Eynde BJ, Morel S. Differential processing of class-I-restricted epitopes by the standard proteasome and the immunoproteasome. *Curr Opin Immunol* 2001;13: 147–153.
60. Barton LF, Cruz M, Rangwala R, Deepe GS Jr, Monaco JJ. Regulation of immunoproteasome subunit expression in vivo following pathogenic fungal infection. *J Immunol* 2002;169:3046–3052.
61. Kuckelkorn U, Ruppert T, Strehl B, Jungblut PR, Zimny-Arndt U, Lamer S, et al. Link between organ-specific antigen processing by 20S proteasomes and CD8 (+) T cell-mediated autoimmunity. *J Exp Med* 2002;195:983–990.
62. Matsui M, Machida S, Itani-Yohda T, Akatsuka T. Downregulation of the proteasome subunits, transporter, and antigen presentation in hepatocellular carcinoma, and their restoration by interferon-gamma. *J Gastroenterol Hepatol* 2002;17:897–907.
63. Delp K, Momburg F, Hilmes C, Huber C, Seliger B. Functional deficiencies of components of the MHC class I antigen pathway in human tumors of epithelial origin. *Bone Marrow Transplant* 2000;25(Suppl 2):S88–S95.
64. Seliger B, Maeurer MJ, Ferrone S. Antigen-processing machinery breakdown and tumor growth. *Immunol Today* 2000;21:455–464.
65. Seliger B, Atkins D, Bock M, Ritz U, Ferrone S, Huber C, et al. Characterization of HLA class I antigen processing machinery defects in renal cell carcinoma lesions with special emphasis on TAP downregulation. *Clin Cancer Res* 2003;9:1721–1727.
66. Wright KL, White LC, Kelly A, Beck S, Trowsdale J, Ting JP. Coordinate regulation of the human TAP1 and LMP2 genes from a shared bidirectional promoter. *J Exp Med* 1995;181:1459–1471.
67. Johnsen AK, Templeton DJ, Sy M, Harding CV. Deficiency of transporter for antigen presentation (TAP) in tumor cells allows evasion of immune surveillance and increases tumorigenesis. *J Immunol* 1999;163:4224–4231.
68. Alimonti J, Zhang QJ, Gabathuler R, Reid G, Chen SS, Jefferies WA. TAP expression provides a general method for improving the recognition of malignant cells in vivo. *Nat Biotechnol* 2000;18:515–520.
69. Murray JL, Hudson JM, Ross MI, Zhang HZ, Ioannides CG. Reduced recognition of metastatic melanoma cells by autologous MART-1 specific CTL: relationship to TAP expression. *J Immunother* 2000;23:28–35.
70. Chen HL, Gabrilovich D, Tampe R, Girgis KR, Nadaf S, Carbone DP. A functionally defective allele of TAP1 results in loss of MHC class I antigen presentation in a human lung cancer. *Nat Genet* 1996;13:210–213.

71. Seliger B, Ritz U, Abele R, Bock M, Tampe R, Sutter G, et al. Immune escape of melanoma: first evidence of structural alterations in two distinct components of the MHC class I antigen processing pathway. *Cancer Res* 2001;61:8647–8650.
72. Corrias MV, Occhino M, Croce M, De Ambrosis A, Pistillo MP, Bocca P, et al. Lack of HLA-class I antigens in human neuroblastoma cells: analysis of its relationship to TAP and tapasin expression. *Tissue Antigens* 2001;57:110–117.
73. Seliger B, Schreiber K, Delp K, Meissner M, Hammers S, Reichert T, et al. Downregulation of the constitutive tapasin expression in human tumor cells of distinct origin and its transcriptional upregulation by cytokines. *Tissue Antigens* 2001;57:39–45.
74. Weinman E, Roche P, Kasperbauer J, Cha S, Sargent D, Cheville J, et al. Characterization of antigen processing machinery and survivin expression in tonsillar squamous cell carcinoma. *Cancer* 2003;97:2203–2211.
75. Ogino T, Bandoh N, Hayashi T, Miyokawa N, Harabuchi Y, Ferrone S. Association of tapasin and HLA class I antigen downregulation in primary maxillary sinus squamous carcinoma lesions with reduced patients' survivial. *Clin Cancer Res* 2003; in press.
76. Brasanac D, Muller CA, Muller GA, Hadzi-Dzokic J, Markovic-Lipkovski J. HLA class I antigens expression in renal cell carcinoma: histopathological and clinical correlation. *J Exp Clin Cancer Res* 1999;18:505–510.
77. Dammrich J, Muller-Hermelink HK, Mattner A, Buchwald J, Ziffer S. Histocompatibility antigen expression in pulmonary carcinomas as indication of differentiation and of special subtypes. *Cancer* 1990;65:1942–1954.
78. Concha A, Esteban F, Cabrera T, Ruiz-Cabello F, Garrido F. Tumor aggressiveness and MHC class I and II antigens in laryngeal and breast cancer. *Semin Cancer Biol* 1991;2:47–54.
79. Jackson PA, Green MA, Marks CG, King RJ, Hubbard R, Cook MG. Lymphocyte subset infiltration patterns and HLA antigen status in colorectal carcinomas and adenomas. *Gut* 1996;38:85–89.
80. Sharpe JC, Abel PD, Gilbertson JA, Brawn P, Foster CS. Modulated expression of human leucocyte antigen class I and class II determinants in hyperplastic and malignant human prostatic epithelium. *Br J Urol* 1994;74:609–616.
81. Levin I, Klein T, Kuperman O, Segal S, Shapira J, Gal R, et al. The expression of HLA class I antigen in prostate cancer in relation to tumor differentiation and patient survival. *Cancer Detect Prev* 1994;18:443–445.
82. Grandis JR, Falkner DM, Melhem MF, Gooding WE, Drenning SD, Morel PA. Human leukocyte antigen class I allelic and haplotype loss in squamous cell carcinoma of the head and neck: clinical and immunogenetic consequences. *Clin Cancer Res* 2000;6:2794–2802.
83. Kamarashev J, Ferrone S, Seifert B, Boni R, Nestle FO, Burg G, et al. TAP1 down-regulation in primary melanoma lesions: an independent marker of poor prognosis. *Int J Cancer* 2001;95:23–28.
84. Levin I, Klein T, Goldstein J, Kuperman O, Kanetti J, Klein B. Expression of class I histocompatibility antigens in transitional cell carcinoma of the urinary bladder in relation to survival. *Cancer* 1991;68:2591–2594.
85. Klein B, Levin I, Klein T. HLA class I antigen expression in human solid tumors. *Isr J Med Sci* 1996;32:1238–1243.
86. Zia A, Schildberg FW, Funke I. MHC class I negative phenotype of disseminated tumor cells in bone marrow is associated with poor survival in R0M0 breast cancer patients. *Int J Cancer* 2001;93:566-570.
87. Jager MJ, Hurks HM, Levitskaya J, Kiessling R. HLA expression in uveal melanoma: there is no rule without some exception. *Hum Immunol* 2002;63:444–451.
88. Menon AG, Morreau H, Tollenaar RA, Alphenaar E, Van Puijenbroek M, Putter H, et al. Down-regulation of HLA-A expression correlates with a better prognosis in colorectal cancer patients. *Lab Investig* 2002;82:1725–1733.

89. Yano T, Fukuyama Y, Yokoyama H, Kuninaka S, Asoh H, Katsuda Y, et al. HLA class I and class II expression of pulmonary adenocarcinoma cells and the influence of interferon gamma. *Lung Cancer* 1998;20:185–190.
90. Garcia-Plata D, Mozos E, Carrasco L, Solana R. HLA molecule expression in cutaneous squamous cell carcinomas: an immunopathological study and clinical-immuno-histopathological correlations. *Histol Histopathol* 1993;8:219–226.
91. Koukourakis MI, Giatromanolaki A, Guddo F, Kaklamanis L, Vignola M, Kakolyris S, et al. c-erbB-2 and episialin challenge host immune response by HLA class I expression in human non-small-cell lung cancer. *J Immunother* 2000;23:104–114.
92. Medeiros LJ, Gelb AB, Wolfson K, Doggett R, McGregor B, Cox RS, et al. Major histocompatibility complex class I and class II antigen expression in diffuse large cell and large cell immunoblastic lymphomas. Absence of a correlation between antigen expression and clinical outcome. *Am J Pathol* 1993;143:1086–1097.
93. Echchakir H, Vergnon I, Dorothee G, Grunenwald D, Chouaib S, Mami-Chouaib F. Evidence for in situ expansion of diverse antitumor-specific cytotoxic T lymphocyte clones in a human large cell carcinoma of the lung. *Int Immunol* 2000;12:537–546.
94. Chaperot L, Manches O, Mi JQ, Moine A, Jacob MC, Gressin R, et al. Differentiation of anti-tumour cytotoxic T lymphocytes from autologous peripheral blood lymphocytes in non-Hodgkin's lymphomas. *Br J Haematol* 2002;119:425–431.
95. Garrido F, Cabrera T, Accolla RS, Bensa JC, Bodmer W, Dohr G, et. al. HLA and cancer: 12th International Histocompatibility Workshop study. In: Genetic Diversity of HLA. Functional and Medical Implication. Proc. Twelfth International Histocompatibility Workshop and Conference. Vol. II. (Charron D, ed.), EDK, Sevres, France, 1997;445–452.
96. Morel S, Levy F, Burlet-Schiltz O, Brasseur F, Probst-Kepper M, Peitrequin AL, et al. Processing of some antigens by the standard proteasome but not by the immunoproteasome results in poor presentation by dendritic cells. *Immunity* 2000;12:107–117.
97. Sun Y, Sijts AJ, Song M, Janek K, Nussbaum AK, Kral S, et al. Expression of the proteasome activator PA28 rescues the presentation of a cytotoxic T lymphocyte epitope on melanoma cells. *Cancer Res* 2002;62:2875–2882.
98. Porgador A, Yewdell JW, Deng Y, Bennink JR, Germain RN. Localization, quantitation, and in situ detection of specific peptide-MHC class I complexes using a monoclonal antibody. *Immunity* 1997;6:715–726.
99. Polakova K, Plaksin D, Chung DH, Belyakov IM, Berzofsky JA, Margulies DH. Antibodies directed against the MHC-I molecule H-2Dd complexed with an antigenic peptide: similarities to a T cell receptor with the same specificity. *J Immunol* 2000;165:5703–5712.
100. Dadaglio G, Nelson CA, Deck MB, Petzol SJ, Unanue ER. Characterization and quantitation of peptide-MHC complexes produced from hen egg lysozyme using a monoclonal antibody. *Immunity* 1997;6:727–738.
101. Anderson PS, Stryhn A, Hansen BE, Fugger L, Engberg J, Buus S. A recombinant antibody with the antigen-specific, major histocompatibility complex-restricted specificity of T cells. *Proc Natl Acad Sci USA* 1996;93:1820–1824.
102. Puri J, Arnon R, Gurevich E, Teitelbaum D. Modulation of the immune response in multiple sclerosis: production of monoclonal antibodies specific to HLA/myelin basic protein. *J Immunol* 1997;158:2471–2476.
103. Eastman S, Deftos M, DeRoos PC, Hsu DH, Teyton L, Braunstein NS, et al. A study of complexes of class II invariant chain peptide: major histocompatibility complex class II molecules using a new complex-specific monoclonal antibody. *Eur J Immunol* 1996;26:385–393.
104. Chames P, Hufton SE, Coulie PG, Uchanska-Ziegler B, Hoogenboom HR. Direct selection of a human antibody fragment directed against the tumor T-cell epitope

HLA-A1-MAGE-A1 from a nonimmunized phage-Fab library. *Proc Natl Acad Sci USA* 2000;97:7969–7974.
105. Denkberg G, Cohen CJ, Lev A, Chames P, Hoogenboom HR, Reiter Y. Direct visualization of distinct T cell epitopes derived from a melanoma tumor-associated antigen by using human recombinant antibodies with MHC-restricted T cell receptor-like specificity. *Proc Natl Acad Sci USA* 2002;99:9421–9426.
106. Lev A, Denkberg G, Cohen CJ, Tzukerman M, Skorecki KL, Chames P, et al. Isolation and characterization of human recombinant antibodies endowed with the antigen-specific, major histocompatibility complex-restricted specificity of T cells directed toward the widely expressed tumor T-cell epitopes of the telomerase catalytic subunit. *Cancer Res* 2002;62:3184–3194.
107. Chames P, Willemsen RA, Rojas G, Dieckmann D, Rem L, Schuler G, et al. TCR-like human antibodies expressed on human CTLs mediate antibody affinity-dependent cytolytic activity. *J Immunol* 2002; 169:1110–1118.
108. Altman JD, Moss PA, Goulder PJ, Barouch DH, McHeyzer-Williams MG, Bell JI, et al. Phenotypic analysis of antigen-specific T lymphocytes. *Science* 1996;274:94–96.
109. Moudgil KD, Sercarz EE. The self-directed T cell repertoire: its creation and activation. *Rev Immunogenet* 2000;2:26–37.
110. Mason D. Some quantitative aspects of T-cell repertoire selection: the requirement for regulatory T cells. *Immunol Rev* 2001;182:80–88.

2 Immune Defects in T Cells From Cancer Patients

Parallels in Infectious Diseases

Augusto C. Ochoa, MD,
Paulo C. Rodriguez, MSc,
Jovanny Zabaleta, MSc, *Pelayo Correa,* MD,
and Arnold H. Zea, PhD

Contents

1. INTRODUCTION

The progressive growth of tumors in cancer and the chronic presence of a pathogenic microorganism reveal the inability of the immune response to eliminate the malignant cells and the chronic infectious agent. This setting is not

From: *Current Clinical Oncology: Cancer Immunotherapy at the Crossroads: How Tumors Evade Immunity and What Can Be Done*
Edited by: J. H. Finke and R. M. Bukowski © Humana Press Inc., Totowa, NJ

uncommon in mice or patients with a congenital or acquired immunodeficiencies. However, this problem is also frequently seen in fully immunocompetent individuals, suggesting that malignant cells and certain microorganisms have developed mechanisms to evade the immune response. The distinct pathophysiology of cancer and chronic infections suggested that the mechanisms by which tumors and infectious agents impair and evade the immune response were different, and therefore, have been studied separately. Recent data however has demonstrated that T lymphocytes in cancer and chronic infections develop similar molecular alterations that lead to a state of unresponsiveness or anergy, suggesting the possibility that these seemingly disparate diseases may use similar pathways to impair the immune response. Here, we discuss some of the mechanisms that support this hypothesis and provide a possible common explanation to this phenomenon.

2. IMMUNE DYSFUNCTION IN CANCER

Seminal studies by Prehn and Main *(1,2)* demonstrated the existence of an immune response against tumor-specific antigens, raising the possibility that the immune response could be used to control tumor growth, and possibly to treat patients with cancer. Multiple studies in mice have confirmed the existence of a "surveillance mechanism" that can destroy tumor cells before they become an established malignancy of clinical significance *(3,4)*. However, studies in cancer patients failed to demonstrate a protective immune response, and instead suggested that the T-cell response was markedly impaired. In 1965, Hersh and Oppenheim *(5)* found that patients with Hodgkin's disease (HD) had a decreased delayed-type hypersensitivity (DTH) response to PPD and DNBC (di-nitrochlorobenzene) and a diminished in vitro response to mitogen stimulation. This immune dysfunction persisted, even in patients who had achieved a complete clinical response to chemotherapy *(6)*. Patients with melanoma also showed a decrease in the cellular immune response, but a marked increase in the levels of serum immunoglobulins. Similarly, patients with other solid tumors including renal cell carcinoma (RCC), prostate and bladder cancer *(7)*, lung cancer *(8)*, breast cancer *(9)*, and gastric cancer *(10)*, consistently showed a decreased cellular response. Several mechanisms were proposed to explain these observations. The high levels of antibodies observed in melanoma patients suggested the possibility that blocking antibodies might interfere with antigen recognition, preventing the priming and activation of T cells *(11,12)*. An alternative explanation suggested instead that the immune system was unable to recognize the original tumor inoculum because of its suboptimal antigenic load *(13)*. A third possibility came from cloning experiments that suggested the existence of T cells or macrophages with suppressor activity in the spleens of tumor-bearing mice *(14)*.

During the early 1980s, North and colleagues *(15–18)* demonstrated the presence of a protective antitumor T-cell response during the first days following tumor implantation, followed by a rapid decline with the appearance of $Ly1^+$ suppressor T cells by the second week. This suppressor function could be transferred into naive animals, and was eliminated with low doses of cyclophosphamide, re-establishing a therapeutic antitumor response. These findings provided insight into a dynamic interaction between tumors and the immune system, which could be manipulated to the benefit of the host. An alternative explanation came from studies on cytokine functions. Mossman and colleagues classified CD4+ T cells according to the cytokines produced. Th1 cells preferentially produced IL-2, IFN-γ, and TNF-α-promoting cellular responses, and Th2 cells secreted IL-4, IL-13, and IL-10, promoting antibody production *(19,20)*. Therefore, it was suggested that the progressive growth of tumor induced a loss of Th1 activity and an increased Th2 function, resulting in a diminished cellular response and an enhanced antibody production. Most of these concepts remained interesting research observations, but had minor relevance for the treatment of patients.

The advent of immunotherapy trials in the 1980s using the adoptive transfer of tumor-infiltrating lymphocytes (TIL) revealed to a greater extent the degree of T-cell dysfunction in patients with cancer. In vitro testing of freshly isolated TIL demonstrated that these cells had a markedly decreased proliferation when stimulated with mitogens or tumor cells, and had a significantly diminished clonogenic potential *(21–24)*. This cellular dysfunction appeared to have a detrimental effect on the therapeutic success of immunotherapy. Loeffler and colleagues *(25)* studied an immunotherapy model of adoptive transfer of T lymphocytes, demonstrating that T cells from mice bearing tumors for >21 d had a markedly diminished antitumor effect. In contrast, T cells from mice bearing tumors for <14 d had a high therapeutic efficacy when transferred into a tumor-bearing recipients. Further studies failed to demonstrate the presence of suppressor cells, yet they confirmed a significant decrease in T-cell cytotoxicity against tumor targets.

3. CHANGES IN T-CELL SIGNAL-TRANSDUCTION MOLECULES AND CANCER

In the mid-1980s, major advances in T-cell biology provided the basis for an understanding of the molecular events that lead to T-cell activation. Among these were the elucidation of the structure and function of T-cell receptor (TCR) and the mechanisms of T-cell signal transduction following antigen stimulation *(26–28)*. Briefly, two polymorphic chains, the α and β chains, confer antigen specificity to the T cell and form the antigen-binding site. These are covalently linked to the CD3 complex formed by the invariant chains γ, δ, ε, and ζ. The latter forms ζζ homodimers (CD3ζ) or ζη heterodimers. Following TCR ligation, Src family tyrosine kinases, *p56*^{lck} (associated with CD4 or CD8) and *p59*^{fyn} phosphorylate CD3ζ and recruit ZAP-70, eventually leading to the activation of nuclear transcription factors such as NF-κB that translocate into the nucleus and activate or repress various genes, including cytokine genes *(29,30)*. Major advances have also been made in understanding the molecular changes that accompany T-cell unresponsiveness or anergy. Quill and colleagues *(31,32)* demonstrated that T cells stimulated by antigens presented on fixed antigen-presenting cells (APC) were anergic—e.g., unresponsive to repeated antigenic stimuli and unable to produce IL-2 *(33,34)*. Furthermore, stimulation of T cells with streptococcus superantigen produced a state of T-cell anergy and resulted in a decreased expression of *p56*^{lck} and *p59*^{fyn} *(31,35)*. Anergic T cells showed several molecular alterations, including the inability to phosphorylate *p21 ras* *(36,37)* and a decreased ability to activate nuclear transcription factors, including NF-κB and AP-1, important in regulating cytokine production *(38)*. These observations provided important tools to study the mechanisms for T-cell dysfunction in cancer.

Mizoguchi and colleagues *(39)* studied molecular changes in dysfunctional T cells from long-term tumor-bearing mice, and found alterations in the expression of several signal-transduction proteins, including a significant decrease in the expression of CD3ζ chain and *p56*^{lck} and *p59*^{fyn} tyrosine kinases. These changes were accompanied by a decreased tyrosine kinase phosphorylation and a diminished Ca^{++} flux. Li *(40)* and Ghosh *(41,42)* later showed that T cells from some patients with RCC and from long-term tumor-bearing mice were unable to translocate NF-κB*p65* nuclear transcription factor, which resulted in a predominance of NF-κB*p*50/50 homodimer in the nucleus, known to act as a repressor of the IFN-γ gene *(43)*. Indeed, cytokine production during the progressive growth of tumors in mice demonstrated a Th1 response (IL-2 and IFN-γ) early after tumor implantation, followed by an increased production of Th2 cytokines (IL-4 and IL-10) after the third week *(41,42)*. These findings provided for the first time a molecular basis to explain T-cell dysfunction in cancer.

Results in cancer patients confirmed the initial observations in tumor-bearing mice. T cells, and natural killer (NK) cells from approximately half of the patients with RCC, colon carcinoma, ovarian carcinoma, gastric cancer, breast cancer, prostate cancer, Hodgkin's disease, acute myelocytic leukemia, and other tumors showed a decreased expression of the CD3ζ chain and a decreased in vitro response to antigens or mitogens *(44–49)*. Alterations in signal-transduction molecules were most markedly observed in T cells that infiltrated tumors or T cells from lymph nodes draining the site of the tumor. In addition, T cells from RCC patients exhibited a diminished ability to translocate NF-κB*p65*. However, changes in signal-transduction molecules were not limited to those associated with the TCR. Kolenko and colleagues demonstrated that Jak-3, a tyrosine kinase associated with the γ chain, a common element to IL-2, IL-4, IL-7, and IL-15 cytokine receptors, was also decreased in T cells from RCC patients *(50)*.

Controversy over these findings arose when Levey and Srivastava *(51)* had difficulty reproducing some of the original observations in mice with transplantable tumors. However, Horiguchi and colleagues *(52)* later demonstrated that de novo tumors (chemically induced) were able to induce all of the alterations in T-cell signal-transduction molecules described initially, yet after repeated passage in mice, the tumors failed to cause T-cell alterations. Thus, it was possible that the tumors used by Levey and Srivastava may have lost their ability to induce immune dysfunction after multiple passages.

Initial work in colon carcinoma *(53)* and RCC *(54)* suggested that patients with more advanced stages of the disease had a higher frequency of T-cell signal-transduction alterations. In addition, TIL in RCC and ovarian carcinoma, as well as T cells from draining lymph nodes, had a more pronounced decrease in the expression of signal-transduction proteins than peripheral-blood T cells. However, in cervical carcinoma *(55)*, some patients with carcinoma *in situ*, an early stage of the disease, already showed a diminished expression of CD3ζ, suggesting that T-cell signal-transduction alterations were not an exclusive characteristic of the advanced stages of cancer. Other reports have also suggested an association between the expression of CD3ζ and survival (*see* Chapter 14). Patients with metastatic melanoma (Stage IV) and patients with head and neck cancer who had normal levels of CD3ζ chain had a significantly longer survival as compared to those who had undetectable levels of the same proteins *(57,58)*.

The expression of CD3ζ changes with treatment. Patients with non-Hodgkin's lymphoma (NHL) and patients with HD *(59,60)* who responded to chemotherapy showed a re-expression of normal levels of ζ chain, which decreased again in patients who had a recurrence of the disease *(61)*. Patients who received immunotherapy were also tested for possible changes in the expression of CD3ζ and other signal-transduction proteins. Farace and colleagues *(62)* initially reported that the decreased expression of CD3ζ chain was not corrected by the infusion of IL-2 alone. In contrast, data from several groups with ovarian carcinoma, melanoma, RCC, and colon carcinoma showed that patients who received IL-2 based therapies had a recovery of the levels of CD3ζ *(47,54)*. It is possible that these contrasting results could be explained by the different doses of IL-2 being infused. Re-expression of normal levels of ζ chain did not always coincide with a full recovery of T-cell function. Tyrosine kinase activity, tyrosine kinase phosphorylation patterns, and the production of cytokines were not always fully restored, suggesting that the expression of tyrosine kinases and/or nuclear transcription factors might not be normalized by IL-2 alone. More recently, Finn and colleagues *(63)* found that patients who received a MUC-1 vaccine and developed a positive DTH to the vaccine recovered the expression of CD3ζ. In a retrospective study, Gratama et al. *(64)* found that RCC patients that achieved a complete response when treated with IL-2 + IFN-α and LAK cells had a complete recovery of both CD3ζ chain and $p56^{lck}$ tyrosine kinase expression. In contrast, <25% of those with progressive disease had a partial re-expression of CD3ζ, and none recovered $p56^{lck}$. These data, although preliminary, suggest that monitoring the expression of signal-transduction proteins may provide a method for evaluating the response to immunotherapy, and could provide prognostic information.

4. MECHANISMS LEADING TO ALTERATIONS IN T-CELL SIGNAL TRANSDUCTION IN CANCER

Most of the studies on mechanisms that cause alterations in T-cell signal transduction have been conducted in murine tumor models. In a series of elegant in vitro experiments, Otsuji et al. *(65)* and Kono et al. *(55,66)* demonstrated that H_2O_2 from macrophages induced the loss of CD3ζ chain in naive T cells, a phenomenon that could be blocked by the depletion of macrophages or the addition of oxygen radical scavengers *(67)*. These observations were extended in patients by Schmielau et al. *(68)*, who suggested that H_2O_2 from neutrophils could induce similar alterations. A second mechanism leading to loss of the CD3ζ chain was found while studying Fas-FasL-induced T-cell apoptosis *(69–73)*. When T cells undergo apoptosis, they lose the expression of CD3ζ as one of the early changes in this process. Therefore, the diminished expression of the CD3ζ chain seen in cancer patients could be partly explained by an increased frequency of apoptotic cells in peripheral blood. However, these mechanisms have not yet been studied in infectious diseases.

5. T-CELL DYSFUNCTION IN CHRONIC INFECTIONS: LESSONS FROM OTHER DISEASES

The development of mechanisms to disrupt the immune response has been an active field of study in chronic infectious diseases. The chronicity of certain infections demonstrates the inability of the immune response alone to eliminate the infectious agent, and therefore suggests that the microorganisms have developed ways of blocking a protective immune response. In some infections, this process is represented by different clinical forms of the disease. Mycobacterial diseases, particularly leprosy, have provided a model for the study of changes in the immune response in chronic infections with different clinical presentations. Leprosy has two major polar forms that are closely associated with differences in the immune response. The tuberculoid form is clinically characterized by the presence of anesthetic and discolored patches of skin,

Table 1
Changes in Signal Transduction in Cancer and Mycobacterial Infections

Changes in Signal Transduction	*Cancer*	*Mycobacterial Infections*
Decreased CD3ζ chain expression	+++	+++
Decreased *p65*^{lck}	+++	+++
Decreased *p59*^{fyn}	+++	?
Inability to translocate NF-κB*p65*	+++	+++
Decreased Ca^{++} flux	++	?

a limited number of bacteria, and the presence of an active T-cell response to lepromin. At the other end of the spectrum are patients with lepromatous leprosy, who have significantly more advanced tissue damage and a large bacterial burden, and have lost the DTH to lepromin antigens. Various studies have demonstrated a predominance of Th_1 response with the production of IFN-γ and TNF-α in tuberculoid leprosy and a predominance of Th2 cytokines in lepromatous leprosy. The injection of IL-2 in the lepromatous nodules reverses this polarization of the immune response and confers an anti-mycobacterial effect *(74)*. Therefore, it has been suggested that the predominance of a Th2 response could provide a partial explanation for the lack of a protective response in lepromatous leprosy. However, despite a strong Th1 response in tuberculoid leprosy, patients still develop the disease, suggesting that other immune alterations might play a role in its pathogenesis. Zea et al. *(56)* studied T-cell signal transduction in these patients and found that, as in cancer patients, patients with lepromatous leprosy had a decreased expression of CD3ζ chain and *p56*^{lck} tyrosine kinase and were unable to translocate NF-κB*p65*. In addition, some of the patients with tuberculoid leprosy also had a decreased expression of *p56*^{lck}, although less frequently than lepromatous patients (Table 1). Similar observations have been made in tuberculosis *(75)* and other non-mycobacterial infections such as *Helicobacter pylori* (Zabaleta, J., et al., submitted).

6. MODULATION OF T-CELL FUNCTION AND CD3ζ EXPRESSION BY ARGININE AVAILABILITY: A COMMON LINK BETWEEN CANCER AND INFECTIOUS DISEASES?

L-arginine is a non-essential amino acid that plays a central role in various biological systems, including the immune response. Taheri et al. and Rodriguez and colleagues *(76,77)*, recently demonstrated that T cells cultured in the absence of arginine lose the expression of CD3ζ, and exhibit a decreased proliferation and a diminished production of IFN-γ. In vivo levels of arginine are maintained by dietary intake and endogenous synthesis, and are decreased by catabolism of the amino acid through three enzymatic pathways, nitric oxide synthase (NOS), and arginase I and II. NOS uses arginine as the substrate to produce nitric oxide (NO), a major cytotoxic mechanism in macrophages and an important mediator of vascular homeostasis. Arginase I (cytoplasmic form) and II (mitochondrial form) use arginine to produce polyamines that are essential for cell proliferation and urea as a method of detoxification. In macrophages, IFN-γ upregulates iNOS, and Th2 cytokines IL-4 and IL-13 upregulate arginase I. Rodriguez et al. *(78)* recently showed that arginase I rapidly depletes L-arginine from the microenvironment, causing the loss of CD3ζ, and resulting in profound T-cell dysfunction. Arginase is produced by macrophages as well as tumor cells that may further enhance the depletion of arginine. Therefore, T cells that infiltrate the tumor and recognize tumor antigens could undergo the loss of CD3ζ chain and other signal-transduction proteins as a result of the arginine depletion, which would effectively prevent the development of an antitumor response.

Arginase is also produced by microorganisms as a means of synthesizing polyamines or other proteins needed for their survival. Some of the microorganisms that produce arginase are also the cause of chronic human disease, including *Helicobacter pylori* and leishmaniasis *(79–82)*. In *H. pylori*, for example, arginase is used to produce urea, which in turn serves as the substrate for the enzyme urease that produces the ammonia needed to neutralize the acidity of the stomach where the bacteria lives. Other examples include leprosy, in which an increased arginase activity has been described in the serum of lepromatous patients *(83)*. However, it is unclear from these reports whether arginase is produced by the microorganism or by infected monocytes. Results from patients with tuberculosis suggest that the increased production of arginase in mycobacterial infections may instead come from arginase produced by macrophages (A. Zea, submitted manuscript). Therefore, arginase produced by microorganisms or by the immune cells of infected patients could provide an important means of evading the immune response through similar mechanisms to tumors.

7. CONCLUSIONS

Tumors and chronic infections induce similar molecular alterations in T cells (Table 1), including the loss of CD3ζ chain, a decreased expression of *p56*^{lck} tyrosine kinase, and the inability to translocate NF-κB*p65*, which lead to a dysfunctional T-cell response and suggest a common mechanism (Fig. 1). Therefore, we have proposed that arginase produced by tumor cells, macrophages, or microorganisms could deplete arginine in tissues, causing the

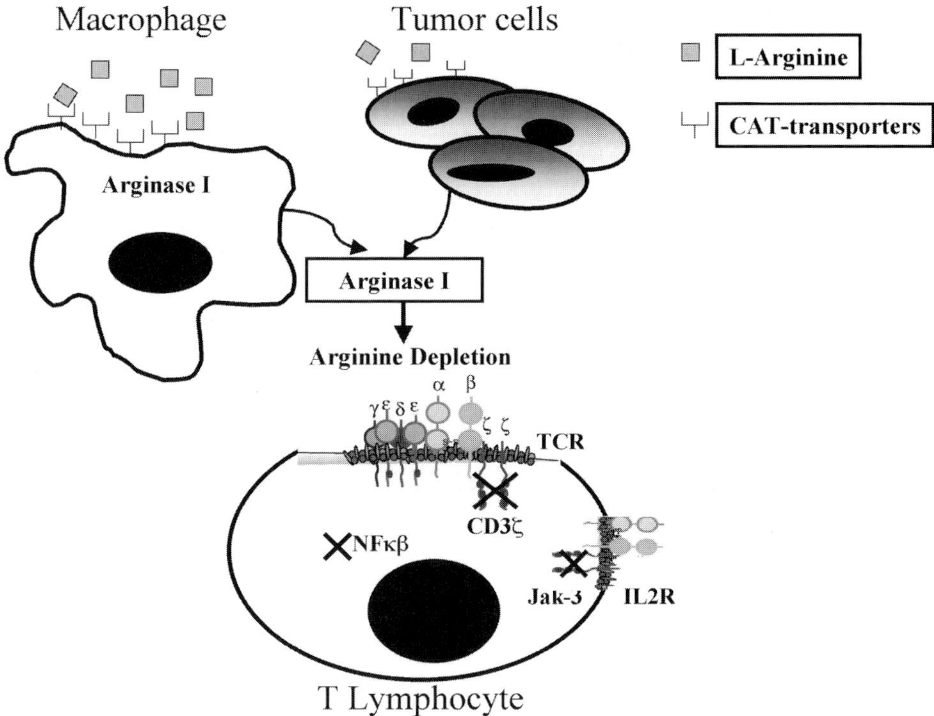

Fig. 1. Arginase produced by macrophages, tumor cells, or microorganisms depletes arginine from the microenvironment and causes alterations in T-cell signal transduction, which results in a state of anergy to the specific antigens.

loss of CD3ζ and inducing a state of anergy in the T cells infiltrating the site. Alternatively, if enough arginase is produced systemically as a result of metastatic tumor or a chronic and disseminated infection (as in miliary tuberculosis), the depletion of arginine could affect the function of specific T cells as well as those that recognize unrelated antigens. Therefore, despite the different pathophysiology of these diseases, a common mechanism leading to these changes appears to be the regulation of arginine availability. Further studies will be required to determine the impact of these changes in the outcome of the disease and the potential for the development of therapies that may prevent and/or reverse the development of T-cell alterations and T-cell anergy.

REFERENCES

1. Pliskin ME, Prehn RT. Are tumor-associated transplantation antigens of chemically induced sarcomas related to alien histocompatibility antigens? *Transplantation* 1978;26:19–24.
2. Prehn RT, Main JM. Immunity to methylcholanthrene-induced sarcomas. *J Natl Cancer Inst* 1957; 18:759–778.

3. Dunn GP, Bruce AT, Ikeda H, Old LJ, Schreiber RD. Cancer immunoediting: from immunosurveillance to tumor escape. *Nat Immunol* 2002;3:991–998.
4. Urban JL, Schreiber H. Host-tumor interactions in immunosurveillance against cancer. *Prog Exp Tumor Res* 1988;32:17–68.
5. Hersh EM, Oppenheim JJ. Impaired in vitro lymphocyte transformation in Hodgkin's disease. *N Engl J Med* 1965;273:1006–1012.
6. Fisher RI, DeVita VT, Jr., Bostick F, Vanhaelen C, Howser DM, Hubbard SM, et al. Persistent immunologic abnormalities in long-term survivors of advanced Hodgkin's disease. *Ann Intern Med* 1980;92:595–599.
7. Catalona WJ, Smolev JK, Harty JI. Prognostic value of host immunocompetence in urologic cancer patients. *J Urol* 1975;114:922–926.
8. Alberola V, Gonzalez-Molina A, Trenor A, San Martin B, Lluch A, Palau F, et al. Mechanism of suppression of the depressed lymphocyte response in lung cancer patients. *Allergol Immunopathol (Madr)* 1985;13:213–219.
9. Jerrells TR, Dean JH, Richardson GL, McCoy JL, Herberman RB. Role of suppressor cells in depression of in vitro lymphoproliferative responses of lung cancer and breast cancer patients. *J Natl Cancer Inst* 1978;61:1001–1009.
10. Iwahashi M, Tanimura H, Yamaue H, Tsunoda T, Tani M, Tamai M, et al. Defective autologous mixed lymphocyte reaction (AMLR) and killer activity generated in the AMLR in cancer patients. *Int J Cancer* 1992;51:67–71.
11. Hellstrom I, Sjogren HO, Warner G, Hellstrom KE. Blocking of cell-mediated tumor immunity by sera from patients with growing neoplasms. *Int J Cancer* 1971;7:226–237.
12. Hellstrom KE, Hellstrom I, Nelson K. Antigen-specific suppressor ("blocking") factors in tumor immunity. *Biomembranes* 1983;11:365–388.
13. Mengersen R, Schick R, Kolsch E. Correlation of "sneaking through" of tumor cells with specific immunological impairment of the host. *Eur J Immunol* 1975;5:532–537.
14. Varesio L, Giovarelli M, Landolfo S, Forni G. Suppression of proliferative response and lymphokine production during the progression of a spontaneous tumor. *Cancer Res* 1979;39:4983–4988.
15. Dye ES, North RJ. Specificity of the T cells that mediate and suppress adoptive immunotherapy of established tumors. *J Leukoc Biol* 1984;36:27–37.
16. Mills CD, North RJ. Ly-1+2- suppressor T cells inhibit the expression of passively transferred antitumor immunity by suppressing the generation of cytolytic T cells. *Transplantation* 1985;39:202–208.
17. North RJ, Bursuker I. Generation and decay of the immune response to a progressive fibrosarcoma. I. Ly-1+2- suppressor T cells down-regulate the generation of Ly-1-2+ effector T cells. *J Exp Med* 1984;159:1295–1311.
18. North RJ. Down-regulation of the antitumor immune response. *Adv Cancer Res* 1985;45:1–43.
19. Mosmann TR, Coffman RL. TH1 and TH2 cells: different patterns of lymphokine secretion lead to different functional properties. *Annu Rev Immunol* 1989;7:145–173.
20. Mosmann TR, Schumacher JH, Street NF, Budd R, O'Garra A, Fong TA, et al. Diversity of cytokine synthesis and function of mouse CD4+ T cells. *Immunol Rev* 1991;123: 209–229.
21. Miescher S, Whiteside TL, Carrel S, von F, V. Functional properties of tumor-infiltrating and blood lymphocytes in patients with solid tumors: effects of tumor cells and their supernatants on proliferative responses of lymphocytes. *J Immunol* 1986;136:1899–1907.
22. Miescher S, Stoeck M, Qiao L, Barras C, Barrelet L, von F, V. Preferential clonogenic deficit of CD8-positive T-lymphocytes infiltrating human solid tumors. *Cancer Res* 1988; 48:6992–6998.

23. Whiteside TL, Miescher S, Moretta L, von F, V. Cloning and proliferating precursor frequencies of tumor-infiltrating lymphocytes from human solid tumors. *Transplant Proc* 1988;20:342–343.
24. Whiteside TL, Rabinowich H. The role of Fas/FasL in immunosuppression induced by human tumors. *Cancer Immunol Immunother* 1998;46:175–184.
25. Loeffler CM. Antitumor effects of interleukin 2 liposomes and anti-CD3-stimulated T-cells against murine MCA-38 hepatic metastasis. *Cancer Res* 1991;51:2127–2132.
26. Frank SJ, Samelson LE, Klausner RD. The structure and signalling functions of the invariant T cell receptor components. *Semin Immunol* 1990;2:89–97.
27. Weiss A, Desai D, Graber M, Picus J, Koretzky G. The regulation of T-cell antigen receptor signal transduction function. *Transplant Proc* 1991;23:32–33.
28. Weissman AM, Baniyash M, Hou D, Samelson LE, Burgess WH, Klausner RD. Molecular cloning of the zeta chain of the T cell antigen receptor. *Science* 1988;239:1018–1021.
29. Bockenstedt LK, Goldsmith MA, Koretzky GA, Weiss A. The activation of T lymphocytes. *Rheum Dis Clin North Am* 1987;13:411–430.
30. Fraser JD, Straus D, Weiss A. Signal transduction events leading to T-cell lymphokine gene expression. *Immunol Today* 1993;14:357–362.
31. Quill H, Schwartz RH. Stimulation of normal inducer T cell clones with antigen presented by purified Ia molecules in planar lipid membranes: specific induction of a long-lived state of proliferative nonresponsiveness. *J Immunol* 1987;138:3704–3712.
32. Quill H, Riley MP, Cho EA, Casnellie JE, Reed JC, Torigoe T. Anergic Th1 cells express altered levels of the protein tyrosine kinases p56lck and p59fyn. *J Immunol* 1992;149:2887–2893.
33. DeSilva DR, Urdahl KB, Jenkins MK. Clonal anergy is induced in vitro by T cell receptor occupancy in the absence of proliferation. *J Immunol* 1991;147:3261–3267.
34. Jenkins MK, Schwartz RH. Antigen presentation by chemically modified splenocytes induces antigen-specific T cell unresponsiveness in vitro and in vivo. *J Exp Med* 1987;165:302–319.
35. Cho EA, Riley MP, Sillman AL, Quill H. Altered protein tyrosine phosphorylation in anergic Th1 cells. *J Immunol* 1993;151:20–28.
36. Fields PE, Gajewski TF, Fitch FW. Blocked Ras activation in anergic CD4+ T cells. *Science* 1996;271:1276–1278.
37. Gajewski TF, Qian D, Fields P, Fitch FW. Anergic T-lymphocyte clones have altered inositol phosphate, calcium, and tyrosine kinase signaling pathways. *Proc Natl Acad Sci USA* 1994;91:38–42.
38. Mondino A, Whaley CD, DeSilva DR, Li W, Jenkins MK, Mueller DL. Defective transcription of the IL-2 gene is associated with impaired expression of c-Fos, FosB, and JunB in anergic T helper 1 cells. *J Immunol* 1996;157:2048–2057.
39. Mizoguchi H, O'Shea JJ, Longo DL, Loeffler CM, McVicar DW, Ochoa AC. Alterations in signal transduction molecules in T lymphocytes from tumor-bearing mice. *Science* 1992;258:1795–1798.
40. Li X, Liu J, Park JK, Hamilton TA, Rayman P, Klein E, et al. T cells from renal cell carcinoma patients exhibit an abnormal pattern of kappa B-specific DNA-binding activity: a preliminary report. *Cancer Res* 1994;54:5424–5429.
41. Ghosh P, Komschlies KL, Cippitelli M, Longo DL, Subleski J, Ye J, et al. Gradual loss of T-helper 1 populations in spleen of mice during progressive tumor growth. *J Natl Cancer Inst* 1995;87:1478–1483.
42. Ghosh P, Sica A, Young HA, Ye J, Franco JL, Wiltrout RH, et al. Alterations in NF kappa B/Rel family proteins in splenic T-cells from tumor-bearing mice and reversal following therapy. *Cancer Res* 1994;54:2969–2972.

43. Young HA, Ghosh P. Molecular regulation of cytokine gene expression: interferon-gamma as a model system. *Prog Nucleic Acid Res Mol Biol* 1997;56:109–127.
44. Buggins AG, Hirst WJ, Pagliuca A, Mufti GJ. Variable expression of CD3-zeta and associated protein tyrosine kinases in lymphocytes from patients with myeloid malignancies. *Br J Haematol* 1998;100:784–792.
45. Finke JH, Zea AH, Stanley J, Longo DL, Mizoguchi H, Tubbs RR, et al. Loss of T-cell receptor zeta chain and p56lck in T-cells infiltrating human renal cell carcinoma. *Cancer Res* 1993;53:5613–5616.
46. Gunji Y, Hori S, Aoe T, Asano T, Ochiai T, Isono K, et al. High frequency of cancer patients with abnormal assembly of the T cell receptor-CD3 complex in peripheral blood T lymphocytes. *Jpn J Cancer Res* 1994;85:1189–1192.
47. Rabinowich H, Suminami Y, Reichert TE, Crowley-Nowick P, Bell M, Edwards R, et al. Expression of cytokine genes or proteins and signaling molecules in lymphocytes associated with human ovarian carcinoma. *Int J Cancer* 1996;68:276–284.
48. Rossi E, Matutes E, Morilla R, Owusu-Ankomah K, Heffernan AM, Catovsky D. Zeta chain and CD28 are poorly expressed on T lymphocytes from chronic lymphocytic leukemia. *Leukemia* 1996;10:494–497.
49. Ungefroren H, Voss M, Bernstorff WV, Schmid A, Kremer B, Kalthoff H. Immunological escape mechanisms in pancreatic carcinoma. *Ann NY Acad Sci* 1999;880:243–251.
50. Kolenko V, Wang Q, Riedy MC, O'Shea J, Ritz J, Cathcart MK, et al. Tumor-induced suppression of T lymphocyte proliferation coincides with inhibition of Jak3 expression and IL-2 receptor signaling: role of soluble products from human renal cell carcinomas. *J Immunol* 1997;159:3057–3067.
51. Levey DL, Srivastava PK. T cells from late tumor-bearing mice express normal levels of p56lck, p59fyn, ZAP-70, and CD3 zeta despite suppressed cytolytic activity. *J Exp Med* 1995;182:1029–1036.
52. Horiguchi S, Petersson M, Nakazawa T, Kanda M, Zea AH, Ochoa AC, et al. Primary chemically induced tumors induce profound immunosuppression concomitant with apoptosis and alterations in signal transduction in T cells and NK cells. *Cancer Res* 1999;59:2950–2956.
53. Nakagomi H, Petersson M, Magnusson I, Juhlin C, Matsuda M, Mellstedt H, et al. Decreased expression of the signal-transducing zeta chains in tumor-infiltrating T-cells and NK cells of patients with colorectal carcinoma. *Cancer Res* 1993;53:5610–5612.
54. Bukowski RM, Rayman P, Uzzo R, Bloom T, Sandstrom K, Peereboom D, et al. Signal transduction abnormalities in T lymphocytes from patients with advanced renal carcinoma: clinical relevance and effects of cytokine therapy. *Clin Cancer Res* 1998;4:2337–2347.
55. Kono K, Ressing ME, Brandt RM, Melief CJ, Potkul RK, Andersson B, et al. Decreased expression of signal-transducing zeta chain in peripheral T cells and natural killer cells in patients with cervical cancer. *Clin Cancer Res* 1996;2:1825–1828.
56. Zea AH, Ochoa MT, Ghosh P, Longo DL, Alvord WG, Valderrama L, et al. Changes in expression of signal transduction proteins in T lymphocytes of patients with leprosy. *Infect Immun* 1998;66:499–504.
57. Zea AH, Corti BD, Longo DL, Alvord WG, Strobl SL, Mizoguchi H, et al. Alterations in T Cell receptor and signal transduction molecules in melanoma patients. *Clin Cancer Res* 1995;1:1327–1335.
58. Reichert TE, Day R, Wagner EM, Whiteside TL. Absent or low expression of the zeta chain in T cells at the tumor site correlates with poor survival in patients with oral carcinoma. *Cancer Res* 1998;58:5344–5347.
59. Massaia M, Attisano C, Beggiato E, Bianchi A, Pileri A. Correlation between disease activity and T-cell CD3 zeta chain expression in a B-cell lymphoma. *Br J Haematol* 1994;88:886–888.

60. Renner C, Ohnesorge S, Held G, Bauer S, Jung W, Pfitzenmeier JP, et al. T cells from patients with Hodgkin's disease have a defective T-cell receptor zeta chain expression that is reversible by T-cell stimulation with CD3 and CD28. *Blood* 1996;88:236–241.
61. Massaia M, Attisano C, Beggiato E, Bianchi A, Pileri A. Correlation between disease activity and T-cell CD3 zeta chain expression in a B-cell lymphoma. *Br J Haematol* 1994;88:886–888.
62. Farace F, Angevin E, Vanderplancke J, Escudier B, Triebel F. The decreased expression of CD3 zeta chains in cancer patients is not reversed by IL-2 administration. *Int J Cancer* 1994;59:752–755.
63. Finn OJ, Lotze MT. A decade in the life of tumor immunology. *Clin Cancer Res* 2001; 7:759s–760s.
64. Gratama JW, Zea AH, Bolhuis RL, Ochoa AC. Restoration of expression of signal-transduction molecules in lymphocytes from patients with metastatic renal cell cancer after combination immunotherapy. *Cancer Immunol Immunother* 1999;48:263–269.
65. Otsuji M, Kimura Y, Aoe T, Okamoto Y, Saito T. Oxidative stress by tumor-derived macrophages suppresses the expression of CD3 zeta chain of T-cell receptor complex and antigen-specific T-cell responses. *Proc Natl Acad Sci USA* 1996;93:13,119–13,124.
66. Kono K, Salazar-Onfray F, Petersson M, Hansson J, Masucci G, Wasserman K, et al. Hydrogen peroxide secreted by tumor-derived macrophages down-modulates signal-transducing zeta molecules and inhibits tumor-specific T cell-and natural killer cell-mediated cytotoxicity. *Eur J Immunol* 1996;26:1308–1313.
67. Corsi MM, Maes HH, Wasserman K, Fulgenzi A, Gaja G, Ferrero ME. Protection by L-2-oxothiazolidine-4-carboxylic acid of hydrogen peroxide-induced CD3zeta and CD16zeta chain down-regulation in human peripheral blood lymphocytes and lymphokine-activated killer cells. *Biochem Pharmacol* 1998;56:657–662.
68. Schmielau J, Finn OJ. Activated granulocytes and granulocyte-derived hydrogen peroxide are the underlying mechanism of suppression of t-cell function in advanced cancer patients. *Cancer Res* 2001;61:4756–4760.
69. Gastman BR, Johnson DE, Whiteside TL, Rabinowich H. Caspase-mediated degradation of T-cell receptor zeta-chain. *Cancer Res* 1999;59:1422–1427.
70. Rabinowich H, Reichert TE, Kashii Y, Gastman BR, Bell MC, Whiteside TL. Lymphocyte apoptosis induced by Fas li. *J Clin Invest* 1998;101:2579–2588.
71. Uzzo RG, Rayman P, Kolenko V, Clark PE, Cathcart MK, Bloom T, et al. Renal cell carcinoma-derived gangliosides suppress nuclear factor-kappaB activation in T cells. *J Clin Investig* 1999;104:769–776.
72. Uzzo RG, Rayman P, Kolenko V, Clark PE, Bloom T, Ward AM, et al. Mechanisms of apoptosis in T cells from patients with renal cell carcinoma. *Clin Cancer Res* 1999;5: 1219–1229.
73. Uzzo RG, Clark PE, Rayman P, Bloom T, Rybicki L, Novick AC, et al. Alterations in NFkappaB activation in T lymphocytes of patients with renal cell carcinoma. *J Natl Cancer Inst* 1999;91:718–721.
74. Kaplan G, Kiessling R, Teklemariam S, Hancock G, Sheftel, Job CK, et al. The reconstitution of cell-mediated immunity in the cutaneous lesions of lepromatous leprosy by recombinant interleukin 2. *J Exp Med* 1989;169:893–907.
75. Zea AH, Culotta K, Ali J, Mason C, Hae-Joon P, Zabaleta J, et al. Alterations in T cell signal transduction proteins in patients with tuberculosis. *FASEB J* 2002; *Exp Biol* 2002;A300.
76. Rodriguez PC, Zea AH, Culotta KS, Zabaleta J, Ochoa JB, Ochoa AC. Regulation of T cell receptor CD3 zeta chain expression by L-arginine. *J Biol Chem* 2002;277:21,123–21,129.
77. Taheri F, Ochoa JB, Faghiri Z, Culotta K, Park HJ, Lan MS, et al. L-Arginine regulates the expression of the T-cell receptor zeta chain (CD3zeta) in Jurkat cells. *Clin Cancer Res* 2001;7:958s–965s.

78. Rodriguez PC, Zea AH, DeSalvo J, Culotta KS, Zabuleta J, Quiceno DG, et al. L-Arginine consumption by macrophages modulates the expression of CD3ζ chain in T lymphocytes. *J Immunol* 2003;17:1232–1239.
79. da Silva ER, Castilho TM, Pioker FC, Tomich de Paula Silva CH, Floeter-Winter LM. Genomic organisation and transcription characterisation of the gene encoding Leishmania (Leishmania) amazonensis arginase and its protein structure prediction. *Int J Parasitol* 2002;32:727–737.
80. Iniesta V, Gomez-Nieto LC, Corraliza I. The inhibition of arginase by N(omega)-hydroxy-l-arginine controls the growth of Leishmania inside macrophages. *J Exp Med* 2001;193:777–784.
81. Iniesta V, Gomez-Nieto LC, Molano I, Mohedano A, Carcelen J, Miron C, et al. Arginase I induction in macrophages, triggered by Th2-type cytokines, supports the growth of intracellular Leishmania parasites. *Parasite Immunol* 2002;24:113–118.
82. Mendz GL, Holmes EM, Ferrero RL. In situ characterization of Helicobacter pylori arginase. *Biochim Biophys Acta* 1998;1388:465–477.
83. Babu CS, Kannan KB, Bharadwaj VP, Katoch VM. Lymphocyte arginase activity in leprosy—a preliminary report. *Indian J Med Res* 1990;91:193–196.

3 Malfunction of the Dendritic Cell System in Cancer

Zoya R. Yurkovetsky, PhD,
Irina L. Tourkova, PhD,
Levent Balkir, MD, PhD, Lori Perez,
Galina V. Shurin, PhD,
Gurkamal S. Chatta, MD,
and Michael R. Shurin, MD, PhD

CONTENTS

1. INTRODUCTION

The induction of antitumor immune responses is a complex sequence of carefully orchestrated events leading to the subsequent activation, migration, and proliferation of different immune cells. Naïve T cells are unable to directly recognize tumor antigens. They require help from specialized cells known as professional antigen-presenting cells (APCs). APCs first interact with tumors, uptake tumor cells/proteins, process them, and present antigenic peptides to T cells in the context of major histocompatibility complex (MHC) class I/II. Dendritic cells (DCs) are the most potent and powerful APCs capable of activating naïve T lymphocytes. The interaction between DCs and tumor cells in the tumor tissue thus plays a crucial role in the induction of specific antitumor immune responses. However, a great number of preclinical and clinical studies provide evidence proving that the immune system is significantly unbalanced in the presence of the tumor. A variety of different processes involved in the immune response have been impaired in the tumor-bearing hosts. For example,

From: *Current Clinical Oncology: Cancer Immunotherapy at the Crossroads: How Tumors Evade Immunity and What Can Be Done*
Edited by: J. H. Finke and R. M. Bukowski © Humana Press Inc., Totowa, NJ

multiple tumor-produced factors exhibit immunomodulatory properties, and play an important role in the regulation of tumor growth and tumor escape from immune recognition and elimination. Some of these molecules inhibit the activity of natural killer (NK) cells and cytotoxic T lymphocytes (CTLs) *(1)*, and impair macrophage and DC functions *(2)*; others induce apoptosis of NK and T cells *(3)*, and cause apoptotic death of DC *(4–6)*.

A major contributor to host immunity and immune surveillance against infection and malignancy is the DC system. Therefore, tumors develop mechanisms that suppress the activity of the DC system in order to evade immune recognition and elimination. A growing body of evidence demonstrates that tumor-derived factors suppress DC generation, function, and resistance to cell death *(6–11)*. In fact, numerous clinical data has demonstrated that the reduced number of DC infiltrating tumors correlates with a poor prognosis for patients *(12–14)*. For instance, analysis of the correlation between the infiltration of DCs and lymphocytes in hepatocellular carcinoma (HCC) tissue and postoperative tumor recurrence and survival rate has demonstrated that tumor recurrence was markedly late in patients with a DC count ≥ 20 and positive lymphocyte infiltration (group A) compared to those who did not meet both criteria simultaneously (group B), with a median interval of 21.6 mo for group A and 4.1 mo for group B *(15)*. The 1-, 3-, and 4-yr survival rates were significantly greater in group A than in group B: 83.5% vs 42.2%, 61.8% vs 28.4%, and 48.7% vs 23.0%, respectively, suggesting that the infiltration of HCC mass by DC and lymphocytes is closely related to a postoperative prognosis. A similar conclusion was made after immunohistochemical analysis of gastric carcinoma tissues. The survival curves show that the prognosis for patients with a low density of DCs was significantly poorer than for patients with high DC density *(14)*.

These findings suggest that DCs present in the tumor microenvironment may be beneficial for generating antitumor immune responses. These data also suggest that the tumor may actively decrease the number of tumor-infiltrating DCs (TIDCs) by inducing their premature death, inhibiting their immigration into the tumor site, and homing within the tumor, or by the general suppression of DC generation. Therefore, it is possible that defects in the DC system in cancer could be responsible for a loss of tumor immunosurveillance.

1.1. Tumor-Mediated Inhibition of DC Generation, Differentiation, and Maturation

Inhibition of hematopoiesis is a common feature in patients with cancer *(16–18)*. The suppressive effect of tumor-derived factors on hematopoiesis significantly increases during metastatic disease, especially in the presence of bone-marrow metastases. However, the effect of tumor-released factors on the differentiation and generation of DCs from hematopoietic precursors was not demonstrated until recently. Gabrilovich et al. first reported that tumor cells released factors that were able to inhibit the production of DCs *(19,20)*. These results were confirmed by other in vitro studies. For instance, we have shown that when the supernatant from murine sarcoma cell line C3 was added to DC cultures derived from murine bone-marrow cells, the proliferation of these cells and their differentiation into functionally active DCs were significantly suppressed *(2)*. Similar results were obtained when we cultured human CD34+ hematopoietic precursor cells with human tumor cells *(5,8,21)*, suggesting that most of the tumor-cell lines tested markedly inhibit or block DC generation and differentiation in in vitro experiments.

These and other studies have demonstrated that production of immunosuppressive factors is one of the mechanisms that enable tumors to evade immunosurveillance *(2,22,23)*. It has been proven that tumor cells produce and release several immunosuppressive factors, including cytokines, growth factors, and other molecules such as nitric oxide (NO), gangliosides, neuropeptides, and prostaglandin E_2 (PgE_2), which can block important functions of immune cells, including DCs (Table 1). In addition, tumor-infiltrating immune cells—for instance, macrophages—can be activated by tumor cells to secrete a number of molecules (H_2O_2, NO, PgE_2), which can decrease the activity of immune effectors. Lymphocytes in the tumor microenvironment may also exhibit unusual effects on DC. For example, transforming growth factor β (TGF-β) may be produced by tumor-infiltrating lymphocytes (TILs) in regional lymph nodes, where it causes a significant immunosuppression of DCs *(24)*. Furthermore, recent in vitro studies suggest that even the efficacy of DC immunization may be impaired by tumor-derived TGF-β *(25)*. The IL-2-mediated proliferation of peripheral lymphocytes may be inhibited by tumor-associated gangliosides and soluble IL-2 receptors. Interestingly, anergic T cells may also serve as strong inhibitors of antigen presentation by DC *(26)*. Granulocyte macrophage colony-stimulating factor (GM-CSF) in some tumors may have an immunosuppressive effect through the induction and expansion of immunosuppressive macrophages. Furthermore, the generation of DCs in the presence of GM-CSF and bacterial endotoxins or interferon-γ may give rise to DCs with strong T-cell inhibitory properties *(27,28)*.

Thus, the escape of malignant cells from the immune response against the tumor may result from a defective differentiation and maturation of DCs, which in turn is associated with impaired function, such as cytokine production, activation of T cells, and migratory potential. In fact, Sombroek et al. recently demonstrated that cyclooxygenase (COX)-1- and COX-2-regulated prostanoids were present in the primary tumor-derived supernatants, and were responsible for the inhibition of monocyte-derived DC differentiation *(29)*. The authors have shown that tumor supernatants inhibit IL-12 production and increased IL-10 production by DCs. Menetrier-Caux et al. have reported that human renal carcinoma cells (RCC) release soluble factors that inhibit the differentiation of

Table 1
Tumor-Derived Factors With Proven or Potential Dendritic Cell (DC) Inhibitory Properties

Tumor-derived factors	*Major functions*	*Effect on DCs*	*References*
VEGF (Vascular endothelial growth factor)	Development of tumor neovasculature	Decrease of tumor-infiltrating DCs Inhibition of DC generation	*19,20,23, 83,84*
TGF-β (Transforming growth factor β)	Suppression of T-cell proliferation, inhibition of TCR signaling Tumor growth factor	Downregulation of CD80 and CD86 expression	*24,25*
M-CSF (macrophage colony-stimulating factor)		Inhibition of DC differentiation from CD34+ precursors	*21*
Gangliosides (sialic acid-containing glycosphingolipids)	Regulation of cellular proliferation and differentiation Immunosuppressive molecule	Inhibition of dendropoiesis from both human and murine hematopoietic precursor cells DC apoptosis	*5*
IL-6	Major plasma-cell growth factor	Inhibition of DC differentiation from CD34+ precursors Switch of differentiation from DCs to macrophages	*29,30, 45,85*
IL-10	Inhibition of activities of immune cells	Block of monocyte differentiation into DCs Downregulation of CD80 and CD86 on DC Downregulation of CD40 expression on DC and CD40-dependent IL-12 production	*24,44,86*
Prostanoids Prostaglandins	COX controls the rate of prostanoid synthesis by catalyzing the conversion of arachidonic acid to PgH_2	Inhibition of differentiation of monocyte-derived DC	*29,35,87*
PgE_2	Downregulates differentiation and activity of immune effectors: increases IL-10 synthesis by macrophages	Prevents the generation of CD1+ DC in cultures	*29,88*
NO	Downregulates activity of immune effectors	May induce apoptosis in DCs	*53,57*
H_2O_2	Downregulates activity of immune effectors	May induce apoptosis in DCs	
Regulatory peptides	May serve as tumor-derived autocrine growth factors	Inhibit dendropoiesis and functional activity of DCs	*36*

CD34+ hematopoietic precursor cells into DCs and redirect their differentiation toward macrophage lineage *(30)*. They concluded that this phenomenon was mediated by IL-6 and microphage colony-stimulating factor (M-CSF).

These data were recently confirmed by other laboratories. For example, it has been demonstrated that coincubation of murine bone-marrow progenitors or human CD34+ progenitor cells with neuroblastoma cells resulted in a significant inhibition of dendropoiesis in vitro up to 90% *(31)*. Furthermore, neuroblastoma-derived gangliosides—as well as purified gangliosides—added to DC cultures also inhibited the generation of functionally active DCs. Similarly, Katsenelson et al. had examined whether human lung-tumor cells produce soluble factors that inhibit differentiation of hematopoietic precursors into mature DC *(10)*. It has been demonstrated that the addition of small-cell lung carcinoma (SCLC)-conditioned medium to CD34+ precursor-cell cultures significantly inhibited colony formation of DC precursors and markedly attenuated DC generation. The authors also revealed that DC generation and differentiation was completely abrogated in CD34+-derived cultures treated with a bronchial carcinoid tumor-conditioned medium, suggesting that carcinoid tumor-derived factors blocked CD34+ cell differentiation into DCs. Similar results were reported by Kiertscher et al., who evaluated the effect of various human tumor-cell lines on DC generation in vitro *(32)*. The effects of tumor-conditioned media appeared to be specific for maturing DCs, and were not reversed by antibodies against known DC regulatory factors including IL-10, vascular endothelial growth factor (VEGF), TGF-β, or PgE_2. Supernatants collected from nonmalignant cell sources had no effect on DC maturation. Using human prostate carcinoma-cell lines, it has been recently demonstrated that soluble tumor-derived factors suppress the generation and maturation of DCs from both CD34+ hematopoietic precursors and CD14+ PBMC-derived adherent monocytes *(8,33)*. PgE_2, known to be produced by different tumor-cell lines or in the tumor microenvironment *(34)*, may also strongly downregulate DC activity and function *(35)*. In fact, Sombroek et al. investigated the presence of soluble antidendropoietic factors in 24-h culture supernatants from freshly excised solid human tumors, including colon, breast, RCC, and melanoma. They found that although COX-1- and COX-2-regulated prostanoids present in the primary tumor supernatants were solely responsible for the observed problems with differentiation of monocyte-derived DCs, both prostanoids and IL-6 contributed to the tumor-induced inhibition of DC differentiation from CD34+ hematopoietic precursor cells *(29)*.

Although several tumor-derived factors with antidendropoietic function have been identified and characterized, the list of new candidates with immunosuppressive properties is constantly growing. We recently reported that bombesin-like peptides released from lung tumor-cell lines dose-dependently inhibit the generation of human DC from monocytic precursors *(36)* (Makarenkova et al., submitted). Bombesin, neuromedin B, and gastrin-releasing peptides all inhibited dendropoiesis and DC activity at varying different degrees. Another interesting finding has been recently reported by Kennedy-Smith et al. Prostate-specific antigen (PSA), which is a diagnostic marker of prostate cancer as well as a serine protease, significantly inhibited mitogen- and antigen-induced proliferation of T cells, suggesting that it may serve as novel tumor-derived immunosuppressant *(37)*. We recently evaluated the effect of PSA on DC generation in vitro and demonstrated that PSA may also inhibit dendropoiesis in a dose-dependent manner *(38)*. Interestingly, Pietra et al. demonstrated that tumor cells in an early phase of apoptosis inhibit DC maturation. In contrast, cells in late apoptosis or even primary necrosis are only able to deliver a partial maturation signal that is not sufficient to accomplish a cross-presentation of tumor antigens to T cells *(39)*. These data may represent an additional mechanism to explain how tumors escape from immune recognition, preventing the development of the antitumor response by blocking maturation of DCs by neoplastic cells in the early phase of apoptosis.

The inhibition of DCs maturation, and particularly downregulation of the expression of costimulatory molecules on DCs, has a decisive impact on the overall development of a specific immune response or tolerance in cancer.

1.2. Functional Impairment of DCs in Cancer

The expression of costimulatory molecules on DCs plays an especially important role in determining whether T-cell survival, apoptosis, anergy, or productive immunity will take place. It is well known that if APCs do not express CD80 or CD86, and thereby fail to provide an appropriate second signal for T cells, tolerance or anergy may develop *(40,41)*. In fact, DCs derived from colon cancer are much less potent inducers of T-cell proliferation in an allogeneic MLR, and indeed induce T-cell anergy *(42)*. A similar toleragenic effect of melanoma-associated DC has also been reported: tumor-derived DCs from progressing metastases may actively induce tolerance in the immune system against tumor tissue. This process may ultimately lead to acceptance of metastatic tumor growth with a "silenced" immune system that is incapable of rejecting the tumor *(43)*. We have recently shown that DCs generated from bone-marrow precursors obtained from tumor-bearing mice and DCs isolated from the spleens of tumor-bearers have a significantly lower expression of CD40, CD80, and CD86 when compared to DCs generated/isolated from tumor-free animals *(44)*. Interestingly, CD40 ligation on DCs generated from tumor-bearing mice did not result in an inducible expression of IL-12 protein or IL-12 *p40* mRNA, as it did in control DCs. This suggests that a decreased level of CD40 expression or impaired CD40 signaling may be responsible for impaired cytokine production by DCs in cancer. This downregulation of CD40 expression no DCs in tumor bearers were caused by tumor-derived IL-10 *(44)*. These findings suggest that tumor-derived factors, including IL-10, inhibit CD40 expression on DCs and DC precursors and suppress their maturation and function. In addition, Brown et al. showed that the number of DCs in the blood of patients with multiple myeloma was normal; however, upregulation of CD80 expression in response to CD40L was significantly reduced on these DCs *(24)*. The author suggested that this functional defect of DCs could be the result of overproduction of TGF-β_1 and IL-10 by tumors. Similarly, Ratta et al. have studied peripheral-blood DCs from patients with multiple myeloma. The data demonstrated that upon maturation, DCs from these patients have significantly lower levels of expression of HLA-DR, CD40, and CD80 *(45)*. These findings suggest that the decreased expression of costimulatory and MHC class II molecules could be responsible for the decreased induction of T-cell proliferation in cancer. The authors theorized that the defect of peripheral-blood DCs isolated from multiple myeloma patients could be partially explained by tumor-derived IL-6. It has also been shown that prostate cancer significantly inhibited the expression of DC markers, such as CD1a and CD83 *(33)*.

Other functions of DCs may also be inhibited by tumor-derived factors. For instance, a decreased ability of peripheral-blood DC to form clusters with T cells in patients with head and neck cancer has been reported *(46)*. DCs obtained from RCC had a reduced ability to capture soluble antigen *(47)*. We demonstrated earlier that murine DCs treated with melanoma supernatant express markedly decreased levels of adhesion molecules, including β2 integrin and intercellular adhesion molecule-1 (ICAM-1) *(48)*. Therefore, the results of several studies clearly illustrate that tumor-derived factors inhibit DC maturation, which in turn could have a tremendous impact on the initiation and activation of immune responses.

Together, these results demonstrate that tumor-derived soluble factors have a significant inhibitory effect on DC generation, maturation, and function in vitro in many different models. Results of in vivo studies have confirmed this conclusion. It has been repeatedly demonstrated that rapidly growing tumors are usually poorly infiltrated by the immune effector cells, and are unable to trigger the activation of DCs. For instance, Troy et al. have shown that DCs extracted from RCC are minimally activated and have reduced allostimulatory activity *(49)*. Similar data were obtained with DCs that infiltrated prostate cancer *(50)* and basal cell carcinomas *(51)*. These DCs express no or very low levels of costimulatory CD80 and CD86 molecules, and had reduced antigen-presenting function. In breast carcinoma tissue, immature DCs reside within the tumor, whereas mature DCs are located in peritumoral areas *(52)*. Thus, it could be concluded that abrogation of DCs maturation is a common feature of tumor-cell DC interaction both in vitro and in vivo. Another common result of this interaction is an induction of premature apoptosis of DCs.

1.3. Induction of DC Apoptosis by Tumors

Apoptosis, together with differentiation, proliferation, and survival, is a highly regulated fundamental biological process that is involved in development, responsiveness, and homeostasis. The cell-death machinery comprises effectors, activators, and negative regulators. Apoptosis of cells of the immune system can be induced by a variety of intracellular and extracellular stimuli, such as growth-factor deprivation, hyperthermia, glucocorticoids, radiation, viruses, chemotherapy, FasL, and TRAIL, and—as recently demonstrated—by a number of tumor-derived factors. A growing body of evidence suggests that apoptosis might play an important role in regulating the DC system in health and disease. DCs have been shown to undergo apoptosis during antigen-specific interaction with T cells. The functional maturation of DCs ends by apoptotic-cell death, and reversion to the immature phenotype cannot be detected. Finally, it is important to note that apoptotic events that occur before terminal maturation play a role in supporting DC lineage selection and homeostasis. Although suppression of apoptosis may prolong the survival of late DC elements, an earlier apoptotic program appears to be required for the selective expansion of DC elements from multipotent progenitor cells *(53)*.

Although the role of apoptosis in the regulation of DC differentiation and elimination in cancer, as well as mechanisms of this regulation, has not been yet systematically addressed, a growing body of evidence suggests that tumor cells cause the eradication of DCs within the tumor microenvironment. In addition, numerous clinical studies demonstrate that the higher number of DCs in the tumor correlates with a better prognosis *(54,55)*. The induction of apoptosis in DCs is one of the key mechanisms that enable tumor cells to escape immune recognition and elimination. In fact, it has been reported that tumors secrete different soluble factors that lead to the induction of a programmed cell death of DCs. The increase of apoptosis in DCs coincubated with tumor cells and in DCs from implanted tumors had been reported in both human and murine systems *(6,9)*.

However, despite increasing interest in the field of physiological and pathological cell death of DCs, the mechanisms of regulated induction and protection of different DC populations and DC precursors from death signals are poorly understood. Kanto et al. studied the mechanisms involved in tumor-induced DC apoptosis using supernatants of murine B16 melanoma and MCA102 and MCA207 fibroblastoma *(56)*. The researchers demonstrated that ceramide mediates tumor-induced apoptosis of DC by downregulation of the PI3K pathway. In addition, Esche et al. have shown that the programmed cell death of DCs was correlated with an upregulation of Bax, a pro-apoptotic protein, and a downregulation of Bcl-2, an anti-apoptotic protein, and was associated with cytochrome c release from mitochondria *(7)*. Also, it has been demonstrated that *S*-nitros-*N*-acetylpenicillamine (SNAP), NO donor, may promote DC apoptosis *(57)*. NO-induced DC apoptosis, which might take place within the tumor mass, is associated with the downregulation of cellular inhibitors of apoptosis proteins (cIAP) expression, which facilitates caspase cascade activation and subsequent poly (ADP-ribose) polymerase (PARP) cleavage *(58)*. These data suggested that tumor-induced NO may influence the number of DC within the tumor mass. Together, these results suggest that the number of active and functional DCs present in the tumor microenvironment is significantly decreased by the tumors themselves.

1.4. Protection of DCs and DC-Based Immunotherapy

Interaction between tumor cells and cells of the immune system appears to be critical for tumor growth and progression. Tumor-derived factors dramatically alter the function and survival of immunocompetent cells in the local tumor microenvironment and systemically *(59)*. This chapter describes numerous inhibitory effects of tumors on the DC system. Many studies clearly demonstrate the importance of developing therapies directed to protect DCs and their precursors from tumor-induced downregulation of cell differentiation, functions, and survival.

For instance, recovery of CD40 signaling, which is decreased in DCs in cancer *(44)*, may potentially increase the efficacy of anticancer immunotherapies. CD40-CD40L interaction plays a crucial role in the generation of antitumor immunity and the regulation of DC generation, maturation, survival, and function *(60–62)*. In fact, it has been demonstrated that CD40L enhances DC efficiency to present antigen to T cells, upregulates the expression of the costimulatory molecules CD80, CD86, CD40, MHC class I/II, and adhesion molecules ICAM, and LFA-3 on DC *(63)*. In addition, CD40 ligation stimulated secretion of different cytokines (IL-12, IL-6, IL-8, TNF-α) by DCs and enhances DC survival *(64,65)*. Furthermore, we demonstrated that the genetically modified DC that overexpresses CD40L cause a complete rejection of TS/A tumors in 80% of mice when administered into the tumor site *(65)*. Similar results were observed by Kikuchi et al., who showed that simultaneous administration of Ad-CD40L and naïve DC induces tumor regression, and that DCs genetically modified to express CD40L elicit strong antitumor effect in B16 melanoma tumors *(66,67)*. As a whole, these data suggest that CD40L might increase the resistance of DC to the tumor-induced inhibition of DC maturation and function.

Other cytokines may also be overcome from tumor-derived inhibition of the DC system in cancer. For example, Menetrier-Caux et al. examined the ability of IL-4 and IL-13 to alter the inhibitory effects of tumor cells and cytokines secreted by tumor cells on the differentiation of DCs from CD34+ progenitors or monocytes *(68)*. The results suggested that both IL-4 and IL-13 were able to reverse the inhibition of DC differentiation induced by RCC by blocking the expression of the IL-6 receptor and M-CSF receptors and preventing the loss of GM-CSF receptor expression. In addition, Hoffmann et al. have evaluated human DC that ingested apoptotic tumor cells after treatment with different cytokines for their ability to present tumor antigen to T cells *(69)*. These data demonstrated that addition of proinflammatory cytokines or CD40L ± IFN-γ improved DC function, particularly the expression of MHC class I/II and costimulatory molecules on the surface of DCs and the induction of IL-12 and IL-15 production. These results confirmed that DCs that have processed tumor antigen generate more effective antitumor-specific T cells when these DCs are activated by cytokines. It has been also demonstrated that administration of DC-overexpressing cytokines, such as TNF-α or IL-12, at the site of the tumor induces strong antitumor responses in the murine tumor models *(70)*. Together, these data demonstrate that DC modification with different cytokines may be beneficial for the development of the antitumor immune response, and may be used as a novel antitumor DC vaccines.

Since DCs play a crucial role in the generation of antitumor immunity, protection of DC from tumor-induced apoptosis might improve the efficiency of DC-based therapies in cancer. It has been recently demonstrated that the cytokine-mediated increase in DC survival was accompanied by an elevated expression of the anti-apoptotic protein Bcl-x_L *(71)* and that intratumoral administration of DCs genetically modified to overexpress the Bcl-x_L gene resulted in a strong inhibition of prostate-tumor growth in mice in vivo. Thus, these data suggested that the protection of DCs from tumor-induced apoptosis may significantly increase the efficacy of DC-based therapies in cancer.

Furthermore, TIDC, which should be considered as DCs treated with tumor-derived factors in vivo, may be also recovered from tumor-induced inhibition and T-cell inhibitory activity. Most interestingly, neutralization of the endogenously derived IL-10 with anti-IL-10, antibodies as well as exposure of the inhibitory DC to CpG oligonucleotides, repolarize them into a stimulatory phenotype *(27)*. Accordingly, these results have important implications in translational research involving DCs. In fact, deficient antitumor immunity could be related to a lack of tumor-antigen presentation by TIDC or to a functional defect of TIDC. Vicari et al. recently reported that TIDC paralysis could be reverted by in vitro or in vivo stimulation with the combination of a CpG immunostimulatory sequence and anti-IL-10-receptor (IL-10R) antibodies *(72)*. Although CpG or anti-IL-10R alone were inactive in TIDC, CpG plus anti-IL-10R enhanced the tumor-specific immune response and triggered *de novo* IL-12 production. Subsequently, CpG plus anti-IL-10R treatment showed robust antitumor therapeutic activity that exceeded by far that of CpG alone, and elicited antitumor immune memory.

Thus, a better understanding of the mechanisms involved in the tumor-mediated inhibition of DC generation, maturation, and function may lead to the development of novel strategies for the prevention of immunosuppression in cancer patients, and the development of novel DC-based immunotherapeutic strategies.

1.5. Limitations of DC-Based Immunotherapy and New Approaches

The absence of characterized tumor-associated antigens (TAA) for many cancers has forced the development of alternative DC-based therapies. The recent pilot study in patients with melanoma and breast carcinoma demonstrated a potent antitumor potential of intratumoral administration of DCs without addition of tumor antigens *(73)*. Combination of intratumoral injection of DCs with cytokines may further increase the efficacy of the therapy. For example, an intratumoral injection of syngeneic naïve DCs in combination with the low dose of adenovector encoding TNF-α elicited marked tumor suppression without toxicity and tumor-specific immune responses in four tumor models *(74)*. Using an adenoviral vector of mCD40L and the number of DCs that by themselves had no effect on tumor growth, Kikuchi et al. reported that the growth of CT26 colon adenocarcinoma and B16 melanoma murine subcutaneous (sc) tumors is significantly suppressed by direct administration of DCs into established tumors that were pretreated with adeno-mCD40L two days previously *(67)*. We recently showed that intratumoral administration of DCs genetically modified to express IL-12 or CD40L significantly inhibits tumor growth, or causes complete tumor rejection in murine prostate, colon, or breast carcinoma models *(65,71)*. These data demonstrate that the combination of intratumoral administration of DCs and cytokines can evoke tumor suppression without systemic toxicity, providing a new paradigm for the use of cytokines and DCs as antitumor therapy.

Intratumoral administration of DCs may offer several advantages: i) it requires no isolation of tumor cells or tumor antigen(s); ii) it also ensures the most appropriate contact between DC and tumor cells, leading to the generation of tumor-specific CD8+ and CD4+ T cells; iii) the use of intratumoral injection of DCs should result in a high level of antigen processing and expression; and iv) finally, intratumoral DC may present previously unidentified epitopes of the tumor antigen in association with different MHC molecules, whereas peptide vaccines are restricted by the HLA haplotype of the patient.

Although definitive evidence is limited, several lines of evidence suggest that intratumoral DCs play an important role in antitumor immune responses. For instance, increased numbers of TIDC are associated with a better outcome in cancer patients with a variety of tumors. For instance, the density of DCs in colorectal cancer primaries was three times lower than that seen in normal colonic mucosa, and DC were rarely observed in metastatic tumors; DC density in metastases was sixfold lower than in colorectal primary tumors *(75)*. The prognosis of lung adenocarcinoma, when it is markedly infiltrated by DCs, is better than that of low infiltrated by DCs *(76)*.

DCs were also found to be cytotoxic for several tumor-cell lines *(77,78)*. Yang et al. demonstrated that immature DCs can kill autologous ovarian carcinoma cells via the Ca^{++}-independent Fas/FasL pathway, and that this may have important consequences for their ability to stimulate tumor-specific CTL *(79)*. These data were confirmed in recent studies, which demonstrated that human immature DC can directly and effectively mediate apoptotic killing against a wide array of cultured and freshly isolated tumor cells without harming normal cells *(80,81)*. Thus, it seems that DCs are fully equipped for an effective direct apoptotic killing of tumor cells, suggesting that this mechanism may play a critical role in both afferent and efferent antitumor immunity.

Now, as clinical trials exploiting the efficacy of DC-based vaccines are underway, there are still many problems to be solved, including the design of broadly applicable clinical protocols, the source of DCs (monocyte, CD34+ precursors, mature or immature DCs), the optimal loading of DC with TAA, and the route and the numbers of DC administration. Further studies are needed to determine the possible role of cytokines such as FLT3L, IL-2, IL-12, IL-15, or CD40L to optimize the efficacy of DC-based therapies. Additional clinical studies should also focus on patients with minimal residual disease or in an adjuvant setting, as these patients may be the most responsive to DC-based vaccination *(82)*.

REFERENCES

1. Whiteside TL. Tumor-induced death of immune cells: its mechanisms and consequences. *Semin Cancer Biol* 2002;12:43–50.
2. Shurin MR, Gabrilovich D. Regulation of dendritic cell system by tumor. *Cancer Research Therapy and Control* 2001;11:65–78.
3. Hoffmann TK, Dworacki G, Tsukihiro T, et al. Spontaneous apoptosis of circulating T lymphocytes in patients with head and neck cancer and its clinical importance. *Clin Cancer Res* 2002;8:2553–2562.
4. Shurin MR, Lu L, Kalinski P, Stewart-Akers AM, Lotze MT. Th1/Th2 balance in cancer, transplantation and pregnancy. *Springer Semin Immunopathol* 1999;21:339–359.
5. Shurin GV, Shurin MR, Bykovskaia S, Shogan J, Lotze MT, Barksdale EM, Jr. Neuroblastoma-derived gangliosides inhibit dendritic cell generation and function. *Cancer Res* 2001;61:363–369.
6. Esche C, Lokshin A, Shurin GV, et al. Tumor's other immune targets: dendritic cells. *J Leukoc Biol* 1999;66:336–344.
7. Esche C, Shurin GV, Kirkwood JM, et al. Tumor necrosis factor-alpha-promoted expression of Bcl-2 and inhibition of mitochondrial cytochrome c release mediate resistance of mature dendritic cells to melanoma-induced apoptosis. *Clin Cancer Res* 2001;7:974s–979s.
8. Shurin GV, Aalamian M, Pirtskhalaishvili G, et al. Human prostate cancer blocks the generation of dendritic cells from CD34+ hematopoietic progenitors. *Eur Urol* 2001;39 Suppl 4:37–40.

9. Pirtskhalaishvili G, Shurin GV, Esche C, et al. Cytokine-mediated protection of human dendritic cells from prostate cancer-induced apoptosis is regulated by the Bcl-2 family of proteins. *Br J Cancer* 2000;83:506–513.
10. Katsenelson NS, Shurin GV, Bykovskaia SN, Shogan J, Shurin MR. Human small cell lung carcinoma and carcinoid tumor regulate dendritic cell maturation and function. *Mod Pathol* 2001;14:40–45.
11. Gabrilovich DI, Cheng P, Fan Y, et al. H1(0) histone and differentiation of dendritic cells. A molecular target for tumor-derived factors. *J Leukoc Biol* 2002;72:285–296.
12. Tsuge T, Yamakawa M, Tsukamoto M. Infiltrating dendritic/Langerhans cells in primary breast cancer. *Breast Cancer Res Treat* 2000;59:141–152.
13. Kikuchi K, Kusama K, Taguchi K, et al. Dendritic cells in human squamous cell carcinoma of the oral cavity. *Anticancer Res* 2002;22:545–557.
14. Takahashi A, Kono K, Itakura J, et al. Correlation of vascular endothelial growth factor-C expression with tumor-infiltrating dendritic cells in gastric cancer. *Oncology* 2002; 62:121–127.
15. Yin X, Lu M, Liang L, Lai Y, Huang J, Li Z. [Infiltration of dendritic cells and lymphocytes in hepatocellular carcinoma tissue]. *Zhonghua Wai Ke Za Zhi* 2002;40:336–343.
16. Corazza F, Beguin Y, Bergmann P, et al. Anemia in children with cancer is associated with decreased erythropoietic activity and not with inadequate erythropoietin production. *Blood* 1998;92:1793–1798.
17. Sietsma H, Nijhof W, Dontje B, Vellenga E, Kamps WA, Kok JW. Inhibition of hemopoiesis in vitro by neuroblastoma-derived gangliosides. *Cancer Res* 1998;58:4840–4844.
18. Meckenstock G, Aul C, Hildebrandt B, et al. Dyshematopoiesis in de novo acute myeloid leukemia: cell biological features and prognostic significance [published erratum appears in *Leuk Lymphoma* 1998 Nov;31(5–6):following 623]. Leuk Lymphoma 1998; 29:523–531.
19. Gabrilovich DI, Ciernik IF, Carbone DP. Dendritic cells in antitumor immune responses. I. Defective antigen presentation in tumor-bearing hosts. *Cell Immunol* 1996;170:101–110.
20. Gabrilovich DI, Nadaf S, Corak J, Berzofsky JA, Carbone DP. Dendritic cells in antitumor immune responses. II. Dendritic cells grown from bone marrow precursors, but not mature DC from tumor-bearing mice, are effective antigen carriers in the therapy of established tumors. *Cell Immunol* 1996;170:111–119.
21. Shurin MR. Regulation of dendropoiesis in cancer. *Clin Immunol Newsletter* 1999; 19:135–139.
22. Chouaib S, Asselin-Paturel C, Mami-Chouaib F, Caignard A, Blay JY. The host-tumor immune conflict: from immunosuppression to resistance and destruction. *Immunol Today* 1997;18:493–497.
23. Gabrilovich D, Ishida T, Oyama T, et al. Vascular endothelial growth factor inhibits the development of dendritic cells and dramatically affects the differentiation of multiple hematopoietic lineages in vivo. *Blood* 1998;92:4150–4166.
24. Brown RD, Pope B, Murray A, et al. Dendritic cells from patients with myeloma are numerically normal but functionally defective as they fail to up-regulate CD80 (B7-1) expression after huCD40LT stimulation because of inhibition by transforming growth factor-beta1 and interleukin-10. *Blood* 2001;98:2992–2998.
25. Lin CM, Wang FH, Lee PK. Activated human CD4+ T cells induced by dendritic cell stimulation are most sensitive to transforming growth factor-beta: implications for dendritic cell immunization against cancer. *Clin Immunol* 2002;102:96–105.
26. Vendetti S, Chai JG, Dyson J, Simpson E, Lombardi G, Lechler R. Anergic T cells inhibit the antigen-presenting function of dendritic cells. *J Immunol* 2000;165:1175–1181.
27. Chakraborty A, Li L, Chakraborty NG, Mukherji B. Stimulatory and inhibitory maturation of human macrophage-derived dendritic cells. *Pathobiology* 1999;67:282–286.

28. Lutz MB, Kukutsch NA, Menges M, Rossner S, Schuler G. Culture of bone marrow cells in GM-CSF plus high doses of lipopolysaccharide generates exclusively immature dendritic cells which induce alloantigen-specific CD4 T cell anergy in vitro. *Eur J Immunol* 2000;30:1048–1052.
29. Sombroek CC, Stam AG, Masterson AJ, et al. Prostanoids play a major role in the primary tumor-induced inhibition of dendritic cell differentiation. *J Immunol* 2002;168:4333–4343.
30. Menetrier-Caux C, Montmain G, Dieu MC, et al. Inhibition of the differentiation of dendritic cells from CD34(+) progenitors by tumor cells: role of interleukin-6 and macrophage colony-stimulating factor. *Blood* 1998;92:4778–4791.
31. Shurin GV, Lotze MT, Barksdale EM. Neuroblastoma inhibits dendritic cell differentiation and function. *Curr Surg* 2000;57:637.
32. Kiertscher SM, Luo J, Dubinett SM, Roth MD. Tumors promote altered maturation and early apoptosis of monocyte- derived dendritic cells. *J Immunol* 2000;164:1269–1276.
33. Aalamian M, Pirtskhalaishvili G, Nunez A, et al. Human prostate cancer regulates generation and maturation of monocyte- derived dendritic cells. *Prostate* 2001;46:68–75.
34. Bishop-Bailey D, Calatayud S, Warner TD, Hla T, Mitchell JA. Prostaglandins and the regulation of tumor growth. *J Environ Pathol Toxicol Oncol* 2002;21:93–101.
35. Harizi H, Juzan M, Pitard V, Moreau JF, Gualde N. Cyclooxygenase-2-issued prostaglandin e(2) enhances the production of endogenous IL-10, which down-regulates dendritic cell functions. *J Immunol* 2002;168:2255–2263.
36. Makarenkova VP, Han B, Shurin GV, Shurin MR. Neuropeptide regulation of dendropoiesis in cancer. *Proc AACR* 2002;49:93.
37. Kennedy-Smith AG, McKenzie JL, Owen MC, Davidson PJ, Vuckovic S, Hart DN. Prostate specific antigen inhibits immune responses in vitro: a potential role in prostate cancer. *J Urol* 2002;168:741–747.
38. Aalamian M, Tourkova IL, Chatta GS, et al. Inhibition of dendropoiesis by tumor-derived and purified PSA. *J Urol,* in press.
39. Pietra G, Mortarini R, Parmiani G, Anichini A. Phases of apoptosis of melanoma cells, but not of normal melanocytes, differently affect maturation of myeloid dendritic cells. *Cancer Res* 2001;61:8218–8226.
40. Harding FA, McArthur JG, Gross JA, Raulet DH, Allison JP. CD28-mediated signalling co-stimulates murine T cells and prevents induction of anergy in T-cell clones. *Nature* 1992;356:607–609.
41. Reiser H, Freeman GJ, Razi-Wolf Z, Gimmi CD, Benacerraf B, Nadler LM. Murine B7 antigen provides an efficient costimulatory signal for activation of murine T lymphocytes via the T-cell receptor/CD3 complex. *Proc Natl Acad Sci USA* 1992;89:271–275.
42. Chaux P, Favre N, Bonnotte B, Moutet M, Martin M, Martin F. Tumor-infiltrating dendritic cells are defective in their antigen-presenting function and inducible B7 expression. A role in the immune tolerance to antigenic tumors. *Adv Exp Med Biol* 1997;417:525–528.
43. Enk AH, Jonuleit H, Saloga J, Knop J. Dendritic cells as mediators of tumor-induced tolerance in metastatic melanoma. *Int J Cancer* 1997;73:309–316.
44. Shurin MR, Yurkovetsky ZR, Tourkova IL, Balkir L, Shurin GV. Inhibition of CD40 expression and CD40-mediated dendritic cell function by tumor-derived IL-10. *Int J Cancer* 2002;101:61–68.
45. Ratta M, Fagnoni F, Curti A, et al. Dendritic cells are functionally defective in multiple myeloma: the role of interleukin-6. *Blood* 2002;100:230–237.
46. Tas M, Simons P, Balm F, Drexhage H. Depressed monocyte polarization and clustering of dendritic cells in patients with head and neck cancer: in vitro restoration of this immunosuppression by thymic hormones. *Cancer Immunol Immunother* 1993;36:108–114.
47. Thurnher M, Radmayar C, Ramoner R, et al. Human renal-cell carcinoma tissue contains dendritic cells. *Int J Cancer* 1996;67:1–7.

48. Esche C, Shurin MR, Lotze MT. B16 melanoma induces downregulation of beta2 integrin and ICAM-1 expression on murine dendritic cells. *J Investig Dermatol* 1997;108:640.
49. Troy A, Davidson P, Atkinson C, Hart D. Phenotypic characterisation of the dendritic cell infiltrate in prostate cancer. *J Urol* 1998;160:214–219.
50. Troy A, Davidson P, Atkinson C, Hart D. Renal cell carcinoma and prostate cancer inhibit dendritic cell activation. *Aust N Z J Surg* 1999;69:A111–A112.
51. Nestle FO, Burg G, Fah J, Wrone-Smith T, Nickoloff BJ. Human sunlight-induced basal-cell-carcinoma-associated dendritic cells are deficient in T cell co-stimulatory molecules and are impaired as antigen-presenting cells. *Am J Pathol* 1997;150:641–651.
52. Bell D, Chomarat P, Broyles D, et al. In breast carcinoma tissue, immature dendritic cells reside within the tumor, whereas mature dendritic cells are located in peritumoral areas. *J Exp Med* 1999;190:1417–1426.
53. Shurin MR, Esche C, Lokshin A, Lotze MT. Apoptosis in Dendritic Cells. In: *Dendritic Cells: Biology and Clinical Applications* (Lotze MT, Thomson AW, eds.), Academic Press, San Diego, CA, pp. 673–692.
54. Becker Y. Anticancer role of dendritic cells (DC) in human and experimental cancers—a review. *Anticancer Res* 1992;12:511–520.
55. Shurin GV, Yurkovetsky ZR, Shurin MR. (2003) Tumor-induced dendritic cell dysfunction. In: *Mechanisms of Tumor Escape* (Ochoa A, ed.), Taylor and Francis, New York, pp. 115–140.
56. Kanto T, Kalinski P, Hunter OC, Lotze MT, Amoscato AA. Ceramide mediates tumor-induced dendritic cell apoptosis. *J Immunol* 2001;167:3773–3784.
57. Lu L, Bonham CA, Chambers FG, et al. Induction of nitric oxide synthase in mouse dendritic cells by IFN- gamma, endotoxin, and interaction with allogeneic T cells: nitric oxide production is associated with dendritic cell apoptosis. *J Immunol* 1996; 157:3577–3586.
58. Stanford A, Chen Y, Zhang XR, Hoffman R, Zamora R, Ford HR. Nitric oxide mediates dendritic cell apoptosis by downregulating inhibitors of apoptosis proteins and upregulating effector caspase activity. *Surgery* 2001;130:326–332.
59. Kavanaugh DY, Carbone DP. Immunologic dysfunction in cancer. *Hematol Oncol Clin North Am* 1996;10:927–951.
60. Mackey MF, Gunn JR, Maliszewsky C, Kikutani H, Noelle RJ, Barth RJ, Jr. Dendritic cells require maturation via CD40 to generate protective antitumor immunity. *J Immunol* 1998;161:2094–2098.
61. Mackey MF, Barth RJ, Jr., Noelle RJ. The role of CD40/CD154 interactions in the priming, differentiation, and effector function of helper and cytotoxic T cells. *J Leukoc Biol* 1998;63:418–428.
62. van Kooten C, Banchereau J. CD40-CD40 ligand. *J Leukoc Biol* 2000;67:2–17.
63. Cella M, Scheidegger D, Palmer-Lehmann K, Lane P, Lanzavecchia A, Alber G. Ligation of CD40 on dendritic cells triggers production of high levels of interleukin-12 and enhances T cell stimulatory capacity: T-T help via APC activation. *J Exp Med* 1996;184:747–752.
64. Esche C, Gambotto A, Satoh Y, et al. CD154 inhibits tumor-induced apoptosis in dendritic cells and tumor growth. *Eur J Immunol* 1999;29:2148–2155.
65. Yurkovetsky ZR, Shurin GV, Gambotto A, Kim SH, Shurin MR, Robbins PD. Intratumoral administration of Ad-CD40L or dendritic cells transduced with Ad-CD40L induces antitumor immunity. *Cancer Gene Ther*, in press.
66. Kikuchi T, Moore MA, Crystal RG. Dendritic cells modified to express CD40 ligand elicit therapeutic immunity against preexisting murine tumors. *Blood* 2000;96:91–99.
67. Kikuchi T, Miyazawa N, Moore MA, Crystal RG. Tumor regression induced by intratumor administration of adenovirus vector expressing CD40 ligand and naive dendritic cells. *Cancer Res* 2000;60:6391–6395.

68. Menetrier-Caux C, Thomachot MC, Alberti L, Montmain G, Blay JY. IL-4 prevents the blockade of dendritic cell differentiation induced by tumor cells. *Cancer Res* 2001;61:3096–3104.
69. Hoffmann TK, Meidenbauer N, Muller-Berghaus J, Storkus WJ, Whiteside TL. Proinflammatory cytokines and CD40 ligand enhance cross-presentation and cross-priming capability of human dendritic cells internalizing apoptotic cancer cells. *J Immunother* 2001;24:162–171.
70. Satoh Y, Esche C, Gambotto A, et al. Local administration of IL-12-transfected dendritic cells induces antitumor immune responses to colon adenocarcinoma in the liver in mice. *J Exp Ther Oncol* 2002;2:337–349.
71. Pirtskhalaishvili G, Shurin GV, Gambotto A, et al. Transduction of dendritic cells with Bcl-xL increases their resistance to prostate cancer-induced apoptosis and antitumor effect in mice. *J Immunol* 2000;165:1956–1964.
72. Vicari AP, Chiodoni C, Vaure C, et al. Reversal of tumor-induced dendritic cell paralysis by CpG immunostimulatory oligonucleotide and anti-interleukin 10 receptor antibody. *J Exp Med* 2002;196:541–549.
73. Triozzi PL, Khurram R, Aldrich WA, Walker MJ, Kim JA, Jaynes S. Intratumoral injection of dendritic cells derived in vitro in patients with metastatic cancer. *Cancer* 2000;89:2646–2654.
74. Kianmanesh A, Hackett NR, Lee JM, Kikuchi T, Korst RJ, Crystal RG. Intratumoral administration of low doses of an adenovirus vector encoding tumor necrosis factor alpha together with naive dendritic cells elicits significant suppression of tumor growth without toxicity. *Hum Gene Ther* 2001;12:2035–2049.
75. Schwaab T, Weiss JE, Schned AR, Barth Jr RJ. Dendritic cell infiltration in colon cancer. *J Immunother* 2001;24:130–137.
76. Gong X, Yan Y, Wu J. [Dendritic cell infiltration in lung adenocarcinoma and its effect on prognosis]. *Zhonghua Jie He He Hu Xi Za Zhi* 2000;23:478–479.
77. Vanderheyde N, Aksoy E, Amraoui Z, Vandenabeele P, Goldman M, Willems F. Tumoricidal activity of monocyte-derived dendritic cells: evidence for a caspase-8-dependent, Fas-associated death domain-independent mechanism. *J Immunol* 2001;167:3565–3569.
78. Sun J, Zhang J, Chen J, Chen H, Chew Y. In vitro study on the morphology of human blood dendritic cells and LPAK cells inducing apoptosis of the hepatoma cell line. *Chin Med J (Engl)* 2001;114:600–605.
79. Yang R, Xu D, Zhang A, Gruber A. Immature dendritic cells kill ovarian carcinoma cells by a FAS/FASL pathway, enabling them to sensitize tumor-specific CTLs. *Int J Cancer* 2001;94:407–413.
80. Janjic BM, Lu G, Pimenov A, Whiteside TL, Storkus WJ, Vujanovic NL. Innate direct anticancer effector function of human immature dendritic cells. I. Involvement of an apoptosis-inducing pathway. *J Immunol* 2002;168:1823–1830.
81. Lu G, Janjic BM, Janjic J, Whiteside TL, Storkus WJ, Vujanovic NL. Innate direct anticancer effector function of human immature dendritic cells. II. Role of TNF, lymphotoxin-?(1)?(2), fas ligand, and TNF-related apoptosis-inducing ligand. *J Immunol* 2002;168:1831–1839.
82. Brossart P, Wirths S, Brugger W, Kanz L. Dendritic cells in cancer vaccines. *Exp Hematol* 2001;29:1247–1255.
83. Saito H, Tsujitani S, Ikeguchi M, Maeta M, Kaibara N. Relationship between the expression of vascular endothelial growth factor and the density of dendritic cells in gastric adenocarcinoma tissue. *Br J Cancer* 1998;78:1573–1577.
84. Ishida T, Oyama T, Carbone DP, Gabrilovich DI. Defective function of Langerhans cells in tumor-bearing animals is the result of defective maturation from hemopoietic progenitors. *J Immunol* 1998;161:4842–4851.

85. Chomarat P, Banchereau J, Davoust J, Palucka AK. IL-6 switches the differentiation of monocytes from dendritic cells to macrophages. *Nat Immunol* 2000;1:510–514.
86. Buelens C, Verhasselt V, De Groote D, Thielemans K, Goldman M, Willems F. Interleukin-10 prevents the generation of dendritic cells from human peripheral blood mononuclear cells cultured with interleukin-4 and granulocyte/macrophage-colony-stimulating factor. *Eur J Immunol* 1997;27:756–762.
87. Miyauchi-Hashimoto H, Kuwamoto K, Urade Y, Tanaka K, Horio T. Carcinogen-induced inflammation and immunosuppression are enhanced in xeroderma pigmentosum group A model mice associated with hyperproduction of prostaglandin E2. *J Immunol* 2001;166:5782–5791.
88. Kalinski P, Hilkens CM, Wierenga EA, et al. Functional maturation of human naive T helper cells in the absence of accessory cells. Generation of IL-4-producing T helper cells does not require exogenous IL-4. *J Immunol* 1995;154:3753–3760.

4 CD4+ T-Cell-Mediated Immunity to Cancer

Tomohide Tatsumi, MD, PhD,
Amy Wesa, PhD, *James H. Finke*, PhD,
Ronald M. Bukowski, MD,
and Walter J. Storkus, PhD

CONTENTS

1. INTRODUCTION

A major clinical focus has been dedicated to the design and application of immunotherapies for the promotion of antitumor cytotoxic T lymphocyte (CTL) responses *(1,2)*. In their purest form, such strategies take the form of adoptively transferred, enriched populations of tumor-reactive CD8+ T cells. These approaches have occasionally been shown to be capable of mediating the regression of lesions in cancer patients *(3)*. However, more often, high circulating

From: *Current Clinical Oncology: Cancer Immunotherapy at the Crossroads: How Tumors Evade Immunity and What Can Be Done*
Edited by: J. H. Finke and R. M. Bukowski © Humana Press Inc., Totowa, NJ

frequencies of such cancer-specific CD8+ T cells fail to provide any demonstrable clinical benefit, despite the co-application of supportive biologic response modifiers, such as interleukin-2 (IL-2) *(4,5)*. Although it is not the purpose of this chapter to survey all of the potential mechanisms that may underlie the ineffectiveness of such immune effector cells *in situ*, one must consider deviation in the functional antitumor CD4+ T "helper" compartment as a major confounding variable.

CD4+ T cells play dominant roles in the initial support of CTL generation, but are also instrumental in directing the infiltration of CD8+ T cells into sites of inflammation, and appear to be critical for the durability of long-term CTL memory *(6–8)*. Without the benefit of functional tumor-specific CD4+ T-cell responses *in situ*, even large numbers of circulating tumoricidal CD8+ T cells are unlikely to be recruited into, or survive within, tumor lesions. Furthermore, if the patient is among the minority of individuals who benefit from immunotherapy, they may be prone to recurrence because of the abbreviated nature of memory within the antitumor CD8+ T-cell repertoire in the absence of appropriate CD4+ T-cell maintenance. CD4+ T effector cells may also mediate direct cytocidal activity against HLA class II-positive tumor cells, or recruit alternate innate immune killer cells to the tumor site.

This chapter explores our current understanding of evolving CD4+ T-cell responses in the cancer setting, and provides some considerations to be addressed in prospective clinical trials of immunotherapy-based strategies.

2. T CELLS AND CANCER: A ROLE FOR CD4+ T CELLS

During the past several decades, clinical studies have provided compelling evidence that T-cell-mediated immunity plays a role in regulating the development, progression, and metastatic spread of cancer. Notably, individuals who undergo systemic immunosuppression for the maintenance of transplanted organ allografts exhibit an increased incidence of developing cancer, suggesting the critical role of a functionally operational immune system in regulating tumor progression *(9–12)*. Furthermore, although they occur in only a small number of patients, spontaneous regressions of cancer lesions have been observed on occasion, and tumors are typically infiltrated with large numbers of lymphocytes *(13,14)*. Within such infiltrates, clonally expanded populations of T-cell-receptor (TCR) α/β+ T cells have been readily demonstrated *(15,16)*, and these have been shown to exhibit tumor-specific reactivity during subsequent in vitro analysis. Interestingly, clones of T cells from primary and metastatic lesions within a single patient frequently appear to be unrelated, and are likely to exhibit differential specificities *(15)*, representing a means to combat disseminated tumor cells that are heterogeneous in their phenotypes. The heterogeneity in T-cell recognition of cancer cells may result from variance in tumor-cell expression of major histocompatibility complex (MHC) antigens that present tumor-derived peptides to T cells, or to changes in the repertoire of tumor-associated peptides that are selected for MHC presentation on the cell surface of a particular tumor cell *(17)*.

CD4+ T cells typically recognize MHC class II-presented peptides *(18)*. Unlike MHC class I molecules that are ubiquitously expressed by most somatic, nucleated cells in the body, the range of cell types that display MHC class II molecule expression is far more restricted in nature *(19)*. Indeed, hematopoietic antigen-presenting cells (APCs such as dendritic cells [DCs], B cells, and macrophages) are the most frequent cell types that constitutively express class II molecules *in situ (19)*. Other types of cells can express MHC class II molecules under inflammatory or "activating" conditions, in which IFN-γ, among other cytokines, can promote the transcriptional activation of these complexes *(20)*. With the exception of certain hematologic malignancies, most carcinomas or other solid tumors express MHC class II molecules in only a minority of cases, and expression is typically heterogeneous in nature within a given lesion *(21,22)*.

Thus, tumor-specific (naïve, effector, or memory) CD4+ T cells may be initially activated *in situ* by autologous APCs that have acquired tumor antigens (as soluble/secreted proteins or glycoproteins or as dead/dying tumor debris) and have "cross-presented" tumor antigen-derived peptides in their MHC class II cell-surface complexes *(23)* (Fig. 1). In those cases in which MHC class II-positive tumor cells may directly present their own peptides to CD4+ T cells, the responding *(24)*, tumor-reactive T cells are likely to be "effector" or "memory" T cells, as naïve CD4+ T cells do not recirculate through tissues *(25)*.

In situations in which tumors qualitatively express MHC class II molecules *in situ*, the literature is equivocal with regard to whether class II expression by the cancer cells is prognostic for clinical outcome. In the majority of publications in which an extensive range of cancer histologies have been evaluated, tumor-cell expression of HLA-DR class II molecules appears to be beneficial, with later-stage, more malignant cancers being class II-deficient *(26–29)* (Table 1). However, there are some reports suggesting that, to the contrary, if the patient bears a class II-positive tumor lesion or expresses certain "susceptibility" HLA-DR alleles, they will have a comparatively poorer clinical prognosis *(30–34)*.

In part, such dichotomous correlations may reflect differences in the functional nature of specific CD4+ T cells that must chronically respond over extended periods of time to their evolving cancer lesions. At some level, expression of MHC class II antigens early in disease progression may be the result of IFN-γ and TNF-α production by infiltrating tumor-specific CD4+ (and/or CD8+) T and NK cells *in situ (13,35)*. Prolonged re-stimulation of these immune effector cells may lead to loss of IFN-γ production *(36)* and the subsequent lack

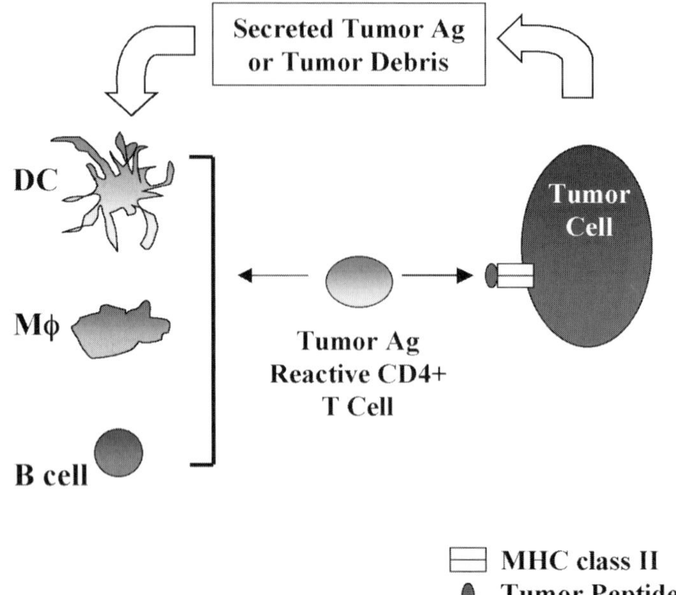

Fig. 1. Tumor-specific CD4+ T cells can recognize both autologous MHC class II+ tumor cells or antigen-presenting cells that have taken up and processed tumor antigens. In the latter case, tumor antigens can take the forms of secreted or shed soluble tumor antigens, or dead or dying tumor cells and their associated debris.

of MHC class II gene transactivation in the locoregional cancer cells. Alternatively, MHC class II gene expression by cancer cells in the absence of costimulatory molecule expression, or chronic presentation of tumor-antigenic peptides by APC, may promote the emergence of anergic, ineffective, or suppressive CD4+ T-cell responses, at least within the local tumor microenvironment, if not systemically. These alternate T-cell functions may ultimately serve to facilitate tumor progression rather than rejection *(37–40)*.

3. FUNCTIONAL CD4+ T-CELL SUBSETS

Mature CD4+ T-helper cells have been typically segregated into three principal functional categories (e.g., Th1-, Th2-, and Th3/Tr-type), based on the nature of their cytokine secretion patterns *(41)*. Although this segregation in T-cell subsets was originally documented in the mouse, recent reports support a similar segregation of such T-cell subpopulations in humans *(42)*. So-called type-1 Th (Th1)-type CD4+ T cells are the main producers of IFN-γ and TNF-α (and IL-2 in mouse), and may be directly cytotoxic against infected or transformed cells *(43)*. Dogmatically, however, their main function is to provide helper signals for cytotoxic CD8+ T-lymphocytes, and nonspecific killer

Table 1
Prognostic Value of MHC Class II Expression in Cancer

Histology	*HLA Class II*	*Prognostic Impact (+/–)*	*Comments*	*Ref.*
Laryngeal	Pan	+	Better survival if lesion <10%+	*26*
Colorectal	Pan	+	Better 5-yr survival if +	*27*
NPC	Pan	+	Better clinical prognosis if +	*28*
Breast Ca.	Pan	+	Better 5-yr survival if node-neg.	*29*
HNC	DR6	–	Poor 5-yr survival	*30*
Melanoma	DR11	–	Predictive of recurrence	*31*
Prostate	DR4	–	Increased (2–3×) risk to develop	*32*
Melanoma	Pan	–	Poor prognosis if primary is +	*33*
Melanoma	Pan	–	Progression linked to level of +	*34*

HNC, head and neck cancer; NPC, nasopharygeal carcinoma.

cells, including NK cells and macrophages *(44)*. Type-2 Th (Th2) cells produce B-cell-stimulatory factors, including IL-4 and IL-5 (and are major producers of IL-10 in the mouse), and promote B-cell proliferation, survival, and Ig production *(41,44)*. Thus, Th1- and Th2-type have been traditionally associated with the promotion of cellular and humoral immunity, respectively (Fig. 2). The Th3/Tr-type CD4+ T-cell subset constitutes an antigen-specific regulatory cell, in part because of its secretion of the immunosuppressive cytokines IL-10 and TGF-β1, which can inhibit both Th1- and Th2-type T-cell responses *(45,46)*. As depicted in Fig. 2, Th1-, Th2- and Th3/Tr-type CD4+ T cells evolve from naïve Th0-type CD4+ T-cell precursors after specific antigenic stimulation. The polarization of the resulting Th-type responses is dictated by the nature and balance of cytokines present within the priming microenvironment *(47)*. Additional factors that may bias the balance of antigen-specific Th1-/Th2-type responses include: the APC: T-cell ratio during induction, the "dose" of MHC-peptide complexes presented to the responder T cells, and the level and type of costimulation available to the stimulated T cells *(48–51)*. There is also evidence that the functional polarization state of DCs (such as DC1 vs DC2) priming antigen-specific T cells can dictate the functional bias of CD4+ T-cell responses to either the Th1- or Th2-type *(52)*.

As indicated in Fig. 2, if IFN-γ constitutes a principal cytokine during the primary response, Th1-type immunity is likely to evolve, whereas if IL-4/IL-5 or IL-10/TGF-β1 predominate during the critical early phases of T-cell activation, Th2- or Th3/Tr-type polarized CD4+ T-cell responses, respectively, may be most common. Although the results of early studies (performed primarily in murine models) supported the terminal "commitment" of polarized CD4+

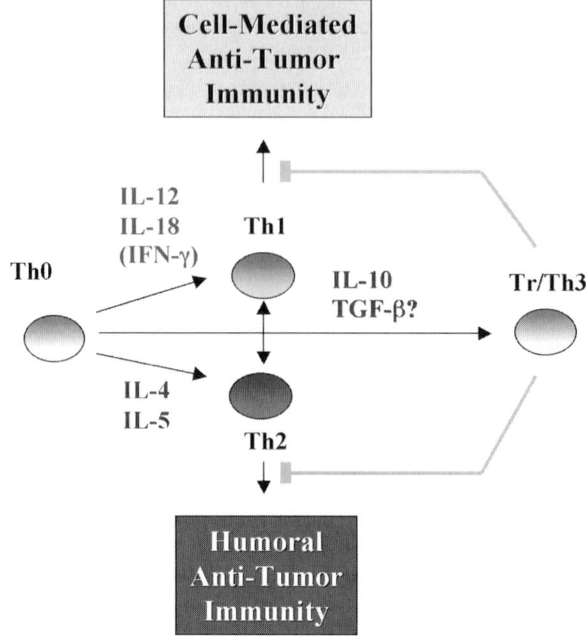

Fig. 2. Functional CD4+ T-cell Subsets. Th1-, Th2-, and Tr/Th3-type CD4+ T cells develop from precursor Th0-type T cells after specific antigen stimulation, with their functional polarizations determined, at least in part, by the balance of biologically dominant cytokines that are present in the microenvironment during the period of antigenic activation. Th1-type polarized CD4+ T-cell responses that drive cell-mediated antitumor immunity, are supported by cytokines such as IL-12, IL-18, and IFN-γ. Th2-type polarized CD4+ T-cell responses that support humoral (antibody-based) antitumor immunity are facilitated by cytokines, such as IL-4 and IL-5, and suppressive Tr/Th3-type responses appear to require the presence of IL-10 and/or TGF-β during the T-cell stimulation period. At the time of each subsequent antigenic restimulation of CD4+ T cells, the balance of different cytokines present in the microenvironment can promote a repolarization of functional T-cell responses *(54)*. For instance, Th2-type CD4+ T-cell responses may be repolarized to Th1-type responses in the presence of IL-12, Th1-type responses may be repolarized to Th3/Tr in the presence of IL-10 and TGF-β.

T-cell responses *(53)*, more recent investigations suggest that the cytokine microenvironment during each subsequent antigen-specific restimulation of CD4+ T cells can modulate the balance of (CD4+ T-cell) cytokines produced *(54)*, and can lead to overt realignment in the types of functional Th responses observed against defined antigens *(55)*. Notably, similar studies should be facilitated by several recent reports that have identified a series of cell-surface membrane markers that can provide a degree of discrimination between the various T-cell subsets (*56–65*; Table 2). For instance, Th1-type CD4+ T cells can be distinguished by a CCR5+/CRTH2-negative phenotype, Th2-type CD4+ T cells

Table 2
CD4+ T-Cell Functional Subsets: Correlative Phenotypic Markers

Type	*Marker*	*Cytokines*	*Effect on CMI*	*Ref.*
Th1	LAG-3, CCR5, CXCR3, IL-12Rβ2, IL-18R	IFN-γ, IL-2	Stimulate++	*56–58*
Th2	CD30, CCR3, ST2L, CRTH2	IL-4, IL-5, IL-10	Suppress	*56, 59–62*
Tr/Th3	CD25, CD45RO, CD62L, CD122, CD152 (CTLA-4), GITR	IL-10, TGF-β1	Suppress++	*63–65*

GITR, glucocorticoid-induced TNFR family-related gene; CMI, cell-mediated immunity

by a CCR5-negative/CRTH2+ phenotype, and Tr-type "suppressor" CD4+ T cells by a CD25+/CD152+ phenotype.

In general, the ability of an organism to mount a Th1-biased immune response has been linked to an enhanced ability to eliminate certain invading pathogens and tumors *(66,67)*. Interleukin-12 (IL-12), produced mainly by DC *(68)*, appears to play an important role in determining whether a Th1- or Th2-biased immune response is mounted to antigenic challenge. Functionally, IL-12 has been demonstrated to bias the immune response toward a Th1 phenotype in vitro and in vivo *(69)*. In addition to promoting Th1 development from naive and memory T-cell populations, IL-12 has also been shown to suppress the development of Th2 cells *(70,71)*. Most recently, IL-12 has also been shown to have the capacity to repolarize committed, human Th2-type CD4+ T cells to produce IFN-γ *(72–74)*. Th2-to-Th1 repolarization requires specific antigenic stimulation, and is associated with increased expression of IL-12βR2 and the Th1-transactivating molecule T-bet and loss of the Th2-associated CRTH2 and transactivating GATA-3 molecules by the responding T cells *(74)*.

4. SPECIFICITY OF TUMOR-REACTIVE CD4+ T CELLS

As previously noted, tumor-reactive CD4+ T cells generally recognize MHC class II complexes that present peptides derived from tumor-cell synthesized proteins and glycoproteins. Based on a significant body of work dedicated to the molecular characterization of tumor-associated antigens (TAA) recognized by CD8+ CTL beginning in the early 1990s *(75)*, hundreds of tumor antigens have now been cloned and catalogued. In most or all cases, a specific TAA can give rise to peptide epitopes recognized by both CD4+ and CD8+ T cells *(76)*. Of relevance to this chapter, a steadily increasing number of CD4+ T-cell-defined peptide epitopes have been defined in the cancer setting (for reviews, *see* refs. *76–78*).

5. IMMUNE MONITORING OF FUNCTIONAL TH RESPONSES

The identification of tumor-peptide epitopes has been facilitated by recent advances in single-cell T-cell screening systems, such as the cytokine ELISPOT, which allow for the identification of tumor-associated peptides using "memory" CD4+ T cells isolated directly from the patient's blood *(79–81)*. By analyzing immune responses to tumor-derived antigens in freshly isolated lymphocytes, one is not prone to any potential artifact associated with extended in vitro culture of effector T cells that may deviate from the repertoire of the bulk antitumor T-cell response. A careful selection of the target cytokines, such as IFN-γ, IL-4/IL-5, and TGF-β1 applied in the ELISPOT and ELISA analyses, allows for the rapid diagnosis of the patient's basal Th1- vs Th2- vs Th3/Tr-type bias in functional CD4+ T-cell response(s) to an autologous tumor. Using this short-term in vitro screening approach, we recently defined a series of tumor-peptide epitopes, and are now in the process of determining the nature of Th1- vs Th2- vs Th3/Tr-type CD4+ T-cell recognition of tumor antigen-derived epitopes in patients who present with diverse cancer histotypes *(82,83)*. These same types of scans of patient peripheral blood-derived CD4+ T-cell responses can be applied during the course of immunotherapy and subsequent follow-up, allowing for the effective monitoring and correlation of tumor-specific immunity with the clinical disease course.

6. DYSFUNCTIONAL CD4+ AND CD8+ T-CELL POLARIZATION IN CANCER?

Despite the frequently observed presence of leukocytes within tumor lesions, a clear correlation with beneficial clinical outcome in immunotherapeutic approaches has not been substantiated *(84)*. Indeed, in many cases, non-regressing lesions may be heavily infiltrated with both CD4+ and CD8+ T lymphocytes *(85)*. Notably, the cell subsets within these immune infiltrates suggest that they may be affiliated with a suboptimal Th1-type antitumor immune response that is unable to slow tumor progression or mediate tumor regression *in situ (86,87)*. However, by considering both the frequency and the function of patient antitumor CD4+ T-cell subset responses *in situ*, it has recently been suggested that prognostic indicators of disease progression and immunotherapeutic responsiveness may be defined *(88–90)*.

Tumor-induced deviation of CD4+ T-cell responses in progressive disease and the role of Th1- and Th2-type CD4+ effector cells have been evaluated in a limited number of murine tumor models and human in vitro analyses *(91–102)*. Studies using the B16 melanoma model have documented a gradual shift of initial Th0-, mixed Th1-/Th2-type CD4+ T-cell response to Th2/Tr-type-dominated responses by 14–20 days of progressive tumor growth *(95,99–101)*. Injection of neutralizing anti-IL-4, -IL-10, or -TGF-β1 antibodies can prevent this tumor-induced functional transition, resulting in enhanced CD8+ CTL generation and protection against tumor growth *(99)*. Depletion of CD4+ T cells in late-stage progressive B16 models, in which the Th2/Tr-type response dominates, restores CTL effector function, and can result in tumor regression and vitiligo, particularly upon administration of rIL-12 *(96)*. Analyses of the antitumor efficacy of Th1- and Th2-type CD4+ T cells have also been evaluated in prophylactic and adoptive transfer tumor models *(91,95,96,98)*. In these latter cases, Th1- and Th2-type can mediate complementary antitumor effector functions, via contrasting mechanims *(102)*. Although Th2-type CD4+ T cells can promote the recruitment of tumoricidal eosinophils and macrophages into the tumor microenvironment and promote acute tumor rejection *(101)*, on a cell-per-cell basis, Th1-type T cells appear to provide a far greater therapeutic index *(94,96,97)*, and only Th1-type CD4+ T cells appear to promote the durable antitumor CTL responses *(97)* that are likely to prove critical to extended disease-free intervals in effectively managed cancer patients.

The occurrence and clinical impact of Th1- vs Th2-type biased immunity in the development and progression of cancer has not been stringently and comprehensively evaluated to date. In the few instances in which studies have been attempted, the data have generally been equivocal *(103–107)*. In some studies, freshly isolated TIL- have been shown to exhibit a predominant Th2-type phenotype associated with the locoregional production of IL-4 and IL-10 *(103–107)*. These cytokines are affiliated with enhanced humoral (e.g., antibody) responses and with inhibition of "professional" APC (e.g., DC) function, respectively, and are often inversely correlated with effective induction, or directly correlated with the dysfunction of cellular T-cell-mediated immunity. However, Angevin et al. *(108)* have shown in 12 patients with primary RCC that isolated TIL- are strongly polarized to a Th1 differentiation pattern (e.g., production of IL-2 and IFN-γ), but may be suppressed in vivo by high levels of IL-6/IL-10 within the tumor microenvironment *(103,104,109)*. These data support a mixed Th1/Th2-type T cell infiltrate that may overall display Th2-type T-cell function. Such results provide some confidence that immunotherapeutic strategies capable of enhancing Th1-type T cell function (in the face of existing Th2- or Th3/Tr-type antitumor immunity) in cancer-bearing patients may provide significant clinical benefit.

Although the specificities of clinically important Th1-, Th2-, and Th3/Tr-type CD4+ T-cell responses have not been comprehensively evaluated at this time, we recently reported that Th1-type CD4+ T cells specific for the MAGE-6 tumor-antigen are functionally deficient in patients with resident RCC *(110)* (Fig. 3). Interestingly, in those patients with active disease, MAGE-6-specific Th2-type CD4+ T-cell responses, characterized by strong production of interleukin-4 and -5, were prevalent *(110)*. In marked contrast, in patients who were rendered disease-free as a result of surgical and/or immunotherapeutic inter-

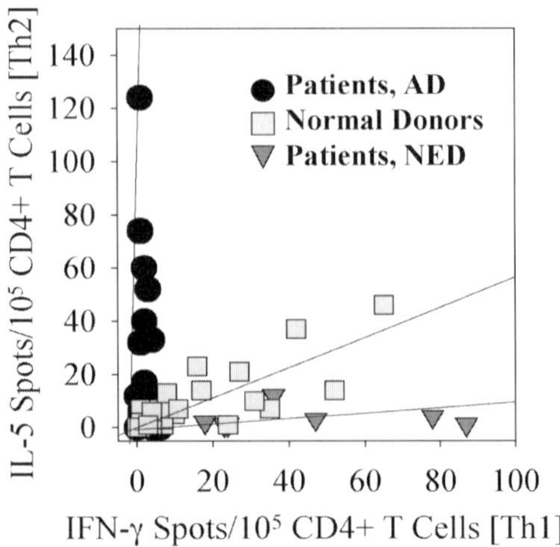

Fig. 3. Cancer-associated CD4+ T-cell functional polarization. Mage-$6_{121-144}$ peptide-specific CD4+ T cells were isolated from the peripheral blood of a series of patients with RCC or normal donors. HLA-DR4+ patients with active disease produced IL-5, but not IFN-γ in response to in vitro restimulation with this peptide (e.g., Th2-type responses), and normal donors displayed mixed Th1/Th2-type responses and patients that were rendered free-of-disease as a result of therapeutic intervention, produced only IFN-γ and no IL-5 (e.g., Th1-type responses) against this MAGE-6 peptide *(110)*.

vention, mixed Th1/Th2- or polarized Th1-type immunity predominated *(110)*. Although evaluated in a longitudinal fashion in very few patients, the functional Th2-to-Th1 shift in MAGE-6 responsiveness could be observed in the peripheral-blood lymphocyte population within 6 wk after intervention with curative therapies, suggesting a potential correlation between these enhanced Th1-type T-cell responses and clinical benefit *(110)*.

7. IMPACT OF CD4+ T-CELL DYSFUNCTION ON PROSPECTIVE THERAPY DESIGN

It is generally believed that Th1-type immunity, and IFN-γ production in particular, favor the generation and support of protective and therapeutic cellular antitumor immunity *(111)*. Recent studies, including our own, indicate that many cancer patients may have a deficiency of systemic tumor-specific Th1-type helper CD4+ T cells and/or a prevalence of tumor-specific Th2-type CD4+ T cells *in situ (110)*. These findings may represent a confounding variable for effective immunotherapy. If these non-Th1-type T cells represent a significant antagonistic barrier *(112)* to the afferent (in lymphoid tissue) or efferent (in tumor) functions of effector Th1-type immunity, therapies should be developed that can functionally neutralize these tumor-reactive Th2/Th3-/Tr-type

T cells (e.g., by deletion, anergizing, or "repolarizating" them to Th1-type responses). Clearly, the destruction of these types of CD4+ T cells is possible through chemotherapeutic drug-treatment regimens, such as cyclophosphamide or depleting anti-CD25 Ab *(113–115)*, but these treatments may also destroy potentially beneficial cellular immunity. Despite this concern, recent clinical trials using non-myeloablative regimens in concert with adoptive immunotherapy using ex vivo-expanded, tumor-specific T cells have yielded surprisingly high objective clinical response rates in patients with melanoma *(116)*.

We have also recently shown that Th2-type CD4+ T-cell responses to MAGE-6 peptides can be populationally "repolarized" to Th1-type responses using conditioned autologous DC (that produce large quantities of IL-12) and specific tumor peptide(s) as an in vitro vaccine (Tatsumi et al., unpublished results). The clinical application of similar vaccines could promote the systemic repolarization of tumor-specific CD4+ T cells in patients with advanced cancer, although this approach may be best suited to patients with a low tumor burden, or as an adjuvant modality for patients with minimal residual disease.

However, it is also possible that the observed Th2-dominated responses are not inhibitory per se, but rather represent a default phenotype. Evidence derived from the study of infectious diseases suggests that Th1-type CD4+ T cells may be differentially sensitive to antigen-induced cell death when compared to antigen-specific Th2-type CD4+ T cells *(117–122)*. Thus, in the setting of chronic tumor antigenic stimulation in the cancer patient, Th1-type, but not Th2-type tumor antigen-specific T cells may be predisposed to apoptosis *(117–122)*, particularly in cases in which IL-12 is deficient *(117)*. Our own recent results suggest that tumor epitope-specific CD4+ T cells may indeed be increasingly prone to undergo programmed cell death (Fig. 4). In these studies, phycoerythrin-labeled HLA-DR4/peptide tetramers containing either an influenza matrix "helper" epitope or the MAGE-$6_{121-144}$ or MAGE-$6_{246-263}$ epitopes (Tatsumi et al., unpublished data) were used to stain peripheral-blood CD4+ T cells isolated from an HLA-DR4+ patient with Stage IV RCC. Fluorescein isothiocyanate (FITC)-labeled Annexin-V was used as a counterstain to determine the frequency of apoptotic/dying cells within the epitope-specific CD4+ T-cell populations, as determined using two-color flow cytometry. As clearly indicated in the right-hand panel of Fig. 4, MAGE-6-specific CD4+ T populations in this patient exhibited elevated frequencies of Annexin-V+ cells, when compared with the influenza-specific CD4+ T cell population or the general CD4+ population (dotted line in Fig. 4, right-hand panel).

We are currently in the process of determining whether these pro-apoptotic T cells preferentially bear a Th1-type phenotype. If they do, this may suggest clinical promise for immunotherapies designed to promote the increased apoptotic resistance of such effector cells *in situ* (Fig. 5). Strategies implementing anti-apoptotic cytokines such as IL-7, IL-12, or IL-15 *(122–124)* in combina-

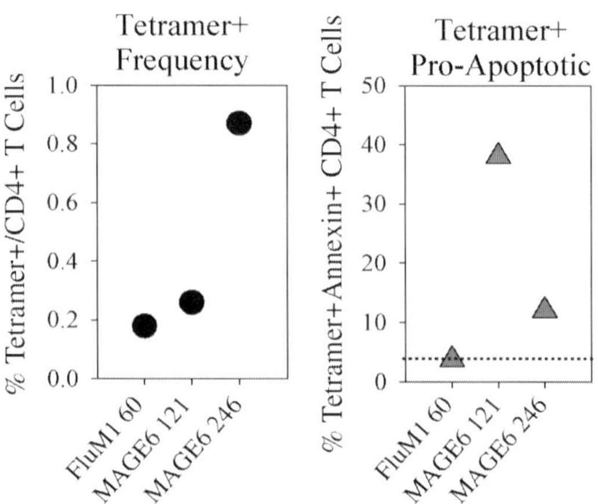

Fig. 4. Tumor-reactive CD4+ T cells isolated from the peripheral blood of cancer patients exhibit a higher incidence of apoptosis. CD4+ T cells were isolated from an HLA-DR4+ patient with RCC and stained using the indicated phycoerythrin (PE)-conjugated HLA-DR4/peptide tetramers and FITC-Annexin-V to mark antigen-specific T cells that were undergoing apoptosis. As indicated in the left panel, viral- or tumor-specific CD4+ T cells occurred at frequencies between approx 0.2–1% of all CD4+ T cells. In the right panel, tumor-reactive CD4+ T cells exhibit elevated frequencies of Annexin-V+ events vs FluM1 (influenza)-reactive T cells. The percent of Annexin-V+ cells among all CD4+ T cells in this individual was 3.1% (as indicated by the dotted line in the right panel).

tion with cancer vaccines or the use of tumor antigen-loaded autologous DC (that have been conditioned or engineered to secrete these cytokines) as vaccines would appear to be logical choices to extend the functional longevity of these clinically important effector cells. The development of therapies with the capability to salvage Th1-type responder T cells and to repolarize non-Th1-type effector cells into Th1-type T cells may prove to be even more clinically beneficial. Lastly, if Th3/Tr-type CD4+ T cells are observed, these may require the application of more drastic lymphoablative therapeutic approaches to allow the patient's immune system to reset itself to a more Th1-dominated pattern of functional antitumor immunity (Fig. 5).

8. SUMMARY

Although rarely studied during the past decade (when compared with CD8+ T cells), recent interest has been focused on achieving a better understanding of how CD4+ T "helper" cells recognize cancer cells, how cancer deviates the numbers and function of specific CD4+ T cell subsets and how clinically preferred CD4+ T-cell-mediated antitumor immunity may be promoted and

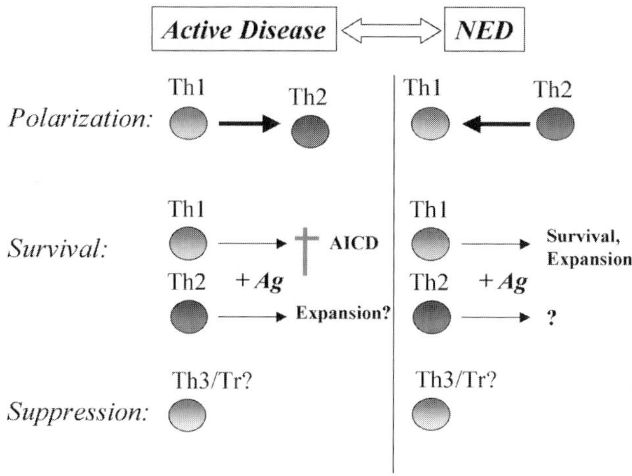

Fig. 5. Hypothetical model of the impact of disease on tumor-reactive CD4+ T-cell polarization. Based on our current understanding, chronic stimulation of the patient's immune system with tumor antigens may promote a gradual polarization of CD4+ T-cell responses away from Th1-type immunity. This may be partly the result of the differential sensitivity of Th1-type responder T cells to activation-induced cell death via apoptotic mechanisms. The observed Th2-type dominance in patients with active disease may represent the default phenotype for immunity under these conditions, although Th2-type responders may also undergo expansion. Tumor-antigen specific Th3/Tr-type CD4+ T-suppressor cells may also occur, although at very rare frequencies. Once the tumor has been removed or rejected by the patient (no evidence of disease, NED), tumor-specific Th1-type responses appear to functionally dominate the patient's CD4+ T-cell repertoire. The mechanism by which previously dominant (during active disease) Th2-type responses are diminished is not well understood, but may involve a repolarization of Th2-to-Th1-type T-cell immunity resulting from increased production of cytokines such as IL-12, IL-18, and IFN-γ. Although the status of tumor-reactive Th3/Tr-type CD4+ T cells in patients that have been rendered disease-free has not been comprehensively evaluated to date, it is likely that these cells are diminished in numbers or potency, since suppression of tumor-antigen specific Th1-type immunity appears to be decreased or absent in these patients.

sustained through therapeutic intervention. In many respects, this research is in its infancy. However, rapid progress is anticipated in the coming years because of the recent molecular identification of tumor antigen-derived peptide epitopes and novel refined methodologies, such as ELISPOT and MHC tetramer-based technologies, which allow for the monitoring of epitope-specific CD4+ T cells from patient peripheral blood, lymph nodes, and the tumor itself. Using such instruments, it will soon be possible to define the most appropriate means to optimally augment clinically beneficial Th1-type CD4+ T-cell responses to cancer and to maintain these responses over extended periods of time in order to sustain durable antitumor CD8+ T effector cells and prevent disease recurrence in patients at high risk for relapse. Furthermore, such studies and clinical trials have led us to a greater understanding of how CD4+

T-cell responses are functionally deviated as a result of the chronic stimulation occurring over extended periods of tumor indolence or slow progression, and may apply this effectively for improved patient diagnosis and treatment.

ACKNOWLEDGMENTS

The authors wish to thank Mrs. Kathy Rakow for excellent secretarial support in the preparation of this chapter and Dr. Cynthia Brissette-Storkus for her careful review and helpful suggestions. This work was supported by National Institutes of Health (NIH) grant CA57840 (W.J.S.).

REFERENCES

1. Jager D, Jager E, Knuth A. Immune responses to tumour antigens: implications for antigen specific immunotherapy of cancer. *J Clin Pathol* 2001;54:669–674.
2. Jager E, Jager D, Knuth A. CTL-defined cancer vaccines: perspectives for active immunotherapeutic interventions in minimal residual disease. *Cancer Metastasis Rev* 1999; 18:143–150.
3. Kawakami Y, Eliyahu S, Jennings C, Sakaguchi K, Kang X, Southwood S, et al. Recognition of multiple epitopes in the human melanoma antigen gp100 by tumor-infiltrating T lymphocytes associated with in vivo tumor regression. *J Immunol* 1995;154:3961–3968.
4. Cohen PA, Peng L, Kjaergaard J, Plautz GE, Finke JH, Koski GK, et al. T-cell adoptive therapy of tumors: mechanisms of improved therapeutic performance. *Crit Rev Immunol* 2001;21:215–248.
5. Labarriere N, Pandolfino MC, Gervois N, Khammari A, Tessier MH, Dreno B, et al. Therapeutic efficacy of melanoma-reactive TIL injected in stage III melanoma patients. *Cancer Immunol Immunother* 2002;51:532–538.
6. Topalian SL. MHC class II restricted tumor antigens and the role of CD4+ T cells in cancer immunotherapy. *Curr Opin Immunol* 1994;6:741–745.
7. Giuntoli RL 2nd, Lu J, Kobayashi H, Kennedy R, Celis E. Direct costimulation of tumor-reactive CTL by helper T cells potentiate their proliferation, survival, and effector function. *Clin Cancer Res* 2002;8:922–931.
8. Marzo AL, Kinnear BF, Lake RA, Frelinger JJ, Collins EJ, Robinson BW, et al. Tumor-specific CD4+ T cells have a major "post-licensing" role in CTL mediated anti-tumor immunity. *J Immunol* 2000;165:6047–6055.
9. Kunische-Hoppe M, Hoppe M, Bohle RM, Rauber K, Weimar B, Friemann S, et al. Metastatic RCC arising in a transplant kidney. *Eur Radiol* 1998;8:1441–1443.
10. Kliem V, Kolditz M, Behrend M, Ehlerding G, Pichlmayr R, Koch KM, et al. Risk of renal cell carcinoma after kidney transplantation. *Clin Transplant* 1997;11:255–258.
11. Jain A, Nalesnik M, Reyes J, Pokharna R, Mazariegos G, Green M, et al. Posttransplant lymphoproliferative disorders in liver transplantation: a 20-year experience. *Ann Surg* 2002;236:429–436.
12. Ramsay HM, Hawley CM, Smith AG, Harden PN. Non-melanoma skin cancer risk in the Queensland renal transplant population. *Br J Dermatol* 2002;147:950–956.
13. Van den Hove LE, Van Gool SW, Van Poppel H, Baert L, Coorrevits L, van Damme B, et al. Phenotype, cytokine production and cytolytic capacity of fresh (uncultured) tumor-infiltrating T lymphocytes in human renal cell carcinoma. *Clin Exp Immunol* 1997;109: 501–509.

14. Finke JH, Rayman P, Hart L, Alexander JP, Edinger MG, Tubbs RR, et al. Characterization of tumor-infiltrating lymphocyte subsets from human renal cell carcinoma: specific reactivity defined by cytotoxicity, interferon-γ secretion, and proliferation. *J Immunother Emphas Tumor Immunol* 1994;15:91–104.
15. Puisieux I, Bain C, Merrouche Y, Malacher P, Kourilsky P, Even J, et al. Restriction of the T-cell repertoire in tumor-infiltrating lymphocytes from nine patients with renal-cell carcinoma. Relevance of the CDR3 length analysis for the identification of in situ clonal T-cell expansions. *Int J Cancer* 1996;66:201–208.
16. Caignard A, Guillard M, Gaudin M, Escudier B, Treibel F, Dietrich PY. In situ demonstration of renal-cell-carcinoma-specific T-cell clones. *Int J Cancer* 1996;66:564–570.
17. Seliger B, Hohne A, Knuth A, Bernhard H, Meyer T, Tampe R, et al. Analysis of major histocompatibility complex class I antigen presentation machinery in normal and malignant renal cells: evidence for deficiencies associated with transformation and progression. *Cancer Res* 1996;56:1756–1760.
18. Irvine DJ, Purbhoo MA, Krogsgaard M, Davis MM. Direct observation of ligand recognition by T cells. *Nature* 2002;419:845–849.
19. Little AM, Parham P. Polymorphism and evolution of HLA class I and II genes and molecules. *Rev Immunogenet* 1999;1:105–123.
20. Ting JP, Trowsdale J. Genetic control of MHC class II expression. *Cell* 2002;109:S21–S33.
21. Ricaniadis N, Kataki A, Agnantis N, Androulakis G, Karakousis CP. Long-term prognostic significance of HSP-70, c-myc and HLA-DR expression in patients with malignant melanoma. *Eur J Surg Oncol* 2001;27:88–93.
22. Cabrera T, Ruiz-Cabello F, Garrido F. Biological implications of HLA-DR expression in tumours. *Scand J Immunol* 1995;41:398–406.
23. Nouri-Shirazi M, Banchereau J, Bell D, Burkeholder S, Kraus ET, Davoust J, et al. Dendritic cells capture killed tumor cells and present their antigens to elicit tumor-specific immune responses. *J Immunol* 2000;165:3797–3803.
24. Qi L, Rojas JM, Ostrand-Rosenberg S. Tumor cells present MHC class II-restricted nuclear and mitochondrial antigens and are the predominant antigen presenting cells in vivo. *J. Immunol.* 2000;165:5451–5461.
25. Dutton RW, Bradley LM, Swain SL. T cell memory. *Annu Rev Immunol* 1998;16:201–223.
26. Sikorska B, Danilewicz M, Wagrowska-Danilewicz M. HLA-DR expression is a significant prognostic factor in laryngeal cancer. A morphometric study. *APMIS* 1999;107:383–388.
27. Kunihiro M, Tanaka S, Haruma K, Yoshihara M, Sumii K, Kajiyama G, et al. Combined expression of HLA-DR antigen and proliferating cell nuclear antigen correlate with colorectal cancer prognosis. *Oncology* 1998;55:326–333.
28. Liu B, Su Z, Chen S. A study of HIA-DR antigen expression in nasopharyngeal carcinoma and its relation with clinical pathology and prognosis. *Zhonghua Bing Li Xue Za Zhi* 1996;25:162–164.
29. Sheen-Chen SM, Chou FF, Eng HL, Chen WJ. An evaluation of the prognostic significance of HLA-DR expression in axillary-node-negative breast cancer. *Surgery* 1994;116:510–515.
30. Tisch M, Kyrberg H, Weidauer H, Mytilineos J, Conradt C, Opelz G, et al. Human leukocyte antigens and prognosis in patients with head and neck cancer: results of a prospective follow-up study. *Laryngoscope* 2002;112:651–657.
31. Lee JE, Abdalla J, Porter GA, Bradford L, Grimm EA, Reveille JD, et al. Presence of the human leukocyte antigen class II gene DRB1*1101 predicts interferon gamma levels and disease recurrence in melanoma patients. *Ann Surg Oncol* 2002;9:587–593.
32. Azuma H, Sada M, Tsuji T, Ueda H, Katsuoka Y. Relationship between HLA-DR antigen and HLA-DRB1 alleles and prostate cancer in Japanese men. *Int Urol Nephrol* 1999; 31:343–349.

33. Ruiter DJ, Mattijssen V, Broecker EB, Ferrone S. MHC antigens in human melanomas. *Semin Cancer Biol* 1991;2:35–45.
34. Colloby PS, West KP, Fletcher A. Is poor prognosis really related to HLA-DR expression by malignant melanoma cells? *Histopathology* 1992;20:411–416.
35. Trieb K, Lechleitner T, Lang S, Windhager R, Kotz R, Dirnhofer S. Evaluation of HLA-DR expression and T-lymphocyte infiltration in osteosarcoma. *Pathol Res Pract* 1998; 194:679–684.
36. Assenmacher M, Lohning M, Scheffold A, Richter A, Miltenyi S, Schmitz J, et al. Commitment of individual Th1-like lymphocytes to expression of IFN-gamma versus IL-4 and IL-10: selective induction of IL-10 by sequential stimulation of naïve Th cells with IL-12 and IL-4. *J Immunol* 1998;161:2825–2832.
37. Tsai SL, Liaw YF, Chen MH, Huang CY, Kuo GC. Detection of type 2-like T-helper cells in hepatitis C virus infection: implications for hepatitis C virus chronicity. *Hepatology* 1997;25:449–458.
38. Chakraborty NG, Li L, Sporn JR, Kurtzman SH, Ergin MT, Mukherji B. Emergence of regulatory CD4+ T cell response to repetitive stimulation with antigen-presenting cells in vitro: implications in designing antigen-presenting cell-based tumor vaccines. *J Immunol* 1999;162:5576–5583.
39. Liyanage UK, Moore TT, Joo HG, Tanaka Y, Herrmann V, Doherty G, et al. Prevalence of regulatory T cells is increased in peripheral blood and tumor microenvironment of patients with pancreas or breast adenocarcinoma. *J Immunol* 2002;169:2756–2761.
40. Lucey DR, Clerici M, Shearer GM. Type 1 and type 2 cytokine dysregulation in human infectious, neoplastic, and inflammatory diseases. *Clin Microbiol Rev* 1996;9:532–562.
41. Mosmann TR, Cherwinski H, Bond MW, Giedlin MA, Coffman RL. Two types of murine helper T cell clones. I. Definition according to profiles of lymphokine activities and secreted proteins. *J Immunol* 1986;136:2348–2357.
42. Mosmann TR, Li L, Hengartner H, Kagi D, Fu W, and Sad S. Differentiation and functions of T cell subsets. *Ciba Found Sym* 1997;204:148–154.
43. Omiya R, Buteau C, Kobayashi H, Paya CV, Celis E. Inhibition of EBV-induced lymphoproliferation by CD4+ T cells specific for an MHC class II promiscuous epitope. *J Immunol* 2002;169:2172–2179.
44. Mosmann TR, Sad S. The expanding universe of T-cell subsets: Th1, Th2 and more. *Immunol Today* 1996;17:138–146.
45. McHugh RS, Shevach EM. The role of suppressor T cells in regulation of immune responses. *J Allergy Clin Immunol* 2002;110:693–702.
46. Weiner HL. Induction and mechanism of action of transforming growth factor-beta-secreting Th3 regulatory cells. *Immunol Rev* 2001;182:207–214.
47. Grakoui A, Donermeyer DL, Kanagawa O, Murphy KM, Allen PM. TCR-independent pathways mediate the effects of antigen dose and altered peptide ligands on Th cell polarization. *J Immunol* 1999;162:1923–1930.
48. Kato T, Nariuchi H. Polarization of naive CD4+ T cells toward the Th1 subset by CTLA-4 costimulation. *J Immunol* 2000;164:3554–3562.
49. Ruedl C, Bachmann MF, Kopf M. The antigen dose determines T helper subset development by regulation of CD40 ligand. *Eur J Immunol* 2000;30:2056–2064.
50. Tanaka H, Demeure CE, Rubio M, Delespesse G, Sarfati M. Human monocyte-derived dendritic cells induce naive T cell differentiation into T helper cell type 2 (Th2) or Th1/Th2 effectors. Role of stimulator/responder ratio. *J Exp Med* 2000;192:405–412.
51. DiMolfetto L, Neal HA, Wu A, Reilly C, Lo D. The density of the class II MHC T cell receptor ligand influences IFN-gamma/IL-4 ratios in immune responses in vivo. *Cell Immunol* 1998;183:70–79.

52. Rissoan MC, Soumelis V, Kadowaki N, Grouard G, Briere F, de Waal Malefyt R, et al. Reciprocal control of T helper cell and dendritic cell differentiation. *Science* 1999; 283:1183–1186.
53. Coffman RL, Mocci S, O'Garra A. The stability and reversibility of Th1 and Th2 populations. *Curr Top Microbiol Immunol* 1999;238:1–12.
54. Kourilsky P, Truffa-Bachi P. Cytokine fields and the polarization of the immune response. *Trends Immunol* 2001 Sep;22(9):502–509.
55. Mitchison NA, Schuhbauer D, Muller B. Natural and induced regulation of Th1/Th2 balance. *Springer Semin Immunopathol* 1999;21:199–210.
56. Annunziato F, Galli G, Cosmi L, Romagnani P, Manetti R, Maggi E, et al. Molecules associated with human Th1 or Th2 cells. *Eur Cytokine Netw* 1998;9:S12–S16.
57. Smeltz RB, Chen J, Ehrhardt R, Shevach EM. Role of IFN-gamma in Th1 differentiation: IFN-γ regulates IL-18Rα expression by preventing the negative effects of IL-4 and by inducing/maintaining IL-12 receptor beta 2 expression. *J Immunol* 2002;168:6165–6172.
58. Shevach EM, Chang JT, Segal BM. The critical role of IL-12 and the IL-12Rβ2 subunit in the generation of pathogenic autoreactive Th1 cells. *Springer Semin Immunopathol* 1999; 21:249–262.
59. Lecart S, Lecointe N, Subramaniam A, Alkan S, Ni D, Chen R, et al. Activated, but not resting human Th2 cells, in contrast to Th1 and T regulatory cells, produce soluble ST2 and express low levels of ST2L at the cell surface. *Eur J Immunol* 2002;32:2979–2987.
60. Yamamoto J, Adachi Y, Onoue Y, Kanegane H, Miyawaki T, Toyoda M, et al. CD30 expression on circulating memory CD4+ T cells as a Th2-dominated situation in patients with atopic dermatitis. *Allergy* 2000;55:1011–1018.
61. Cosmi L, Annunziato F, Galli G, Manetti R, Maggi E, Romagnani S. CRTH2: marker for the detection of human Th2 and Tc2 cells. *Adv Exp Med Biol* 2001;495:25–29.
62. Scotet E, Schroeder S, Lanzavecchia A. Molecular regulation of CC-chemokine receptor 3 expression in human T helper 2 cells. *Blood* 2001;98:2568–2570.
63. Levings MK, Sangregorio R, Roncarolo MG. Human CD25+CD4+ T regulatory cells suppress naive and memory T cell proliferation and can be expanded in vitro without loss of function. *J Exp Med* 2001;193:1295–1302.
64. Wing K, Ekmark A, Karlsson H, Rudin A, Suri-Payer E. Characterization of human CD25+ CD4+ T cells in thymus, cord and adult blood. *Immunology* 2002;106:190–199.
65. Antony PA, Restifo NP. Do CD4+ CD25+ immunoregulatory T cells hinder tumor immunotherapy? *J Immunother* 2002;25:202–206.
66. Gately MK, Gubler U, Brunda MJ, Nadeau RR, Anderson TD, Lipman JM, et al. Interleukin-12: a cytokine with therapeutic potential in oncology and infectious diseases. *Ther Immunol* 1994;1:187–196.
67. Qin Z, Blankenstein T. CD4+ T cell-mediated tumor rejection involves inhibition of angiogenesis that is dependent on IFN gamma receptor expression by nonhematopoietic cells. *Immunity* 2000;12:677–686.
68. O'Garra A, Hosken N, Macatonia S, Wenner CA, Murphy K. The role of macrophage- and dendritic cell-derived IL-12 in Th1 phenotype development. *Res Immunol* 1995;146:466–472.
69. Trinchieri G. Role of IL-12 in human Th1 response. *Chem Immunol* 1996;63:14–29.
70. Hussell T, Khan U, Openshaw P. IL-12 treatment attentuates T helper type 2 and B cell responses but does not improve vaccine-enhanced lung illness. *J Immunol* 1997; 159:328–334.
71. Scott P, Hondowicz B, Eatron A, Scharton-Kersten T. The role of IL-12 in regulation of T helper cell subsets in vivo. Lessons from experimental cutaneous leishmaniasis. *Ann NY Acad Sci* 1996;795:250–256.

72. Annunziano F, Cosmi L, Manetti R, Brugnolo F, Parronchi P, Maggi E, et al. Reversal of human allergen-specific CRTH2+ Th2 T cells by IL-12 or the PS-DSP30 oligodeoxynucleotide. *J Allergy Clin Immunol* 2001;108:815–821.
73. Kalinski P, Smits HH, Schuitemaker JH, Vieira PL, van Eijk M, de Jong EC, et al. IL-4 is a mediator of IL-12p70 induction by human Th2 cells: reversal of polarized Th2 phenotype by dendritic cells. *J Immunol* 2000;165:1877–1881.
74. Smits HH, van Rietschoten JG, Hilkens CM, Sayilir R, Stiekema F, Kapsenberg ML, et al. IL-12-induced reversal of human Th2 cells is accompanied by full restoration of IL-12 responsiveness and loss of GATA-3 expression. *Eur J Immunol* 2001;31:1055–1065.
75. van der Bruggen P, Traversari C, Chomez P, Lurquin C, De Plaen E, Van den Eynde B, et al. A gene encoding an antigen recognized by cytolytic T lymphocytes on a human melanoma. *Science* 1991;254:1643–1647.
76. Sloan JM, Kershaw MH, Touloukian CE, Lapointe R, Robbins PF, Restifo NP, et al. MHC class I and class II presentation of tumor antigen in retrovirally and adenovirally transduced dendritic cells. *Cancer Gene Ther* 2002;9:946–950.
77. Storkus WJ, Zarour HM. Melanoma antigens recognised by CD8+ and CD4+ T cells. *Forum (Genova)* 2000;10:256–270.
78. Wang RF, Rosenberg SA. Human tumor antigens for cancer vaccine development. *Immunol Rev* 1999;170:85–100.
79. Asai T, Storkus WJ, Whiteside TL. Evaluation of the modified ELISPOT assay for gamma interferon production in cancer patients receiving antitumor vaccines. *Clin Diagn Lab Immunol* 2000;7:145–154.
80. Keilholz U, Weber J, Finke JH, Gabrilovich DI, Kast WM, Disis ML, et al. Immunologic monitoring of cancer vaccine therapy: results of a workshop sponsored by the Society for Biological Therapy. *J Immunother* 2002;25:97–138.
81. Herr W, Ranieri E, Gambotto A, Kierstead LS, Amoscato AA, Gesualdo L, et al. Identification of naturally-processed HLA-presented Epstein-Barr virus peptides recognized by ex vivo CD4+ or CD8+ T lymphocytes from human blood. *Proc Natl Acad Sci USA* 1999;96:12,033–12,038.
82. Kierstead LS, Ranieri E, Olson W, Brusic V, Sidney J, Sette A, et al. gp100/pmel17 and tyrosinase encode multiple epitopes recognized by Th1-type CD4+ T cells. *Br J Cancer* 2001;85:1738–1745.
83. Tatsumi T, Kierstead LS, Ranieri E, Gesualdo L, Schena FP, Finke JH, et al. MAGE-6 encodes DR?1*0401-presented epitopes recognized by CD4+ T cells derived from patients with melanoma or renal cell carcinoma. *Clin Cancer Res* 2003;9:947–954.
84. Kolbeck PC, Kaveggia FF, Johansson SL, Grune MT, Taylor RJ. The relationships among tumor-infiltrating lymphocytes, histopathologic findings, and long-term clinical follow-up in renal cell carcinoma. *Mod Pathol* 1992;5:420–425.
85. Storkel S, Keymer R, Steinbach F, Thoenes W. Reaction pattern of tumor infiltrating lymphocytes in different renal cell carcinomas and oncocytomas. *Prog Clin Biol Res* 1992; 378:217–223.
86. Burger UL, Chang MP, Nagoshi M, Goedegebuure PS, Eberlein TJ. Improved in vivo efficacy of tumor-infiltrating lymphocytes after restimulation with irradiated tumor cells in vitro. *Ann Surg Oncol* 1996;3:580–587.
87. Schirrmacher V, Schild HJ, Guckel B, von Hoegen P. Tumour-specific CTL response requiring interactions of four different cell types and recognition of MHC class I and class II restricted tumour antigens. *Immunol Cell Biol* 1993;71:311–326.
88. To WC, Seeley BM, Barthel SW, Shu S. Therapeutic efficacy of Th1 and Th2 L-selectin- CD4+ tumor-reactive T cells. *Laryngoscope* 2000;110:1648–1654.
89. Ossendorp F, Mengede E, Camps M, Filius R, Melief CJ. Specific T helper cell requirement for optimal induction of cytotoxic T lymphocytes against major histocompatibility complex II negative tumors. *J Exp Med* 1998;187:693–702.

90. Surman DR, Dudley ME, Overwijk WW, Restifo NP. Cutting edge: CD4+ T cell control of CD8+ T cell reactivity to a model tumor antigen. *J Immunol* 2000;164:562–565.
91. Hung K, Hayashi R, Lafond-Walker A, Lowenstein C, Pardoll D, Levitsky H. The central role of CD4+ T cells in the antitumor immune response. *J Exp Med* 1998;188:2357–2368.
92. Levitsky HI, Lazenby A, Hayashi RJ, Pardoll DM. In vivo priming of two distinct antitumor effector populations: the role of MHC class I expression. *J Exp Med* 1994;179:1215–1224.
93. Dranoff G, Jaffee E, Lazenby A, Golumbek P, Levitsky H, Brose K, et al. Vaccination with irradiated tumor cells engineered to secrete murine granulocyte-macrophage colony-stimulating factor stimulates potent, specific, and long-lasting anti-tumor immunity. *Proc Natl Acad Sci USA* 1993;90:3539–3543.
94. Fallarino F, Grohmann U, Bianchi R, Vacca C, Fioretti MC, Puccetti P. Th1 and Th2 cell clones to a poorly immunogenic tumor antigen initiate CD8+ T cell-dependent tumor eradication in vivo. *J Immunol* 2000;165:5495–5501.
95. Nagai H, Hara I, Horikawa T, Oka M, Kamidono S, Ichihashi M. Elimination of CD4+ T cells enhances anti-tumor effect of locally secreted interleukin-12 on B16 mouse melanoma and induces vitiligo-like coat color alteration. *J Investig Dermatol* 2000;115:1059–1064.
96. Nishimura T, Iwakabe K, Sekimoto M, Ohmi Y, Yahata T, Nakui M, et al. Distinct role of antigen-specific T helper type 1 (Th1) and Th2 cells in tumor eradication in vivo. *J Exp Med* 1999;190:617–627.
97. Nishimura T, Nakui M, Sato M, Iwakabe K, Kitamura H, Sekimoto M, et al. The critical role of Th1-dominant immunity in tumor immunology. *Cancer Chemother Pharmacol* 2000;46:S52–S61.
98. Gorelik L, Flavell RA. Immune-mediated eradication of tumors through the blockade of transforming growth factor-beta signaling in T cells. *Nat Med* 2001;7:1118–1122.
99. Seo N, Hayakawa S, Takigawa M, Tokura Y. Interleukin-10 expressed at early tumour sites induces subsequent generation of CD4+ T-regulatory cells and systemic collapse of antitumour immunity. *Immunology* 2001;103:449–457.
100. Oka H, Emori Y, Hayashi Y, Nomoto K. Breakdown of Th cell immune responses and steroidogenic CYP11A1 expression in CD4+ T cells in a murine model implanted with B16 melanoma. *Cell Immunol* 2000;206:7–15.
101. Kobayashi M, Kobayashi H, Pollard RB, Suzuki F. A pathogenic role of Th2 cells and their cytokine products on the pulmonary metastasis of murine B16 melanoma. *J Immunol* 1998;160:5869–5873.
102. Ito N, Nakamura H, Tanaka Y, Ohgi S. Lung carcinoma: analysis of T helper type 1 and 2 cells and T cytotoxic type 1 and 2 cells by intracellular cytokine detection with flow cytometry. *Cancer* 1999;85:2359–2367.
103. Maeurer MJ, Martin DM, Castelli C, Elder E, Leder G, Storkus WJ, et al. Host immune response in renal cell cancer: interleukin-4 (IL-4) and IL-10 mRNA are frequently detected in freshly collected tumor-infiltrating lymphocytes. *Cancer Immunol Immunother* 1995;41:111–121.
104. Schoof DD, Terashima Y, Peoples GE, Goedegebuure PS, Andrews JV, Richie JP, et al. CD4+ T cell clones isolated from human renal cell carcinoma possess the functional characteristics of Th2 helper cells. *Cell Immunol* 1993;150:114–123.
105. Goldman M, Druet P. The Th1/Th2 concept and its relevance to renal disorders and transplantation immunity. *Nephrol Dial Transplant* 1995;10:1282–1284.
106. Elsasser-Beile U, Kolble N, Grussenmeyer T, Schultze-Seemann W, Wetterauer U, Gallati H, et al. Th1 and Th2 cytokine response patterns in leukocyte cultures of patients with urinary bladder, renal cell and prostate carcinomas. *Tumour Biol* 1998;19:470–476.
107. Fridman WH, Tartour E. Macrophage- and lymphocyte-produced Th1 and Th2 cytokines in the tumour microenvironment. *Res Immunol* 1998;149:651–653.

108. Angevin E, Kremer F, Gaudin C, Hercend T, Triebel F. Analysis of T-cell immune response in renal cell carcinoma: polarization to type 1-like differentiation pattern, clonal T-cell expansion and tumor-specific cytotoxicity. *Int J Cancer* 1997;72:431–440.
109. Knoefel B, Nuske K, Steiner T, Junker K, Kosmehl H, Rebstock K, et al. Renal cell carcinomas produce IL-6, IL-10, IL-11, and TGF-β1 in primary cultures and modulate T lymphocyte blast transformation. *J Interferon Cytokine Res* 1997;17:95–102.
110. Tatsumi T, Kierstead LS, Ranieri E, Gesualdo L, Schena FP, Finke JH, et al. Disease-associated bias in T helper type 1 (Th1)/Th2 CD4+ T cell responses against MAGE-6 in HLA-DRB1*0401+ patients with renal cell carcinoma or melanoma. *J Exp Med* 2002;196:619–628.
111. Kaplan DH, Shankaran V, Dighe AS, Stockert E, Aguet M, Old LJ, et al. Demonstration of an interferon gamma-dependent tumor surveillance system in immunocompetent mice. *Proc Natl Acad Sci USA* 1998;95:7556–7561.
112. Biedremann T, Mailhammer R, Mai A, Sander C, Ogilvie A, Brombacher F, et al. Reversal of established delayed type hypersensitivity reactions following therapy with IL-4 or antigen-specific Th2 cells. *Eur J Immunol* 2001;31:1582–1591.
113. Bass KK, Mastrangelo MJ. Immunopotentiation with low-dose cyclophosphamide in the active specific immunotherapy of cancer. *Cancer Immunol Immunother* 1998;47:1–12.
114. Tanaka H, Tanaka J, Kjaergaard J, Shu S. Depletion of CD4+ CD25+ regulatory cells ugments the generation of specific immune T cells in tumor-draining lymph nodes. *J Immunother* 2002;25:207–217.
115. Matar P, Rozados VR, Gervasoni SI, Scharovsky GO. Th2/Th1 switch induced by a single low dose of cyclophosphamide in a rat metastatic lymphoma model. *Cancer Immunol Immunother* 2002;50:588–596.
116. Dudley ME, Wunderlich JR, Robbins PF, Yang JC, Hwu P, Schwartzentruber DJ, et al. Cancer regression and autoimmunity in patients after clonal repopulation with antitumor lymphocytes. *Science* 2002;298:850–854.
117. Marth T, Zeitz M, Ludviksson BR, Strober W, Kelsall BL. Extinction of IL-12 signaling promotes Fas-mediated apoptosis of antigen-specific T cells. *J Immunol* 1999; 162:7233–7240.
118. Yu XZ, Anasetti C. Enhancement of susceptibility to Fas-mediated apoptosis of Th1 cells by nonmitogenic anti-CD3εF(ab′)$_2$. *Transplantation* 2000;69:104–112.
119. Reinhard G, Noll A, Schlebusch H, Mallmann P, Ruecker AV. Shifts in the Th1/Th2 balance during human pregnancy correlate with apoptotic changes. *Biochem Biophys Res Commun* 1998;245:933–938.
120. Varadhachary AS, Perdow SN, Hu C, Ramanarayanan M, Salgame P. Differential ability of T cell subsets to undergo activation-induced cell death. *Proc Natl Acad Sci USA* 1997;94:5778–5783.
121. Zhang X, Brunner T, Carter L, Dutton RW, Rogers P, Bradley L, et al. Unequal death in T helper cell (Th1) and Th2 effectors: Th1, but not Th2, effectors undergo rapid Fas/FasL-mediated apoptosis. *J Exp Med* 1997;185:1837–1849.
122. Estaquier J, Idziorek T, Zou W, Emilie D, Farber CM, Bourez JM, et al. T helper type 1/type 2 cytokines and T cell death: preventative effect of interleukin 12 on activation-induced and CD95 (Fas/APO-1)-mediated apoptosis of CD4+ T cells from human immunodeficiency virus-infected persons. *J Exp Med* 1995;182:1759–1767.
123. Waldmann T. The contrasting roles of IL-2 and IL-15 in the life and death of lymphocytes: implications for the immunotherapy of rheumatological diseases. *Arthritis Res* 2002;4:S161–S167.
124. Amos CL, Woetmann A, Nielsen M, Geisler C, Odum N, Brown BL, et al. The role of caspase 3 and BclxL in the action of interleukin 7 (IL-7): a survival factor in activated human T cells. *Cytokine* 1998;10:662–668.

5 Immunological Ignorance in Cancer

Koji Tamada, MD, PhD
and Lieping Chen, MD, PhD

Contents

1. INTRODUCTION

Recognition of an antigen by specific T lymphocytes carrying the appropriate antigen receptor does not always lead to activation or inactivation. Many studies have found that such lymphocytes could remain in resting status after exposure to the antigen, a phenomenon described as "ignorance" or "indifference." Immunological ignorance, although first introduced more than 10 years ago, remains a poorly understood phenomenon in the field of lymphocyte biology. Experimental data indicates that many tumor antigens are ignored by tumor-specific T cells in tumor-bearing animals and in cancer patients. In this chapter, we summarize the current status of research and the methods that may be utilized to overcome T-cell ignorance with the goal of achieving more effective antitumor T-cell responses.

1.1. Definition

Immunological ignorance is defined as a phenomenon in which fully competent T cells fail to mount productive immune responses in vivo despite

From: *Current Clinical Oncology: Cancer Immunotherapy at the Crossroads: How Tumors Evade Immunity and What Can Be Done*
Edited by: J. H. Finke and R. M. Bukowski © Humana Press Inc., Totowa, NJ

the presence of reactive antigens (Ag), although they respond normally when stimulated with those Ag in vitro. T-cell ignorance is thus recognized only in vivo, and could therefore be distinguished from T-cell anergy, in which prior exposure to antigen leads to unresponsiveness of T cells to corresponding Ag in the presence of appropriate antigen-presenting cells (APCs). Ignorance is also different from suppression, in which the T-cell response is inhibited, usually in an antigen nonspecific fashion. Withdrawal of suppressive factors is sufficient to recover the response. In addition, anergy and suppression could be readily established in vitro in the cell-culture system, yet the reproducible in vitro system for T-cell ignorance is not yet available.

T-cell ignorance may occur in both the priming and effector stage. In the former case, Ag-reactive T cells are not primed, and thus remain a naïve phenotype. In the latter case, however, primed T cells are incapable of performing effector functions against the target that expresses reactive Ag in vivo. A narrow definition of immunological ignorance sometimes excludes the latter, and therefore it is alternatively known as immunological incompetence.

1.2. Experimental Models Demonstrating T-Cell Ignorance to Self-Ag

In 1991, T-cell ignorance were first described in two reports by Ohashi et al. and Oldstone et al. *(1,2)*. In these studies, expression of viral Ag in pancreatic islet cells under rat insulin promoter did not elicit detectable CD8+ cytotoxic T lymphocyte (CTL) responses in vivo and islet tissues remained intact, even in the presence of frequent Ag-specific T cells. These T cells are fully functional in vitro, indicating that deletion and anergy of Ag-specific T cells are not responsible for tolerance shown in vivo. Systemic infection of Ag-expressing virus in these mice led to the rapid onset of autoimmune diabetes because of a breakdown of T-cell tolerance, suggesting that inappropriate priming of T cells—e.g., ignorance of Ag—accounts for the tolerance shown in these experimental systems.

A number of experimental models other than autoimmune diabetes also demonstrated T-cell ignorance as a mechanism for peripheral tolerance. Viral Ag expressed in hepatocytes under the control of mouse albumin promoter is ignored by Ag-specific T-cell receptor (TCR) transgenic T cells, whereas infection of Ag-expressing virus has led to the onset of autoimmune hepatitis *(3)*. Similarly, transgenic mice that express E6 and E7 of human papillomaviruses (HPV) in keratinized epithelia driven by keratin-14 promoter harbor ignorant T cells *(4)*. CTL reactive to antigenic E7 peptide were not primed in these mice. However, active immunization with E7 peptide stimulated CTL generation at a comparable level to non-transgenic mice, indicating that E7-reactive CTL are not deleted or anergized. Interestingly, immunization of E7 peptide in these transgenic mice induced no pathological changes in epithelial tissues, which express the HPV-16 E7 gene, although they acquired resistance to a subsequent challenge of E7-expressing tumor. These data suggest that T-cell ignorance in this model is governed at both the priming and effector stages, and that a breakdown of T-cell ignorance at the priming stage does not guarantee overall destruction of T-cell tolerance, which results in autoimmune diseases.

2. IMMUNOLOGICAL IGNORANCE AS A MECHANISM OF IMMUNE EVASION BY CANCER

There is ample evidence that immunological ignorance affects self-reactive T cells as well as T cells that are specific to tumor-associated antigen (TAA), and therefore may account for ineffective immunological responses against cancer. To characterize and overcome T-cell ignorance through the manipulation of immune systems thus provides important strategies for the advance of tumor immunotherapy. It has been reported that, as in T-cell ignorance to self-Ag, TAA-reactive T cells ignore Ag at the priming or effector stage or both, as described here.

2.1. Ignorance at the Priming Stage of Tumor-Specific T Cells

Transgenic expression of simian virus 40 large T antigen (SV40 Tag) under the control of rat insulin promoter spontaneously causes pancreatic β-cell tumors to produce insulin, leading to progressive hypoglycemia *(5)*. By co-expression of another viral Ag in β cells as a surrogate tumor Ag, antitumor T-cell responses may be monitored along with tumor growth and immunological manipulations *(6)*. In this model, tumor Ag-specific T cells were not spontaneously activated or tolerized by anergy or deletion, but maintained as the unprimed condition. Systemic infection of virus expressing tumor Ag activated otherwise ignorant T cells, leading to the temporal retardation of tumor growth.

Zinkernagel et al. also provided strong evidence for the presence of ignorant T cells in a tumor-bearing host *(7,8)*. Highly immunogenic tumors that expressed virus-derived protein as surrogate tumor Ag progressively grew when implanted as a small tissue fragment, whereas they were spontaneously rejected when inoculated in a cell-suspension form. In the host with growing tumor, CTL specific to tumor Ag were devoid of priming, but were readily activated by the vaccination of Ag-expressing viruses, indicating that they were not deleted or anergized. The remarkable findings in these studies indicated that generation of ignorant T cells strictly correlated with the inability of tumor cells to migrate and interact with T cells at the secondary lymphoid organs. Thus, these studies suggest that the location of antigen presentation affects the generation of ignorant T cells at the priming stage.

Using tetrameric complexes of peptide/major histocompatibility complex (MHC), human T cells specific to tumor Ag could be enumerated and characterized in cancer patients and healthy individuals. In 7 of 10 melanoma patients examined, CTLs specific to Melan-A/MART-1 tumor Ag in circulating peripheral-blood mononuclear cells (PBMC) express naïve phenotype, whereas those in tumor-draining lymph node show Ag-experienced memory phenotype *(9,10)*. Similarly, T cells specific to the telomerase catalytic subunit—a self-derived tumor Ag shared in most types of cancers—were detected as ignorant status in peripheral blood from the patients with melanoma, prostate cancer, bladder cancer, and lung cancer *(11)*. In contrast to these studies, several reports indicate the presence of Ag-experienced tumor-specific CTLs in cancer patients *(12,13)*. Together, these findings indicate that immunological ignorance is prevalent in experimental tumor models and in cancer patients, whereas other mechanisms such as anergy, deletion, or suppression of TAA-reactive CTLs also take place.

2.2. Ignorance at the Effector Stage of Tumor-Specific T Cells

It is frequently observed that the efficient priming of tumor-reactive T cells does not correlate with the control of tumor outgrowth *(14)*. For example, clinical trials using TAA with or without dendritic cells (DC) are capable of activating tumor-reactive CTLs in most cases, as evidenced by detection of these T cells in PBMC and at the site of vaccination. Nevertheless, these responses often do not parallel significant clinical responses such as complete regression of tumor *(15–17)*. Furthermore, adoptive immunotherapy based on transfer of fully activated tumor-reactive T cells—in which T cells are primed by optimal stimulation ex vivo—have not been shown to be highly therapeutic for cancer. Whereas various tumor evasion mechanisms, including impaired migration and insufficient survival of CTL, tumor-derived immunosuppressive factors, and the counterattack mechanism by the tumor, have been proposed to interpret these findings, ignorance of T cells for tumor antigens at the effector phase should be seriously considered.

Immunological ignorance of tumor-specific T cells at the effector stage is also evident in several experimental tumor models. For example, using 2C transgenic mice that harbored T cells specific to L^d of MHC class I, Wick et al. demonstrated that tumor cells expressing transfected L^d gene grew in these mice, whereas L^d-expressing skin graft were readily rejected *(18)*, suggesting that an ongoing CTL response selectively spares tumor cells from destruction. Furthermore, Sarma et al. showed that P1A Ag-positive tumor cells grow in transgenic mice that express TCR specific to P1A *(19)*. Importantly, in this model, B7-transfected—but not mock—tumor was eliminated when these tumors are inoculated in a single transgenic mouse, but in different anatomic locations. In addition, there are sublines of transgenic mice expressing oncogene SV40 Tag in islet β cells starting from 8–10 wk of age *(20)*. Subsequently, after Ag expression, these mice develop autoimmune insulitis accompanied by lymphocytic infiltration. Nevertheless, pancreatic β-cell tumors expressing Tag progressively grew in these mice, and no infiltrating lymphocytes were observed at the site of the tumor. These studies thus suggest that the optimization of effector function of CTL "at the site of tumor" is essential to achieve the effective treatment of cancer.

3. MECHANISMS LEADING TO T-CELL IGNORANCE

Recent studies suggest that immunological ignorance is controlled at several levels, including expression levels of tumor antigens, strength of the costimulatory signal, frequency of antigen-reactive T cells, and accessibility of lymphoid organs, as discussed here. However, these mechanisms may not be mutually exclusive.

3.1. Expression Levels of Tumor Antigens

Studies by Kurts et al. highlight the importance of expression levels of Ag in the generation of peripheral T-cell tolerance *(21)*. They have demonstrated that peripheral T cells are tolerized to OVA antigens in two transgenic mouse lineages that express either high or low levels of ovalbumin (OVA) in pancreatic β cells. By evaluating the activation status of OVA-specific T cells, it was revealed that the mice expressing OVA at high levels induced deletion of specific T cells, whereas T cells in the mice expressing lower levels of Ag remain ignorant. Peripheral deletion of OVA-specific T cells was associated with cross-presentation of OVA by bone marrow-derived APC *(21,22)*, suggesting that T cells ignore Ag when APC lack cross-presentation as a result of insufficient doses of Ag. In a tumor-bearing setting, this notion has been elegantly demonstrated in a recent study using a tumor harboring drug-mediated inducible TAA *(23)*. Tumors that expressed a high level of TAA generated specific CTL responses accompanied with tumor eradication, whereas those with lower levels of TAA were ignored by T cells. It was further demonstrated that induction of TAA-specific CTLs requires cross-presentation of TAA by bone marrow-derived host stroma cells.

In addition to the levels of antigen expression, certain features associated with antigens appear to be an important determinant for immunological ignorance. Various types of Ag including SV40 Tag, influenza virus hemagglutinin (HA), and glycoprotein (GP) of lymphocytic choriomeningitis virus (LCMV), have been introduced into pancreatic β cells under the control of identical rat insulin promoter *(1,2,24,25)*. Interestingly, among these mice, T cells reactive to SV40 Tag and HA antigen are either deleted or anergized, whereas T cells specific to LCMV GP ignore Ag and remain unprimed. Furthermore, transgenic expression of costimulator B7-1 along with LCMV GP antigen in pancreatic β cells induces spontaneous development of autoimmune diabetes, whereas expression of B7-1 alone is not sufficient to break ignorance against naturally expressing islet antigens *(26)*. These studies suggest that the immunogenicity of Ag also affects the generation of T-cell ignorance.

3.2. Strength of T-Cell Costimulation

To achieve optimal activation of T-cell responses, two distinct signals delivered by professional APC are required. Signal one is transmitted by the interaction between MHC/peptide and TCR, and the second signal is mediated by costimulatory receptor-ligand interactions *(27)*. The generation of unresponsive T cells by TCR stimulation in the absence of major costimulatory signals supports its essential role in peripheral T-cell tolerance *(28)*. Costimulation also plays a critical role in the development of immunological ignorance. Transgenic expression of B7-1 costimulator—along with either viral Ag, inflammatory cytokines, or MHC molecules on pancreatic islet cells—is capable of breaking T-cell ignorance, and leads to autoimmune diabetes *(26,29,30)*. These studies also indicate that single transgenic expression of B7-1 is insufficient to develop autoimmune phenotypes. Interestingly, Johnston et al. demonstrated that vaccination of EL4 tumor expressing B7-1 elicits CTL responses against subdominant (silent) epitopes of tumor Ag, which are otherwise ignored by T cells *(31)*. It is thus likely that the strength of costimulatory signal may regulate a threshold of T cells to become activated, ignorant, or anergic *(32)*. Expression of the costimulatory molecule on tumor cells may break T-cell ignorance upon priming stage, and converts silent Ag to become immunogenic.

Expression of costimulatory molecules has also been shown to be effective in breaking immunological ignorance in the effector stage of tumor-reactive CTL. T-cell ignorance observed in 2C transgenic mice in which CTL ignore L^d-expressing tumor, but not grafted L^d-positive skin, was abrogated when tumor cells expressed the costimulatory molecules B7-1 and CD48 *(18)*. In addition, B7-positive, but not B7-negative, tumor expressing P1A tumor Ag was readily rejected in the P1A-reactive TCR transgenic mice *(19)*. These results are in agreement with studies indicating that B7 expression on tumor cells plays an important role in recruiting and maturing CTL at the site of the tumor *(33,34)*. In addition to the definite participation of B7-1 molecule, other molecules in the expanding B7-CD28 family also contribute to T-cell ignorance *(35)*. In addition to B7-CD28 interaction, a negative costimulatory pathway through CTLA-4 may also regulate T-cell ignorance. Perez et al. showed that blockade of CTLA-4 signal by monoclonal antibody (MAb) rendered T cells activated, whereas blockade of both CD28 and CTLA-4 signals led to T-cells ignorant *(36)*, suggesting that a balance of positive vs negative costimulatory signals contributes to the generation of T-cell ignorance.

3.3. Frequency of T Cells Reactive to Ag

The mice that express LCMV GP antigen and SV40 Tag under the control of rat insulin promoter spontaneously develop pancreatic β-cell tumor accompanied with ignorant T cells to GP Ag *(6)*. Nguyen et al. further crossed these mice with transgenic mice harboring T cells with GP-specific TCR, and found that in the triple transgenic mice, the ignorant status of GP-specific T cells was broken and the outgrowth of tumor was partially controlled *(37)*. This study thus offers a hypothesis that immunological ignorance is maintained only when the frequency of Ag-specific T cells is lower than a certain threshold. However, it is unclear whether these findings are physiologically relevant because the frequency of Ag-specific T cells in these mice is very high. In addition, initiation of T-cell priming in the triple transgenic mice largely depends on bone marrow-derived APC located in the draining lymph nodes, but not GP-expressing islet cells, supporting an important role for cross-presentation in breaking T-cell ignorance.

3.4. Role of Lymphoid Organs

Ochsenbein et al. demonstrated that T-cell ignorance to a model tumor Ag is closely associated with an insufficient interaction between tumor cells and CTL at the secondary lymphoid organs *(7,8)*. Encapsulation of tumor cells resident in lymphoid organs also contributes to the generation of ignorant T cells. In alymphoplastic *(aly/aly)* mice lacking lymph nodes, tumor-reactive CTL ignore Ag and allow the outgrowth of cancer, even if tumor cells are vaccinated as an immunogenic form. Interestingly, B7-1 expression on tumor cells does not affect the priming of tumor-reactive CTL, but rather enhances infiltration of CTL into the tumor, suggesting a predominant role of B7-1 on the effector stage of T-cell responses. In these experimental models, the use of highly immunogenic viral Ag as a surrogate tumor Ag might decrease the costimulatory effect of B7 on T-cell priming. Presentation of Ag "at the secondary lymphoid organs" is also critical for the activation of allo-reactive T cells in a setting of organ transplantation. Splenectomized *aly/aly* mice, which are devoid of all secondary lymphoid organs, accept fully allogeneic cardiac grafts, although the ignorant T cells from these mice are fully competent, as evidenced by readily rejecting grafts when transferred into T cell-deficient mice with competent lymphoid organs *(38)*. As a whole, these data indicate that lymphoid organs play a critical role in the control of immunological ignorance.

4. STRATEGIES TO OVERCOME T-CELL IGNORANCE IN CANCER

Molecular cloning and identification of tumor antigens recognized by T cells have opened a new avenue for Ag-specific immunotherapy of cancer

(39). Studies on the mechanisms of antigen processing and presentation by professional APC have provided invaluable information that reveals how a tumor antigen can gain access to specific T cells. However, the majority of studies focus on dominant tumor antigens—e.g., those antigens that could elicit strong T-cell responses at the host with a normal immune system. However, in tumor-bearing animals and cancer patients, T cells that react to the dominant epitopes of TAA appear to be functionally impaired. For example, TAA-specific CTL observed in melanoma patients are unresponsive to Ag, and even to mitogen stimulation, suggesting the development of anergy in these T cells *(13)*. Therefore, immunotherapy targeted to boost T cells against dominant TAA epitopes requires the restoration of the intrinsic defects and the need to overcome the anergic phenotype. This appears to be a very difficult task. In sharp contrast, T cells specific to silent TAA epitopes, which are probably similar to those known as subdominant or cryptic epitopes, are in ignorant status and retain their responsiveness to Ag. These cells may be stimulated and differentiate into effector cells by appropriate methods of stimulation. Cancer immunotherapies that target these silent epitopes of TAA thus encompass immunological benefits, and therefore, effective strategies to break T-cell ignorance should be seriously considered as a strategy for cancer immunotherapy.

4.1. Provision of Costimulatory Signals

As discussed in Subheading 3.2, provision of costimulatory signals by the expression of B7-1 on tumor or pancreatic islet cells is capable of breaking immunological ignorance, and results in the rejection of tumor or autoimmune diabetes, respectively. Augmentation of B7-CD28 interaction is effective in breaking ignorance at priming, effector, or both stages of T-cell responses. This is probably achieved by multiple mechanisms, including conversion of silent Ag to dominant Ag by a decreasing threshold of TCR signals, increase of direct presentation capacity of APC, increased effector function of CTL, and enhancement of cross-presentation through an increased release of TAA *(31,34,40,41)*.

Several other costimulators, such as CD137 and CD40, are proposed to enable T cells to overcome ignorant status. Signaling to CD137 by CD137 ligand or agonistic MAb costimulates T-cell growth and prevents activation-induced cell death (AICD) *(42)*. Therapeutic efficacy of anti-CD137 MAb in various types of tumor mouse models suggests that activation of CTL by CD137 may overcome the tolerant status observed in tumor-bearing animals *(43,44)*. In this regard, Wilcox et al. recently demonstrated that ignorant T cells resident in the mice with poorly immunogenic tumors can be activated by immunization of tumor antigen combined with anti-CD137 MAb administrations, helping to eradicate established tumors *(45)*. The rationale of this strategy is that vaccination with tumor antigen induces CD137 expression on CTL, which are otherwise negative for CD137 because of an ignorant status, and subsequent treatment with anti-CD137 MAb further stimulates and empowers tumor-reactive CTL to kill tumor. Interestingly, DC and natural killer (NK) cells also express CD137, and signaling through CD137 enhances their functions *(46–48)*. Thus, it is possible that activation of innate immunity facilitate stimulation of T cells, leading to break ignorance, in addition to the direct effect of CD137 on T cells.

CD40 may play a critical role in the maturation and conditioning of APC in order to initiate T-cell responses *(49)*. Consistent with this theory, Garza et al. demonstrated that administration of agonistic anti-CD40 MAbs along with the vaccination of LCMV GP peptide breaks T-cell ignorance in the transgenic mice expressing GP on islet cells and GP-specific TCR on T cells *(50)*.

4.2. Introduction of Ag Into the Secondary Lymphoid Organs

It has been proposed that T cells are rendered as ignorant status unless they are exposed to the reactive Ag at the secondary lymphoid organs, as described in Subheading 3.4. This concept is supported by evidence that Ag-expressing fibroblasts, which do not express B7 costimulatory ligands, can activate Ag-specific T cells when inoculated into the spleen *(51)*. Based on these studies, Maloy et al. evaluated the efficacy of DNA vaccination administered either inside or outside of secondary lymphoid organs *(52)*. Compared with intradermal or intramuscular injection of naked DNA, intrasplenic or intra-lymph node vaccination of the same DNA is 100- to 1000-fold more efficient in generating CTL activity against encoded Ag. Accordingly, intra-lymph node, but not intramuscular, administration of naked DNA containing virus Ag gave rise to significant protection against subsequent challenge with live viruses or tumor cells expressing the same Ag. Thus, these data suggest intra-lymphatic vaccination as a novel strategy to break T-cell ignorance. All these studies employed viral model antigen that may be highly immunogenic. Its practical value for cancer immunotherapy has not yet been accessed in poorly immunogenic tumors or established tumors.

4.3. Modification of Ag Immunization

Immunization using DC pulsed with antigenic peptide is a powerful tool to elicit T-cell responses, and therefore, is applied to various immune-related diseases, including cancer *(53)*. This strategy was also employed to break T-cell ignorance in several models. In the mice bearing OVA-expressing EL4 tumor, OT-I T cells, which are specific to OVA in context of H-2 K^b, fall into ignorant status and allow tumor cells to grow *(54)*. Immunization of DC pulsed with OVA peptide break ignorance of OT-I T cells and elicit antitumor responses, even in the absence of T helper cells. Similarly, Ochsenbein et al. also demonstrated that vaccination with DC broke T-cell ignorance observed in mice implanted with tumor, although repeated vaccination is required to achieve the effective tumor eradication *(7)*.

5. CONCLUSION

Unresponsiveness or tolerance of T cells observed in the host with cancer constitutes a major obstacle to achieve effective immunotherapy. Understanding the mechanisms behind the unresponsiveness is a critical issue in the field of tumor immunology. Multiple mechanisms may co-exist or work in sequence to induce tolerance of T-cell responses, leading to an uncontrolled growth of cancer. Nevertheless, ignorant T cells appear to be an opportune target. Thus, regulation of immunological ignorance may be the next frontier in tumor immunotherapy.

ACKNOWLEDGMENT

This work is supported by the Mayo Foundation, the National Cancer Institute grant CA79915, CA85721, CA97085, American Cancer Society, Department of Defense, and by the Fraternal Order of Eagles Foundation.

REFERENCES

1. Ohashi PS, Oehen S, Buerki K, et al. Ablation of "tolerance" and induction of diabetes by virus infection in viral antigen transgenic mice. *Cell* 1991;65:305–317.
2. Oldstone MB, Nerenberg M, Southern P, Price J, Lewicki H. Virus infection triggers insulin-dependent diabetes mellitus in a transgenic model: role of anti-self (virus) immune response. *Cell* 1991;65:319–331.
3. Voehringer D, Blaser C, Grawitz AB, Chisari FV, Buerki K, Pircher H. Break of T cell ignorance to a viral antigen in the liver induces hepatitis. *J Immunol* 2000;165:2415–2422.
4. Melero I, Singhal MC, McGowan P, et al. Immunological ignorance of an E7-encoded cytolytic T-lymphocyte epitope in transgenic mice expressing the E7 and E6 oncogenes of human papillomavirus type 16. *J Virol* 1997;71:3998–4004.
5. Hanahan D. Heritable formation of pancreatic beta-cell tumours in transgenic mice expressing recombinant insulin/simian virus 40 oncogenes. *Nature* 1985;315:115–122.
6. Speiser DE, Miranda R, Zakarian A, et al. Self antigens expressed by solid tumors do not efficiently stimulate naive or activated T cells: implications for immunotherapy. *J Exp Med* 1997;186:645–653.
7. Ochsenbein AF, Klenerman P, Karrer U, et al. Immune surveillance against a solid tumor fails because of immunological ignorance. *Proc Natl Acad Sci USA* 1999;96:2233–2238.
8. Ochsenbein AF, Sierro S, Odermatt B, et al. Roles of tumour localization, second signals and cross priming in cytotoxic T-cell induction. *Nature* 2001;411:1058–1064.
9. Pittet MJ, Valmori D, Dunbar PR, et al. High frequencies of naive Melan-A/MART-1-specific CD8(+) T cells in a large proportion of human histocompatibility leukocyte antigen (HLA)-A2 individuals. *J Exp Med* 1999;190:705–715.
10. Romero P, Dunbar PR, Valmori D, et al. Ex vivo staining of metastatic lymph nodes by class I major histocompatibility complex tetramers reveals high numbers of antigen-experienced tumor-specific cytolytic T lymphocytes. *J Exp Med* 1998;188:1641–1650.
11. Vonderheide RH, Schultze JL, Anderson KS, et al. Equivalent induction of telomerase-specific cytotoxic T lymphocytes from tumor-bearing patients and healthy individuals. *Cancer Res* 2001;61:8366–8370.

12. D'Souza S, Rimoldi D, Lienard D, Lejeune F, Cerottini JC, Romero P. Circulating Melan-A/Mart-1 specific cytolytic T lymphocyte precursors in HLA-A2+ melanoma patients have a memory phenotype. *Int J Cancer* 1998;78:699–706.
13. Lee PP, Yee C, Savage PA, et al. Characterization of circulating T cells specific for tumor-associated antigens in melanoma patients. *Nat Med* 1999;5:677–685.
14. Srivastava PK. Immunotherapy of human cancer: lessons from mice. *Nat Immunol* 2000;1:363–366.
15. Rosenberg SA, Yang JC, Schwartzentruber DJ, et al. Immunologic and therapeutic evaluation of a synthetic peptide vaccine for the treatment of patients with metastatic melanoma. *Nat Med* 1998;4:321–327.
16. Marchand M, van Baren N, Weynants P, et al. Tumor regressions observed in patients with metastatic melanoma treated with an antigenic peptide encoded by gene MAGE-3 and presented by HLA-A1. *Int J Cancer* 1999;80:219–230.
17. Anichini A, Molla A, Mortarini R, et al. An expanded peripheral T cell population to a cytotoxic T lymphocyte (CTL)-defined, melanocyte-specific antigen in metastatic melanoma patients impacts on generation of peptide-specific CTLs but does not overcome tumor escape from immune surveillance in metastatic lesions. *J Exp Med* 1999;190:651–667.
18. Wick M, Dubey P, Koeppen H, et al. Antigenic cancer cells grow progressively in immune hosts without evidence for T cell exhaustion or systemic anergy. *J Exp Med* 1997;186:229–238.
19. Sarma S, Guo Y, Guilloux Y, Lee C, Bai XF, Liu Y. Cytotoxic T lymphocytes to an unmutated tumor rejection antigen P1A: normal development but restrained effector function in vivo. *J Exp Med* 1999;189:811–820.
20. Ganss R, Hanahan D. Tumor microenvironment can restrict the effectiveness of activated antitumor lymphocytes. *Cancer Res* 1998;58:4673–4681.
21. Kurts C, Sutherland RM, Davey G, et al. CD8 T cell ignorance or tolerance to islet antigens depends on antigen dose. *Proc Natl Acad Sci USA* 1999;96:12,703–12,707.
22. Kurts C, Heath WR, Kosaka H, Miller JF, Carbone FR. The peripheral deletion of autoreactive CD8+ T cells induced by cross-presentation of self-antigens involves signaling through CD95 (Fas, Apo-1). *J Exp Med* 1998;188:415–420.
23. Spiotto MT, Yu P, Rowley DA, et al. Increasing tumor antigen expression overcomes ignorance to solid tumors via cross presentation by bone marrow-derived stromal cells. *Immunity* 2002;17:737–747.
24. Forster I, Hirose R, Arbeit JM, Clausen BE, Hanahan D. Limited capacity for tolerization of CD4+ T cells specific for a pancreatic beta cell neo-antigen. *Immunity* 1995;2:573–585.
25. Lo D, Freedman J, Hesse S, Palmiter RD, Brinster RL, Sherman LA. Peripheral tolerance to an islet cell-specific hemagglutinin transgene affects both CD4+ and CD8+ T cells. *Eur J Immunol* 1992;22:1013–1022.
26. von Herrath MG, Guerder S, Lewicki H, Flavell RA, Oldstone MB. Coexpression of B7-1 and viral ("self") transgenes in pancreatic beta cells can break peripheral ignorance and lead to spontaneous autoimmune diabetes. *Immunity* 1995;3:727–738.
27. Lenschow DJ, Walunas TL, Bluestone JA. CD28/B7 system of T cell costimulation. *Annu Rev Immunol* 1996;14:233–258.
28. Mueller DL, Jenkins MK, Schwartz RH. Clonal expansion versus functional clonal inactivation: a costimulatory signalling pathway determines the outcome of T cell antigen receptor occupancy. *Annu Rev Immunol* 1989;7:445–480.
29. Guerder S, Picarella DE, Linsley PS, Flavell RA. Costimulator B7-1 confers antigen-presenting-cell function to parenchymal tissue and in conjunction with tumor necrosis factor alpha leads to autoimmunity in transgenic mice. *Proc Natl Acad Sci USA* 1994; 91:5138–5142.

30. Guerder S, Meyerhoff J, Flavell R. The role of the T cell costimulator B7-1 in autoimmunity and the induction and maintenance of tolerance to peripheral antigen. *Immunity* 1994;1:155–166.
31. Johnston JV, Malacko AR, Mizuno MT, et al. B7-CD28 costimulation unveils the hierarchy of tumor epitopes recognized by major histocompatibility complex class I-restricted CD8+ cytolytic T lymphocytes. *J Exp Med* 1996;183:791–800.
32. Chen L. Immunological ignorance of silent antigens as an explanation of tumor evasion. *Immunol Today* 1998;19:27–30.
33. Maric M, Chen L, Sherry B, Liu Y. A mechanism for selective recruitment of CD8 T cells into B7-1-transfected plasmacytoma: role of macrophage-inflammatory protein 1-alpha. *J Immunol* 1997;159:360–368.
34. Bai XF, Bender J, Liu J, et al. Local costimulation reinvigorates tumor-specific cytolytic T lymphocytes for experimental therapy in mice with large tumor burdens. *J Immunol* 2001;167:3936–3943.
35. Liu X, Bai XF, Wen J, et al. B7H costimulates clonal expansion of, and cognate destruction of tumor cells by, CD8(+) T lymphocytes in vivo. *J Exp Med* 2001;194:1339–1348.
36. Perez VL, Van Parijs L, Biuckians A, Zheng XX, Strom TB, Abbas AK. Induction of peripheral T cell tolerance in vivo requires CTLA-4 engagement. *Immunity* 1997;6:411–417.
37. Nguyen LT, Elford AR, Murakami K, et al. Tumor growth enhances cross-presentation leading to limited T cell activation without tolerance. *J Exp Med* 2002;195:423–435.
38. Lakkis FG, Arakelov A, Konieczny BT, Inoue Y. Immunologic "ignorance" of vascularized organ transplants in the absence of secondary lymphoid tissue. *Nat Med* 2000;6:686–688.
39. Boon T, Coulie PG, Van den Eynde B. Tumor antigens recognized by T cells. *Immunol Today* 1997;18:267–268.
40. Chen L, Ashe S, Brady WA, et al. Costimulation of antitumor immunity by the B7 counterreceptor for the T lymphocyte molecules CD28 and CTLA-4. *Cell* 1992;71:1093–1102.
41. Huang AY, Bruce AT, Pardoll DM, Levitsky HI. Does B7-1 expression confer antigen-presenting cell capacity to tumors in vivo? *J Exp Med* 1996;183:769–776.
42. Sica G, Chen L. Modulation of the immune response through 4-1BB. *Adv Exp Med Biol* 2000;465:355–362.
43. Melero I, Shuford WW, Newby SA, et al. Monoclonal antibodies against the 4-1BB T-cell activation molecule eradicate established tumors. *Nat Med* 1997;3:682–685.
44. Ye Z, Hellstrom I, Hayden-Ledbetter M, Dahlin A, Ledbetter JA, Hellstrom KE. Gene therapy for cancer using single-chain Fv fragments specific for 4-1BB. *Nat Med* 2002; 8:343–348.
45. Wilcox RA, Flies DB, Zhu G, et al. Provision of antigen and CD137 signaling breaks immunological ignorance, promoting regression of poorly immunogenic tumors. *J Clin Invest* 2002;109:651–659.
46. Melero I, Johnston JV, Shufford WW, Mittler RS, Chen L. NK1.1 cells express 4-1BB (CDw137) costimulatory molecule and are required for tumor immunity elicited by anti-4-1BB monoclonal antibodies. *Cell Immunol* 1998;190:167–172.
47. Wilcox RA, Chapoval AI, Gorski KS, et al. Cutting edge: expression of functional CD137 receptor by dendritic cells. *J Immunol* 2002;168:4262–4267.
48. Wilcox RA, Tamada K, Strome SE, Chen L. Signaling through NK cell-associated CD137 promotes both helper function for CD8(+) cytolytic T cells and responsiveness to IL-2 but not cytolytic activity. *J Immunol* 2002;169:4230–4236.
49. Ridge JP, Di Rosa F, Matzinger P. A conditioned dendritic cell can be a temporal bridge between a CD4+ T-helper and a T-killer cell. *Nature* 1998;393:474–478.
50. Garza KM, Chan SM, Suri R, et al. Role of antigen-presenting cells in mediating tolerance and autoimmunity. *J Exp Med* 2000;191:2021–2027.

51. Kundig TM, Bachmann MF, DiPaolo C, et al. Fibroblasts as efficient antigen-presenting cells in lymphoid organs. *Science* 1995;268:1343–1347.
52. Maloy KJ, Erdmann I, Basch V, et al. Intralymphatic immunization enhances DNA vaccination. *Proc Natl Acad Sci USA* 2001;98:3299–3303.
53. Banchereau J, Steinman RM. Dendritic cells and the control of immunity. *Nature* 1998;392:245–252.
54. Dalyot-Herman N, Bathe OF, Malek TR. Reversal of CD8+ T cell ignorance and induction of anti-tumor immunity by peptide-pulsed APC. *J Immunol* 2000;165:6731–6737.

6 The Role of Receptor-Mediated Apoptosis in T-Cell Dysfunction

Hannah Rabinowich, PhD
and Brian R. Gastman, MD

Contents

1. INTRODUCTION

Many escape mechanisms have been proposed to explain the failure of the immune system to detect and reject tumor cells. The identification of Fas ligands on the surface of multiple types of tumor cells has led to the recognition that tumor cells may escape destruction by immune effector cells, and may be actively involved in the killing of Fas-expressing lymphocytes. Thus, the Fas/Fas ligand (Fas/FasL) interaction serves both as a mechanism of cytotoxicity for T and natural killer (NK) cells, and as a tumor "counterattack" mechanism against lymphocytes. This mechanism of tumor-induced death of infiltrating lymphocytes complements the concept of FasL-mediating immune-privilege to certain organs, such as the eye, testes, or ovary, where histocompatibility differences are partially tolerated. Despite the wealth of data

From: *Current Clinical Oncology: Cancer Immunotherapy at the Crossroads: How Tumors Evade Immunity and What Can Be Done*
Edited by: J. H. Finke and R. M. Bukowski © Humana Press Inc., Totowa, NJ

supporting the role of the Fas/FasL system in mediating immune-privilege and tumor counterattack, these concepts have recently been challenged by many contradictory reports. Here, we review the evidence for and against a role for the Fas/FasL system in immune escape mechanisms.

2. FAS/FASL APOPTOTIC PATHWAY

Fas is a member of the TNF-receptor family that contains 2–6 cysteine-rich domains in their extracellular regions, a single transmembrane domain, and variably sized intracytoplasmic domains. It is a type I membrane-bound glycoprotein that is expressed on activated T and NK lymphocytes, as well as on various tissues, including the thymus, heart, liver, and kidney *(1)*. FasL is a type II membrane-bound ligand for Fas that is also a member of the tumor necrosis factor (TNF) family. The extracellular portion of FasL shares significant homology with TNF-α, CD30 ligand, CD40 ligand, lymphotoxin, and TRAIL. The expression of FasL is regulated at the transcriptional level as well as by metalloproteinase cleavage. As compared to cell-surface FasL, the soluble form of this ligand, sFasL, has reduced efficacy in inducing apoptosis. FasL is expressed on numerous cell types and organs, including the eye, testes, ovary, and placenta. FasL is biologically active as a homotrimer. Receptor binding has been localized to the C-terminus of the trimer. A self-association motif is located at the N-terminus of the ligand's extracellular domain. Upon binding of the homotrimer ligand, Fas receptor oligomerizes and initiates a complex signal-transduction cascade. The binding of FasL or agonistic anti-Fas antibody results in recruitment of the death-inducing signaling complex (DISC). Fas carries a death domain (DD) near the carboxy-terminal region of the molecule, which binds to a C-terminal DD in the adaptor molecule, FADD. The N-terminal part of FADD, the death effector domain (DED), is responsible for recruiting procaspase-8. Following oligomerization at the plasma membrane, procaspase-8 is autoactivated to a mature enzyme *(1–4)*.

Two pathways have been elucidated for the signal transduction that occurs downstream of caspase-8, which are used in various cell types *(5,6)*. In type I cells, caspase-8 directly activates procaspase-3. In type II cells, direct activation of procaspase-3 by caspase-8 is inefficient. Instead, caspase-8 cleaves Bid, a BH3-only proapoptotic member of the Bcl-2 family. Truncated Bid translocates to the mitochondria, and through its activation of mitochondrial Bax and/or Bak, stimulates the release of cytochrome c. Cytochrome c, together with APAF-1, activates procaspase-9, which leads to the downstream processing of procaspase-3.

Because the Fas/FasL system is involved in deletion of activated lymphocytes, defects in this pathway predispose to autoimmune disorders *(7)*. Two mutant mice with defects in either Fas or FasL have been identified and successfully used in studies investigating the in vivo role of this death-receptor apoptotic mechanism *(8)*. These mice display a phenotype of uncontrolled accumulation of $CD4^-CD8^-$ T cells associated with lymphoadenopathy, splenomegaly, and autoimmunity. The Fas-deficient mice, *lpr*, and the FasL-deficient mice, *gld*, present multiple features of accelerated autoimmune syndrome.

3. THE ROLE OF FAS/FASL IN IMMUNE-PRIVILEGE OF NORMAL TISSUES

Several sites in the body have been recognized as "immune-privileged," in which the immune response is limited. Immune-privileged tissues, including the brain, ovary, testes, placenta, and the eye, have demonstrated a relative tolerance to histocompatibility differences. The immune-privileged status of the eye is best exemplified by the high rate of acceptance of corneal transplants that do not require tissue matching or immunosuppressive treatments. Griffith et al. *(9)* were the first to demonstrate that Fas/FasL interactions were involved in the inhibition of the destructive inflammatory response in the eye. Inflammatory cells entering the anterior chamber of the eye in response to viral infection underwent Fas-mediated apoptosis. In contrast, viral infection in *gld* mice, which lack functional FasL, resulted in inflammation and invasion of the ocular tissue without apoptosis. Also, Fas-positive but not Fas-negative tumor cells underwent apoptosis when placed within isolated anterior segments of the eyes of normal, but not FasL-negative, mice. Subsequent studies provided further support to the concept of Fas-mediated immune-privilege to the eye. FasL-expressing allogeneic corneas transplanted under the kidney capsule maintained clarity for weeks, whereas those obtained from *gld* mice were rapidly rejected *(10,11)*. Corneal endothelial cells that constitutively express FasL were found to be involved in the protection of grafted corneas *(12,13)*. In the eye, the ability of FasL to eliminate Fas-positive lymphocytes was also demonstrated following a direct introduction of toxoplasma *(14)*, or injection of hapten-conjugated splenocytes *(11)*.

Several studies have also detected an increase in the levels of soluble FasL in vitreous fluid of patients with ocular uveitis during ocular inflammation *(15,16)*. The individual roles of membrane-bound and soluble forms of FasL in regulating immune-privilege of the eye were recently examined in an ocular tumor model *(17)*. Following injection into the eye, tumors that expressed only soluble FasL failed to trigger inflammation and grew progressively. By contrast, tumors that expressed only membrane FasL initiated vigorous neutrophil-mediated inflammation, terminated immune-privilege, and were rejected. However, a higher threshold level of membrane FasL on the tumor was required to initiate inflammation within the immune-privileged eye, as compared with nonprivileged sites. The higher threshold may be a result of the suppressive microenvironment found within aqueous humor that blocks membrane FasL activation of neutrophils. This concept has been further supported by studies demonstrating that the cytokine milieu in the microenvironment determines whether FasL is immunoprotective or immunodestructive *(18,19)*. Chen et al. *(18)* demonstrated that FasL-expressing colon carcinoma cells were rejected if injected subcutaneously in the flank (a nonprivileged site). However, when these tumor cells were injected into the anterior chamber of the eye, they grew progressively, as expected in an immune-privileged site. Co-expression of TGF-β and FasL conferred protection to these cells when transplanted under the skin. Also, TNF-α, a proinflammatory cytokine, has been reported to sensitize cells to apoptosis mediated by ocular FasL *(19)*. These studies suggest that local cytokines, with either immunosuppressive or regulatory effects, determine the function of the Fas/FasL apoptotic mechanism in preventing an inflammatory response in the eye.

4. THE ROLE OF FAS/FASL IN ALLOGRAFT SURVIVAL

Despite the substantial evidence supporting the role of FasL in mediating the immune-privilege status of the eye, applying this phenomenon to the field of transplantation using nonocular tissues has produced conflicting results *(20–22)*. Allografts of testes under the kidney capsule were accepted unless they were derived from *gld* or *lpr* mice *(20)*. FasL-expressing Sertoli cells from rat or pig xeno-transplanted in rat survived at least 2 mo with no immunosuppressive therapy *(22)*. However, subsequent studies with testes or Sertoli cell xenografts challenged the original findings *(21)*. Furthermore, enforced expression of FasL in pancreatic islets *(23–25)* or myoblasts *(26)* triggered neutrophil infiltration and graft rejection. In addition, co-transplantation of FasL-transfected myoblasts with islet cells resulted in a predominant neutrophil-mediated apoptosis of the islet cells *(27)*. These conflicting findings suggested that FasL expression is associated with different immune responses in various tissues. It appears that enforced expression of FasL, which results in a high level of expression, is associated with rejection of either pancreatic islets or myoblasts. However, in other normal tissues, including the liver *(28)*, kidney *(29)*, lung *(30)*, and thyroid *(31)*, enforced expression of FasL protected the grafts from immune rejection. These findings further emphasize the role of the local microenvironment and immunosuppressive cytokines in regulating the outcome of FasL-expressing allografts.

5. THE ROLE OF FAS/FASL IN ACTIVATION-INDUCED CELL DEATH

Activation-induced cell death involves apoptosis of activated T cells upon a subsequent encounter with antigen *(32,33)*. This mechanism of elimination of T lymphocytes plays a significant role in downregulation of the immune response, negative T-cell selection in the thymus, and clonal deletion of activated T cells in order to maintain T-cell homeostasis. The term "activation-induced cell death" (AICD) was coined to describe the apoptotic cascade induced in T-lymphocytes in response to antigenic signaling *(34)*. Resting mature T lymphocytes are activated when triggered via their antigen-specific T-cell receptor to elicit an appropriate immune response. In contrast, pre-activated T cells may undergo AICD in response to the same signal. In the process of AICD, T-cell stimulation results in upregulated expression of surface death ligands, which in turn engage their counter receptors on the same or a neighboring cell. AICD is mediated mainly by the Fas/FasL death cascade, but the involvement of the TNF- and TRAIL systems has also been reported *(35,36)*. T-cell susceptibility to AICD is regulated by the stage of T-cell maturity, the previous activation history of T cells, and the presence of antigen-presenting cells (APC) *(34,37,38)*. The majority of developing T cells in the thymus are eliminated by AICD following reaction with self-antigens. The role of Fas/FasL in thymocyte AICD is controversial as negative intrathymic T-cell selection proceeds normally in Fas-deficient *lpr* or FasL-deficient *gld* mice *(39,40)*. In pre-activated mature T cells, AICD can be triggered via the TCR/CD3 complex or via other receptors known to activate T cells, such as the CD2 *(41)*. Most of the studies regarding AICD were performed with anti-CD3 or anti-TCR crosslinking antibodies that induce AICD in mature pre-activated, but not resting, T cells. Crosslinking of the TCR/CD3 complex induces AICD in T cells expressing either $\alpha\beta$ or $\gamma\delta$ TCR *(42)*. AICD is dependent on those signal-transduction molecules known to trigger effector function in T cells, including the TCR-ζ chain and protein tyrosine kinases, such as Lck, Fyn, and ZAP-70 *(43,44)*. The molecular regulation of AICD is still unclear. Exposure to IL-2 has been reported to prime mature T lymphocytes for AICD *(45,46)*. This increased susceptibility may be the result of upregulation of Fas expression and downregulation of FLIP, an endogenous inhibitor of the Fas cascade *(47)*. In contrast, various costimulatory signals such as ligation of CD4 or CD28 protect T cells from AICD *(48,49)*. Crosslinking of CD28 by B7.1 or B7.2 expressed on APC stimulates cytokine production, upregulates expression of Bcl-XL and FLIP, and downregulates FasL. AICD seems to be differentially regulated in T-helper subsets. Upon stimulation with phorbolester and ionomycin or anti-TCR/CD3 Ab, Th1 clones express significantly higher levels of surface FasL than Th2 clones *(50)*. Although Th1 clones are considered to be more AICD sensitive than Th2 cells, the mechanisms regulating the relative resistance of Th2 clones are unclear. It has been suggested that a negative regulator of the Fas-cascade, such as the Fas-inhibitor Fap-1, may be induced in Th2 cells stimulated by anti-TCR/CD3 *(51,52)*. AICD is considered to be one of the mechanisms responsible for the increased apoptotic rate among tumor-infiltrating lymphocytes (TIL) *(53–56)*. Thus, antigenic stimulation within the tumor microenvironment may be involved in the enhanced expression and function of FasL on T cells resulting in activation of autocrine or paracrine mechanisms of apoptosis. Such a scenario has been reported for human melanoma, in which tumor cells caused apoptotic death of tumor-specific T cells only upon specific major histocompatibility complex (MHC) class I-restricted antigen recognition *(54)*. This apoptotic death of anti-tumor T cells was blocked by anti-Fas MAb, but mediated by FasL on activated T cells, as the melanoma tumor cells did not express either protein or mRNA for FasL.

6. THE ROLE OF FAS/FASL IN TUMOR COUNTERATTACK

A mechanism of tumor counterattack on Fas expressing T lymphocytes has been proposed to explain the Fas-mediated apoptotic death of TIL. The Fas counterattack model proposes that FasL expressed on various types of tumor cells is utilized to mediate the death of Fas-expressing TILs *(57,58*; Fig. 1). According to this model, FasL expressing tumor cells counterattack the T lymphocytes, utilizing the T cells' own principal mechanism of cytotoxicity. Various types of tumors were reported to express FasL and induce apoptosis in T cells expressing Fas, including colorectal carcinoma *(59)*, colonic adenocarcinoma *(59)*, head and neck squamous cell carcinoma (HNSCC) *(60)*, ovarian carcinoma *(61)*, gastric carcinoma *(62,63)*, hepatocellular carcinoma (HCC) *(64)*, lung carcinoma *(65)*, glioblastoma *(66)*, esophageal tumors *(67)*, melanoma *(68)*, and angiosarcomas *(69)*.

Multiple studies utilized in vitro experimental systems to demonstrate the tumor activity against cultured T lymphocytes. For example, Shiraki et al. *(59)* utilized human colon adenocarcinoma cell lines to demonstrate by immunohistochemistry the expression of cell-surface FasL on these cells. They also demonstrated that Jurkat T lymphocytes underwent Fas-mediated apoptosis upon incubation with FasL expressing colon carcinoma cells. However, as in many other in vitro studies, the possibility of involvement of activation-induced expression of FasL on Jurkat cells in this type of tumor-induced T-cell death has not been excluded. Other studies reported that a significant increase in TIL apoptosis occurred in areas of FasL-expressing tumors *(62,63)* or was consistently more frequent in FasL-positive tumors. Okada et al. *(70)* demonstrated that FasL was detected on the cell surface as well as in cytoplasm of human colorectal carcinoma cells in 61% of the cases. They also demonstrated that apoptosis of TIL was consistently more frequent in FasL-positive tumors than in FasL-negative ones. A similar correlation between FasL expression on tumor cells and apoptosis of TIL has been demonstrated for gastric cancer *(63)* and esophageal cancer *(62)*. Likewise, in angiosarcomas, low FasL expression was associated with a high level of T-cell infiltration and high FasL expression with significantly reduced infiltration *(69)*.

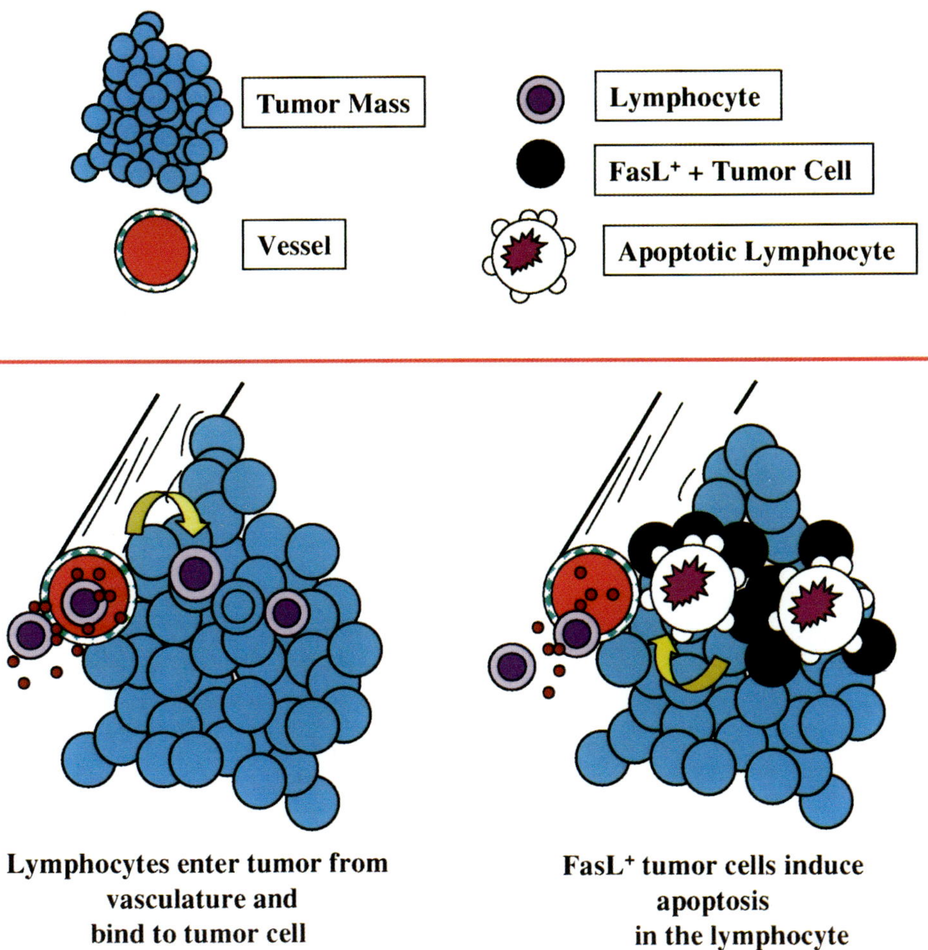

Fig. 1. Cartoon of the proposed Fas counterattack model for the induction of apoptosis in T cells by tumors. Lymphocytes enter the tumor via the vasculature and bind to tumor cells (left). The infiltrating lymphocytes that express Fas receptor are potentially sensitive to apoptosis mediated by the tumor cells that express the FasL. Following Fas engagement on the T cells, they undergo death-receptor mediated apoptosis (right).

Various animal models have been used to demonstrate the ability of FasL-expressing tumors to downregulate antitumor immune responses. Tumor growth of a subcutaneously injected FasL-positive murine melanoma cell line was faster in wild-type or *gld* (FasL-deficient) mice than in *lpr* (Fas-receptor deficient) mice *(68)*. Also, growth of a murine renal cell carcinoma (RCC) transfected with FasL and implanted under the kidney capsule of syngeneic mice was significantly better than that of control cells *(71)*. Fas expressed on rat histocytoma tumors, which were injected into the peritoneum of mice, killed a population of NK cells that would otherwise destroy the tumor *(72)*. Fas/FasL involvement in in vivo immunosuppression was also demonstrated in allogeneic mice transplanted with FasL-transfected colon carcinoma cells *(73)*.

6.1. Sources of Controversy

6.1.1. Usage on Nonspecific FasL Antibodies

Despite the numerous reports and growing evidence in support of the tumor counterattack model, the validity of the experimental data is highly controversial. Studies have found that several of the anti-FasL antibodies used for detection of FasL on tumor cells were not specific, leading to the report of false-positive results in multiple publications *(74,75)*. Rabbit antibodies raised by Santa Cruz Biotechnology (Santa Cruz, CA) against a C-terminus peptide of FasL (C-20) were utilized in multiple studies to demonstrate FasL expression by immunoblotting, immunofluorescence, immunohistochemistry, and flow cytometry. In contrast to FasL-specific MAbs NOK-1 and Alf1.2, the C-20 antibodies could not detect by flow cytometry the expression of FasL on a transfected cell line *(74)*. Also, clone 33 MAb (Transduction Laboratories, Lexington, KY) has been shown to detect by immunoblotting unidentified proteins with different mobilities than that of FasL *(76,77)*. Clone G247-4 anti-FasL MAb (PharMingen, San Diego, CA) has been found to be most suitable for immunoblotting and immunofluorescence detection of FasL *(76)*. A recent study examined the reliability of 12 anti-FasL Abs for immunohistochemistry studies using FasL-transfected cells *(75)*. This study determined that G247-4, NOK-1, NOK-2, 4H9 and MIKE-1 Abs stained FasL-transfected cells, but not control cells. Clones 33 (Transduction), C-20 and N-20 (Santa Cruz) stained both transfected and control cells. It was concluded that G247-4 MAb is the most appropriate to use for immunohistochemistry studies, as FasL detection by this MAb matched the distribution of FasL mRNA, as analyzed by *in situ* hybridization.

6.1.2. Induction of Inflammation by Fas/FasL Interaction

Further controversy regarding the relevance of the FasL-mediated tumor counterattack in vivo was contributed by the conflicting results obtained in an animal model for survival of FasL-transfected tumor cells. In most of the experimental systems, overexpression of FasL in murine tumor cells that are resistant to Fas-mediated apoptosis led to rapid tumor rejection mediated by neutrophils *(78–83)*. Several mechanisms for the recruitment of the tumor rejecting neutrophils have been proposed. Two studies suggested that soluble FasL serves as a chemotactic factor for neutrophils *(84,85)*. However, other studies could not detect such chemotactic activity for sFasL in vivo or in vitro *(86,87)*. Furthermore, membrane-bound FasL, rather than sFasL was found to be responsible for the observed inflammation. Shudo et al. *(87)* utilized tumor-cell lines that express one or both forms of human FasL. When cells that express both forms or only the membrane-bound form were transplanted into the peritoneal cavity of syngeneic mice, neutrophil response was elicited. Conversely, tumor cells that express only sFasL did not induce neutrophil infiltration. Accelerated rejection of the tumor was associated with neutrophil response to the membrane-bound form of the ligand, but not sFasL. Alternatively, it has been proposed that FasL serves to trigger the production of granulocyte chemoattractants by surrounding cells *(88)*. Engagement of Fas on resident macrophages or dendritic cells (DC) induces the secretion of proinflammatory cytokines, such as IL-1β and IL-18 *(89,90)*.

Granulocytosis may also be explained as a response to a supra-physiologic expression of FasL, as naturally expressed FasL does not induce granulocytosis under physiologic conditions. The expression of Fas on neutrophils was required to induce the proinflammatory response *(18,91)*. Thus, it is possible that under certain conditions neutrophils respond to Fas triggering by production of inflammatory cytokines, rather than apoptosis. The non-apoptotic response of neutrophils to FasL may be mediated by activation of caspases known to be involved in the generation of pro-inflammatory cytokines. Caspase-1 is responsible for processing of IL-1β into its mature form *(92)*, whereas caspase-3 is involved in activation of the IL-16 and IL-18, two potent pro-inflammatory cytokines *(93,94)*.

6.1.3. Lack of Distinction Between AICD and TICD (Tumor-Induced Cell Death)

In many of the studies that evaluate the inhibition of tumor counterattack by neutralizing anti-FasL antibodies or by Fas-Fc fusion protein, there is no attempt to differentiate between tumor cells or T cells expressing FasL as the initiators of the attack. Therefore, such studies could not possibly distinguish between AICD and tumor counterattack as the mechanism responsible for the induction of the Fas cascade. In the same vein, Zaks et al. *(54)* reported that melanoma cells could induce apoptotic death of tumor-specific T cells only upon specific MHC class I-restricted recognition. Thus, contrary to the prevailing view that tumor cells cause the death of antitumor T cells by expressing FasL, this study suggested that FasL was instead expressed by T-lymphocytes upon activation. Furthermore, in conflict with other studies performed with melanoma cells *(68)*, those performed by Restifo's group did not detect FasL expression (including reverse transcriptase-polymerase chain reaction [RT-PCR]) in any of the 26 melanoma cell lines tested *(54–56)*. The contradictory findings obtained with

RT-PCR for FasL may be a result of the detection of immature mRNA that does not give rise to a functional protein, and thus must be resolved by confirming the identity of the PCR products by either sequencing or appropriate hybridization.

The sensitivity of T cells to Fas-mediated apoptosis has been shown to significantly increase following activation. Thus, T cells that are susceptible to AICD mediated by FasL expressed on the same or neighboring T cells will also be susceptible to those tumor cells expressing functional FasL. In addition, differential sensitivity to Fas-mediated apoptosis has been reported for CD4 and CD8 T cells *(44,95,96)*. CD4 Th1 cells were found to be more sensitive than CD4 Th2 or CD8 cells. These findings imply that in the presence of AICD or tumor counterattack, an antitumor response can still be mediated by cytotoxic CD8 or CD4 Th2 T cells.

7. INVOLVEMENT OF TRAIL AND TNF IN IMMUNE ESCAPE MECHANISMS

The death ligand TRAIL has also been demonstrated to downregulate the antitumor effect of T lymphoctes *(97)*. Mouse mammary adenocarcinoma cells engineered to express TRAIL on their membranes were better suited to overcome tumor-specific immunity and grow across minor and major histocompatibility barriers than wild-type parental cells. The resistance of these tumor cells appeared to be mainly the result of TRAIL's ability to induce apoptosis in interacting activated lymphocytes. Also, ex vivo morphological evaluations of the TRAIL-transfected tumors showed a much lower inflammatory reaction than that elicited by wild-type cells. The expression of TRAIL on tumor cells has been documented *(98)*, but its involvement in the tumor counterattack mechanism has not been as exhaustively investigated as that of FasL.

The cytokine TNF-α and its receptor TNF-R1 *(p55)* are involved in deletion of activated lymphocytes *(36,99–101)*. Although this type of T-cell deletion may be mediated by AICD, recent studies suggest that it may be mediated by an induced expression of FasL on nonlymphoid cells *(102,103)*. Staphylococcal enterotoxin B (SEB) was shown to induce upregulation of FasL expression and function in nonlymphoid cells of the liver and small intestine. In severe combined immunodeficiency (SCID) animals, nonlymphoid tissues did not express FasL in response to SEB, unless transplanted lymphocytes were present *(102)*. These findings suggest that certain immune responses induce FasL expression in nonlymphoid tissues, which in turn induce apoptosis of Fas-expressing lymphocytes. A recent study examined the role of TNF-α in this feedback regulation *(103)*. Injection of TNF-α into mice caused rapid upregulation of FasL mRNA in intestinal epithelial cells via an NFκB-dependent mechanism. In contrast to wild-type animals, TNF-$\alpha^{-/-}$ and TNFR$1^{-/-}$ mice did not demonstrate an increase in FasL expression on intestinal epithelial cells following superantigen-induced activation. These observations suggest a novel mechanism for regulation of the expression of one member of the TNF superfamily (FasL) by another (TNF-α). Inducible expression of FasL on nonlymphoid cells may potentially serve as a feedback mechanism for controlling lymphocyte infiltration and inflammation in certain tissues.

8. CONCLUDING REMARKS

The debate over the exact role of Fas/FasL system in immune-privilege, inflammation, and tumor counterattack has not yet been resolved. The current controversy regarding the relevance of Fas/FasL relates not only to the utilization of nonspecific anti-FasL Ab in multiple studies, but also to other factors involved in the regulation of expression and function of Fas/FasL that have not yet been elucidated. For example, enforced overexpression of FasL may be associated with a different immune response from that induced by the naturally occurring FasL level. It has been suggested that overexpression of FasL is associated with neutrophil-mediated inflammation, whereas a physiological level of FasL mediates the deletion of immune effector cells as a part of a counterattack mechanism. The Fas/FasL response may also be regulated by specific microenvironmental factors, such as the cytokine milieu. The presence of immunosuppressive cytokines, such as TGF-β or IL-10, appears to be conducive to immune counterattack via Fas/FasL, as demonstrated in the anterior chamber of the eye. Release of pro-inflammatory cytokines, such as TNF-α, by activated lymphocytes may also have a backfire effect on the lymphocytes themselves. Similar to its effect on intestinal epithelium, TNF-α may induce FasL expression on tumors. Induction of FasL expression on tumors has been documented following chemotherapeutic treatments, and therefore, the function of Fas/FasL may depend on the tumor status in relation to previous therapies. The function of Fas/FasL is also dependent on the susceptibility of T lymphocytes to such mechanisms of immune evasion. As indicated, T-cell sensitivity to Fas-mediated apoptosis varies widely with the activation status of these cells, as well as their classification as CD4 or CD8, Th1, or Th2. In summary, the escape of immune-privileged tissues or tumors from the immune response involves multiple immunoregulatory factors other than FasL, which may represent independent immune evasion mechanisms, or alternatively serve to modulate the function of Fas/FasL.

REFERENCES

1. Nagata S. Fas and Fas ligand: a death factor and its receptor. *Adv Immunol* 1994;57:129–144.
2. Nagata S. Fas ligand-induced apoptosis. *Annu Rev Genet* 1999;33:29–55.
3. Orlinick JR, Vaishnaw AK, Elkon KB. Structure and function of Fas/Fas ligand. *Int Rev Immunol* 1999;18:293–308.
4. Pinkoski MJ, Green DR. Fas ligand, death gene. *Cell Death Differ* 1999;6:1174–1181.

5. Scaffidi C, Fulda S, Srinivasan A, Friesen C, Li F, Tomaselli KJ, et al. Two CD95 (APO-1/Fas) signaling pathways. *EMBO J* 1998;17:1675–1687.
6. Scaffidi C, Schmitz I, Zha J, Korsmeyer SJ, Krammer PH, Peter ME. Differential modulation of apoptosis sensitivity in CD95 type I and type II cells. *J Biol Chem* 1999;274: 22,532–22,538.
7. Suda T, Nagata S. Why do defects in the Fas-Fas ligand system cause autoimmunity? *J Allergy Clin Immunol* 1997;100:S97–S101.
8. Nagata S, Suda T. Fas and Fas ligand: lpr and gld mutations. *Immunol Today* 1995;16: 39–43.
9. Griffith TS, Brunner T, Fletcher SM, Green DR, Ferguson TA. Fas ligand-induced apoptosis as a mechanism of immune privilege. *Science* 1995;270:1189–1192.
10. Hori J, Joyce N, Streilein JW. Epithelium-deficient corneal allografts display immune privilege beneath the kidney capsule. *Investig Ophthalmol Vis Sci* 2000;41:443–452.
11. Griffith TS, Yu X, Herndon JM, Green DR, Ferguson TA. CD95-induced apoptosis of lymphocytes in an immune privileged site induces immunological tolerance. *Immunity* 1996;5:7–16.
12. Jorgensen A, Wiencke AK, la Cour M, Kaestel CG, Madsen HO, Hamann S, et al. Human retinal pigment epithelial cell-induced apoptosis in activated T cells. *Investig Ophthalmol Vis Sci* 1998;39:1590–1599.
13. Zhang J, Ma B, Marshak-Rothstein A, Fine A. Characterization of a novel cis-element that regulates Fas ligand expression in corneal endothelial cells. *J Biol Chem* 1999;274:26,537–26,542.
14. Hu MS, Schwartzman JD, Yeaman GR, Collins J, Seguin R, Khan IA, et al. Fas-FasL interaction involved in pathogenesis of ocular toxoplasmosis in mice. *Infect Immun* 1999;67:928–935.
15. Sotozono C, Sano Y, Suzuki T, Tada R, Ikeda T, Nagata S, et al. Soluble Fas ligand expression in the ocular fluids of uveitis patients. *Curr Eye Res* 2000;20:54–57.
16. Sugita S, Taguchi C, Takase H, Sagawa K, Sueda J, Fukushi K, et al. Soluble Fas ligand and soluble Fas in ocular fluid of patients with uveitis. *Br J Ophthalmol* 2000;84: 1130–1134.
17. Gregory MS, Repp AC, Holhbaum AM, Saff RR, Marshak-Rothstein A, Ksander BR. Membrane fas ligand activates innate immunity and terminates ocular immune privilege. *J Immunol* 2002;169:2727–2735.
18. Chen JJ, Sun Y, Nabel GJ. Regulation of the proinflammatory effects of Fas ligand (CD95L). *Science* 1998;282:1714–1717.
19. Elzey BD, Griffith TS, Herndon JM, Barreiro R, Tschopp J, Ferguson TA. Regulation of Fas ligand-induced apoptosis by TNF. *J Immunol* 2001;167:3049–3056.
20. Bellgrau D, Gold D, Selawry H, Moore J, Franzusoff A, Duke RC. A role for CD95 ligand in preventing graft rejection. *Nature* 1995;377:630–632.
21. Allison J, Georgiou HM, Strasser A, Vaux DL. Transgenic expression of CD95 ligand on islet beta cells induces a granulocytic infiltration but does not confer immune privilege upon islet allografts. *Proc Natl Acad Sci USA* 1997;94:3943–3947.
22. Saporta S, Cameron DF, Borlongan CV, Sanberg PR. Survival of rat and porcine Sertoli cell transplants in the rat striatum without cyclosporine-A immunosuppression. *Exp Neurol* 1997;146:299–304.
23. Kang SM, Schneider DB, Lin Z, Hanahan D, Dichek DA, Stock PG, et al. Fas ligand expression in islets of Langerhans does not confer immune privilege and instead targets them for rapid destruction. *Nat Med* 1997;3:738–743.
24. Chervonsky AV, Wang Y, Wong FS, Visintin I, Flavell RA, Janeway CA, Jr., et al. The role of Fas in autoimmune diabetes. *Cell* 1997;89:17–24.

25. Hsu PN, Lin HH, Tu CF, Chen NJ, Wu KM, Tsai HF, et al. Expression of human Fas ligand on mouse beta islet cells does not induce insulitis but is insufficient to confer immune privilege for islet grafts. *J Biomed Sci* 2001;8:262–269.
26. Takeuchi T, Ueki T, Nishimatsu H, Kajiwara T, Ishida T, Jishage K, et al. Accelerated rejection of Fas ligand-expressing heart grafts. *J Immunol* 1999;162:518–522.
27. Turvey SE, Gonzalez-Nicolini V, Kingsley CI, Larregina AT, Morris PJ, Castro MG, et al. Fas ligand-transfected myoblasts and islet cell transplantation. *Transplantation* 2000; 69:1972–1976.
28. Li XK, Okuyama T, Tamura A, Enosawa S, Kaneda Y, Takahara S, et al. Prolonged survival of rat liver allografts transfected with Fas ligand- expressing plasmid. *Transplantation* 1998;66:1416–1423.
29. Swenson KM, Ke B, Wang T, Markowitz JS, Maggard MA, Spear GS, et al. Fas ligand gene transfer to renal allografts in rats: effects on allograft survival. *Transplantation* 1998;65:155–160.
30. Schmid RA, Stammberger U, Hillinger S, Gaspert A, Boasquevisque CH, Malipiero U, et al. Fas ligand gene transfer combined with low dose cyclosporine A reduces acute lung allograft rejection. *Transpl Int* 2000;13:S324–S328.
31. Tourneur L, Malassagne B, Batteux F, Fabre M, Mistou S, Lallemand E, et al. Transgenic expression of CD95 ligand on thyroid follicular cells confers immune privilege upon thyroid allografts. *J Immunol* 2001;167:1338–1346.
32. Green DR, Bissonnette RP, Glynn JM, Shi Y. Activation-induced apoptosis in lymphoid systems. *Semin Immunol* 1992;4:379–388.
33. Kabelitz D, Pohl T, Pechhold K. Activation-induced cell death (apoptosis) of mature peripheral T lymphocytes. *Immunol Today* 1993;14:338–339.
34. Janssen O, Sanzenbacher R, Kabelitz D. Regulation of activation-induced cell death of mature T-lymphocyte populations. *Cell Tissue Res* 2000;301:85–99.
35. Martinez-Lorenzo MJ, Alava MA, Gamen S, Kim KJ, Chuntharapai A, Pineiro A, et al. Involvement of APO2 ligand/TRAIL in activation-induced death of Jurkat and human peripheral blood T cells. *Eur J Immunol* 1998;28:2714–2725.
36. Zheng L, Fisher G, Miller RE, Peschon J, Lynch DH, Lenardo MJ. Induction of apoptosis in mature T cells by tumour necrosis factor. *Nature* 1995;377:348–351.
37. Budd RC. Activation-induced cell death. *Curr Opin Immunol* 2001;13:356–362.
38. Russell JH. Activation-induced death of mature T cells in the regulation of immune responses. *Curr Opin Immunol* 1995;7:382–388.
39. Singer GG, Abbas AK. The fas antigen is involved in peripheral but not thymic deletion of T lymphocytes in T cell receptor transgenic mice. *Immunity* 1994;1:365–371.
40. Sidman CL, Marshall JD, Von Boehmer H. Transgenic T cell receptor interactions in the lymphoproliferative and autoimmune syndromes of lpr and gld mutant mice. *Eur J Immunol* 1992;22:499–504.
41. Mollereau B, Deckert M, Deas O, Rieux-Laucat F, Hirsch F, Bernard A, et al. CD2-induced apoptosis in activated human peripheral T cells: a Fas- independent pathway that requires early protein tyrosine phosphorylation. *J Immunol* 1996;156:3184–3190.
42. Wesselborg S, Janssen O, Kabelitz D. Induction of activation-driven death (apoptosis) in activated but not resting peripheral blood T cells. *J Immunol* 1993;150:4338–4345.
43. Combadiere B, Freedman M, Chen L, Shores EW, Love P, Lenardo MJ. Qualitative and quantitative contributions of the T cell receptor zeta chain to mature T cell apoptosis. *J Exp Med* 1996;183:2109–2117.
44. Oberg HH, Lengl-Janssen B, Kabelitz D, Janssen O. Activation-induced T cell death: resistance or susceptibility correlate with cell surface fas ligand expression and T helper phenotype. *Cell Immunol* 1997;181:93–100.

45. Lenardo MJ. Interleukin-2 programs mouse alpha beta T lymphocytes for apoptosis. *Nature* 1991;353:858–861.
46. Van Parijs L, Refaeli Y, Lord JD, Nelson BH, Abbas AK, Baltimore D. Uncoupling IL-2 signals that regulate T cell proliferation, survival, and Fas-mediated activation-induced cell death. *Immunity* 1999;11:281–288.
47. Refaeli Y, Van Parijs L, London CA, Tschopp J, Abbas AK. Biochemical mechanisms of IL-2-regulated Fas-mediated T cell apoptosis. *Immunity* 1998;8:615–623.
48. Collette Y, Benziane A, Razanajaona D, Olive D. Distinct regulation of T-cell death by CD28 depending on both its aggregation and T-cell receptor triggering: a role for Fas-FasL. *Blood* 1998;92:1350–1363.
49. Radvanyi LG, Shi Y, Vaziri H, Sharma A, Dhala R, Mills GB, et al. CD28 costimulation inhibits TCR-induced apoptosis during a primary T cell response. *J Immunol* 1996; 156:1788–1798.
50. Ramsdell F, Seaman MS, Miller RE, Picha KS, Kennedy MK, Lynch DH. Differential ability of Th1 and Th2 T cells to express Fas ligand and to undergo activation-induced cell death. *Int Immunol* 1994;6:1545–1553.
51. Sato T, Irie S, Kitada S, Reed JC. FAP-1: a protein tyrosine phosphatase that associates with Fas. *Science* 1995;268:411–415.
52. Varadhachary AS, Perdow SN, Hu C, Ramanarayanan M, Salgame P. Differential ability of T cell subsets to undergo activation-induced cell death. *Proc Natl Acad Sci USA* 1997;94:5778–5783.
53. Radoja S, Saio M, Frey AB. CD8+ tumor-infiltrating lymphocytes are primed for Fas-mediated activation-induced cell death but are not apoptotic in situ. *J Immunol* 2001; 166:6074–6083.
54. Zaks TZ, Chappell DB, Rosenberg SA, Restifo NP. Fas-mediated suicide of tumor-reactive T cells following activation by specific tumor: selective rescue by caspase inhibition. *J Immunol* 1999;162:3273–3279.
55. Restifo NP. Not so Fas: re-evaluating the mechanisms of immune privilege and tumor escape. *Nat Med* 2000;6:493–495.
56. Chappell DB, Restifo NP. T cell-tumor cell: a fatal interaction? *Cancer Immunol Immunother* 1998;47:65–71.
57. O'Connell J, O'Sullivan GC, Collins JK, Shanahan F. The Fas counterattack: Fas-mediated T cell killing by colon cancer cells expressing Fas ligand. *J Exp Med* 1996;184:1075–1082.
58. O'Connell J, Bennett MW, O'Sullivan GC, Collins JK, Shanahan F. The Fas counterattack: cancer as a site of immune privilege. *Immunol Today* 1999;20:46–52.
59. Shiraki K, Tsuji N, Shioda T, Isselbacher KJ, Takahashi H. Expression of Fas ligand in liver metastases of human colonic adenocarcinomas. *Proc Natl Acad Sci USA* 1997;94: 6420–6425.
60. Gastman BR, Atarshi Y, Reichert TE, Saito T, Balkir L, Rabinowich H, et al. Fas ligand is expressed on human squamous cell carcinomas of the head and neck, and it promotes apoptosis of T lymphocytes. *Cancer Res* 1999;59:5356–5364.
61. Rabinowich H, Reichert TE, Kashii Y, Gastman BR, Bell MC, Whiteside TL. Lymphocyte apoptosis induced by Fas ligand- expressing ovarian carcinoma cells. Implications for altered expression of T cell receptor in tumor-associated lymphocytes. *J Clin Investig* 1998;101:2579–2588.
62. Bennett MW, O'Connell J, O'Sullivan GC, Brady C, Roche D, Collins JK, et al. The Fas counterattack in vivo: apoptotic depletion of tumor- infiltrating lymphocytes associated with Fas ligand expression by human esophageal carcinoma. *J Immunol* 1998;160:5669–5675.
63. Koyama S, Koike N, Adachi S. Fas receptor counterattack against tumor-infiltrating lymphocytes in vivo as a mechanism of immune escape in gastric carcinoma. *J Cancer Res Clin Oncol* 2001;127:20–26.

64. Strand S, Hofmann WJ, Hug H, Muller M, Otto G, Strand D, et al. Lymphocyte apoptosis induced by CD95 (APO-1/Fas) ligand-expressing tumor cells—a mechanism of immune evasion? *Nat Med* 1996;2:1361–1366.
65. Niehans GA, Brunner T, Frizelle SP, Liston JC, Salerno CT, Knapp DJ, et al. Human lung carcinomas express Fas ligand. *Cancer Res* 1997;57:1007–1012.
66. Gratas C, Tohma Y, Van Meir EG, Klein M, Tenan M, Ishii N, et al. Fas ligand expression in glioblastoma cell lines and primary astrocytic brain tumors. *Brain Pathol* 1997;7: 863–869.
67. Shibakita M, Tachibana M, Dhar DK, Kotoh T, Kinugasa S, Kubota H, et al. Prognostic significance of Fas and Fas ligand expressions in human esophageal cancer. *Clin Cancer Res* 1999;5:2464–2469.
68. Hahne M, Rimoldi D, Schroter M, Romero P, Schreier M, French LE, et al. Melanoma cell expression of Fas(Apo-1/CD95) ligand: implications for tumor immune escape. *Science* 1996;274:1363–1366.
69. Zietz C, Rumpler U, Sturzl M, Lohrs U. Inverse relation of Fas-ligand and tumor-infiltrating lymphocytes in angiosarcoma: indications of apoptotic tumor counterattack. *Am J Pathol* 2001;159:963–970.
70. Okada K, Komuta K, Hashimoto S, Matsuzaki S, Kanematsu T, Koji T. Frequency of apoptosis of tumor-infiltrating lymphocytes induced by fas counterattack in human colorectal carcinoma and its correlation with prognosis. *Clin Cancer Res* 2000;6:3560–3564.
71. Nishimatsu H, Takeuchi T, Ueki T, Kajiwara T, Moriyama N, Ishida T, et al. CD95 ligand expression enhances growth of murine renal cell carcinoma in vivo. *Cancer Immunol Immunother* 1999;48:56–61.
72. Khar A, Varalakshmi C, Pardhasaradhi BV, Mubarak Ali A, Kumari AL. Depletion of the natural killer cell population in the peritoneum by AK- 5 tumor cells overexpressing fas-ligand: a mechanism of immune evasion. *Cell Immunol* 1998;189:85–91.
73. Arai H, Chan SY, Bishop DK, Nabel GJ. Inhibition of the alloantibody response by CD95 ligand. *Nat Med* 1997;3:843–848.
74. Smith D, Sieg S, Kaplan D. Technical note: Aberrant detection of cell surface Fas ligand with anti- peptide antibodies. *J Immunol* 1998;160:4159–4160.
75. Strater J, Walczak H, Hasel C, Melzner I, Leithauser F, Moller P. CD95 ligand (CD95L) immunohistochemistry: a critical study on 12 antibodies. *Cell Death Differ* 2001;8:273–278.
76. Fiedler P, Schaetzlein C, Eibel H. Technical comment: Constitutive expression of FasL in thyrocytes. *Science* 1998;279:2015 online.
77. Stokes T, Rymaszewski M, Arscott P, Wang SH, Bretz JD, Barton J, et al. Technical comment: constitutive expression of FasL in thyrocytes. *Science* 1998;279:2015 online.
78. Behrens CK, Igney FH, Arnold B, Moller P, Krammer PH. CD95 ligand-expressing tumors are rejected in anti-tumor TCR transgenic perforin knockout mice. *J Immunol* 2001;166:3240–3247.
79. Seino K, Kayagaki N, Fukao K, Okumura K, Yagita H. Rejection of Fas ligand-expressing grafts. *Transplant Proc* 1997;29:1092–1093.
80. Seino K, Kayagaki N, Okumura K, Yagita H. Antitumor effect of locally produced CD95 ligand. *Nat Med* 1997;3:165–170.
81. Shimizu M, Fontana A, Takeda Y, Yagita H, Yoshimoto T, Matsuzawa A. Induction of anti-tumor immunity with Fas/APO-1 ligand (CD95L)-transfected neuroblastoma neuro-2a cells. *J Immunol* 1999;162:7350–7357.
82. Okamoto S, Takamizawa S, Bishop W, Wen J, Kimura K, Sandler A. Overexpression of Fas ligand does not confer immune privilege to a pancreatic beta tumor cell line (betaTC-3). *J Surg Res* 1999;84:77–81.
83. Yagita H, Seino K, Kayagaki N, Okumura K. CD95 ligand in graft rejection. *Nature* 1996;379:682.

84. Seino K, Iwabuchi K, Kayagaki N, Miyata R, Nagaoka I, Matsuzawa A, et al. Chemotactic activity of soluble Fas ligand against phagocytes. *J Immunol* 1998;161:4484–4488.
85. Ottonello L, Tortolina G, Amelotti M, Dallegri F. Soluble Fas ligand is chemotactic for human neutrophilic polymorphonuclear leukocytes. *J Immunol* 1999;162:3601–3606.
86. Hohlbaum AM, Moe S, Marshak-Rothstein A. Opposing effects of transmembrane and soluble Fas ligand expression on inflammation and tumor cell survival. *J Exp Med* 2000;191:1209–1220.
87. Shudo K, Kinoshita K, Imamura R, Fan H, Hasumoto K, Tanaka M, et al. The membrane-bound but not the soluble form of human Fas ligand is responsible for its inflammatory activity. *Eur J Immunol* 2001;31:2504–2511.
88. Miwa K, Asano M, Horai R, Iwakura Y, Nagata S, Suda T. Caspase 1-independent IL-1beta release and inflammation induced by the apoptosis inducer Fas ligand. *Nat Med* 1998;4:1287–1292.
89. Hohlbaum AM, Gregory MS, Ju ST, Marshak-Rothstein A. Fas ligand engagement of resident peritoneal macrophages in vivo induces apoptosis and the production of neutrophil chemotactic factors. *J Immunol* 2001;167:6217–6224.
90. Rescigno M, Piguet V, Valzasina B, Lens S, Zubler R, French L, et al. Fas engagement induces the maturation of dendritic cells (DCs), the release of interleukin (IL)-1beta, and the production of interferon gamma in the absence of IL-12 during DC-T cell cognate interaction: a new role for Fas ligand in inflammatory responses. *J Exp Med* 2000;192: 1661–1668.
91. Kang SM, Braat D, Schneider DB, O'Rourke RW, Lin Z, Ascher NL, et al. A non-cleavable mutant of Fas ligand does not prevent neutrophilic destruction of islet transplants. *Transplantation* 2000;69:1813–1817.
92. Thornberry NA, Bull HG, Calaycay JR, Chapman KT, Howard AD, Kostura MJ, et al. A novel heterodimeric cysteine protease is required for interleukin-1 beta processing in monocytes. *Nature* 1992;356:768–774.
93. Akita K, Ohtsuki T, Nukada Y, Tanimoto T, Namba M, Okura T, et al. Involvement of caspase-1 and caspase-3 in the production and processing of mature human interleukin 18 in monocytic THP.1 cells. *J Biol Chem* 1997;272:26,595–26,603.
94. Zhang Y, Center DM, Wu DM, Cruikshank WW, Yuan J, Andrews DW, et al. Processing and activation of pro-interleukin-16 by caspase-3. *J Biol Chem* 1998;273:1144–1149.
95. Ehl S, Hoffmann-Rohrer U, Nagata S, Hengartner H, Zinkernagel R. Different susceptibility of cytotoxic T cells to CD95 (Fas/Apo-1) ligand-mediated cell death after activation in vitro versus in vivo. *J Immunol* 1996;156:2357–2360.
96. Janssen O, Stocker A, Sanzenbacher R, Oberg HH, Siddiqi MA, Kabelitz D. Differential regulation of activation-induced cell death in individual human T cell clones. *Int Arch Allergy Immunol* 2000;121:183–193.
97. Giovarelli M, Musiani P, Garotta G, Ebner R, Di Carlo E, Kim Y, et al. A "stealth effect": adenocarcinoma cells engineered to express TRAIL elude tumor-specific and allogeneic T cell reactions. *J Immunol* 1999;163:4886–4893.
98. Koyama S, Koike N, Adachi S. Expression of TNF-related apoptosis-inducing ligand (TRAIL) and its receptors in gastric carcinoma and tumor-infiltrating lymphocytes: a possible mechanism of immune evasion of the tumor. *J Cancer Res Clin Oncol* 2002;128: 73–79.
99. Mogil RJ, Radvanyi L, Gonzalez-Quintial R, Miller R, Mills G, Theofilopoulos AN, et al. Fas (CD95) participates in peripheral T cell deletion and associated apoptosis in vivo. *Int Immunol* 1995;7:1451–1458.
100. Brunner T, Mogil RJ, LaFace D, Yoo NJ, Mahboubi A, Echeverri F, et al. Cell-autonomous Fas (CD95)/Fas-ligand interaction mediates activation-induced apoptosis in T-cell hybridomas. *Nature* 1995;373:441–444.

101. Sytwu HK, Liblau RS, McDevitt HO. The roles of Fas/APO-1 (CD95) and TNF in antigen-induced programmed cell death in T cell receptor transgenic mice. *Immunity* 1996;5:17–30.
102. Bonfoco E, Stuart PM, Brunner T, Lin T, Griffith TS, Gao Y, et al. Inducible nonlymphoid expression of Fas ligand is responsible for superantigen-induced peripheral deletion of T cells. *Immunity* 1998;9:711–720.
103. Pinkoski MJ, Droin NM, Green DR. TNF-α upregulates non-lymphoid Fas-ligand following superantigen-induced peripheral lymphocyte activation. *J Biol Chem* 2002;277: 42,380–42,385.

7 Alterations in T-Cell Signaling Pathways and Increased Sensitivity to Apoptosis

Ithaar H. Derweesh, MD,
Luis Molto, MD, PhD,
Charles Tannenbaum, PhD,
Patricia Rayman, MS, *Christina Moon,* BS,
Cynthia Combs, BS, *Thomas Olencki,* DO,
Paul Elson, ScD, *Ronald M. Bukowski,* MD,
and James H. Finke, PhD

CONTENTS

From: *Current Clinical Oncology: Cancer Immunotherapy at the Crossroads: How Tumors Evade Immunity and What Can Be Done*
Edited by: J. H. Finke and R. M. Bukowski © Humana Press Inc., Totowa, NJ

1. INTRODUCTION: T-CELL RESPONSES ARE DIMINISHED IN CANCER PATIENTS

Despite the presence of antigens on tumors, studies suggest that that the antitumor immune response is attenuated. Well-recognized immune dysfunction in T cells of tumor-bearing hosts is most pronounced in tumor-infiltrating lymphocytes (TIL), and is characterized by impaired proliferation and reduced cytotoxic effector function *(1)*. Some in vivo gene expression studies suggest that in the tumor microenvironment, there is minimal induction of inflammatory responses involving the expression of IFN-γ and IL-2 mRNA *(2,3)*. In a subset of patients, diminished T-cell function has also been observed in the peripheral blood, which is mostly associated with reduced production of TH1 type cytokines (e.g., IFN-γ) following stimulation of peripheral-blood T cells with mitogens or anti-CD3 antibody *(4)*.

A more global immune dysfunction has been well-described in animal tumor models and in cancer patients, which is typically associated with more advanced tumor burden. This dysfunction is characterized by a hyporesponsiveness to challenge with common recall antigens *(5)*. Associated with the occurrence of global immune dysfunction in T cells from cancer patients are changes in the function and expression of the T-cell receptor (TCR), defects in downstream TCR signaling, and attenuation of the lytic activity of T-cell lines associated with suppression of NF-κB translocation. Recent studies by several laboratories provide evidence for the presence of apoptotic T cells within the tumor microenvironment, and even within the peripheral blood of some patients.

The goal of this chapter is to review recent findings that support the concept that tumors and their products induce immune dysfunction by altering the sensitivity of T cells to apoptosis. This chapter focuses on the mechanisms by which the tumor microenvironment can either sensitize T cells to activation-induced cell death (AICD) or directly induce apoptosis via the mitochondrial pathway of apoptosis. Chapter 6 of this book covers the role of receptor-mediated apoptosis in T-cell dysfunction.

2. INCREASED SENSITIVITY OF T CELLS TO APOPTOSIS IN TUMOR-BEARING HOSTS

Apoptosis is one mechanism that regulates several facets of the immune response. Apoptosis plays an essential role in maintaining cellular homeostasis during development, differentiation, and pathophysiological processes. Recent investigations reveal that during the course of T-cell development in the thymus, negative selection of autoreactive immature T cells occurs via a typical apoptotic process *(6)*. Apoptosis is also involved in the regulation of lymphocyte homeostasis during immune responses *(7)*. Apoptosis of antigen-specific T cells is considered to be a major mechanism by which T-cell responses are downregulated following repeated antigen stimulation *(7–9)*. In this setting, downregulation of lymphocyte expansion occurs via cell–cell interaction in which T cells expressing Fas receptor undergo apoptosis induced by other T cells that display FasL *(10,11)*. Apoptosis is also involved in the formation of immune sanctuaries *(10)*.

Tumor cells appear to take advantage of apoptotic mechanisms to escape immune detection and destruction. There is growing evidence that apoptosis of T lymphocytes may be enhanced in tumor-bearing hosts, which can in turn impair the development of an effective immune response to tumors *(12–14)*. Apoptotic T cells have been detected *in situ* in several tumor types, including renal cell carcinoma (RCC). The measurement of DNA breaks by the terminal deoxynucleotidyl transferase-mediated nick-end labeling (TUNEL) assay using RCC tissue sections revealed that approximately one-half of the tumors have a significant number of apoptotic T cells, within the 5–15% range. Although apoptotic T cells have been reported in several different tumor types, it is unclear whether the level of apoptosis relates to stage, grade, or clinical outcome. The majority of the tumor-infiltrating T cells (TIL) do not display DNA breaks, yet these cells are very sensitive to AICD following stimulation in vitro *(13)*. Similar findings have been reported in CD8+ T cells infiltrating murine adenocarcinoma, MCA-38 *(12)*. Although the frequency of apoptotic TIL after initial isolation was low, stimulating these cells in vitro with anti-CD3 antibody induced Fas-dependent AICD. Likewise, injection of MCA-38 tumor with antibodies to the TCR *in situ* also caused the TILs to undergo AICD in vivo *(12)*.

The heightened sensitivity of T cells to apoptosis in cancer patients is not limited to the T cells that infiltrate the tumor. Indeed, spontaneous apoptosis of a subset of T cells in the peripheral blood of patients with advanced melanoma and gastric cancer has been observed *(15,16)*. The apoptosis appears to be Fas-mediated, since the majority of the cells expressing DNA breaks were CD8+ T cells that express FasR *(15)*. In analyzing T cells from RCC patients, no evidence for spontaneous apoptosis in the bulk peripheral-blood lymphocyte population was observed; however, patient T cells showed a heightened sensitivity to AICD following in vitro stimulation for 24/48 h with either PMA/ionomycin or anti-CD3 antibody *(17)*.

3. APOPTOTIC PATHWAYS (FIG. 1)

Apoptosis of cells can be mediated by engagement of the TNF family of receptors or by initiation of the mitochondrial pathway. The caspases, a family of cysteine proteases, play a critical role in the execution phase of apoptosis

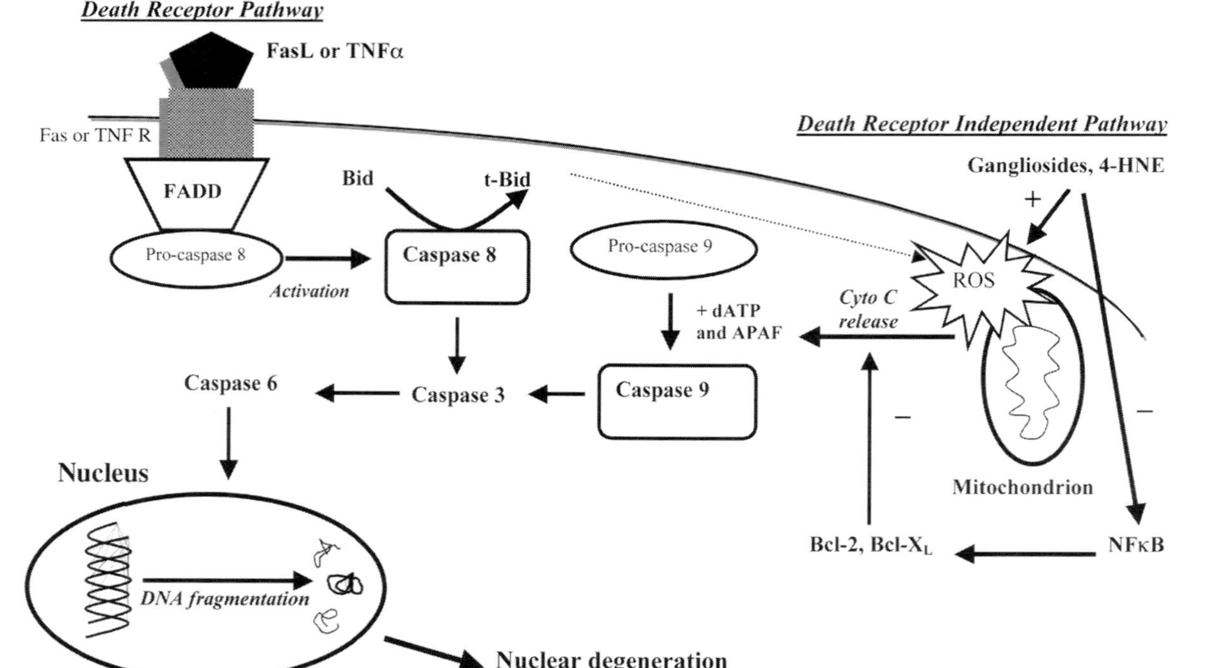

Fig. 1. In the death-receptor pathway, apoptosis is triggered by ligation of death receptors of the TNF family such as Fas and TNFR1. Fas-associated death domain (FADD) is directly or indirectly recruited to ligated Fas or TNFR1, leading to procaspase-8 recruitment and autoactivation of caspase-8. Active caspase-8 activates downstream caspases, initiating the caspase cascade. Caspase 8 activates caspase 3 and BID. Caspase 3 in turn activates caspase 6. Caspases 3 and 6 have specific roles in the nuclear changes accompanying apoptosis, while truncated BID translocates to mitochondria, where it disrupts mitochondrial membrane potential, leading to release of cytochrome-*c*. The death-receptor independent pathway is controlled by mitochondria. Induction of cell death in response to a variety of apoptotic stimuli, including gangliosides, and 4-HNE is associated with the generation of reactive oxygen species (ROS), which promotes mitochondrial damage and release of cytochrome-*c*, an event that is blocked by antiapoptotic members of the Bcl-2 family. In the cytosol, cytochrome-*c*, together with dATP, form a complex with APAF-1 that results in activation of caspase-9 and downstream effector caspases –3 and –6. This figure shows that gangliosides and 4-HNE cannot only induce ROS formation, but also inhibit NF-κB that downregulates the expression of Bcl-2. The induction of ROS along with the loss of Bcl-2 likely promotes apoptosis.

for both of these pathways, and are responsible for many of the biochemical and morphological changes associated with apoptosis *(18)*. Two distinct pathways of caspase activation have been delineated—one involving caspase-8 as the apical caspase for the death-receptor pathway, and the other involving caspase-9 as the most apical caspase for the mitochondrial pathway.

In the death-receptor pathway, activation of the initiator caspase-8 is triggered upon ligation of death receptors of the TNF family of immune effectors, including Fas, TNFR1, or death receptor 3, by their respective ligands (FasL, TNF, TRAIL). Fas-associated death domain (FADD) *(19)* is recruited directly to ligated Fas or indirectly to ligated TNFR1, leading to death-receptor oligomerization and recruitment of a death-inducing complex (DISC) *(20–22)* formed by assembly of FADD with procaspase-8, resulting in autoactivation of caspase-8 *(19)*. Active caspase-8 cleaves and activates downstream caspases, initiating the caspase cascade. Caspase-8 activates caspase-3 *(23)* and BID, a cytosolic proapoptotic member of the Bcl-2 family *(24)*. In turn, caspase-3 activates caspase-6. Caspases-3 and -6 play specific roles in the nuclear changes accompanying apoptosis *(23)*, and truncated BID translocates to mitochondria, where it alters mitochondrial membrane potential *(24)*, leading to release of caspase activators such as cytochrome-c and a caspase-independent death effector known as apoptosis-inducing factor (AIF) *(25)*.

The second pathway, a death-receptor independent pathway, is essentially controlled by mitochondria in which caspase-9 has been proposed as the initiating caspase in this pathway *(26,27)*. Induction of cell death in response to a variety of apoptotic stimuli is associated with mitochondrial release of cytochrome-c, an event that is blocked by antiapoptotic members of the Bcl-2 family and promoted by proapoptotic members such as Bax and Bak *(28–30)*. In the cytosol, cytochrome-*c*, together with deoxyadenosine triphosphate (dATP), forms a complex with APAF-1 that results in activation of caspase-9 and downstream effector caspases-3, -6, and -7 *(26,27,31)*. Potential mechanisms for the release of cytochrome-*c* include opening of mitochondrial PT pores, the presence of specific channels for cytochrome-*c* release, or mitochondrial swelling and rupture of the outer membrane, but without loss of mitochondrial membrane potential *(32)*. Another group of death-promoting molecules sequestered by the mitochondria has been identified. The second group of mitochondria-derived caspase activators (Smac/DIABLO) work by disrupting the linkage between the antiapoptotic proteins known as inhibitors of apoptosis (IAP, named XIAP, c-IAP1, cIAP2) and effector caspases. Smac/DIABLO can interfere with the ability of the IAPs to neutralize the caspases, which in turn facilitates both autoproteolytic cleavage of caspases and caspase-mediated cleavage of IAP *(33,34)*.

4. MECHANISMS RESPONSIBLE FOR HEIGHTENED SENSITIVITY TO APOPTOSIS IN T CELLS

A number of different mechanisms have been observed and described that could increase the sensitivity of T cells in cancer patients to apoptosis. Because receptor-mediated apoptosis of the T cell is covered in Chapter 6, we will only briefly discuss chronic stimulation leading to AICD. The major focus of this chapter is receptor-independent mechanisms, including the role of oxidative stress and tumor-derived products such as gangliosides in stimulating the mitochondrial pathway of T cell death.

4.1. Chronic Stimulation by Antigen

Generation of an immune response involves a process of activation, proliferation, differentiation, and ultimately, death of effector T cells. Following TCR ligation, T cells respond in functionally different ways to death signals, depending on their state of activation and the surrounding circumstances of inflammation or its absence *(35–38)*. At the peak of an immune response following multiple restimulations, the majority of T cells can undergo AICD *(39,40)*. CD4+ T cells become more sensitive to Fas-mediated apoptosis, while at the same time, their counterpart CD8+ T cells are rendered anergic under similar circumstances *(46)*. However, under the appropriate conditions, CD8+ cells are also sensitized to AICD *(41–46)*. AICD is driven by repetitive antigen exposure as well as high doses of persisting antigen or antigens expressed systemically *(43–45)*. Most of AICD is mediated by Fas receptors, but there is evidence that TNF-α receptors can also be involved *(41,42)*. T-cell activation also includes upregulation of Fas and FasL, and this interaction then activates the apoptosis program *(35,47–50)*.

FLIP (FLICE-inhibitory protein) is an inhibitor of Fas-mediated apoptosis, since it is homologous to caspase-8 but without proteolytically active domains and can regulate the sensitivity of T cells to AICD *(38)*. Memory or primed T cells are more resistant to apoptosis than naïve T cells, possibly because of their increased levels of FLIP protein in the earlier hours following antigen restimulation *(37)*. Algeciras-Schimnich et al. *(22)* demonstrated that sensitization of resting peripheral T cells to Fas-mediated apoptosis following TCR activation is caused by a decrease in c-FLIP. They noted that activated T cells arrested in G_1 phase contain high levels of c-FLIP, whereas T cells arrested in S phase show decreased c-FLIP protein levels. This links regulation of FLIP protein levels with cell-cycle progression and provides an explanation for the increase in TCR-induced apoptosis observed during the S phase of the cell cycle *(51,52)*.

Chronic antigen stimulation observed in various disease states is believed to cause T cells to become increasingly sensitive to apoptosis. Repeated stimulation during chronic viral infection is known to lead to either T-cell anergy or the induction of apoptosis, depending on the nature of the epitopes *(53)*. Chronic stimulation by tumor-associated antigens (TAAs) in cancer patients may contribute to immune dysfunction. It seems likely that cancer patients are chronically exposed to tumor antigens, resulting in chronic antigen presentation and ultimately, increased sensitivity to AICD. Such a mechanism may be relevant, considering the evidence from Hoffman et al. that demonstrates increased spontaneous apoptosis of CD8+ T cells in patients with head and neck cancer, and the finding that the most affected populations also express FasR *(54)*. Future studies using tetramers combined with staining for apoptosis events to identify tumor-specific T cells and their sensitivity to apoptosis should provide some insight into this issue.

4.2. Oxidative Stress

There is growing evidence to suggest that oxidative stress can promote apoptosis, or at least sensitize cells to apoptosis. Many agents that induce apoptosis are either oxidants or stimulators of cellular oxidative metabolism. Conversely, many inhibitors of apoptosis have antioxidant activities or enhance cellular antioxidant defenses. Cells within the tumor microenvironment often exist in a state of oxidative siege, in which survival requires an appropriate balance of oxidants and antioxidants *(55)*. Free radicals or reactive oxygen species (ROS), including superoxide anion (O_2^-), hydrogen peroxide (H_2O_2), and hydroxyl radical (OH^-), play an important role in carcinogenesis. Primary antioxidant enzymes such as superoxide dismutase, glutathione peroxidase, and catalase, protect against cellular and molecular damage caused by ROS production *(56)*. When the antioxidant defense system is no longer capable of eliminating free radicals, they cause lipid and protein oxidation. 4-hydroxy-2-nonenal (HNE) and malondialdehyde (MDA) *(57)* are markers of oxidative stress, and represent aldehyde products of oxidative breakdown of unsaturated fatty acids, and may thus reflect oxidative membrane breakdown *(57)*. It is generally believed that following the generation of free radicals, fatty acid hydroperoxides form as primary products, and decompose to HNE. Lipid peroxidation products such as HNE also bind to and from adducts with proteins that can modify their function. These products can cause cellular damage, including apoptosis *(57)*.

Oxidative stress develops in tumors, and probably plays a role in malignant growth *(58,59)*. Evidence of ROS formation and the generation of lipid peroxidized products has been demonstrated in primary tumors including RCC *(60)*. Blood samples collected from colon cancer patients and healthy controls demonstrated decreased levels of antioxidant vitamins *(61,62)* and increased levels of lymphocyte 8-oxo-2′-deoxyguanosine *(62)*, a marker for oxidative stress seen in colon cancer patients but not in the healthy controls. In addition, the determination of total antioxidant status and plasma levels of the lipid per-

Table 1
Decreased Antioxidative Enzymes in RCC *(64)*

glutathione *S*-transferase
aldo-keto reductase family 1, member A1
flavin-containing monooxygenase
glutathione peroxidase 3 (plasma)
glutathione transferases GSTT1, GSTT2
gluathione *S*-transferase A3
thioredoxin
liver microsomal UDP-glucuronosyltransferase
monoamine oxidase A
carbonyl reductase 1
thioredoxin-dependent peroxide reductase 1
glutathione transferase M3

oxidation products MDA and 4-HNE in colon cancer patients demonstrated that total antioxidant status was significantly decreased and lipid peroxidation products were increased *(63)*. In breast cancer patients, ROS production and lipid peroxidation were observed to be significantly higher than in a matched cancer-free cohort *(56)*. Furthermore, the activity level of the antioxidant enzyme catalase was noted to be significantly depressed in the serum of breast-cancer patients compared to the levels in the cancer-free cohort. This study linked elevated ROS production and lipid peroxidation with decreased antioxidant activity *(56)*. Decreased antioxidant vitamin concentrations and enzyme activity may thus be responsible for the formation of the pro-oxidative environment in the blood of cancer patients *(61,62)*. Furthermore, cDNA microarray studies comparing the level of mRNA expression in tumor tissue to that in normal tissues have demonstrated decreased expression of a number of antioxidative enzymes in RCC *(64)* (Table 1).

There is evidence that although cancers elaborate ROS and peroxidized lipids to create oxidative stress in their microenvironment, select tumors can express elevated levels of some antioxidant enzymes as a means of response to ROS formation. Human cancers such as mesothelioma *(65)*, malignant central nervous system (CNS) tumors *(66)*, gastric and esophageal cancer *(67)*, as well as a subset of RCCs, *(64)* have been reported to express high levels of MnSOD. Manganese superoxide dismutase (MnSOD) is a superoxide anion scavenger located in mitochondria. Increased expression of MnSOD can diminish oxygen radical-mediated injuries and the cytotoxic effects of tumor necrosis factor alpha (TNF-α), ionizing radiation, and certain chemotherapeutic agents *(65,66)*. Upregulation of MnSOD in cancer tissue most likely serves as a protective mechanism against endogenous anti-carcinogenic agents such as hepatocyte growth factor or IL-1, as well as anticancer therapies known to produce superoxide radicals as a key component of their tumor-killing activity *(67,68)*.

In various cellular models, ROS formation has been associated with apoptosis induced through the mitochondrial pathway. For example, treatment of undifferentiated pheochromocytoma line PC12 cells with H_2O_2 resulted in apoptotic changes, including the induction of cytochrome-*c* release, the processing of procaspase-9 and subsequent activation of caspase-3 *(69,70)*. On the other hand, Bcl-2 overexpression attenuated apoptosis and decreased caspase-9 and -3 activation as well as cytochrome-*c* release *(70)*. Treatment of the Jurkat T-cell leukemia line with H_2O_2 also resulted in the dissipation of mitochondrial potential, followed by the appearance of cytochrome-*c* in the cytosol and subsequent caspase activation *(71)*. Pretreatment with the thiol antioxidant *N*-acetylcysteine (NAC), which after uptake, deacylation, and conversion to lutathione functions as both a redox buffer and a ROS scavanger *(55)*, rendered Jurkat cells resistant to apoptosis by agonistic anti-Fas antibody *(72)*. These findings suggest that in some cell types, the death-receptor pathway may also involve ROS formation through the mitochondria.

In contrast to some tumor types that are somewhat resistant to the toxic effects of ROS formation, lymphocytes such as T cells are rather sensitive to their effects, which have been shown to promote apoptosis *(73,74)*. Recent data from our laboratory indicate that lipid peroxidation products such as HNE that are present in the tumor microenvironment may be involved in tumor-induced apoptosis of T cells. Our findings demonstrate that HNE and HNE adducts are present in renal tumor lines and in supernatants from renal tumor explants cultured in vitro (Derweesh et al., manuscript in preparation; Rayman et al., manuscript in preparation). Moreover, out studies and others have shown that HNE can induce apoptosis in T lymphocytes (Rayman et al., manuscript in preparation; Kalinich et al., 2000) *(75)*. Data from our laboratory indicates that preincubation of resting T cells from healthy donors with the antioxidants amifostine or NAC significantly attenuated apoptosis produced by a variety of HNE containing RCC supernatants, thus suggesting that antioxidants can protect T cells from the toxic effects of HNE and possibly other oxidized lipid products that are present in the tumor environment (Rayman and Finke, unpublished data) (Fig. 2).

Tumors may be a source of HNE and other oxidized lipids, and macrophages may be a source of free radicals such as H_2O_2 that can impair the function of immune cells by promoting cellular damage and lipid peroxidation *(73)*. ROS production is known to attenuate cytokine-induced activation and antitumor cytotoxicity of effector lymphocytes such as natural killer (NK) cells at the site of tumor growth *(76)*. Histamine inhibits ROS formation in macrophages via H2-receptors, and may therefore protect NK cells from ROS-mediated inhibition *(76)* and restore their tumor cytotoxicity. Indeed, histamine synergizes with

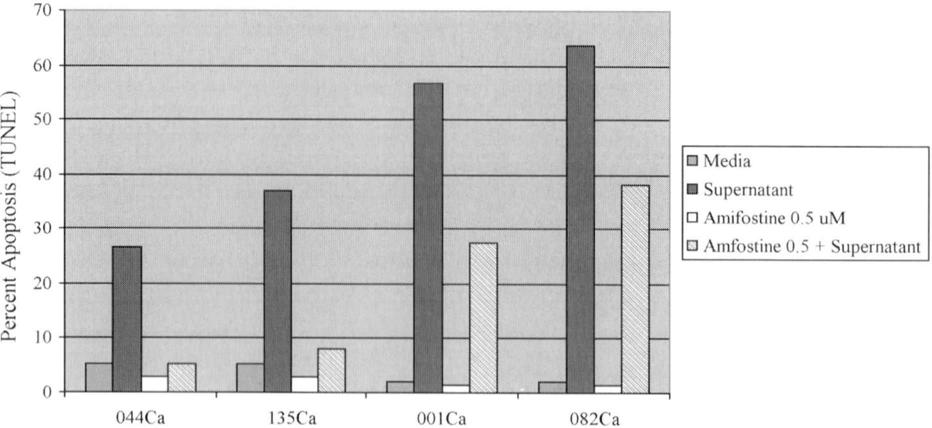

Fig. 2. Amifostine can partially block T-cell apoptosis induced by RCC supernatants. T cells isolated from the peripheral blood of healthy volunteers (>97% CD3+) were co-cultured with RCC supernatant (40–50% volume) in the presence and absence of amifostine (0.5 μ*M*). Amifostine was added to T cells 1 h prior to the addition of tumor supernatant. After 48 h, T cells were evaluated for DNA breaks with the TUNEL assay. RCC supernatants (001 Ca, 044 Ca, 082 Ca, and 135 Ca) were prepared by culturing tumor explants (3 × 3 mm fragment) for 2–3 d in Dulbecco's Modified Eagle's Medium (DMEM) media without serum. The supernatants were filtered and stored at –70°C. Viability of the tissue fragments was assessed by the MTT assay.

IL-2 and IFN-α to induce killing of NK cell-sensitive human tumor cells in vitro, and also optimizes cytokine-induced activation of several subsets of T cells by affording protection against macrophage-inflicted oxidative inhibition *(77)*. The putative clinical benefit of histamine as an adjunct to immunotherapy with IL-2 and/or IFN-α is currently being evaluated in clinical trials in metastatic malignant melanoma and acute myelogenous leukemia. A recently completed Phase III trial of IL-2 vs IL-2/histamine in patients with melanoma demonstrated a trend toward superior survival benefits for patients with hepatic metastases IL-2/histamine vs IL-2 alone. Currently, a similar trial is being developed for acute myelogenous leukemia (AML) patients *(77)*.

4.3. Gangliosides

Another proposed mechanism of tumor escape is the release by tumor cells of soluble products into their microenvironment, leading to suppression of the immune response *(78)*. Several groups have suggested that the gangliosides, a class of biologically active cell-surface glycolipids, may function as soluble modulators of the immune response in tumor-bearing hosts. Upregulated levels of ganglioside expression have been identified in several human epithelial cancers *(79)*, including neuroblastoma, melanoma, retinoblastoma, and hepatoma, as well as RCC *(80)*. Tumor cells that synthesize and shed gangliosides into their microenvironment have been shown to be highly immunosuppressive in vitro *(78,81–84)*.

Gangliosides inhibit many steps in the cellular immune response, including antigen (Ag) processing and presentation *(85)*, lymphocyte proliferation *(86,87)*, IL-2-induced T-cell proliferation *(88)*, CD4 expression *(89)*, and the generation of a cytotoxic response *(90)*. Most recently, it has been shown that gangliosides may shift the balance of the antitumor immune response from a type 1 cytokine response (IFN-γ) toward a type 2 response (IL-4, IL-5), possibly leading to a reduction in the cellular antitumor immune response that is critical for tumor elimination *(91)*. More details regarding the impact of gangliosides on immune dysfunction are presented by Dr. Ladish in Chapter 8 of this book.

4.3.1. Gangliosides Alter Sensitivity to Apoptosis

There is increasing evidence that select gangliosides are involved in sensitizing cells to undergo apoptosis following subsequent activation. We found that the product in RCC supernatants that sensitizes T cells to AICD is less than 3000 Daltons in size, a molecular weight consistent with the size of the monomeric form of gangliosides *(92)*. Moreover, pretreatment of supernatants with neuraminidase abrogates the sensitizing activity because ganglosides contain a sialic acid residue *(13,92)*. Furthermore, gangliosides isolated from specific RCC supernatants mimic the ability of those tumor-conditioned media to sensitize T cells to AICD *(13)*. Alone, these isolated gangliosides do not induce a significant level of apoptosis. Only when subsequently activated with PMA/ionomycin do the sensitized ganglioside-treated cells become TUNEL-positive. Similar findings (Fig. 3) have been observed with select bovine brain-derived gangliosides (GD3, GM1, and GD1a), which, when added to T-cell cultures at 50–200 μg/mL, also sensitize the lymphocytes to AICD (Finke et al., manuscript in preparation). Even at the elevated concentrations of 200 μg/mL, those gangliosides that sensitize T cells to AICD did not directly induce apoptosis within 48 h. The ability to sensitize cells to AICD is not a common property of all gangliosides, since GM3 is not effective at priming T cells for AICD.

Recent evidence in a rat hepatocyte model has identified GD3 as an emerging ganglioside involved in apoptosis, activating the mitochondrial-dependent apoptosome by sequential induction of mitochondrial ROS formation, followed by the mitochondrial permeability transition (MPT), cytochrome-*c* release, and caspase activation *(93–97)*. In this model, both ceramide precursor and ganglioside GD3 were noted to stimulate a burst of ROS formation at the mitochondrial level, which is the distinguishing feature of mitochondrial-induced apoptosis. Yet hepatocytes were killed only by GD3, which, unlike ceramides, was able to suppress NF-κB, suggesting that the promotion of hepatocyte-cell

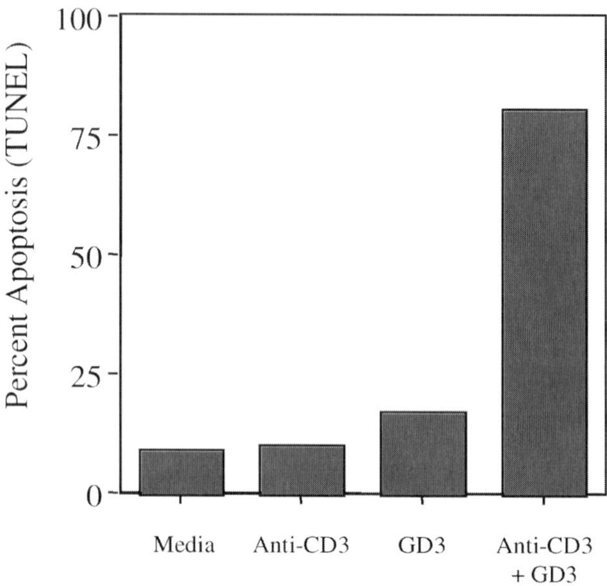

Fig. 3. GD3 can sensitize T cells to activation-induced cell death (AICD). Peripheral-blood T cells (>97% CD3+) were incubated with either media or bovine brain-derived GD3 (200 μg/mL) for 24 h prior to stimulating T cells with crosslinked anti-CD3 antibody for an additional 48 h. As controls, T cells were stimulated with anti-CD3 antibody or GD3 alone. T cells were then tested for DNA breaks by the TUNEL assay. Representative data from one of five experiments is shown.

death involves the lethal combination of mitochondrial ROS generation, followed by the subsequent release of apoptotic factors (cytochrome-*c*) and the suppression of the NF-κB-dependent survival pathway *(97)*. This same group has found that TNF-α will synergize with GD3 to induce apoptosis in hepatocytes. These investigators demonstrated that TNF may function in transporting GD3 from the membrane to the mitochondria via actin cytoskeleton vesicular trafficking. In the presence of latrunculin A, an actin-disrupting agent, GD3 remains at the cell surface. This blockage of the TNF-α stimulated loss of GD3 from the plasma membrane and its movement to mitochondria attenuates TNF-α induced apoptosis *(74)*, suggesting a synergistic role for a death ligand with an activator of the mitochondrial pathway in the induction of apoptosis in hepatocytes.

Recent investigations from our laboratory have demonstrated the ganglioside GD3 can induce apoptosis in T cells following activation with either phorbol myristate acetate and ionomycin (PMA/Iono) or anti-CD3 antibody. This ability of GD3 to synergize with PMA/Iono stimulation to induce T-cell apoptosis is attenuated by the pan-caspase inhibitor Z-VAD.fmk and the antioxidant *N*-acetyl cysteine, suggesting that the mechanism of initiating apoptosis by this combination is a caspase-dependent process that requires ROS formation

(Derweesh et al., manuscript in preparation). Furthermore, the apoptogenic effects of GD3 were abrogated in a dose-dependent manner by the addition of a neutralizing anti-TNF-α antibody. Although TNF-α or GD3 alone could not induce apoptosis in resting T cells, the combination of TNF-α and GD3 induced apoptosis in resting T cells, by a process that is caspase-dependent and involves ROS generation (Derweesh et al., manuscript in preparation). This work in progress demonstrates the collaborative role of death ligands and gangliosides in inducing T-cell apoptosis.

We also have evidence that gangliosides from some RCC are apoptogenic. Isolated gangliosides from several RCC tumors induced DNA breaks in normal T cells without the need for stimulation. Gangliosides derived from supernatants of uninvolved kidney tissue did not induce or sensitize T cells to apoptosis. The inability of the extract derived from the supernatant of uninvolved kidney to induce apoptosis was not the result of a decreased level of gangliosides isolated as noted by high-performance thin layer chromagraphy (HPTLC) analysis, but may be caused by a difference in the types of gangliosides expressed (Finke et al., unpublished data). Further studies in our lab with the glucosylceramide synthase inhibitor DL-threo-1-phenyl-2-hexadecanoylamino-3-pyrrolidino-1-propanol (PPPP) demonstrated abrogation of RCC tumor-induced apoptosis of activated T cells, as well as the Jurkat T cell line, mediated by reducing cellular ganglioside content within the tumors (80%). These findings, using a well-established RCC line (SK-RC-45, provided by Dr. Bander, Cornell University School of Medicine), provide evidence that gangliosides expressed by the tumor cells themselves can participate in T-cell-mediated apoptosis, and that downregulating the expression of gangliosides can prevent apoptosis of lymphocytes *(98)*.

5. TUMORS CAN ALTER NF-κB ACTIVATION IN T CELLS

5.1. NF-κB

NF-κB regulates transcription of a diverse set of genes with products that play a significant role in T-lymphocyte activation and the development of immunity *(99–101)*. NF-κB consists of multiple proteins that belong to the Rel family, which include *p105/p50*(NFκB1), *p65*(RelA), *p100/p52*(Lyt10, NFkB2), c-Rel, and RelB *(99,100)*. Different family members associate in various homo- and heterodimeric forms through a highly conserved N-terminal sequence referred to as the Rel homology region *(100,101)*. The RelA/*p50* heterodimer has been most extensively studied, and is known to have transactivating function, whereas the *p50* homodimer appears to function most often as a transcriptional suppressor *(99,100)*.

NF-κB complexes are sequestered in an inactive form in the cytoplasm through interaction with one or more inhibitory proteins known as IκBs

(100,101). The IκBs bind to the Rel homology region, masking the nuclear localization sequences (NLS) and preventing Rel translocation to the nucleus. IκBα, IκBβ, and IκBε appear to be the main regulators of NF-κB, since their degradation parallels NF-κB nuclear translocation *(100,101)*. Localization of NF-κB to the nucleus is dependent on the phosphorylation and subsequent degradation of the IκBs *(100,101)*. Phosphorylation of IκBα on serine residues at positions 32 and 36 mark this protein for ubiquitination and degradation by the 26S proteasome pathway *(100–102)*. The enzyme responsible for phosphorylation is a kinase termed IKK, which contains two catalytic subunits, IKKα (85 kDa) and IKKβ (87 kDa) *(100–102)*. Following degradation of IκBs, the active Rel dimers are rapidly transported to the nucleus through heterodimeric NLS-receptor complexes *(100)*.

5.2. NF-κB Regulation of Apoptosis

The importance of NF-κB in host survival has been elucidated from studies using knockout mice with deletions of individual NF-κB family members. Cells that are deficient in RelA are much more sensitive to TNF-α mediated apoptosis as compared to the wild-type *(99,103)*. This increased sensitivity to apoptosis is reversed by overexpression of RelA *(103)*. The inhibition of NF-κB activation in T cells from mice that express a dominant/negative form of IκBα also leads to a dramatic increase in apoptosis *(104)*. Sensitivity to Fas-mediated apoptosis is also enhanced in T cells in which NF-κB activation is impaired *(105)*.

The increased susceptibility of NF-κB-defective cells to apoptosis probably results from the fact that NF-κB regulates the expression of anti-apoptotic genes *(106–109)*. This includes TRAFs -1 and -2, which associate with the cytoplasmic regions of TNF-R family members *(106)*. TRAF-2 interacts with downstream signal transducers that activate NF-κB, and TRAF-1 is required for the recruitment of the NF-κB-inducible cellular inhibitors of apoptosis proteins (cIAP-1, cIAP-2, XIAP) *(110–113)*. The cIAPs can directly bind and neutralize caspases-3, -7, and -9, and are believed to have other downstream anti-apoptotic roles as signal transducers *(106,112,113)*. Interestingly, the relative expression levels of these proteins can also impact on cell survival. Once bound, TRAF-2 can recruit either TRAF-1 and cIAP for protective responses, or other pro- apoptotic molecules that are capable of inhibiting TRAF-2-mediated NF-κB activation *(114)*. Thus, inhibited TRAF-1 expression, notwithstanding abundant TRAF-2 levels, could itself render T cells sensitive to AICD. Overexpression of TRAF-1, TRAF-2, cIAP-1, and cIAP-2 can together inhibit the apoptosis observed when NF-κB activation is suppressed in TNF-sensitive cells *(106)*. IEX-1L is another NF-κB-dependent gene, whose transfection into NF-κB- defective mutants also provides protection against apoptosis in some systems *(108)*. Other anti-apoptotic molecules with NF-κB-dependent expression include the Bcl-X_L *(107)* and Bfl-1/A1 *(109)*, members of the Bcl family of proteins. These molecules are known to protect against apoptosis induced by mediators of the mitochondrial permeability transition, and have also been found to inhibit the activation of caspase-9 *(115)*.

5.3. Tumor Alteration of NF-κB in Lymphocytes

Impaired activation of NF-κB has been documented in tumor-bearing hosts. Studies in animal models *(116)* have demonstrated that as the tumor progressed, the ability to activate NF-κB in splenic T cells from these animals was lost. This impaired activation of NF-κB coincided with decreased production of IFN-γ from these T cells. Defective NF-κB activation has also been observed in T cells isolated from patients with renal cancer *(92)* and breast cancer *(117)*. Impaired κB-binding activity after T-cell stimulation was noted in TIL and peripheral-blood-derived T cells. Furthermore, we previously reported that T cells from less than 5% of patients with no evidence of disease (NED) had defective NF-κB activation compared to more than 50% with active disease, suggesting that the presence of a tumor has a negative impact on NF-κB activation *(118)*. The major problem is in the nuclear accumulation of RelA/*p50* dimers following T-cell activation, as determined by Western blotting and by κB-binding activity (gel mobility shift assays).

Data from several different laboratories have demonstrated that tumors or tumor-derived products are responsible for the defective NF-κB in T cells within the tumor microenvironment (Table 2). In co-culture experiments, tumor cells were found to inhibit the lytic activity of tumor-reactive T cells, correlating with the suppression of NF-κB in these cells *(119)*. We also recently noted in co-culture experiments that the renal tumor line SK-RC-45 can inhibit NF-κB activation in peripheral-blood T cells (Thornton et al., manuscript submitted). Supernatants from renal-tumor explants were found to suppress the activation of NF-κB in normal peripheral-blood T cells, and one of the products responsible for this suppression appears to be gangliosides *(92)*. Recent findings also suggest that HNE, at concentrations present in supernatants from renal tumor explants, can also inhibit the activation of NF-κB in T cells. Further studies by Batra et al. demonstrated that supernatants from lung-tumor lines would inhibit NF-κB activation in T cells, although the responsible molecule has not been identified *(120)*. Finally, Malmberg et al. (2001) suggest that oxidative stress within the tumor microenvironment may play a role in blocking NF-κB activation in infiltrating T cells. Increased production of ROS from tumor-infiltrating macrophages or granulocytes may be responsible for NF-κB suppression. They demonstrated that hydrogen peroxide inhibited NF-κB primarily in memory T cells, which correlated with reduced expression of TH1 cytokines *(73)*.

There are at least two mechanisms by which tumors or their products can inhibit the activation of NF-κB. In one case, IκBα degradation is impaired, resulting in retention of Rel dimers in the cytoplasm. Supernatants from non-

Table 2
Potential Mechanisms for Tumor-Induced NF-κB Defect in Immune Cells

- Hydrogen peroxide inhibition of NF-κB correlated with reduced expression of TH1 cytokines *(73)*
- Ganglioside suppressed NF-κB activation in T cells *(92)*
- 4-hydroxyneonal suppresses NF-κB by blocking IκBα degradation (*122*, Finke et al., unpublished)

small-cell lung cancer (NSCLC) suppressed NF-κB activation by blocking the stimulus-dependent degradation of the inhibitor IκB. Furthermore, lung tumor supernatants block IκBα degradation by inhibiting the activation of IKKα via an unknown mechanism *(120)*. We have found that supernatants from some renal-tumor explants also suppress NF-κB by blocking IκBα phosphorylation and the subsequent degradation of the inhibitor *(121)*. Although the tumor-derived product that can inhibit NF-κB activation by blocking IκBα degradation has not been identified, HNE present in renal-tumor supernatants may be partly responsible for this phenotype. HNE has been shown to bind to IKKα, forming an adduct that can block IκBα degradation and impair NF-κB binding activity *(122)*. In contrast, other tumor products can suppress NF-κB activation without affecting the normal stimulus-dependent degradation of IκBα. We have reported that some RCC tumor supernatants do not impair events upstream of IκBα degradation, but do prevent the accumulation of NF-κB complexes in the nucleus. One of the products responsible for this phenotype of NF-κB inhibition is the gangliosides. We *(92)* and others *(91)* have shown that gangliosides isolated from RCC supernatant or commercial sources of bovine brain-derived gangliosides (GD3, GM1, and GD1a) can suppress NF-κB in T cells without blocking IκBα degradation.

Recent reports suggest that NF-κB suppression in hepatocytes by the ganglioside GD3 may be mechanistically distinct in comparison to what we have observed in T cells with gangliosides expressed by tumor supernatants or by the tumor line, SK-RC-45 *(123)*. Exposing hepatocytes to GD3 alone induced IκBα to degrade; however, κB binding in the nucleus was not detected. Data gathered by confocal microscopy confirmed that NF-κB was retained in the cytoplasm following stimulation by GD3. Thus, in hepatocytes, exogenous GD3 blocks NF-κB activation by inhibiting the nuclear import of RelA/*p50*, preventing NF-κB-dependent transcription *(97)*. We have also investigated the effects of RCC-derived gangliosides upon T cells, and unlike hepatocytes, gangliosides present in tumor supernatants or expressed by SK-RC-45 alone did not induce IκBα degradation, and did not induce activation of NF-κB (Finke, unpublished data). Similar results were observed when T cells were exposed to GD3 (Ng et al., manuscript in preparation). Additional studies suggest that suppression of NF-κB in T cells by GD3 and RCC-derived gangliosides involves RelA degradation. These findings suggest that ganglioside-induced inhibition of NF-κB activation in T cells results from degradation of RelA/*p50* rather than a nuclear import problem.

5.4. Tumor Microenvironment Products Can Induce Decreased Expression of Antiapoptotic Genes in T Cells That May Contribute to Increased Sensitivity of T Cells to Apoptosis

As discussed previously, a number of intracellular proteins may negatively regulate apoptosis by interfering with the caspase cascade, or alternatively, by blocking the mitochondrial damage that causes cytochrome-*c* release. However, very few studies have been done to document that the T cells within the tumor microenvironment that are sensitive to apoptotic stimuli are deficient in the expression of NF-κB-regulated anti-apoptotic genes. Recent work by Johnson et al. demonstrated that tumor-associated T lymphocytes harvested from patients with ovarian cancer expressed fragmented XIAP/hIL-P that was not detected in control T cells purified from the peripheral blood of normal donors *(33)*. This same group has also shown that the XIAP is cleaved in apoptotic T lymphocytes, suggesting that the heightened sensitivity of T cells from ovarian cancer patients may be related to depressed levels of XIAP. In renal cancer patients, we have noted that infiltrating T cells from some patients are deficient in the expression of cIAP1, Bcl-2, and XIAP (Kudo et al., manuscript submitted). We have also noted a reduced expression of XIAP in RCC patient peripheral-blood T cells when compared to XIAP levels in normal healthy volunteers (Combs, C. et al., unpublished data). Additional studies examining Bcl-2 expression in T cells from RCC patients using immunohistochemistry and immunocytometry have demonstrated that TIL from a subset of patients express reduced levels of Bcl-2 compared to T cells in the peripheral blood (Richmond et al., unpublished data). Tumor-derived products appear to be responsible for the down-regulation of select anti-apoptotic proteins in T cells isolated from RCC patients. Supernatant fluids from in vitro cultured RCC explants can decrease the expression of Bcl-2, XIAP, cIAP-1, and cIAP-2 in normal peripheral-blood-derived T cells. Gangliosides isolated from these tumor supernatants can also inhibit the expression of these anti-apoptotic proteins in T cells. We have theorized that the ability of gangliosides to inhibit the expression of the anti-apoptotic proteins is related to the suppression of NF-κB by this tumor-derived product *(98,123)*. Whether other products in the tumor microenvironment that can inhibit NF-κB are involved in suppressing in vivo anti-apoptotic gene expression has not yet been determined.

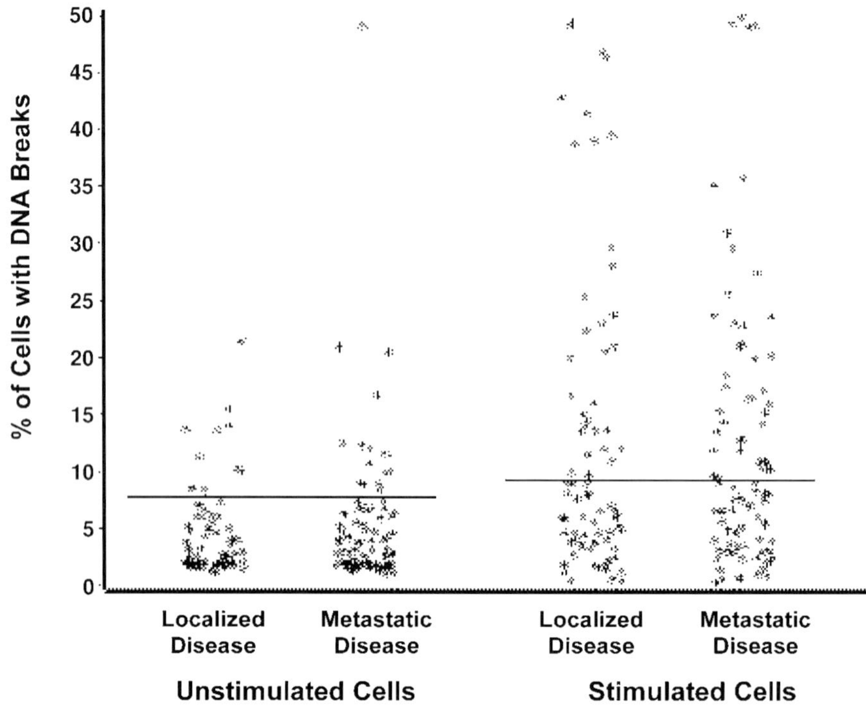

Fig. 4. Peripheral-blood-derived T cells from RCC patients show heightened sensitivity to AICD. T cells, isolated from the peripheral blood of RCC patients (metastatic and localized) and normal volunteers were stimulated or not for 24/48 h with PMA (10 ng/mL) and ionomycin (0.75 μg/mL). Thereafter, T cells were evaluated for DNA breaks (TUNEL assay). Each point on the graph represents the percent of T cells from individual patients that display DNA breaks after in vitro stimulation. The solid horizontal line in each group (unstimulated cells and stimulated cells) represent the mean plus 2 standard errors of 51 control patients.

5.5. Clinical Correlative Studies in RCC Patients With Defective NF-κB and Increased AICD Activity

We recently determined whether impaired NF-κB activation and altered sensitivity of T cells to AICD observed in peripheral-blood T cells of RCC patients is significantly different than the frequency of these defects observed in T cells from healthy, normal volunteers (Fig. 4). Patients were tested for AICD as follows: peripheral-blood T cells were cultured for 24/48 h with or without stimulus (PMA/ionomycin) prior to testing cells for DNA breaks by TUNEL analysis. TUNEL assay data were available for 51 normal controls, 79 localized RCC patients, and 93 metastatic RCC patients. T cells from normal individuals displayed little AICD, with less than 5% of the cells displaying DNA breaks after 24/48 h of stimulation. Whether activation was for 24 or 48 h, the

AICD was statistically significantly greater in patients with RCC as compared to controls ($p < 0.001$); however, there was no significant difference in AICD between localized and metastatic patients ($p = 0.91$). Overall, 59% of RCC patients had elevated activation-induced apoptosis, defined as TUNEL-positive results: 2 SD above the normal control values (Fig. 4). Attempts to determine whether AICD in patient T cells correlated with histology and grade demonstrated no correlation with histologic type of RCC. However, preliminary findings with a relatively small sample size suggested that AICD may correlate with grade I and II, $p = 0.05$, since grade III/IV tumors had significantly less AICD than patients with lower grades. These findings suggest that T cells from less aggressive tumors are more sensitive to AICD than those from more aggressive dedifferentiated tumors.

Although these results are somewhat surprising, it may be that decreased sensitivity to AICD in higher-grade tumors is a function of the overall global immune hyporesponsiveness that is seen in patients with advanced or aggressive disease. Conversely, T cells from low-grade, less aggressive tumors may have a greater ability to develop an immune response compared to those from more aggressive tumors. The ability to mount an immune response to a tumor may be associated with increased AICD activity by T cells recognizing and responding to antigens expressed by tumors. Whether more aggressive tumors are less effective at inducing a T-cell response, as a result of a more effective immunosuppressive mechanisms, is a focus of further investigation for our lab group.

NF-κB binding activity was also measured in T cells by evaluating the ability of nuclear extracts from resting and stimulated T cells (2 h with PMA/ionomycin) to bind to radiolabeled κB probe (electrophoretic mobility shift assay, EMSA). To semiquantitate the EMSA data for analysis, the RelA/*p50* transactivating band was desensitized for both unstimulated and stimulated T cells, and the data for patient T cells was compared to that of a normal individual run at the same time. NF-κB data was available for 74 localized and 95 metastatic RCC patients. NF-κB activation was significantly less in patients with RCC, regardless of localized or metastatic state ($p < 0.001$), when compared to normal controls. Correlating EMSA data to histology and grade demonstrated no relationship to grade, but was linked to histology, with clear-cell tumors showing a marked 66% abnormal NF-κB activity ($p = 0.06$).

Further questions to address include whether impaired NF-κB activation in patient T cells correlates with reduced expression of various anti-apoptotic genes that are regulated by NF-κB, such as Bfl-1/A1, Bcl-2, cIAP-1, c-IAP-2, and XIAP. It is also unknown whether the heightened sensitivity to AICD in patient T cells is related to altered expression of either pro-apoptotic or anti-apoptotic genes. We also plan to test whether the defect in NF-κB activation and increased sensitivity of patient T cells to AICD correlates with decreased patient survival. However, this analysis remains preliminary.

ACKNOWLEDGMENT

Sources of Support: NIH grants RO1 CA56937, RO1 CA87644; The Kidney Cancer Association; American Foundation of Urological Disease.

REFERENCES

1. Finke JH, Rayman P, Hart L, Alexander JP, Edinger MG, Tubbs RR, et. al. Characterization of TIL subsets from human renal cell carcinoma: specific reactivity defined by cytotoxicity IFN-γ secretion and proliferation. *J Immunother* 1994;15:91–104.
2. Wang Q, Redovan C, Tubbs R, Olencki T, Klein E, Kudoh S, et al. Selective cytokine gene expression in renal cell carcinoma tumor cells and tumor-infiltrating lymphocytes. *Int J Cancer* 1995;61:780–785.
3. Olive C, Cheung C, Nicol D, and Falk MC. Expression of cytokine mRNA transcripts in renal cell carcinoma. *Immunol Cell Biol* 1998;76:357–362.
4. Ochoa AC, Longo DL. (1995) Alteration of signal transduction in T cells from cancer patients. In *Important Advances in Oncology* (Devita VD, Hellman S, and Rosenberg SA, eds.), J. B. Lipponcott, Philadelphia, PA, pp. 43–54.
5. Klugo RC. Diagnostic and therapeutic immunology of renal cell cancer. *Henry Ford Med J* 1979;27:106–109.
6. Sun EW, Shi YF. Apoptosis: the quiet death silences the immune system. *Pharmacol Ther* 2001;92:135–145.
7. Estaquier J, Ameisen JC. A role for T-helper type-1 and type-2 cytokines in the regulation of human monocyte apoptosis. *Blood* 1997;90:1618–1625.
8. Dhein J, Walczak H, Baumler C, Debatin KM, and Krammer PH. Autocrine T-cell suicide mediated by APO-1/(Fas/CD95). *Nature* 1995;373:438–441.
9. Telford WG, Miller RA. Aging increases CD8 T cell apoptosis induced by hyperstimulation but decreases apoptosis induced by agonist withdrawal in mice. *Cell Immunol* 1999;191:131–138.
10. Griffith TS, Brunner T, Fletcher SM, Green DR, and Gerguson TA. Fas ligand-induced apoptosis as a mechanism of immune privilege. *Science* 1995;270:1189–1191.
11. van Parijs L, Abbas A. Role of Fas-mediated cell death in the regulation of immune responses. *Curr Opin Immunol* 1996;8:355–361.
12. Radoja S, Saio M, Frey AB. CD8+ tumor-infiltrating lymphocytes are primed for Fas-mediated activation-induced cell death but are not apoptotic in situ. *J Immunol* 2001; 166:6074–6083.
13. Finke JH, Rayman P, George R, Tannenbaum CS, Kolenko V, Uzzo R, et al. Tumor-induced sensitivity to apoptosis in T cells from patients with renal cell carcinoma: role of nuclear factor-kappaB suppression. *Clin Cancer Res* 2001;7:940s–946s.
14. Whiteside TL, Rabinowich H. The role of Fas/FasL in immunosuppression induced by human tumors. *Cancer Immunol Immunother* 1998;46:175–184.
15. Saito T, Dworacki G, Gooding W, Lotze MT, Whiteside TL. Spontaneous apoptosis of CD8+ T lymphocytes in peripheral blood of patients with advanced melanoma. *Clin Cancer Res* 2000;6:1351–1364.
16. Takahashi R, Deveraux Q, Tamm I, Welsh K, Assa-Munt N, Salvesen GS, et al. A single BIR domain of XIAP sufficient for inhibiting caspases. *J Biol Chem* 1998;273:7787–7790.
17. Uzzo RG, Rayman P, Kolenko V, Ckarj OE, Bloom T, Ward AM, et al. Mechanisms of Apoptosis in T cells from patients with renal cell carcinoma. *Clin Cancer Res* 1999; 5:1219–1229.
18. Nunez G, Benedict MA, Hu Y, Inohara N. Caspases: the proteases of thea poptotic pathway. *Oncogene* 1998;17:3237–3245.

19. Ashkenazi A, Dixit VM. Death receptors: signaling and modulation. *Science* 1998; 281:1305–1308.
20. Chinnaiyan AM, O'Rourke K, Tewari M, Dixit VM. FADD, a novel death domain-containing protein, interacts with the death domain of Fas and initiates apoptosis. *Cell* 1995; 81:505–512.
21. Muzio M. Signalling by proteolysis: death receptors induce apoptosis. *Int J Clin Lab Res* 1998;28:141–147.
22. Algeciras-Schimnich A, Shen L, Barnhart BC, Murmann AE, Burkhardt JK, Peter ME. Molecular ordering of the initial signaling events of CD95. *Mol Cell Biol* 2002;22:207–220.
23. Hirata H, Takahashi A, Kobayashi S, Yonebara S, Sawai H, Okazaki T, et al. Caspases are activated in a branched protease cascade and control distinct downstream processes in Fas-induced apoptosis. *J Exp Med* 1998;187:587–600.
24. Li H, Zhu H, Xu CJ, Yuan J. Cleavage of BID by caspase 8 mediates the mitochondrial damage in the Fas pathway of apoptosis. *Cell* 1998;94:491–501.
25. Loeffler M, Kroemer G. The mitochondrion in cell death control: certainties and incognita. *Exp Cell Res* 2000;256:19–26.
26. Li P, Nijhawan D, Budihardjo I, Srinivasula SM, Ahmad M, Alnemri ES, et al. Cytochrome *c* and dATP-dependent formation of Apaf-1/caspase-9 complex initiate an apoptotic protease cascade. *Cell* 1997;91:479–489.
27. Zou H, Henzel WJ, Liu X, Lutschg A, Wang X. Apaf-1, a human protein homologous to C. elegans CED-4, participates in cytochrome c-dependent activation of caspase-3. *Cell* 1997;90:405–413.
28. Yang J, Liu X, Bhalla K, Kim CN, Ibrado AM, Cai J, et al. Prevention of apoptosis by Bcl-2: release of cytochrome *c* from mitochondria blocked. *Science* 1997;1129–1132.
29. Kluck RM, Bossy-Wetzel E, Green DR, Newmeyer DD. The release of cytochrome *c* from mitochondria: a primary site for Bcl-2 regulation of apoptosis. *Science* 1997;275:1132–1136.
30. Jurgensmeier JM, Xie Z, Deveraux Q, Ellerby L, Bredesen D, Reed JC. Bax directly induces release of cytochrome c from isolated mitochondria. *Proc Natl Acad Sci USA* 1998; 95:4997–5002.
31. Srinivasula SM, Ahmad M, Fernandes-Alnemri T, and Alnemri ES. Autoactivation of procaspase-9 by Apaf-1-mediated oligomerization. *Mol Cell* 1998;1:949–957.
32. Reed JC. Cytochrome c— can't live with it—can't live without it. *Cell* 1997;91:559–562.
33. Johnson DE, Gastman BR, Wieckowski E, Wang GQ, Amoscato A, Delach SM, et al. Inhibitor of apoptosis protein hILP undergoes caspase-mediated cleavage during T lymphocyte apoptosis. *Cancer Res* 2000;60:1818–1823.
34. Yang YL, Lee XM. The IAP family: endogenous caspase inhibitors with multiple biological activities. *Cell Res* 2000;10:169–177.
35. Dhein J, Walczak H, Baumler C, Debatin KM, and Krammer PH. Autocrine T-cell suicide mediated by APO-1/(Fas/CD95). *Nature* 1995;373:438–441.
36. O'Connell J, Bennett MW, O'Sullivan GC, Shanahan F. The Fas counterattack: cancer as a site of immune privilege. *Immunol Today* 1999;20:46–52.
37. Inaba M, Kurasawa K, Mamura M, Kumano K, Saito Y, Iwamoto I. Primed T cells are more resistant to Fas-mediated activation-induced cell death than naive T cells. *J Immunol* 1999;163:1315–1320.
38. Irmler M, Thome M, Hahne M, Schneider P, Hofmann K, Steiner V, et al. Inhibition of death receptor signals by cellular FLIP. *Nature* 1997;388:190–195.
39. Bonfoco F, Stuart PM, Brunner T, Lin T, Griffith TS, Gao Y, et al. Inducible non-lymphoid expression of Fas Ligand is responsible for superantigen-induced peripheral deletion of T cells. *Immunity* 1998;9:711–720.
40. Hildeman DA, Zhu Y, Mitchell TC, Kappler J, Marrack P. Molecular mechanisms of activated T cell death in vivo. *Curr Opin Immunol* 2002;14:354–359.

41. Zheng L, Fisher G, Miller RE, Peschon J, Lynch DH, Lenardo MJ. Induction of apoptosis in mature T cells by tumour necrosis factor. *Nature* 1995;377:348–351.
42. Lenardo M, Chan KM, Hornung F, McFarland H, Siegel R, Wang J, et al. Mature T lymphocyte apoptosis—immune regulation in a dynamic and unpredictable antigenic environment. *Annu Rev Immunol* 1999;17:221–253.
43. van Parijs L, Peterson DA, Abbas AK. The Fas/Fas ligand pathway and Bcl-2 regulate T cell responses to model self and foreign antigens. *Immunity* 1998;8:265–274.
44. Derby MA, Snyder JT, Tse R, Alexander-Miller MA, Berzofsky JA. An abrupt and concordant initiation of apoptosis: antigen-dependent death of CD8+ CTL. *Eur J Immunol* 2001;31:2951–2959.
45. Zhou S, Ou R, Huang L, Moskophidis D. Critical role for perforin-, Fas/FasL-, and TNFR1-mediated cytotoxic pathways in down-regulation of antigen-specific T cells during persistent viral infection. *J Virol* 2002;76:829–840.
46. Tham EL, Mescher MF. The poststimulation program of CD4 versus CD8 T cells (death versus activation-induced nonresponsiveness). *J Immunol* 2002;169:1822–1828.
47. Ju ST, Panka DJ, Cui H, Ettinger R, el-Khatib M, Sherr DH, et al. Fas(CD95)/FasL interactions required for programmed cell death after T-cell activation. *Nature* 1995; 373:444–448.
48. Wang R, Zhang L, Yin D, Mufson RA, Shi Y. Protein kinase C regulates Fas (CD95/APO-1) expression. *J Immunol* 1998;161:2201–2207.
49. Gonzalez-Garcia A, R-Borlado L, Leonardo E, Merida I, Martinez-A C, Carrera AC. Lck is necessary and sufficient for Fas-ligand expression and apoptotic cell death in mature cycling T cells. *J Immunol* 1997;158:4104–4112.
50. Carrera AC, Calvo V, Borlado LR, Paradis H, Alemany S, Roberts TM, et al. The catalytic domain of pp56(lck), but not its regulatory domain, is sufficient for inducing IL-2 production. *J Immunol* 1996;157:3775–3782.
51. Algeciras-Schimnich A, Griffith TS, Lynch DH, Paya CV. Cell cycle-dependent regulation of FLIP levels and susceptibility to Fas-mediated apoptosis. *J Immunol* 1999; 162:5205–5211.
52. Kirchhoff S, Muller WW, Krueger A, Schmitz I, Krammer PH. TCR-mediated up-regulation of c-FLIPshort correlates with resistance toward CD95-mediated apoptosis by blocking death-inducing signaling complex activity. *J Immunol* 2000;165:6293–6300.
53. Zhou S, Ou R, Huang L, Moskophidis D. Critical role for perforin-, Fas/FasL-, and TNFR1-mediated cytotoxic pathways in down-regulation of antigen-specific T cells during persistent viral infection. *J Virol* 2002;76:829–840.
54. Hoffmann TK, Dworacki G, Tsukihiro T, Meidenbauer N, Gooding W, Johnson JT, et al. Spontaneous apoptosis of circulating T lymphocytes in patients with head and neck cancer and its clinical importance. *Clin Cancer Res* 2002;8:2553–2562.
55. Sandstrom PA, Mannie MD, Buttke TM. Inhibition of activation-induced death in T cell hybridomas by thiol antioxidants: oxidative stress as a mediator of apoptosis. *J Leukoc Biol* 1994;55:221–226.
56. Ray G, Batra S, Shukla NK, Deo S, Raina V, Ashok S, et al. Lipid peroxidation, free radical production and antioxidant status in breast cancer. *Breast Cancer Res Treat* 2000;59:163–170.
57. Parola M, Bellomo G, Robino G, Barrera G, Dianzani MU. 4-Hydroxynonenal as a biological signal: molecular basis and pathophysiological implications. *Antioxid Redox Signal* 1999;1:255–284.
58. Brown NS, Bicknell R. Hypoxia and oxidative stress in breast cancer. Oxidative stress: its effects on the growth, metastatic potential and response to therapy of breast cancer. *Breast Cancer Res* 2001;3:323–327.

59. Lusini L, Tripodi SA, Rossi R, Giannerini F, Giustarini D, del Vecchio MT, et al. Altered glutathione anti-oxidant metabolism during tumor progression in human renal-cell carcinoma. *Int J Cancer* 2001;91:55–59.
60. Okamoto K, Toyokuni S, Uchida K, Ogawa O, Takenewa J, Kakehi Y, et al. Formation of 8-hydroxy-2′-deoxyguanosine and 4-hydroxy-2-nonenal-modified proteins in human renal-cell carcinoma. *Int J Cancer* 1994;58:825–829.
61. Hronek M, Zadak Z, Solichova D, Jandik P, Melichar B. The association between specific nutritional antioxidants and manifestation of colorectal cancer. *Nutrition* 2000;16: 189–191.
62. Gackowski D, Banaszkiewicz Z, Rozalski R, Jawien A, Olinski R. Persistent oxidative stress in colorectal carcinoma patients. *Int J Cancer* 2002;101:395–397.
63. Skrzydewska E, Stankiewicz A, Michalak K, Sulkowska M, Zalewski B, Piotrowski Z. Antioxidant status and proteolytic-antiproteolytic balance in colorectal cancer. *Folia Histochem Cytobiol* 2001;39 Suppl 2:98–99.
64. Boer JM, Huber WK, Sultmann H, Wilmer F, von Heydebreck A, Haas S, et al. Identification and classification of differentially expressed genes in renal cell carcinoma by expression profiling on a global human 31,500-element cDNA array. *Genome Res* 2001;11: 1861–1870.
65. Kinnula VL, Pietarinen-Runtti P, Raivio K, Kahlos K, Pelin K, Mattson K, et al. Manganese superoxide dismutase in human pleural mesothelioma cell lines. *Free Radic Biol Med* 1996;21:527–532.
66. Cobbs CS, Levi DS, Aldape K, Israel MA. Manganese superoxide dismutase expression in human central nervous system tumors. *Cancer Res* 1996;56:3192–3195.
67. Izutani R, Asano S, Imano M, Kuroda D, Kato M, Ohyanagi H.Expression of manganese superoxide dismutase in esophageal and gastric cancers. *J Gastroenterol* 1998;33: 816–822.
68. Arakaki N, Kajihara T, Arakaki R, Ohnishi T, Kazi JA, Nakashima H, et al. Involvement of oxidative stress in tumor cytotoxic activity of hepatocyte growth factor/scatter factor. *J Biol Chem* 274:13,541–13,546, 1999.
69. Pias EK, Ekshyyan OY, Rhoads CA, Fuseler J, Harrison L, Aw TY. Differential effects of superoxide dismutase isoform expression on hydroperoxide-induced apoptosis in PC-12 cells. *J Biol Chem* 2003 Apr 11;278(15):13,294–13,301.
70. Yamakawa H, Ito Y, Naganawa T, Banno Y, Nakashima S, Yoshimura S, et al. Activation of caspase-9 and -3 during H2O2-induced apoptosis of PC12 cells independent of ceramide formation. *Neurol Res* 2000;22:556–564.
71. Stridh H, Kimland M, Jones DP, Orrenius S, Hampton MB. Cytochrome c release and caspase activation in hydrogen peroxide- and tributyltin-induced apoptosis. *FEBS Lett* 1998;429:351–355.
72. Gastman BR, Yin XM, Johnson DE, Wieckowski E, Wang GQ, Watkins SC, et al. Tumor-induced apoptosis of T cells: amplification by a mitochondrial cascade. *Cancer Res* 2000; 60:6811–6817.
73. Malmberg KJ, Arulampalam V, Ichihara F, Petersson M, Seki K, Andersson T, et al. Inhibition of activated/memory (CD45RO(+)) T cells by oxidative stress associated with block of NF-kappaB activation. *J Immunol* 2001;167:2595–2601.
74. Garcia-Ruiz C, Colell A, Morales A, Calvo M, Enrich C, Fernandez-Checa JC. Trafficking of ganglioside GD3 to mitochondria by tumor necrosis factor-alpha. *J Biol Chem* 2002; 277:36,443–36,448.
75. Kalinich JF, Ramakrishnan R, McClain DE, Ramakrishnan N. 4-Hydroxynonenal, an end-product of lipid peroxidation, induces apoptosis in human leukemic T- and B-cell lines. *Free Radic Res* 2000;33:349–358.

76. Hellstrand K, Brune M, Naredi P, Mellqvist UH, Hansson M, Gehlsen KR, et al. Histamine: a novel approach to cancer immunotherapy. *Cancer Investig* 2001;18:347–355.
77. Agarwala SS, Sabbagh MH. Histamine dihydrochloride: inhibiting oxidants and synergising IL-2-mediated immune activation in the tumour microenvironment. *Expert Opin Biol Ther* 2001;1:869–879.
78. Black PH. Shedding from the cell surface of normal and cancer cells. *Adv Cancer Res* 1980;32:75–199.
79. Hakomori S. Tumor-associated carbohydrate antigens. *Annu Rev Immunol* 1984;2: 103–126.
80. Hoon DS, Okun E, Neuwirth H, Morton DL, Irie RF. Aberrant expression of gangliosides in human renal cell carcinomas. *J Urol* 1993;150:2013–2018.
81. Ladisch S, Gillard B, Wong C, Ulsh L. Shedding and immunoregulatory activity of YAC-1 lymphoma cell gangliosides. *Cancer Res* 1983;43:3808–3813.
82. Skipksi VP, Katopodis N, Prendergast JS, Stock CC. Gangliosides in blood serum of normal rats and Morris hepatoma 5123tc-bearing rats. *Biochem Biophys Res Commun* 67: 1975;1122–1127.
83. Kloppel TM, Keenan TW, Freeman MJ, Morre DJ. Glycolipid-bound sialic acid in serum: increased levels in mice and humans bearing mammary carcinomas. *Proc Natl Acad Sci USA* 1977;74:3011–3013.
84. Li R, Ladisch S. Shedding of human neuroblastoma gangliosides. *Biochim Biophys Acta* 1991;1083:57–64.
85. Heitger A, Ladisch S. Gangliosides block antigen presentation by human monocytes. *Biochim Biophys Acta* 1303:1996;161–168.
86. Miller HC, Esselman WJ. Modulation of the immune response by antigen reactive lymphocytes after cultivation with gangliosides. *J Immunol* 1975;115:839–843.
87. Lu P, Sharom FJ. Immunosuppression by YAC-1 lymphoma: role of shed gangliosides. *Cell Immunol* 1996;173:22–32.
88. Sharom FJ, Chiu AL, Chu JW. Membrane gangliosides modulate interleukin-2-stimulated T-lymphocyte proliferation. *Biochim Biophys Acta* 1991;1094:35–42.
89. Garofalo T, Sorice M, Misasi R, Cinque B, Giammatteo M, Pontieri GM, et al. A novel mechanism of CD4 down-modulation induced by monosialoganglioside GM3: involvement of serine phosphorylation and protein kinase Cd translocation. *J Biol Chem* 1998;273: 35,153–35,160.
90. Grayson G, Ladisch S. Immunosuppression by human gangliosides. II. Carbohydrate structure and inhibition of human NK activity. *Cell Immunol* 1992;139:18–29.
91. Irani DN. The susceptibility of mice to immune-mediated neurologic disease correlates with the degree to which their lymphocytes resist the effects of brain-derived gangliosides. *J Immunol* 1998;161:2746–2752.
92. Uzzo RG, Rayman P, Klenko V, Clark PE, Cathcart MK, Bloom T, et al. Renal cell carcinoma-derived galgliosides suppress nuclear factor-κB activation in T cells. *J Clin Investig* 1999;104:769–776.
93. García-Ruiz C, Colell A, París R, Fernández-Checa J. C.Direct interaction of GD3 ganglioside with mitochondria generates reactive oxygen species followed by mitochondrial permeability transition, cytochrome c release, and caspase activation. *FASEB J* 2000; 14:847–858.
94. Scorrano L, Petronilli P, DiLisa F, Bernardi P. Commitment to apoptosis by GD3 ganglioside depends on opening of the mitochondrial permeability transition pore. *J Biol Chem* 1999;274:22,581–22,585.
95. Kristal BS, Brown AM. Apoptogenic ganglioside GD3 directly induces the mitochondrial permeability transition. *J Biol Chem* 1999;274:23,169–23,175.

96. Rippo MR, Malisan F, Rayagnan L, Tomassini B, Condo I, Costantini P, et al. GD3 ganglioside directly targets mitochondria in a bcl-2-controlled fashion. *FASEB J* 2000;14: 2047–2054.
97. Colell A, Garcia-Ruiz C, Roman J, Ballesta A, Fernandez-Checa JC. Ganglioside GD3 enhances apoptosis by suppressing the nuclear factor-kappa B-dependent survival pathway. *FASEB J* 2001;15:1068–1070.
98. Kudo D, Rayman P, Horton C, Cathcart M, Bukowski RM, Thornton M, et al. Gangliosides expressed by the renal cell carcinoma cell line SK-RC-45 are involved in tumor-induced apoptosis of T cells. *Cancer Res* 2003;63:1676–1683.
99. Baeuerle PA, Baltimore D. NF-kappa B: ten years after. *Cell* 1996;87:13–20.
100. May MJ, and Ghosh S. Signal transduction through NF-kappa B. *Immunol Today* 1998;19: 80–88.
101. Jacobs MD, Harrison SC. Structure of an IkappaBalpha/NF-kappaB complex. *Cell* 1998; 95:749–758.
102. DiDonato JA, Hayakawa M, Rothwarf DM, Zandi E, Karin M. A cytokine-responsive IkappaB kinase that activates the transcription factor NF-kappaB. *Nature* 1997;388:548–554.
103. Beg AA, Baltimore D. An essential role for NF-kappaB in preventing TNF-alpha-induced cell death. *Science* 1996;274:782–784.
104. Ferreira V, Sidenius N, Tarantino N, Hubert P, Chatenoud L, Blasi F, et al. In vivo inhibition of NF-kappa B in T-lineage cells leads to a dramatic decrease in cell proliferation and cytokine production and to increased cell apoptosis in response to mitogenic stimuli, but not to abnormal thymopoiesis. *J Immunol* 1999;162:6442–6450.
105. Dudley E, Hornung F, Zheng L, Scherer D, Ballard D, Lenardo M. NF-kappaB regulates Fas/APO-1/CD95- and TCR-mediated apoptosis of T lymphocytes. *Eur J Immunol* 1999; 29:878–886.
106. Wang CY, Mayo MW, Komeluk RG, Goeddel DV, Baldwin AS Jr. NF-kappaB antiapoptosis: induction of TRAF1 and TRAF2 and c-IAP1 and c-IAP2 to suppress caspase-8 activation. *Science* 1998;281:1680–1683.
107. Tamatani M, Che YH, Matsuzaki H, Ogawa S, Okado H, Miyake S, et al. Tumor necrosis factor induces Bcl-2 and Bcl-x expression through NFkappaB activation in primary hippocampal neurons. *J Biol Chem* 1999;274:8531–8638.
108. Wu MX, Ao Z, Prasad KV, Wu R, Schlossman SF. IEX-1L, an apoptosis inhibitor involved in NF-kappaB-mediated cell survival. *Science* 1998;281:998–1001.
109. Zong WX, Edelstein LC, Chen C, Bash J, Gelinas C. The prosurvival Bcl-2 homolog Bfl-1/A1 is a direct transcriptional target of NF-kappaB that blocks TNFalpha-induced apoptosis. *Genes Dev* 1999;13:382–387.
110. Rothe M, Pan MG, Henzel WJ, Ayres TM, Goeddel DV. The TNFR2-TRAF signaling complex contains two novel proteins related to baculoviral inhibitor of apoptosis proteins. *Cell* 1995;83:1243–1252.
111. Shu HB, Takeuchi M, Goeddel DV. The tumor necrosis factor receptor 2 signal transducers TRAF2 and c-IAP1 are components of the tumor necrosis factor receptor 1 signaling complex. *Proc Natl Acad Sci USA* 1996;93:13,973–13,978.
112. Chu ZL, McKinsey TA, Liu L, Gentry JJ, Malim MH, Ballard DW. Suppression of tumor necrosis factor-induced cell death by inhibitor of apoptosis c-IAP2 is under NF-kappaB control. *Proc Natl Acad Sci USA* 1997;94:10,057–10,062.
113. Deveraux QL, Reed JC. IAP family proteins: suppressors of apoptosis. *Genes Dev* 1999; 13:239–252.
114. Lee SY, Lee SY, Choi Y. TRAF-interacting protein (TRIP): a novel component of the tumor necrosis factor receptor (TNFR)- and CD30-TRAF signaling complexes that inhibits TRAF2-mediated NF-kappaB activation. *J Exp Med* 1997,185:1275–1285.

115. Nagata S. Apoptosis by death factor. *Cell* 1997;88:355–365.
116. Franco JL, Ghosh P, Wiltrout RH, Carter CR, Zea AH, Momozaki N, et al. Partial degradation of T-cell signal transduction molecules by contaminating granulocytes during protein extraction of splenic T cells from tumor-bearing mice. *Cancer Res* 1995; 55:3840–3846.
117. Kurt RA, Urba WJ, Smith JW, Schoof DD. Peripheral T lymphocytes from women with breast cancer exhibit abnormal protein expression of several signaling molecules. *Int J Cancer* 1998;78:16–20.
118. Uzzo RG, Clark PE, Rayman P, Bloom T, Rybicki L, Novick AC, et al. Alterations in NFkappaB activation in T lymphocytes of patients with renal cell carcinoma. *J Natl Cancer Inst* 1999;91:718–721.
119. Gati A, Guerra N, Giron-Michel J, Azzarone B, Angevin E, Moretta A, et al. Tumor cells regulate the lytic activity of tumor-specific cytotoxic T lymphocytes by modulating the inhibitory natural killer receptor function. *Cancer Res* 2001;61:3240–3244.
120. Batra RK, Lin Y, Sharma S, Dohadwala M, Luo J, Pold M, et al. Non-small cell lung cancer-derived soluble mediators enhance apoptosis in activated T lymphocytes through an I kappa B kinase-dependent mechanism. *Cancer Res* 2003;63:642–646.
121. Ling W, Rayman P, Uzzo R, Clark P, Kim HJ, Tubbs R, et al. Impaired activation of NFkappaB in T cells from a subset of renal cell carcinoma patients is mediated by inhibition of phosphorylation and degradation of the inhibitor, IkappaBalpha. *Blood* 1998;92:1334–1341.
122. Page S, Fischer C, Baumgartner B, Haas M, Kreusel U, Loidl G, et al. 4-Hydroxynonenal prevents NF-kappaB activation and tumor necrosis factor expression by inhibiting IkappaB phosphorylation and subsequent proteolysis. *J Biol Chem* 1999;274:11,611–11,618.
123. Ng CS, Novick AC, Tannenbaum CS, Bukowski RM, Finke JH. Mechanisms of immune evasion by renal cell carcinoma: tumor-induced T-lymphocyte apoptosis and NFkappaB suppression. *Urology* 2002;1:9–14.

8 The Role of Tumor Gangliosides in the Immune Dysfunction of Cancer

Stephan Ladisch, MD

CONTENTS

1. INTRODUCTION

Tumor formation is a complex multi-step process that is influenced by many factors. Among these, transformation and tumorigenicity are two phenotypic characteristics of cells that are under separate genetic control *(1)*. Transformation indicates that a cell line is immortalized, and capable of proliferating independently and indefinitely in vitro. In contrast, tumorigenicity demands that transformed cells proliferate in vivo, resist elimination by the syngeneic normal host, and form progressively growing tumors. It is highly likely—and increasingly recognized—that local tumor cell–host interactions influence the initial steps of tumor formation.

From: *Current Clinical Oncology: Cancer Immunotherapy at the Crossroads: How Tumors Evade Immunity and What Can Be Done*
Edited by: J. H. Finke and R. M. Bukowski © Humana Press Inc., Totowa, NJ

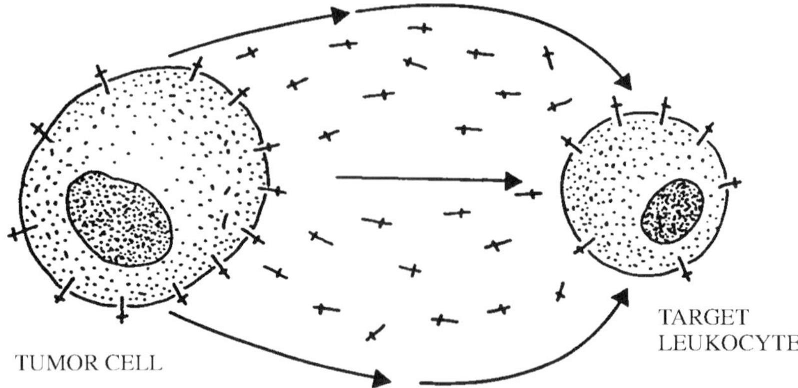

Fig. 1. The dynamic process of ganglioside shedding-tumor release, microenvironmental localization, and target-cell binding.

These interactions take place in the tumor-cell microenvironment. Although much progress has been made in understanding the process of transformation, less is known about the complex tumor cell–host interactions in the in vivo microenvironment of the tumor, which must result in resistance to elimination by the syngeneic normal host. An evolution in thought has been the recognition that the release of soluble circulating factors by tumors can markedly alter the host immune system *(2)*. The specific tumor–host interaction that is the subject of this chapter is the process of release, or shedding, of certain soluble immunosuppressive membrane molecules known as gangliosides. The initial hypothesis underlying work in this field, schematically depicted in Fig. 1, is that tumor gangliosides are released into the immediate extracellular microenvironment of the tumor cell, where they can bind to infiltrating leukocytes and inhibit their function (*3*; Fig. 1).

Evidence from several experimental approaches supports this concept of inhibition of the cellular immune response by tumor gangliosides. Many laboratories have contributed to developing the concept that tumor gangliosides are biologically relevant immunomodulatory molecules, and this chapter highlights only several selected recent studies, with the goal of presenting some evidence for each of the different individual steps depicted by the schema in Fig. 1.

2. GANGLIOSIDE STRUCTURE

Prior to addressing immunomodulatory properties of these tumor-derived molecules, an understanding of their structure is useful. Marked structural differences characterize many gangliosides of tumor origin—a diverse group of molecules—in comparison with gangliosides of normal tissues *(4)*. Further-

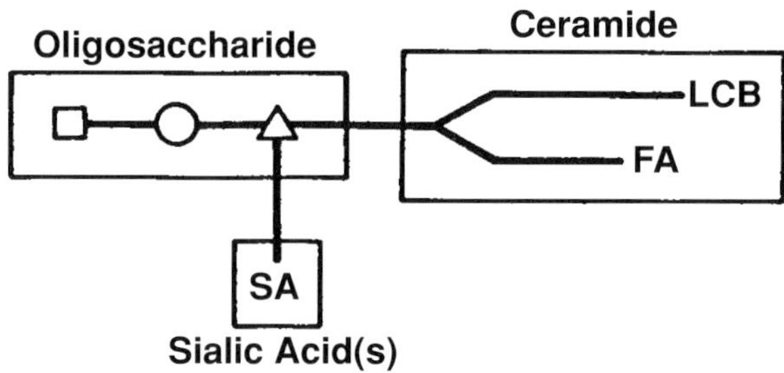

Fig. 2. Schematic depiction of ganglioside structure.

more, ganglioside immunosuppressive activity is highly dependent upon ganglioside molecular structure *(5,6)*.

The ganglioside molecule consists of three elements (Fig. 2): an oligosaccharide core to which one or more sialic acids and a hydrophobic lipid (ceramide) are attached, consisting of a long-chain base (LCB) and a fatty acid (FA). Oligosaccharide heterogeneity and sialic acid diversity (either *N*-glycolyl or *N*-acetyl neuraminic acid) are known. Less appreciated has been the structural diversity of the ceramide portion of the molecule, especially of tumor gangliosides.

Ceramide structural differences may occur both in LCB and in the FA, and consist of three types of variations: length of the carbon chain, degree of unsaturation, and substitution by hydroxyl groups. All these have been shown to influence ganglioside immunosuppressive activity. The major LBC structures of normal human brain gangliosides are d18:1 and d20:1, and the major FA structures are 18:0 and 20:0. The major alteration in tumor ganglioside ceramide structure is significant variation in fatty acyl chain length *(7)*. This complexity of structure, especially in tumor gangliosides, has implications for immunological activity, and the particular importance of ceramide structure is suggested by studies showing differential immunosuppressive effects of ceramide subspecies of tumor gangliosides *(6)*.

3. SHEDDING OF TUMOR GANGLIOSIDES

The first step in the interaction of soluble tumor-derived gangliosides with normal leukocytes is their release by the tumor cell. This is consistent with the general concept proposed a number of years ago, that the release of molecules by tumor cells may be important in the evasion of host immune responses by tumors *(8)*. Shedding of cell-surface gangliosides is a prominent component of tumor ganglioside metabolism characteristic of numerous types of tumor cells, including neuroblastoma *(9,10)*, lymphoma *(3)*, melanoma *(8)*, and leukemia *(11)*. Brain tumor cells have also recently been found to shed gangliosides

(12,13). In humans, shedding has been documented in the peripheral circulation (e.g., in neuroblastoma) and most recently in the cerebrospinal fluid of patients with medulloblastoma and astrocytomas, where a mean threefold elevation of the brain tumor-associated ganglioside GD3 was found *(13)*. The biological significance of tumor ganglioside shedding has been widely recognized *(14)* as shedding of tumor-derived gangliosides have been shown to influence tumor progression. In patients with neuroblastoma, for example, shedding of tumor GD2 ganglioside is strongly correlated with the incidence and rate of tumor progression. Patients with the highest circulating levels (≥568 pmol/mL) had a shorter median progression-free survival time (9 mo) than patients with the lowest GD2 levels (103 pmol/mL; 28 mo), demonstrating a direct relationship between quantitative aspects of ganglioside shedding in human neuroblastoma and tumor progression in vivo *(15)*. Other studies are consistent with earlier observations of a correlation between increased circulating ganglioside concentrations and tumor burden *(16)* and the presence of specific tumor-derived gangliosides in the circulation *(9,17)*. Although correlative, these studies further support the possibility that tumor gangliosides, because of their intrinsic immunological properties, have a high potential to develop a mechanism by which tumors escape host immune responses.

4. TRANSPORT OF TUMOR GANGLIOSIDES

Once released by tumor cells, how are shed tumor gangliosides found in vivo? To address this question, the serum localization of shed G_{D2}, a major ganglioside of human neuroblastoma, was traced. Sera from patients with neuroblastoma tumors were separated into the lipoprotein fractions (very low-density lipoproteins [VLDL], low-density lipoproteins [LDL], high-density lipoproteins [HDL]) and lipoprotein-depleted serum. 73% of the total G_{D2} was present in the LDL fraction, VLDL and HDL contained 21% and 6%, respectively. Significantly, lipoprotein-depleted serum was devoid of G_{D2}. Thus, shed neuroblastoma tumor gangliosides are exclusively associated with the serum lipoprotein (and predominantly LDL) fractions in vivo *(18)*. These findings have implications for the immunological detection of these molecules, and ultimately for the development of approaches to their removal from the circulation of patients with cancer. However, ganglioside–lipoprotein binding is relatively weak, with most of the LDL-bound gangliosides (the major lipoprotein to which gangliosides are bound) being loosely associated—e.g., adsorbed to rather than inserted in the lipoprotein particle *(19)*. This makes them easily available to target cells. Further, melanoma-tumor gangliosides associated with LDL were as active in suppressing human lymphoproliferative responses as the same gangliosides presented in micellar (unbound) form *(20)*. Thus, both lipoprotein-associated tumor gangliosides and free tumor gangliosides can inhibit cellular immune responses in vitro.

5. HISTORICAL PERSPECTIVE ON IMMUNOSUPPRESSION BY TUMOR GANGLIOSIDES

The consideration of gangliosides as molecules that may regulate the cellular immune response originated more than two decades ago with studies of brain gangliosides. The initial studies documented the inhibition of mitogen and antigen-induced lymphoproliferative responses by normal brain gangliosides *(21–23)*. The first studies of the immunosuppressive activity of tumor-derived gangliosides of the murine YAC-1 lymphoma demonstrated that tumor gangliosides strongly suppressed the antitumor-induced cellular immune response in vitro *(3)*. These findings were confirmed by others *(24)*, leading to further development of the concept *(3)* that tumor-derived gangliosides may adversely affect host immune responses in vivo *(25,26)*. Once again, this immunosuppressive activity is greatly influenced by ganglioside structure *(5,6)*, and certain ganglioside structures that are only minor components in normal tissue but are frequently major species in tumors are in fact biologically very active ganglioside species *(5)*.

6. MECHANISMS OF IMMUNOSUPPRESSION

Characteristic effects on two leukocyte-cell populations have been reported: the accessory-cell and the lymphocyte. Briefly, gangliosides inhibit the accessory function *(27)* tumor necrosis factor (TNF) production *(28)*, and other functions *(29)* of adherent macrophage-enriched peripheral-blood mononuclear cells (PBMC). Gangliosides induce a reversible state of unresponsiveness of antigen-processing cells to antigenic stimulation, and such a mechanism is likely to be operative in the local environment of the tumor in vivo *(27)*. Gangliosides impair the responsiveness of human lymphocytes to activation by a direct interference with the proliferation of mitogen-activated lymphocytes *(30,31)*. This has been demonstrated to be the result of interference with IL-2-dependent cell proliferation, probably by direct binding of gangliosides to IL-2 *(32)*, and by blocking the IL-2/IL-2-receptor interaction *(33)*. Gangliosides also inhibit cytotoxic effector function *(34)* and B-cell immunoglobulin production *(35)*. Recently, modulatory effects of gangliosides on the expression of T-cell-surface membrane proteins have been described—e.g., the modulation of CD4 by exogenous gangliosides *(36,37)*.

Considering the first step in the cellular immune response, the antigen-presenting cell (APC) function of monocytes consists of effective antigen processing (intracellular) and presentation (intercellular). Preincubation of purified human monocytes with gangliosides in vitro, either in free form or in liposomes, reversibly blocks human PBMC proliferative responses to tetanus toxoid *(27)*, and this was shown to be by an effect on monocyte antigen processing/presentation. To elucidate the cellular mechanism of inhibition, the

APC function of human monocytes preincubated with human gangliosides was evaluated in several assays of MHC class II-restricted T-cell proliferation *(27)*. Monocytes exposed to 100-μ*M* gangliosides for 48 h and then pulsed with tetanus toxoid (TT) were unable to trigger T-cell proliferation. However, ganglioside-exposed monocytes did not act as suppressor cells, since they did not inhibit T-cell proliferative responses to immobilized anti-CD3 or to antigen-pulsed control monocytes. If monocytes were first pulsed with TT to allow antigen processing and then exposed to gangliosides, they still failed to trigger T-cell proliferation, indicating that inhibition was occurring after antigen processing was complete. Stimulation by a TT peptide fragment that does not require processing was also inhibited by exposure of monocytes to gangliosides, as was the proliferative response of purified T cells to purified ganglioside-exposed allogeneic monocytes. These results show that exogenous gangliosides bind to monocytes and interfere with a step in the intercellular process of presentation (adhesion, antigen-specific recognition, and costimulation) of fully formed stimulating antigens by monocytes. Flow cytometric analysis revealed that gangliosides completely inhibit antigen-induced monocyte expression of CD80, but not of HLA-DR or of the adhesion molecules ICAM-1 or LFA-3 (unpublished results). This suggests that gangliosides, shed by tumor cells and binding to tumor-infiltrating monocytes in vivo, may inhibit monocyte APC function in part by interfering with delivery of the costimulatory signal. This concept is supported by recent findings that neuroblastoma-derived gangliosides inhibit the generation of the potent APC, dendritic cells (DC), from murine bone-marrow precursors *(38)*, and that lipopolysaccharide (LPS)-stiumulated DCs exposed to purified ganglioside GD1a also demonstrate inhibited expression of costimulatory molecules *(39)*.

Gangliosides also affect cytokine production, and activation of cells by cytokines. The initial studies in this area were those that identified a relationship between gangliosides and IL-2 *(30–32)*. Subsequently, gangliosides were found to suppress TNF production by human monocytes *(28)*, and brain-derived gangliosides have been shown to regulate the cytokine production and proliferation of activated T cells *(40)*. Specifically in this latter case, IL-2 and interferon gamma gene transcription were blocked, without inhibition of production of IL-4 and IL-10 mRNA. These findings were believed to be attributed to an interference of gangliosides with the activation of NF-κB in mitogen-stimulated T cells *(40)*.

The fascinating link between tumor-derived gangliosides and impaired T-cell activation has been amplified by the exciting recent work of Uzzo et al. *(41,42)*, which built upon an earlier observation that impaired NF-κB activation characterizes the circulating T cells of patients with renal cell carcinoma (RCC). The ability to reproduce this impairment by tumor-derived soluble products, and specifically by purified gangliosides, has linked suppressed NF-κB binding in

T cells to ganglioside-induced inhibition of expression of IL-2 and interferon gamma. These findings in RCC (reported in detail in Chapter 7) have thus identified a specific antitumor immune response in humans to be affected by gangliosides *(41,42)*, further underscoring the biological importance of shed tumor-derived gangliosides.

Finally, there is some evidence that certain gangliosides may stimulate, rather than suppress, some immune responses. For example, enhancement of tumor necrosis factor-alpha (TNF-α) production, by the ganglioside GM2, was observed in human monocyte cultures *(43)*. This is in contrast to an inhibitory effect of the same ganglioside on spontaneous immunoglobulin production *(44)*. Specific gangliosides, at very low concentrations, have also been shown to enhance the production of certain cytokines. In human peripheral-blood T cells, the gangliosides GDlb, GTlb, and GQlb (100 nm), but not other gangliosides, enhanced PHA-induced IL-2 and IFN-γ secretion of peripheral-blood T cells several-fold compared with controls, while they decreased PHA-induced IL-4 secretion and IL-5, again compared with controls *(45)*. How these findings relate to the general observation of suppressive—not stimulatory—activity of higher concentrations of gangliosides, as well as to the issues of structure/function relationships has not yet been elucidated, but it is clear that there may be widely divergent effects of different gangliosides on production and action of different cytokines, a subject that is currently under intense investigation.

7. BIOLOGICAL SIGNIFICANCE OF TUMOR GANGLIOSIDE IMMUNOSUPPRESSION

Because of their multiple biological effects, gangliosides can be viewed as a new class of intercellular signaling molecules. As intercellular signaling molecules, gangliosides released by tumor cells act through several mechanisms: they can associate with antigen-processing/presenting cells to inhibit antigen presentation, interact with lymphokines to inhibit cytokine-mediated lymphocyte proliferation, alter the expression of cell-surface-receptor molecules so that the cell becomes less responsive to proliferative stimuli, or—as most recently suggested—also affect intracellular signal transduction after insertion into the target-cell membrane *(4)*. All these lines of evidence make it increasingly likely that gangliosides that are shed by tumor cells affect host immunologic responses in vivo. The lack of an unequivocal demonstration of tumor ganglioside-induced immunosuppression in vivo, and specifically of inhibition of host antitumor immune responses to a syngeneic tumor, are not fully understood.

The importance of the intact cellular immune response in vivo in the process of tumor rejection is widely accepted, and underscored by the demonstration that cytotoxic T lymphocytes (CTL) generated in response to immunization with specific tumor antigens are capable of eliminating tumor cells in vivo *(46)*.

Attempts to augment the immune response, such as by the pharmacologic use of cytokines *(47)*, further emphasize the significance attached to an intact cellular immune response in patients with cancer. Interference with the proliferative and cytotoxic phases of the cellular immune response at the site of tumor-cell growth in vivo, such as that caused by gangliosides shed by tumor cells, may be important in disrupting the local host response and thereby allowing further tumor growth. Thus, in vivo studies of ganglioside inhibition of immune responses to syngeneic tumor cells, are a critical next step in determining the specific role of gangliosides in the alteration of tumor immunity in the host.

8. GANGLIOSIDE IMMUNOSUPPRESSION IN VIVO

The potent in vitro inhibition of human cellular immune responses by tumor gangliosides has led to studies that determine the inhibitory effects of tumor gangliosides on the allogeneic immune response in vivo. These studies used a murine model of the allogeneic immune response developed by Kroczek et al. *(48)*. This experimental system measures the cellular immune response in the lymph node draining the injection site of a foreign antigen in the form of allogeneic cells. In this model, 4 d after injection of allogeneic (C3H) spleen cells into the hind footpad of Balb/c mice, the cellular immune response in the draining popliteal lymph nodes was evidenced as an increase in lymph-node mass (twofold), lymphocyte number (sixfold) and lymphocyte DNA synthesis (sixfold). Purified human neuroblastoma gangliosides (10 nmol) co-injected with the stimulating allogeneic cells significantly suppressed this in vivo immune response: the increase in the lymph-node mass was reduced by 65%, the increase in lymphocyte number (4.0×10^6 cells/node) was almost completely inhibited (1.1×10^6 cells/node), and in vitro [^{3}H]thymidine uptake by the lymphocytes recovered in vivo was reduced by 80% *(49)*.

The demonstration of the effect of purified neuroblastoma gangliosides on the allogeneic response led to further studies of the role of tumor gangliosides in inhibiting host antitumor immune responses in experimental models in vivo, and two lines of supporting evidence have been developed. The first was provided by a comprehensive study to evaluate the role of tumor-derived gangliosides in modifying the host immune response to a tumor in a fully syngeneic murine tumor model, the FBL-3 lymphoma. The impact of shed gangliosides on the in vivo antitumor immune response was tested in this fully autochthonous system (FBL-3 erythroleukemia cells, C57BL/6 mice, and highly purified FBL-3-cell gangliosides). The major FBL-3 ganglioside was identified as GMIb by mass spectrometry. Substantial ganglioside shedding (90 pmol/108 cells/h), a requisite for their inhibition of the immune function of tumor-infiltrating leukocytes (TIL), was detected. Immunosuppression by FBL-3 gangliosides was potent; 5–20 m*M* inhibited the tumor-specific secondary proliferative response (80–100%) and suppressed the generation of tumor-specific CTLs (97% reduction of FBL-3 cell lysis at an E:T ratio of 100:1). In vivo, coinjection of 10 nmol of FBL-3 gangliosides with a primary FBL-3 cell immunization led to a reduced response to a secondary challenge (the increase in the draining popliteal lymph-node mass, cell number, and lymphocyte thymidine incorporation were lowered by 70%, 69%, and 72%, respectively). Coinjection of gangliosides with a secondary tumor challenge led to a 61%, 74%, and 42% reduction of the increase in lymph-node mass, cell number, and thymidine uptake and a 63–74% inhibition of the increase of draining lymph-node T cells (CD3+), B cells (CD19+), and dendritic cells [DC]/macrophages (Mac-3+). Overall, these experiments provided the first in vivo evidence that tumor-derived gangliosides inhibit syngeneic antitumor immune responses, and they implicated these molecules as a potent factors in promoting tumor formation and progression *(50)*.

The second recent approach has been to attempt to directly link changes in glycosphingolipid metabolism to tumor formation. This has become possible with the recent development of inhibitors of glycosphingolipid synthesis, which have been shown to decrease ganglioside synthesis and shedding *(51)*. Although they do not directly address the issue of tumor ganglioside induction of immunosuppression, these studies tested the hypothesis that the interaction of shed tumor gangliosides with host cells, in the tumor microenvironment, influences tumor development. Once again, a syngeneic tumor system was studied *(52)*.

In this study, the ability of tumor cells that were pharmacologically depleted of gangliosides to form tumors in mice was tested using a ganglioside-rich line subline of B16 murine melanoma, MEB4. PPPP (D-1-threo-1-phenyl-2-hexadecanoylamino-3-pyrrolidino-1-propanol-HCl) *(53)* was used to deplete the cells of endogenous gangliosides by inhibiting glucosylceramide synthase. Tumor formation was evaluated twice a week for 10 wk after the intradermal injection of tumor cells, and metastatic potential 4 wk after tail-vein injection of tumor cells. Reduction of the ganglioside content of MEB4 cells (which was not cytotoxic to cells and did not inhibit cell proliferation in vitro) markedly reduced the ability of these cells to form tumors; only 40% of mice injected intradermally with 10^5 ganglioside-depleted MEB4 cells developed tumors, compared with 100% of mice injected with 10^5 control MEB4 cells. In addition, unmanipulated MEB4 cells were highly metastatic, compared to ganglioside-depleted MEB4. When 2×10^5 ganglioside-depleted MEB4 cells were injected intravenously, a mean of 5 pulmonary metastases were detected per mouse, vs a mean of 25 for control MEB4 cells *(52)*. Thus, although a link between inhibition of tumor formation by tumor-cell ganglioside depletion and a subsequent reduction in ganglioside-induced suppression of the antitumor immune response has not been definitely established in these studies, the evidence strongly links ganglioside metabolism to tumor formation.

In conclusion, the compelling evidence from many laboratories implicating tumor gangliosides in inhibiting host immune responses, and the demonstration of in vivo immunosuppression by human tumor gangliosides, suggests that future studies should be undertaken to eliminate these molecules in vivo (e.g., removal from the circulation, neutralization by monoclonal antibodies, or therapeutic modification of ganglioside biosynthesis and shedding, as described previously) as a potential therapeutic approach to the treatment of cancer.

ACKNOWLEDGMENT

This work was supported by grants ROI CA42361 and ROI CA61010 from the National Cancer Institute, and by The Children's Cancer Foundation and the Phi Beta Psi sorority.

REFERENCES

1. Stanbridge EJ, Der CJ, Doersen CJ, et al. Human cell hybrids: analysis of transformation and tumorigenicity. *Science* 1982;215:252–259.
2. Black PH. Shedding from the cell surface of normal and cancer cells. *Adv Cancer Res* 1980;32:75–199.
3. Ladisch S, Gillard B, Wong C, Ulsh L. Shedding and immunoregulatory activity of YAC-1 lymphoma cell gangliosides. *Cancer Res* 1983;43:3808–3813.
4. Hakomori S. New directions in cancer therapy based on aberrant expression of glycosphingolipids: anti-adhesion and ortho-signaling therapy. *Cancer Cells* 1991;3:461–470.
5. Ladisch S, Becker H, Ulsh L. Immunosuppression by human gangliosides: I. Relationship of carbohydrate structure to the inhibition of T cell responses. *Biochim Biophys Acta* 1992;1125:180–188.
6. Ladisch S, Li R, Olson E. Ceramide structure predicts tumor ganglioside immunosuppressive activity. *Proc Natl Acad Sci USA* 1994;91:1974–1978.
7. Ladisch S, Sweeley CC, Becker H, Gage D. Aberrant fatty acyl alpha-hydroxylation in human neuroblastoma tumor gangliosides. *J Biol Chem* 1989;264:12,097–12,105.
8. Bernhard H, Meyer zum Buschenfelde KH, Dippold WG. Ganglioside GD3 shedding by human malignant melanoma cells. *Int J Cancer* 1989;44:155–160.
9. Ladisch S, Wu ZL. Detection of a tumour-associated ganglioside in plasma of patients with neuroblastoma. *Lancet* 1985;1:136–138.
10. Ladisch S, Wu ZL, Feig S, et al. Shedding of GD2 ganglioside by human neuroblastoma. *Int J Cancer* 1987;39:73–76.
11. Merritt WD, Der-Minassian V, Reaman GH. Increased GD3 ganglioside in plasma of children with T-cell acute lymphoblastic leukemia. *Leukemia* 1994;8:816–822.
12. Chang F, Li R, Ladisch S. Shedding of gangliosides by human medulloblastoma cells. *Exp Cell Res* 1997;234:341–346.
13. Ladisch S, Chang F, Li R, et al. Detection of medulloblastoma and astrocytoma-associated ganglioside GD3 in cerebrospinal fluid. *Cancer Lett* 1997;120:71–78.
14. Hakomori S. Tumor malignancy defined by aberrant glycosylation and sphingo(glyco)lipid metabolism. *Cancer Res* 1996;56:5309–5318.
15. Valentino L, Moss T, Olson E, et al. Shed tumor gangliosides and progression of human neuroblastoma. *Blood* 1990;75:1564–1567.

16. Kloppel TM, Keenan TW, Freeman MJ, Morre DJ. Glycolipid-bound sialic acid in serum: increased levels in mice and humans bearing mammary carcinomas. *Proc Natl Acad Sci USA* 1977;74:3011–3013.
17. Portoukalian J, Zwingelstein G, Abdul-Malak N, Dore JF. Alteration of gangliosides in plasma and red cells of humans bearing melanoma tumors. *Biochem Biophys Res Commun* 1978;85:916–920.
18. Valentino LA, Ladisch S. Localization of shed human tumor gangliosides: association with serum lipoproteins. *Cancer Res* 1992;52:810–814.
19. Mikhailenko IA, Dubrovskaya SA, Korepanova OB, et al. Interaction of low-density lipoproteins with gangliosides. *Biochim Biophys Acta* 1991;1085:299–305.
20. Dumontet C, Rebbaa A, Bienvenu J, Portoukalian J. Inhibition of immune cell proliferation and cytokine production by lipoprotein-bound gangliosides. *Cancer Immunol Immunother* 1994;38:311–316.
21. Miller HC, Esselman WJ. Modulation of the immune response by antigen-reactive lymphocytes after cultivation with gangliosides. *J Immunol* 1975;115:839–843.
22. Ryan JL, Shinitzky M. Possible role for glycosphingolipids in the control of immune responses. *Eur J Immunol* 1979;9:171–175.
23. Whisler RL, Yates AJ. Regulation of lymphocyte responses by human gangliosides. I. Characteristics of inhibitory effects and the induction of impaired activation. *J Immunol* 1980;125:2106–2111.
24. Gonwa TA, Westrick MA, Macher BA. Inhibition of mitogen- and antigen-induced lymphocyte activation by human leukemia cell gangliosides. *Cancer Res* 1984;44:3467–3470.
25. Ladisch S, Kitada S, Hays EF. Gangliosides shed by tumor cells enhance tumor formation in mice. *J Clin Investig* 1987;79:1879–1882.
26. Hachida M, Irie R, Morton DL. Significant immunosuppressive effect of ganglioside GM3 in organ transplantation. *Transplant Proc* 1990;22:1663–1665.
27. Ladisch S, Ulsh L, Gillard B, Wong C. Modulation of the immune response by gangliosides. Inhibition of adherent monocyte accessory function in vitro. *J Clin Investig* 1984; 74:2074–2081.
28. Ziegler-Heitbrock HW, Kafferlein E, Haas JG, et al. Gangliosides suppress tumor necrosis factor production in human monocytes. *J Immunol* 1992;148:1753–1758.
29. Hoon DS, Jung T, Naungayan J, et al. Modulation of human macrophage functions by gangliosides. *Immunol Lett* 1989;20:269–275.
30. Merritt WD, Bailey JM, Pluznik DH. Inhibition of interleukin-2-dependent cytotoxic T-lymphocyte growth by gangliosides. *Cell Immunol* 1984;89:1–10.
31. Sharom FJ, Chiu AL, Chu JW. Membrane gangliosides modulate interleukin-2-stimulated T-lymphocyte proliferation. *Biochim Biophys Acta* 1991;1094:35–42.
32. Robb RJ. The suppressive effect of gangliosides upon IL 2-dependent proliferation as a function of inhibition of IL 2-receptor association. *J Immunol* 1986;136:971–976.
33. Lu P, Sharom FJ. Immunosuppression by YAC-1 lymphoma: role of shed gangliosides. *Cell Immunol* 1996;173:22–32.
34. Prokazova NV, Dyatlovitskaya EV, Bergelson LD. Sialylated lactosylceramides. Possible inducers of non-specific immunosuppression and atherosclerotic lesions. *Eur J Biochem* 1988;172:1–6.
35. Kimata H, Yoshida A. Differential effects of gangliosides on Ig production and proliferation by human B cells. *Blood* 1994;84:1193–1200.
36. Repke H, Barber E, Ulbricht S, et al. Ganglioside-induced CD4 endocytosis occurs independent of serine phosphorylation and is accompanied by dissociation of P56lck. *J Immunol* 1992;149:2585–2591.
37. Offner H, Thieme T, Vandenbark AA. Gangliosides induce selective modulation of CD4 from helper T lymphocytes. *J Immunol* 1987;139:3295–3305.

38. Shurin GV, Shurin MR, Bykovskaia S, et al. Neuroblastoma-derived gangliosides inhibit dendritic cell generation and function. *Cancer Res* 2001;61:363–369.
39. Shen W, Ladisch S. Ganglioside GD1a impedes lipopolysacchride-induced maturation of human dendritic cells. *Cellular Immunology* 2003, in press.
40. Irani DN, Lin KI, Griffin DE. Brain-derived gangliosides regulate the cytokine production and proliferation of activated T cells. *J Immunol* 1996;157:4333–4340.
41. Uzzo RG, Rayman P, Kolenko V, et al. Renal cell carcinoma-derived gangliosides suppress nuclear factor-kappaB activation in T cells. *J Clin Investig* 1999;104:769–776.
42. Ng CS, Novick AC, Tannenbaum CS, et al. Mechanisms of immune evasion by renal cell carcinoma: tumor-induced T-lymphocyte apoptosis and NFkappaB suppression. *Urology* 2002;59:9–14.
43. Mizutani K, Oka N, Akiguchi I, et al. Enhancement of TNF-alpha production by ganglioside GM2 in human mononuclear cell culture. *Neuroreport* 1999;10:703–706.
44. Kimata H, Yoshida A. Inhibition of spontaneous immunoglobulin production by ganglioside GM2 in human B cells. *Clin Immunol Immunopathol* 1996;79:197–202.
45. Kanda N, Watanabe S. Gangliosides GD1b, GT1b, and GQ1b enhance IL-2 and IFN-gamma production and suppress IL-4 and IL-5 production in phytohemagglutinin-stimulated human T cells. *J Immunol* 2001;166:72–80.
46. Engers HD, Sorenson GD, Terres G, et al. Functional activity in vivo of effector T cell populations. I. Antitumor activity exhibited by allogeneic mixed leukocyte culture cells. *J Immunol* 1982;129:1292–1298.
47. Borden EC, Sondel PM. Lymphokines and cytokines as cancer treatment. Immunotherapy realized. *Cancer* 1990;65:800–814.
48. Kroczek RA, Black CD, Barbet J, et al. Induction of IL-2 receptor expression in vivo. Response to allogeneic cells. *Transplantation* 1987;44:547–553.
49. Li R, Villacreses N, Ladisch S. Human tumor gangliosides inhibit murine immune responses in vivo. *Cancer Res* 1995;55:211–214.
50. McKallip R, Li R, Ladisch S. Tumor gangliosides inhibit the tumor-specific immune response. *J Immunol* 1999;163:3718–3726.
51. Inokuchi J, Jimbo M, Momosaki K, et al. Inhibition of experimental metastasis of murine Lewis lung carcinoma by an inhibitor of glucosylceramide synthase and its possible mechanism of action. *Cancer Res* 1990;50:6731–6737.
52. Deng W, Li R, Ladisch S. Influence of cellular ganglioside depletion on tumor formation. *J Natl Cancer Inst* 2000;92:912–917.
53. Lee L, Abe A, Shayman JA. Improved inhibitors of glucosylceramide synthase. *J Biol Chem* 1999;274:14,662–14,669.

9 Interleukin-10-Induced Immune Suppression in Cancer

Arvin S. Yang, PhD
and Edmund C. Lattime, PhD

CONTENTS

1. INTRODUCTION

The generation of an effective immune response to tumors and/or non-tumor antigens requires the presence of an appropriate and recognizable antigen, antigen-presenting cells (APC) such as dendritic cells (DC), and a supportive cytokine milieu. Cytokines present at the immunization site—or in the case of tumors, the tumor site—have been shown to have a marked effect on the magnitude as well as the nature of the response. They play a role in recruiting appropriate cells to the site, activating APCs, and directing whether the resultant T-cell response generates a cell-mediated or humoral event *(1,2)*. Therefore, the combination of cytokines naturally present or provided by immunotherapeutic intervention can be a major factor in determining the success of the resultant immune response in eliminating tumor or pathogens. In addition to their use in immune interventions to positively effect immune responses, tumors have exploited the regulatory actions of certain cytokines such as interleukin (IL)-10, transforming growth factor (TGF)-β, and vascular endothelial growth factor (VEGF) to escape effective immune recognition. This chapter focuses on tumor-induced IL-10 and its immunosuppressive effects on adaptive T-cell antitumor responses. IL-10 was originally described as cytokine synthesis inhibitory factor (CSIF),

From: *Current Clinical Oncology: Cancer Immunotherapy at the Crossroads: How Tumors Evade Immunity and What Can Be Done*
Edited by: J. H. Finke and R. M. Bukowski © Humana Press Inc., Totowa, NJ

which was produced by mouse Th2 cells and inhibited activation and cytokine production by Th1 cells *(3)*. IL-10 is known to have multiple mechanisms of action, which either enhance or inhibit effective antitumor immune responses—and as our studies and others have demonstrated, the presence of IL-10 at the tumor site can dramatically effect immune recognition and subsequent development of antitumor effector function.

1.1. Cytokines and the Regulation of Cell-Mediated Immunity

There are two basic types of immune responses, which vary in efficacy in an antitumor response. The humoral or type 2-mediated responses are associated with defense against extracellular and soluble pathogens, and type 1 or cell-mediated responses are developed to protect against intracellular pathogens and malignant cells. Two polarized sets of mouse T-helper (Th) cells, Th1, and Th2, secrete distinct cytokine patterns that correspond to their associated function in directing cellular or humoral responses *(4)*. Furthermore, the type 1 and type 2 cytokines are mutually inhibitory for the differentiation and effector function of the reciprocal phenotype. Although best described and perhaps more mutually exclusive in murine systems, humans have similar function-associated cytokine expression. Th1 cells secrete IL-2, IL-12, IL-18, and interferon (IFN)-γ, which promote cellular immunity. Th2 cells are associated with IL-4, IL-5, and IL-10 secretion, which promote B-cell proliferation, differentiation, and Ig class switching. IL-12 is also produced by APCs, including DC and monocytes, which are inducers of IFN-γ production by T cells *(5)*. Th1 cell-secreted IL-12-induced IFN-γ suppresses IL-4 and effectively suppresses Th2 cells from proliferating. In contrast, Th2-associated IL-10, also produced by T cells, monocytes, and macrophages, has antiinflammatory and potent anti-IFN-γ and anti-IL-12 effects *(6,7)*.

The impact of the modulation of Th1 vs Th2 is arguably best shown in the *Leishmania* parasite system in mice. Inbred mouse strains can be divided into resistant strains that mount an effective cell-mediated response and susceptible strains that predominantly generate a humoral response and succumb to the disease. Following infection with the parasite, Th1 cells from resistant mice were shown to generate IFN-γ associated with the development of host protection, and in susceptible mouse strains, an ineffective type 2 immune response characterized by IL-4 and IL-10 production resulted in a terminal infection *(8)*. Relevant to our goal of "redirecting" antitumor responses, studies from the Scott laboratory demonstrated that administration of IFN-γ at the time of inoculation of the parasite in susceptible mice converted them to the resistant phenotype, and administration of anti-IFN-γ to resistant mice converted them to the susceptible phenotype *(9)*. Similar to the murine *Leishmania* findings, *Mycobacterium leprae* infection in man also reflects the dichotomy between mounting a type 1 or type 2 immune response. Individuals who mount a type 1 response to *Mycobacterium leprae* develop a milder tuberculoid form of the disease, and those who generate a type 2 immune response develop the aggressive lepromatomous form *(10)*.

Type 1 cytokines also support the generation of CD8+ cytotoxic T lymphocytes (CTL), which are believed to be one of the critical effector cells that mediate antitumor effects. The adoptive transfer of tumor-specific CTL has been shown to be effective in treating relevant tumor-bearing syngeneic animals *(11)*. Furthermore, depletion of CD8+ T cells has been shown to prevent immunotherapeutic vaccine-induced antitumor immunity in a number of systems *(12,13)*. Just as CD4 T-helper cells have been shown to have a Th1 and Th2 phenotype, CD8 cytotoxic T cell (Tc) populations can also be distinguished by their ability to secrete cytokines. Tc1 populations secrete IFN-γ and TNF-α, and the Tc2 population secretes IL-4, IL-5, and IL-10 *(14)*. Whereas the in vitro cytotoxicity of Tc1 and Tc2 cells may be similar, only adoptive transfer of Tc1 cells allows antitumor protective immunity *(15)*. CTL populations generated in tumor-bearing hosts can present a Tc2 cell profile. In a mouse model, tumor draining LN cells were separated by their TCR-Vβ expression. A population of TIL that expressed TCR-Vβ5, 7, and 11 were found to secrete IL-10 and have no in vivo antitumor activity *(16)*. Thus, although the generation of a tumor-specific cell-mediated immune response is efficacious in tumor therapy, there is a demonstrable ability for the tumor to skew it toward less effective mediators. These results, together with those from a number of other systems, have resulted in the goal of cancer immunotherapy to induce type 1 cell-mediated immune responses.

1.2. Tumor-Associated IL-10 Expression

Studies performed in our laboratory have focused on the role of Th2 cytokines—and IL-10 in particular—on host antitumor responses following our initial demonstration that tumor biopsies from patients with melanoma *(17,18)* followed by bladder carcinoma *(19)* expressed high levels of IL-10 mRNA, as did the growth of the murine bladder tumor MB49 that was associated with the *in situ* expression of Th2 cytokines *(20)*. Coincident with our biopsy findings, studies from a number of laboratories that have focused primarily on the analysis of tumor-cell lines demonstrated IL-10 mRNA expression in a wide range of human tumors *(21–26)*.

Levels of IL-10 in tumors have been reported to be associated with tumor aggressiveness and survival. As examples, IL-10 was found in basal-cell carcinoma lesions, but IFN-γ and TNF-β were found in benign skin lesions *(27)* and in melanoma, the amount of IL-10 production was reported to correlate with progression vs regression *(28)*. Prolonged survival of patients with IL-10-negative nasopharyngeal carcinomas was nearly 90%, yet only 15% in IL-10-positive groups *(29)*.

Subsequent to our demonstration of IL-10 mRNA in tumor tissue and others, studies from a number of laboratories have examined patient serum for IL-10, and attempted to correlate tissue and/or serum expression with stage of disease and/or prognosis. Studies found increased serum IL-10 levels in patients with various solid tumors, including ovarian, pancreatic, melanoma, and gastric adenocarcinomas *(30–32)*. Although a number of investigators have reported a prognostic value for serum IL-10 levels, such as the increased serum IL-10 and decreased IL-2 found to be associated with progression of adenoma to colorectal carcinoma *(33)*, and a correlation of serum IL-10 with prognosis in renal cell carcinoma *(34,35)*, other studies found no such correlations *(36)*.

Although it is possible that large tumor burdens may indeed be associated with increased IL-10 serum levels that may in turn have systemic immune manifestations, the production of IL-10 in the local tumor environment—e.g., at the interface between tumor and the immune response—is more likely to occur early, and we would suggest a pivotal role in the regulation of antitumor responses.

1.3. IL-10 and the Modulation of Antitumor Immunity

In light of the association of Th2 cytokines, particularly IL-10 with tumors, studies by our laboratory and others have focused on the hypothesis that production of such cytokines in the local tumor environment could result in the inhibition of an effective antitumor response. Our studies addressed the IL-10 question by comparing tumor growth and the induction of tumor-specific immunity in the presence and absence of IL-10. This was made possible by our finding in the MB49 murine bladder model that although MB49 did not produce IL-10 or IL-10 mRNA itself, growth in vivo was associated with IL-10 production at the tumor site by host cells *(37)*. When grown in syngeneic mice, MB49 uniformly progressed and failed to prime for immunity to the expressed tumor-associated HY antigen, as measured in splenic responders. Blockade and/or elimination of IL-10 production using anti-IL-10- or IL-10-knockout mice respectively resulted in the generation of a Th1 IFN-γ-producing response to HY, and in the case of the IL-10 knockouts, rejection of tumor in approx 40% of mice *(37)*, thus demonstrating the profound effect of IL-10 in suppressing the development of antitumor immunity. We further demonstrated that the MB49-associated IL-10 production effected the generation of an immune response to soluble antigens presented at the tumor site. Although β-galactosidase is a potent Th1 response-inducing antigen in C57BL/6 mice, immunization at the IL-10$^+$ MB49 tumor site resulted in a shift to Th2, which was restored in IL-10-knockout mice *(37)*. These findings are consistent with those from the Dubinett group using a transgenic mouse with IL-10 driven by the IL-2 promotor, which demonstrated a similar IL-10-based suppression of immunity to the Lewis lung carcinoma *(38)*. An additional link between Th2 cytokines and tumor progression was found in studies using the murine B-cell leukemia/

lymphoma BCL1 that progressed to lethality in mice responding with a Th2 cytokine profile, but was rejected by those expressing a Th1 profile *(39)*.

As depicted in Fig. 1, IL-10 has effects at the APC as well as T-cell compartments that are active in the generation of immune responses. The principal function of IL-10 as an antiinflammatory molecule *(40)* may be crucial in allowing tumors to escape immune recognition. The danger theory emphasizes the need for danger signals such as those generated in inflammatory responses for the generation of an immune response *(41)*. IL-10 suppresses the production of inflammatory cytokines in activated monocytes and macrophages *(42,43)*. Macrophage release of tumor necrosis factor alpha (TNF-α), IL-1, IL-6, reactive oxygen intermediates, and nitric oxide (NO) have all been shown to be suppressed by IL-10 *(44–46)*. In addition to downregulating production of the pro-inflammatory cytokines, IL-10 also upregulates the release of IL-1-receptor antagonists and soluble TNF-receptor proteins from mononuclear cells and fibroblasts, which may contribute to the suppression of the inflammatory response *(47)*.

1.4. Effects of IL-10 on DCs

Dendritic cells (DCs) are professional APCs that are capable of inducing and modulating adaptive immune responses *(48)*. Although more closely associated with their potent induction ability, DCs also play a role in generating tolerance. This capability of DCs to either induce or tolerize during an immune response makes them pivotal factors in determining the effectiveness of the response. In the case of tumors in which immune escape is critical, the effect of tumors and their products on DC function may be central to the development or lack of development of effective anti-tumor responses. Multiple tumor-induced cytokines, including VEGF, PGE_2, and TGF-β, have been shown to suppress DC function in tumor systems *(49–52)*.

DCs typically reside in tissues in an immature form, where they phagocytize antigens. Danger signals in the form of pro-inflammatory cytokines, cells, and microorganisms then induce the maturation of the DCs that lose the capacity for phagocytosis and migrate to lymph nodes, where they manifest potent antigen-presenting activity. IL-10 has been shown to suppress DC maturation and activation as well as migration. IL-10 has been reported to selectively inhibit maturation of immature DCs, yet it does not affect mature DCs *(53)*. In vitro studies have shown that IL-10 skews the granulocyte-macrophage colony-stimulating factor (GM-CSF)-induced differentiation of monocytes from DC to macrophage-like cells *(53)* and that pre-incubation with IL-10 inhibits the GM-CSF maturation of Langerhans cells, thus blocking their ability to prime for a response to tumor-associated antigens (TAA) *(54)*. In addition, IL-10 selectively induces the apoptosis of CD8α-positive DCs, which are the IL-12-producing DC subset *(55)*, and impairs the ability of DC to produce IL-12 and induce a Th1 response in vivo *(56)*.

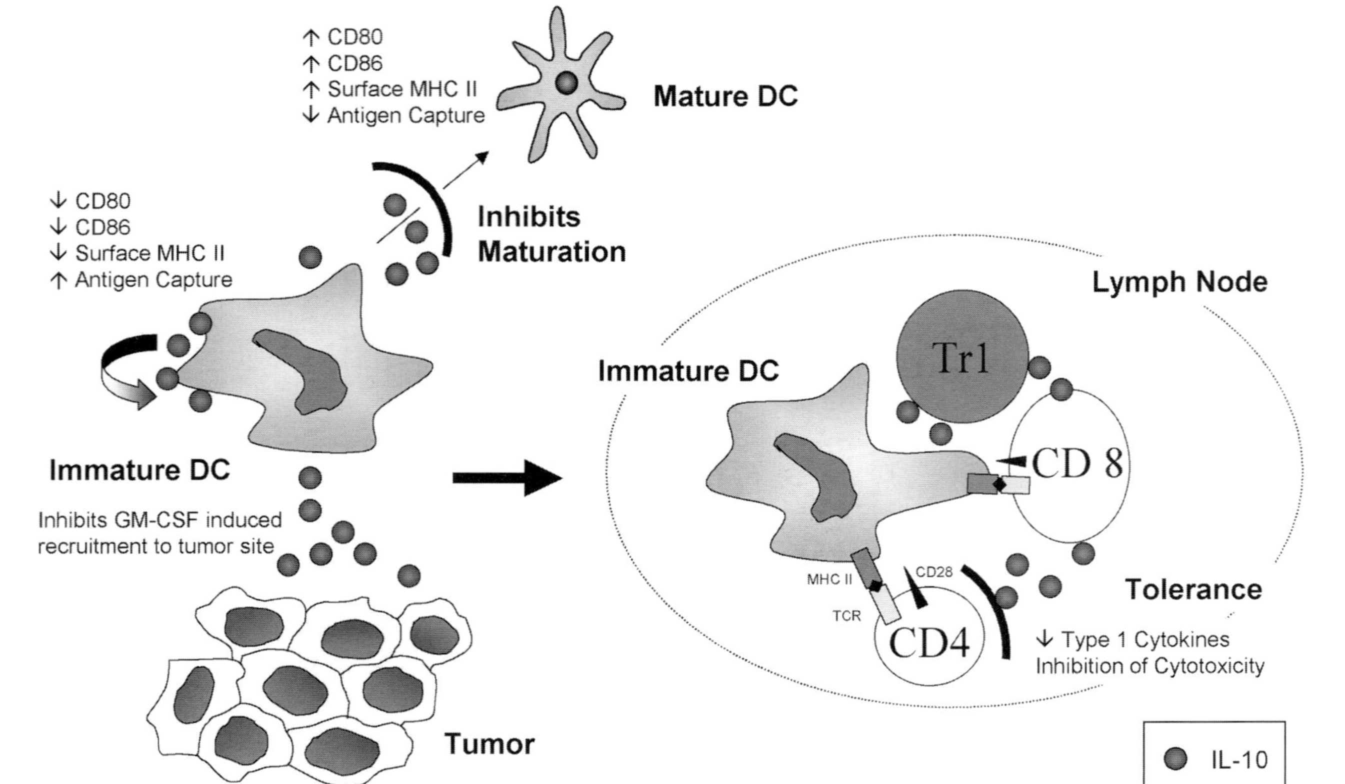

Fig. 1. Tumor-associated immunosuppressive effects of IL-10. Tumor-associated IL-10 inhibits the recruitment of DCs to the tumor site. Both tumor-generated and autocrine levels of IL-10 are involved in the suppression of DC maturation. This prevents the upregulation of costimulatory molecules that are critical for the activation of T lymphocytes. The lack of costimulatory molecules by production of IL-10 and other suppressive cytokines are involved in the tolerization of T lymphocytes, inhibition of Th1 cytokine secretion, and the generation of T regulatory cells (Tr1), which produce both IL-10 and TGF-β.

An integral part of DC maturation involves the upregulation of the potent costimulatory molecules CD80 and CD86. IL-10 has been demonstrated to inhibit this upregulation *(57–59)*. Exposure to IL-10 has also been shown to decrease expression of major histocompatibility complex (MHC) class II and CD11c, while increasing phagocytosis *(60)*. The downregulation of the MHC class II molecule is described to involve an accumulation of the internalized MHC class II complexes and not inhibition of transciption, protein synthesis, or assembly of the molecules. This blockade of the upregulation of receptors required for effective antigen presentation, coupled with a continued ability to phagocytize, would be consistent with the role of IL-10 in maintaining the immature form of DCs *(61)*. Lack of expression of such costimulatory molecules has been associated with lack of responsiveness, and in some cases, anergy to tumor and non-tumor antigens. Exposure to antigen without the proper costimulatory molecules can result in long-term non-responsiveness, and is considered a mechanism of tumor immune escape. Recognizing the importance and value of costimulatory molecules, vaccine strategies have incorporated such molecules in their design to potentially overcome the downregulatory effects of IL-10 *(62–64)*.

Although the majority of studies into the regulation of DC by IL-10 have been reported in non-tumor systems, our studies and others have linked tumor-associated IL-10 production with decreased DC function. Studies from our laboratory using the previously-described MB49 system have shown that in the presence of IL-10, harvested DCs have a significantly reduced ability to stimulate both allogeneic and tumor antigen-specific responses, and in the absence of IL-10 (MB49 bearing IL-10-knockout mice), normal levels of DC function are measured *(64a)*. In addition, Shurin et al. recently demonstrated that ex vivo generated BM-DCs from colon adenocarcinoma (producing IL-10)-bearing mice had decreased CD40 expression and IL-12 production *(65)*. Further evidence of the inhibitory effects of IL-10 is the demonstration that overexpression of IL-10 under control of an IL-2 promoter results in a decreased DC function phenotype and enhanced growth of the Lewis lung carcinoma *(38)*.

The status of intratumoral DCs may also be relevant to the efficacy of antitumor therapies. The infiltration of DCs in tumors has been reported to have positive prognostic value in lung, gastric, and breast cancer *(66–68)*. Access to the tumor may be essential to generate tumor-specific responses. IL-10 was shown to inhibit the GM-CSF-induced recruitment and accumulation of DCs to the tumor site *(69)*. Clinically, a lack of DCs in some tumors, including renal carcinoma *(70)*, has been observed. In addition to inhibition of DC recruitment, IL-10 has also been shown to promote DC apoptosis, which may also explain the lack of DCs at the tumor site *(71)*.

Although DC infiltration of tumors is essential for the generation of the response, the subset of DC-recruited influences the type of immune response that is developed. Experiments by Mukherji et al. suggest the presence of both a stimulatory and inhibitory population of DCs in humans, in which autocrine levels of IL-10 may bias toward development of functionally inhibitory DCs *(72)*. In summary, IL-10 clearly impacts the induction of antitumor immune responses through inhibited development of mature DCs, decreased recruitment to the tumor site, and the development of inhibitory DC populations.

1.5. IL-10 Effects on T Cells

IL-10-mediated regulation of maturation-associated APC secretion of cytokines and chemokines ultimately influences T-cell differentiation, proliferation, and migration. Tolerogenic DCs may drive the differentiation of regulatory rather than effector T cells from naïve T-cell precursors *(73,74)*. Immature DCs have also been shown to prime human CD4 or CD8 T cells toward an IL-10-producing population with suppressive properties *(75,76)*. T-cell proliferation and cytokine production, including IL-2, IFN-γ, IL-6, GM-CSF, and TNF-α, were all reduced by IL-10 in a human allo-MLR *(77)*. Decreased cytokine production and reduced frequency of alloantigen-specific cytotoxic precursors have been associated with IL-10 *(78)*. There is also evidence that IL-10 directly inhibits proliferation and effector function of peripheral-blood T lymphocytes by inhibiting IL-2 production at the mRNA level *(79,80)*.

Human CD4 T cells have been shown to maintain long-term antigen-specific anergy induced by IL-10 *(81)*. Although this anergy could not be reversed by IL-2 or stimulation by anti-CD3 and anti-CD28 *(81)*, the unresponsiveness of IL-10-exposed anergic CD4 T cells could be overcome by mature DC stimulation *(82)*. Anergic T cells stimulated by IL-10-treated DCs were found to upregulate CTLA-4, a negative regulator of T-cell responses *(83)*.

In addition to its putative indirect and direct effects on T-cell function, IL-10 has been associated with the immune-suppressive TGF-β. In mice, IL-10 inhibits primary allogeneic responses, an effect associated with the production of TGF-β *(84)*. Tumor-derived TGF-β can induce the production of IL-10, resulting in suppression of Th1-dependent antitumor responses *(85)*. The potentially synergistic effects of IL-10 and TGF-β are also evident in the function of regulatory T cells (Tr), which play a role in immunological tolerance and suppress Th1-mediated immune responses *(86)*. IL-10 has been reported to play a role in both the generation and effector function of Tr1 cells *(87,88)*. Tr1 cells secrete both TGF-β and IL-10 and in at least one system in vivo, anti-IL-10 blocking Abs completely prevented their regulatory function *(89)*. Tr1 cells have also been demonstrated to inhibit Th1-cell-dependent activation of antitumor CTLs *(90)*.

1.6. IL-10-Induced Antitumor Responses

IL-10 is not solely associated with impaired antitumor responses, as studies from a number of laboratories have demonstrated positive antitumor effects of

IL-10. IL-10 administration through tumor transfection or systemic administration of protein has been reported to inhibit tumor growth in models of breast cancer, mastocytoma, melanoma, prostate, and colon cancer *(91–96)*. These antitumor responses have been linked to natural killer (NK) activity, CD8 T cells, and neutrophils *(95,97)*.

The in vivo effects of local IL-10 expression on tumor rejection may depend on the balance between NK-mediated and CTL-mediated effects. IL-10 decreases the expression of MHC class I presentation potentially through downregulation of TAP-1/2 proteins *(98)*. This downregulation of MHC I levels results in resistance to CTL and increases susceptibility to NK-mediated cytotoxicity *(99–101)*. Many of the experiments showing IL-10 gene transfection to inhibit tumor growth have been conducted in severe combined immunodeficiency (SCID) or nude mouse models that demonstrate that a component of the IL-10-mediated tumor rejection is T-cell-independent *(93,102–104)*, and in many cases secondary to the production of IFN-γ *(105)*.

In comparing studies such as ours—which demonstrate IL-10-dependent immune suppression—with the studies showing enhanced antitumor effects, we have found that the systems that demonstrate enhanced antitumor activity usually used tumor/tissue transfection or the administration of high levels of IL-10 protein, and we hypothesize that both of these would result in higher levels of IL-10 than found as a result of the localized physiologic response to tumor. To address this question, we have transfected our MB49 tumor with the cDNA for IL-10, and compared the growth and immune response to the parental and IL-10 transfectant head to head. As hypothesized, we found that the levels of IL-10 derived from the tumor transfectants were significantly higher than the levels found to be associated with the growth of the parental MB49, and consistent with other studies showing that the IL-10 transfected MB49 was rejected by the majority of mice, which then manifested immunity to the parental tumor *(106)*. These studies demonstrate that in well-defined and controlled systems, one is able to elucidate the activities of cytokines such as IL-10, yet their activity may be dependent on a number of variables and mediated through a number of mechanisms.

1.7. Implications for Immunotherapy

The suppressive effects of tumor-associated IL-10 on the development of antitumor immune responses, and particularly the mechanistic characterization of this activity, support a number of putative immunotherapeutic strategies. As noted here, the best-characterized effects of IL-10 are in the area of suppression of antigen presentation and the skewing of responses toward Th2. Thus, approaches aimed at enhancing APC function and stimulating Th1 T-cell responses may be effective in overcoming the negative effects of IL-10 production.

To this end, a number of laboratories have focused their efforts on modulating the cytokine environment at the tumor or vaccine immunization site with the overall goal of enhancing the recruitment of APC and stimulating Th1 responses. Studies using antigen-encoding vaccines have found that the addition of cytokines such as GM-CSF, IFN-γ, IL-12, and others of this type significantly enhance vaccine responsiveness in both preclinical *(64,107,108)* and clinical systems *(109)*. Preclinical studies have also shown that tumor transfection with GM-CSF and/or costimulatory molecules enhances the immunogenicity of non- or weakly immunogenic tumors *(13,110)*. When taken to the clinic, this approach has been reported in both renal and prostate patients to enhance tumor-specific immunity *(111,112)*.

Along these lines, we have examined the effects of *in situ* tumor transfection using genes for GM-CSF and other regulatory molecules through localized administration of vaccinia virus recombinants *(113)*. In addition to our clinical studies, which demonstrate that intratumor (melanoma) and intravesical (bladder) administration of poxvirus was safe and able to transfer virally encoded genes to the tumor *(114,115)*, using recombinant vaccinia encoding human GM-CSF, we have demonstrated long-term remission of melanoma in a number of treated patients *(116)*. Whether these strategies are capable of overcoming the tumor-associated production of IL-10 and similar cytokines has not been determined; however, they do represent first steps in achieving this goal.

2. CONCLUSION

The studies described in this chapter clearly demonstrate that IL-10 production is associated with a wide range of tumor types, both preclinical and clinical, and that it has the ability to exert significant regulatory activity both in the nature and magnitude of immune responses to tumor and non-tumor antigens. Although studies on the regulatory function of IL-10 demonstrate that its predominant role is one of immune suppression, a number of systems are characterized by enhancement of discrete cellular function(s). These pleiotropic effects of IL-10 may be a result of many variables, including the levels of IL-10, whether the exposure is systemic or local, and finally, whether it occurs during induction or effector phase of the immune response. With further understanding of the diverse actions of tumor-associated IL-10, future immunotherapeutic strategies will be designed to overcome the IL-10-associated immunosuppressive effects, and potentially, to take advantage of possible IL-10-associated antitumor effects.

REFERENCES

1. Schiller JH, Pugh M, Kirkwood JM, Karp D, Larson M, Borden E. Eastern cooperative group trial of interferon gamma in metastatic melanoma: an innovative study design. *Clin Cancer Res* 1996;2:29–36.

2. Mocellin S, Wang E, Marincola FM. Cytokines and immune response in the tumor microenvironment. *J Immunother* 2001;24:392–407.
3. Fiorentino DF, Bond MW, Mosmann TR. Two types of mouse T helper cell. IV. Th2 clones secrete a factor that inhibits cytokine production by Th1 clones. *J Exp Med* 1989; 170:2081–2095.
4. Mosmann TR, Sad S. The expanding universe of T-cell subsets: Th1, Th2 and more. *Immunol Today* 1996;17:138–146.
5. Trinchieri G. Interleukin-12: a cytokine at the interface of inflammation and immunity. *Adv Immunol* 1998;70:83–243.
6. Huang M, Wang J, Lee P, et al. Human non-small cell lung cancer cells express a type 2 cytokine pattern. *Cancer Res* 1995;55:3847–3853.
7. O'Hara RJ, Greenman J, MacDonald AW, et al. Advanced colorectal cancer is associated with impaired interleukin 12 and enhanced interleukin 10 production. *Clin Cancer Res* 1998; 4:1943–1948.
8. Howard JG, Nicklin S, Hale C, Liew FY. Prophylactic immunization against experimental leishmaniasis: I. Protection induced in mice genetically vulnerable to fatal Leishmania tropica infection. *J Immunol* 1982;129:2206–2212.
9. Scott P, Pearce E, Cheever AW, Coffman RL, Sher A. Role of cytokines and CD4+ T-cell subsets in the regulation of parasite immunity and disease. [Review]. *Immunol Rev* 1989; 112:161–182.
10. Yamamura M, Uyemura K, Deans RJ, et al. Defining protective responses to pathogens: cytokine profiles in leprosy lesions. *Science* 1991;254:277–279.
11. Melief CJ. Tumor eradication by adoptive transfer of cytotoxic T lymphocytes. *Adv Cancer Res* 1992;58:143–175.
12. Fearon ER, Pardoll DM, Itaya T, et al. Interleukin-2 production by tumor cells bypasses T helper function in the generation of an antitumor response. *Cell* 1990;60:397–403.
13. Dranoff G, Jaffee E, Lazenby A, et al. Vaccination with irradiated tumor cells engineered to secrete murine granulocyte-macrophage colony-stimulating factor stimulates potent, specific, and long-lasting anti-tumor immunity. *Proc Natl Acad Sci USA* 1993;90: 3539–3543.
14. Sad S, Marcotte R, Mosmann TR. Cytokine-induced differentiation of precursor mouse CD8+ T cells into cytotoxic CD8+ T cells secreting Th1 or Th2 cytokines. *Immunity* 1995;2:271–279.
15. Kemp RA, Ronchese F. Tumor-specific tc1, but not tc2, cells deliver protective antitumor immunity. *J Immunol* 2001;167:6497–6502.
16. Aruga A, Aruga E, Tanigawa K, Bishop DK, Sondak VK, Chang AE. Type 1 versus type 2 cytokine release by Vbeta T cell subpopulations determines in vivo antitumor reactivity: IL-10 mediates a suppressive role. *J Immunol* 1997;159:664–673.
17. Lattime EC, Mastrangelo MJ, Berd D. Human metastatic melanoma lesions and cell lines express mRNA for IL-10. *Proc Am Assoc Cancer Res* 1994;35:489.
18. Lattime EC, Mastrangelo MJ, Bagasra O, Li W, Berd D. Expression of cytokine mRNA in human melanoma tissues. *Cancer Immunol Immunother* 1995;41:151–156.
19. Lattime EC, McCue PA, Keeley FX, Li W, Gomella LG. Expression of IL10 mRNA in biopsies of superficial and invasive TCC of the human bladder. *Proc Am Assoc Cancer Res* 1995; 36:462.
20. McAveney KM, Gomella LG, Lattime EC. Induction of TH1 and TH2 associated cytokine mRNA in mouse bladder following intravesical growth of the murine bladder tumor MB49 and BCG immunotherapy. *Cancer Immunol Immunother* 1994;39:401–406.
21. Chen Q, Daniel V, Maher DW, Hersey P. Production of IL-10 by melanoma cells: examination of its role in immunosuppression mediated by melanoma. *Int J Cancer* 1994; 56:755–760.

22. Huang M, Wang J, Lee P, et al. Human non-small cell lung cancer cells express a Type 2 cytokine pattern. *Cancer Res* 1995;55:3847–3853.
23. Nakagomi H, Pisa P, Pisa EK, et al. Lack of interleukin-2 (IL-2) expression and selective expression of IL-10 mRNA in human renal cell carcinoma. *Int J Cancer* 1995;63:366–371.
24. Venetsanakos E, Beckman I, Bradley J, Skinner JM. High incidence of interleukin 10 mRNA but not interleukin 2 mRNA detected in human breast tumours. *Br J Cancer* 1997; 75:1826–1830.
25. Hishii M, Nitta T, Ishida H, et al. Human glioma-derived interleukin-10 inhibits antitumor immune responses in vitro. *Neurosurgery* 1995;37:1160–1166; discussion 1166–1167.
26. Young MR, Wright MA, Lozano Y, Matthews JP, Benefield J, Prechel MM. Mechanisms of immune suppression in patients with head and neck cancer: influence on the immune infiltrate of the cancer. *Int J Cancer* 1996;67:333–338.
27. Yamamura M, Modlin RL, Ohmen JD, Moy RL. Local expression of antiinflammatory cytokines in cancer. *J Clin Investig* 1993;91:1005–1010.
28. Conrad CT, Ernst NR, Dummer W, Brocker EB, Becker JC. Differential expression of transforming growth factor beta 1 and interleukin 10 in progressing and regressing areas of primary melanoma. *J Exp Clin Cancer Res* 1999;18:225–232.
29. Fujieda S, Lee K, Sunaga H, et al. Staining of interleukin-10 predicts clinical outcome in patients with nasopharyngeal carcinoma. *Cancer* 1999;85:1439–1445.
30. Pisa P, Halapi E, Pisa EK, et al. Selective expression of interleukin 10, interferon gamma, and granulocyte-macrophage colony-stimulating factor in ovarian cancer biopsies. *Proc Natl Acad Sci USA* 1992;89:7708–7712.
31. Fortis C, Foppoli M, Gianotti L, et al. Increased interleukin-10 serum levels in patients with solid tumours. *Cancer Lett* 1996;104:1–5.
32. Bellone G, Turletti A, Artusio E, et al. Tumor-associated transforming growth factor-beta and interleukin-10 contribute to a systemic Th2 immune phenotype in pancreatic carcinoma patients. *Am J Pathol* 1999;155:537–547.
33. Berghella AM, Pellegrini P, Del Beato T, Adorno D, Casciani CU. IL-10 and sIL-2R serum levels as possible peripheral blood prognostic markers in the passage from adenoma to colorectal cancer. *Cancer Biother Radiopharm* 1997;12:265–272.
34. Philip T, Negrier S, Lasset C, et al. Patients with metastatic renal carcinoma candidate for immunotherapy with cytokines. Analysis of a single institution study on 181 patients. *Br J Cancer* 1993;68:1036–1042.
35. Vassilakopoulos TP, Nadali G, Angelopoulou MK, et al. Serum interleukin-10 levels are an independent prognostic factor for patients with Hodgkin's lymphoma. *Haematologica* 2001;86:274–281.
36. Cortes JE, Talpaz M, Cabanillas F, Seymour JF, Kurzrock R. Serum levels of interleukin-10 in patients with diffuse large cell lymphoma: lack of correlation with prognosis. *Blood* 1995;85:2516–2520.
37. Halak BK, Maguire HC, Jr., Lattime EC. Tumor-induced interleukin-10 inhibits type 1 immune responses directed at a tumor antigen as well as a non-tumor antigen present at the tumor site. *Cancer Res* 1999;59:911–917.
38. Sharma S, Stolina M, Lin Y, et al. T cell-derived IL-10 promotes lung cancer growth by suppressing both T cell and APC function. *J Immunol* 1999;163:5020–5028.
39. Lee PP, Zeng D, McCaulay AE, et al. T helper 2-dominant antilymphoma immune response is associated with fatal outcome. *Blood* 1997;90:1611–1617.
40. Moore KW, de Waal Malefyt R, Coffman RL, O'Garra A. Interleukin-10 and the interleukin-10 receptor. *Annu Rev Immunol* 2001;19:683–765.
41. Gallucci S, Matzinger P. Danger signals: SOS to the immune system. *Curr Opin Immunol* 2001;13:114–119.

42. Kambayashi T, Alexander HR, Fong M, Strassmann G. Potential involvement of IL-10 in suppressing tumor-associated macrophages. Colon-26-derived prostaglandin E2 inhibits TNF-alpha release via a mechanism involving IL-10. *J Immunol* 1995;154:3383–3390.
43. de Waal Malefyt R, Abrams J, Bennett B, Figdor CG, de Vries JE. Interleukin 10(IL-10) inhibits cytokine synthesis by human monocytes: an autoregulatory role of IL-10 produced by monocytes. *J Exp Med* 1991;174:1209–1220.
44. Bogdan C, Vodovotz Y, Nathan C. Macrophage deactivation by interleukin 10. *J Exp Med* 1991;174:1549–1555.
45. Cunha FQ, Moncada S, Liew FY. Interleukin-10 (IL-10) inhibits the induction of nitric oxide synthase by interferon-gamma in murine macrophages. *Biochem Biophys Res Commun* 1992;182:1155–1159.
46. Howard M, O'Garra A, Ishida H, de Waal Malefyt R, de Vries J. Biological properties of interleukin 10. *J Clin Immunol* 1992;12:239–247.
47. Seitz M, Loetscher P, Dewald B, Towbin H, Gallati H, Baggiolini M. Interleukin-10 differentially regulates cytokine inhibitor and chemokine release from blood mononuclear cells and fibroblasts. *Eur J Immunol* 1995;25:1129–1132.
48. Banchereau J, Steinman RM. Dendritic cells and the control of immunity. *Nature* 1998;392:245–252.
49. Halliday GM, Le S. Transforming growth factor-beta produced by progressor tumors inhibits, while IL-10 produced by regressor tumors enhances, Langerhans cell migration from skin. *Int Immunol* 2001;13:1147–1154.
50. Gabrilovich DI, Chen HL, Girgis KR, et al. Production of vascular endothelial growth factor by human tumors inhibits the functional maturation of dendritic cells [published erratum appears in *Nat Med* 1996 Nov;2(11):1267]. *Nat Med* 1996;2:1096–1103.
51. Kalinski P, Schuitemaker JH, Hilkens CM, Kapsenberg ML. Prostaglandin E2 induces the final maturation of IL-12-deficient CD1a+CD83+ dendritic cells: the levels of IL-12 are determined during the final dendritic cell maturation and are resistant to further modulation. *J Immunol* 1998;161:2804–2809.
52. Vieira PL, de Jong EC, Wierenga EA, Kapsenberg ML, Kalinski P. Development of Th1-inducing capacity in myeloid dendritic cells requires environmental instruction. *J Immunol* 2000;164:4507–4512.
53. Allavena P, Piemonti L, Longoni D, et al. IL-10 prevents the differentiation of monocytes to dendritic cells but promotes their maturation to macrophages. *Eur J Immunol* 1998;28:359–369.
54. Beissert S, Hosoi J, Grabbe S, Asahina A, Granstein RD. IL-10 inhibits tumor antigen presentation by epidermal antigen-presenting cells. *J Immunol* 1995;154:1280–1286.
55. Maldonado-Lopez R, Maliszewski C, Urbain J, Moser M. Cytokines regulate the capacity of CD8alpha(+) and CD8alpha(–) dendritic cells to prime Th1/Th2 cells in vivo. *J Immunol* 2001;167:4345–4350.
56. De Smedt T, Van Mechelen M, De Becker G, Urbain J, Leo O, Moser M. Effect of interleukin-10 on dendritic cell maturation and function. *Eur J Immunol* 1997;27:1229–1235.
57. Caux C, Massacrier C, Vanbervliet B, Barthelemy C, Liu YJ, Banchereau J. Interleukin 10 inhibits T cell alloreaction induced by human dendritic cells. *Int Immunol* 1994;6:1177–1185.
58. Steinbrink K, Wolfl M, Jonuleit H, Knop J, Enk AH. Induction of tolerance by IL-10-treated dendritic cells. *J Immunol* 1997;159:4772–4780.
59. Chang CH, Furue M, Tamaki K. B7-1 expression of Langerhans cells is up-regulated by proinflammatory cytokines, and is down-regulated by interferon-gamma or by interleukin-10. *Eur J Immunol* 1995;25:394–398.
60. Faulkner L, Buchan G, Baird M. Interleukin-10 does not affect phagocytosis of particulate antigen by bone marrow-derived dendritic cells but does impair antigen presentation. *Immunology* 2000;99:523–531.

61. Koppelman B, Neefjes JJ, de Vries JE, de Waal Malefyt R. Interleukin-10 down-regulates MHC class II alphabeta peptide complexes at the plasma membrane of monocytes by affecting arrival and recycling. *Immunity* 1997;7:861–871.
62. Chamberlain RS, Carroll MW, Bronte V, et al. Costimulation enhances the active immunotherapy effect of recombinant anticancer vaccines. *Cancer Res* 1996;56:2832–2836.
63. Bai XF, Bender J, Liu J, et al. Local costimulation reinvigorates tumor-specific cytolytic T lymphocytes for experimental therapy in mice with large tumor burdens. *J Immunol* 2001; 167:3936–3943.
64. Hodge JW, Grosenbach DW, Rad AN, Giuliano M, Sabzevari H, Schlom J. Enhancing the potency of peptide-pulsed antigen presenting cells by vector-driven hyperexpression of a triad of costimulatory molecules. *Vaccine* 2001;19:3552–3567.
64a. Yang AS, Lattime EC. Tumor-induced IL-10 suppresses the ability of splenic dendritic cells to stimulate CD4 and CD8 T-cell responses. *Cancer Res* 2003;63:2150–2157.
65. Shurin MR, Yurkovetsky ZR, Tourkova IL, Balkir L, Shurin GV. Inhibition of CD40 expre sion and CD40-mediated dendritic cell function by tumor-derived IL-10. *Int J Cancer* 2002;101:61–68.
66. Lespagnard L, Gancberg D, Rouas G, et al. Tumor-infiltrating dendritic cells in adenocarcinomas of the breast: a study of 143 neoplasms with a correlation to usual prognostic factors and to clinical outcome. *Int J Cancer* 1999;84:309–314.
67. Zeid NA, Muller HK. S100 positive dendritic cells in human lung tumors associated with cell differentiation and enhanced survival. *Pathology* 1993;25:338–343.
68. Tsujitani S, Kakeji Y, Watanabe A, Kohnoe S, Maehara Y, Sugimachi K. Infiltration of dendritic cells in relation to tumor invasion and lymph node metastasis in human gastric cancer. *Cancer* 1990;66:2012–2016.
69. Qin Z, Noffz G, Mohaupt M, Blankenstein T. Interleukin-10 prevents dendritic cell accumulation and vaccination with granulocyte-macrophage colony-stimulating factor gene-modified tumor cells. *J Immunol* 1997;159:770–776.
70. Troy AJ, Summers KL, Davidson PJ, Atkinson CH, Hart DN. Minimal recruitment and activation of dendritic cells within renal cell carcinoma. *Clin Cancer Res* 1998;4:585–593.
71. Ludewig B, Graf D, Gelderblom HR, Becker Y, Kroczek RA, Pauli G. Spontaneous apoptosis of dendritic cells is efficiently inhibited by TRAP (CD40-ligand) and TNF-alpha, but strongly enhanced by interleukin-10. *Eur J Immunol* 1995;25:1943–1950.
72. Chakraborty A, Li L, Chakraborty NG, Mukherji B. Stimulatory and inhibitory differentiation of human myeloid dendritic cells. *Clin Immunol* 2000;94:88–98.
73. Reid SD, Penna G, Adorini L. The control of T cell responses by dendritic cell subsets. *Curr Opin Immunol* 2000;12:114–121.
74. Roncarolo MG, Levings MK, Traversari C. Differentiation of T regulatory cells by immature dendritic cells. *J Exp Med* 2001;193:F5–F9.
75. Jonuleit H, Schmitt E, Schuler G, Knop J, Enk AH. Induction of interleukin 10-producing, nonproliferating CD4(+) T cells with regulatory properties by repetitive stimulation with allogeneic immature human dendritic cells. *J Exp Med* 2000;192:1213–1222.
76. Dhodapkar MV, Steinman RM, Krasovsky J, Munz C, Bhardwaj N. Antigen-specific inhibition of effector T cell function in humans after injection of immature dendritic cells. *J Exp Med* 2001;193:233–238.
77. Bejarano MT, de Waal Malefyt R, Abrams JS, et al. Interleukin 10 inhibits allogeneic proliferative and cytotoxic T cell responses generated in primary mixed lymphocyte cultures. *Int Immunol* 1992;4:1389–1397.
78. Roncarolo MG, Bacchetta R, Bordignon C, Narula S, Levings MK. Type 1 T regulatory cells. *Immunol Rev* 2001;182:68–79.
79. Taga K, Mostowski H, Tosato G. Human interleukin-10 can directly inhibit T-cell growth. *Blood* 1993;81:2964–2971.

80. de Waal Malefyt R, Yssel H, de Vries JE. Direct effects of IL-10 on subsets of human CD4+ T cell clones and resting T cells. Specific inhibition of IL-2 production and proliferation. *J Immunol* 1993;150:4754–4765.
81. Groux H, Bigler M, de Vries JE, Roncarolo MG. Interleukin-10 induces a long-term antigen-specific anergic state in human CD4+ T cells. *J Exp Med* 1996;184:19–29.
82. Chen M, Wang F, Lee P, Lin C. Interleukin-10-induced T cell unresponsiveness can be reversed by dendritic cell stimulation. *Immunol Lett* 2001;75:91–96.
83. Chambers CA, Kuhns MS, Egen JG, Allison JP. Ctla-4-mediated inhibition in regulation of t cell responses: mechanisms and manipulation in tumor immunotherapy. *Annu Rev Immunol* 2001;19:565–594.
84. Zeller JC, Panoskaltsis-Mortari A, Murphy WJ, et al. Induction of CD4+ T cell alloantigen-specific hyporesponsiveness by IL-10 and TGF-beta. *J Immunol* 1999;163:3684–3691.
85. Maeda H, Shiraishi A. TGF-beta contributes to the shift toward Th2-type responses through direct and IL-10-mediated pathways in tumor-bearing mice. *J Immunol* 1996;156: 73–78.
86. Chatenoud L, Salomon B, Bluestone JA. Suppressor T cells—they're back and critical for regulation of autoimmunity! *Immunol Rev* 2001;182:149–163.
87. Groux H, O'Garra A, Bigler M, et al. A CD4+ T-cell subset inhibits antigen-specific T-cell responses and prevents colitis. *Nature* 1997;389:737–742.
88. Asseman C, Powrie F. Interleukin 10 is a growth factor for a population of regulatory T cells. *Gut* 1998;42:157–158.
89. Groux H, Powrie F. Regulatory T cells and inflammatory bowel disease. *Immunol Today* 1999;20:442–445.
90. Seo N, Hayakawa S, Takigawa M, Tokura Y. Interleukin-10 expressed at early tumour sites induces subsequent generation of CD4(+) T-regulatory cells and systemic collapse of anti-tumour immunity. *Immunology* 2001;103:449–457.
91. Berman RM, Suzuki T, Tahara H, Robbins PD, Narula SK, Lotze MT. Systemic administration of cellular IL-10 induces an effective, specific, and long-lived immune response against established tumors in mice. *J Immunol* 1996;157:231–238.
92. Grohmann U, Silla S, Belladonna ML, et al. Circulating levels of IL-10 are critically related to growth and rejection patterns of murine mastocytoma cells. *Cell Immunol* 1997;181:109–119.
93. Stearns ME, Fudge K, Garcia F, Wang M. IL-10 inhibition of human prostate PC-3 ML cell metastases in SCID mice: IL-10 stimulation of TIMP-1 and inhibition of MMP-2/MMP-9 expression. *Invasion Metastasis* 1997;17:62–74.
94. Gerard CM, Bruyns C, Delvaux A, et al. Loss of tumorigenicity and increased immunogenicity induced by interleukin-10 gene transfer in B16 melanoma cells. *Hum Gene Ther* 1996;7:23–31.
95. Giovarelli M, Musiani P, Modesti A, et al. Local release of IL-10 by transfected mouse mammary adenocarcinoma cells does not suppress but enhances antitumor reaction and elicits a strong cytotoxic lymphocyte and antibody-dependent immune memory. *J Immunol* 1995;155:3112–3123.
96. Huang S, Xie K, Bucana CD, Ullrich SE, Bar-Eli M. Interleukin 10 suppresses tumor growth and metastasis of human melanoma cells: potential inhibition of angiogenesis. *Clin Cancer Res* 1996;2:1969–1979.
97. Richter G, Kruger-Krasagakes S, Hein G, et al. Interleukin 10 transfected into Chinese hamster ovary cells prevents tumor growth and macrophage infiltration. *Cancer Res* 1993; 53:4134–4137.
98. Salazar-Onfray F, Charo J, Petersson M, et al. Down-regulation of the expression and function of the transporter associated with antigen processing in murine tumor cell lines expressing IL-10. *J Immunol* 1997;159:3195–3202.

99. Salazar-Onfray F, Petersson M, Franksson L, et al. IL-10 converts mouse lymphoma cells to a CTL-resistant, NK-sensitive phenotype with low but peptide-inducible MHC class I expression. *J Immunol* 1995;154:6291–6298.
100. Kundu N, Fulton AM. Interleukin-10 inhibits tumor metastasis, downregulates MHC class I, and enhances NK lysis. *Cell Immunol* 1997;180:55–61.
101. Schwarz MA, Hamilton LD, Tardelli L, Narula SK, Sullivan LM. Stimulation of cytolytic activity by interleukin-10. *J Immunother Emphasis Tumor Immunol* 1994;16:95–104.
102. Huang S, Ullrich SE, Bar-Eli M. Regulation of tumor growth and metastasis by interleukin-10: the melanoma experience. *J Interferon Cytokine Res* 1999;19:697–703.
103. Huang S, Xie K, Bucana CD, Ullrich SE, Bar-Eli M. Interleukin 10 suppresses tumor growth and metastasis of human melanoma cells: potential inhibition of angiogenesis. *Clin Cancer Res* 1996;2:1969–1979.
104. Zheng LM, Ojcius DM, Garaud F, et al. Interleukin-10 inhibits tumor metastasis through an NK cell-dependent mechanism. *J Exp Med* 1996;184:579–584.
105. Sun H, Jackson MJ, Kundu N, Fulton AM. Interleukin-10 gene transfer activates interferon-gamma and the interferon-gamma-inducible genes Gbp-1/Mag-1 and Mig-1 in mammary tumors. *Int J Cancer* 1999;80:624–629.
106. Halak B, Lattime EC. Disparate effects of interleukin-10 (IL10) on tumor immunity are determined by gene-transfected vs. physiologic IL10 production. *Proc Am Assoc Cancer Res* 2000;41:111.
107. Kass E, Panicali DL, Mazzara G, Schlom J, Greiner JW. Granulocyte/macrophage-colony stimulating factor produced by recombinant avian poxviruses enriches the regional lymph nodes with antigen-presenting cells and acts as an immunoadjuvant. *Cancer Res* 2001;61:206–214.
108. Kass E, Parker J, Schlom J, Greiner JW. Comparative studies of the effects of recombinant GM-CSF and GM-CSF administered via a poxvirus to enhance the concentration of antigen-presenting cells in regional lymph nodes. *Cytokine* 2000;12:960–971.
109. Horig H, Lee DS, Conkright W, et al. Phase I clinical trial of a recombinant canarypoxvirus (ALVAC) vaccine expressing human carcinoembryonic antigen and the B7.1 co-stimulatory molecule. *Cancer Immunol Immunother* 2000;49:504–514.
110. Hodge JW, Schlom J. Comparative studies of a retrovirus versus a poxvirus vector in whole tumor-cell vaccines. *Cancer Res* 1999;59:5106–5111.
111. Simons JW, Mikhak B, Chang JF, et al. Induction of immunity to prostate cancer antigens: results of a clinical trial of vaccination with irradiated autologous prostate tumor cells engineered to secrete granulocyte-macrophage colony-stimulating factor using ex vivo gene transfer. *Cancer Res* 1999;59:5160–5168.
112. Simons JW, Jaffee EM, Weber CE, et al. Bioactivity of autologous irradiated renal cell carcinoma vaccines generated by ex vivo granulocyte-macrophage colony-stimulating factor gene transfer. *Cancer Res* 1997;57:1537–1546.
113. Mastrangelo MJ, Eisenlohr LC, Gomella L, Lattime EC. Poxvirus vectors: orphaned and underappreciated. *J Clin Investig* 2000;105:1031–1034.
114. Gomella LG, Mastrangelo MJ, McCue PA, Maguire HC, Mulholland SG, Lattime EC. Phase I study of intravesical vaccinia virus as a vector for gene therapy of bladder cancer. *J Urol* 2001;166:1291–1295.
115. Mastrangelo MJ, Maguire HC, Jr, McCue PA, et al. A pilot study demonstrating the feasibility of using intratumoral vaccinia injections as a vector for gene transfer. Vaccine Research 1995;4:55–69.
116. Mastrangelo MJ, Maguire HC, Jr, Eisenlohr LC, et al. Intratumoral recombinant GM-CSF-encoding virus as gene therapy in patients with cutaneous melanoma. *Cancer Gene Ther* 1999;6:409–422.

10 Accentuating Tumor Immunity Through Costimulation

A Detailed Analysis of OX40 Engagement and CTLA-4 Blockade

Andrew D. Weinberg, PhD,
Dean E. Evans, PhD,
and Arthur A. Hurwitz, PhD

CONTENTS

1. REVIEW OF T-CELL COSTIMULATION: ITS IMPORTANCE AND USE IN PROMOTING ANTITUMOR IMMUNITY

T cells recognize foreign- and/or self-antigens through the T-cell receptor (TCR) interaction with a peptide in the context of "self" major histocompatibility complex (MHC) molecules. However, the TCR : MHC interaction is insufficient to trigger productive activation of T cells. It is now widely recognized that a second signal known as costimulation is required for the productive acti-

From: *Current Clinical Oncology: Cancer Immunotherapy at the Crossroads: How Tumors Evade Immunity and What Can Be Done*
Edited by: J. H. Finke and R. M. Bukowski © Humana Press Inc., Totowa, NJ

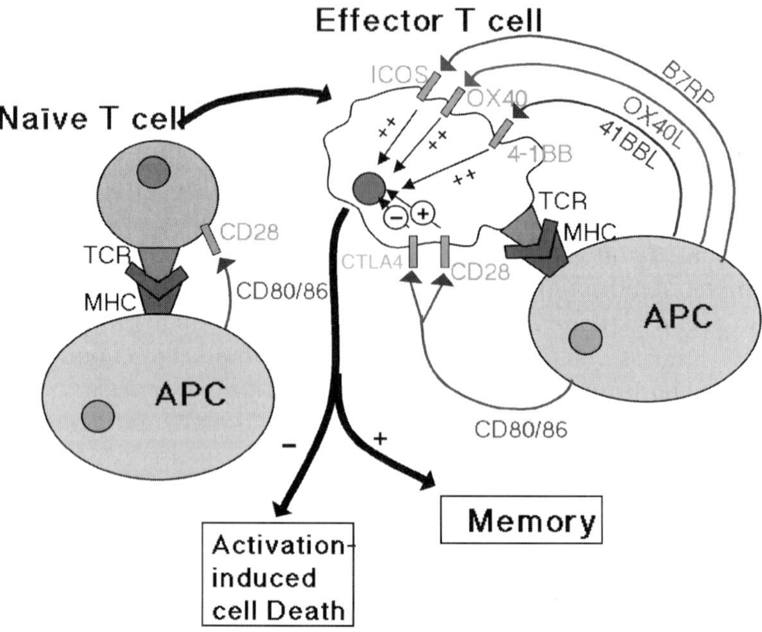

Fig. 1. Overview of the molecules involved with costimulation on naïve and effector T cells. Costimulation is considered the second signal required for T-cell activation, proliferation, and cytokine production following TCR engagement. The costimulatory requirements to activate naïve T cells are primarily mediated through CD28 and CD80/86 interaction. Once a naïve T cell becomes activated and divides 2–4 times, it advances to the effector T-cell stage. During the effector stage, the T cell recognizes antigen, and depending on the costimulatory signals delivered by the antigen-presenting cell (APC) will become a memory T cells and survive or undergo activation-induced cell death (AICD). The majority of effector T cells will downregulate their function through CD80/86 engagement of CTLA-4 and will undergo AICD unless survival signals are delivered to the effector T cells (e.g., OX40, 4-1BB). Upon engagement of the "survival" costimulatory receptors, the T cells increase their lifespan, ultimately becoming long-lived memory T cells.

vation of antigen (Ag)-specific T cells. The interactions between costimulatory molecules and their ligands are multifaceted, and the outcome depends on the stage of T-cell maturation. Figure 1 schematically represents some of the costimulatory molecules that are discussed in this chapter, and their expression and function on naïve and effector T cells. Naïve T cells require a signal delivered through CD28 via CD80 or CD86 expressed on antigen-presenting cells (APC) to induce cell-cycle progression, leading to DNA synthesis and replication *(1)*. Once the T cell has begun to divide, an activation molecule known as CTLA-4 is expressed on the surface of T cells that binds CD80 and CD86 with 50-fold greater affinity than CD28 *(2)*. When CTLA-4 is engaged by its ligand on the cycling T cells, it causes decreased activation, leading to downregulation of effector T-cell function and proliferation *(3,4)*. Several T-cell costimulatory proteins that are independent of the CD28 pathway are also expressed after activation of CD4 and CD8 T cells. When engaged, these cell-surface proteins can lead to enhanced effector T-cell cytokine production, increased cell-cycle progression, and an increase in memory T-cell development and survival *(5,6)*. Currently, there are strategies in place to enhance individual costimulatory pathways or combinations of the pathways to accentuate antitumor immunity in mouse models and for cancer-specific clinical trials. This chapter reviews costimulation in tumor-bearing hosts with a focus on engagement of CD134 (OX40) and blockade of CTLA-4 to enhance antitumor immunity.

Although antibodies to both OX40 and CTLA-4 have been shown to increase antitumor immunity, augmenting other costimulatory pathways can also have potent immune-enhancing effects against cancer. Other molecular costimulatory pathways include CD28 or CTLA-4/CD80 and/or CD86, 4-1BB/4-1BBL, CD27/CD70, and ICOS/B7RP-1 *(7–9)*. CD80 and CD86 are expressed predominantly on cells known as "professional" APCs, such as dendritic cells (DC), macrophages, and B cells. They are not typically expressed on cells such as epithelial cells, and as a result, only "professional" APCs (e.g., DC) are believed to be capable of fully activating naive T cells. Many solid tumors are of epithelial origin, and therefore express few or no costimulatory molecules. This phenotype has been shown to induce T-cell anergy/tolerance by limiting T-cell activation upon TCR signaling *(1)*. Therefore, attempts have been made to enhance activation of tumor-reactive T cells by inoculating animals with tumors that have been modified to express CD80 and/or CD86. This approach has been used with mixed success. Both CD80 and CD86 have been transfected into tumor cells in an attempt to make them more effective in activating tumor-specific T cells. Transfection of CD80/86 has been effective for enhancing immune responses to immunogenic tumors in a prophylactic vaccine setting *(10–14)*; however, this strategy has not been effective against tumors of low immunogenicity *(10,12,13)*. Current evidence suggests that most tumor-reactive T cells are not stimulated directly by the tumor cells, but by DC-presenting tumor peptides within tumor-draining lymph nodes (e.g., cross-priming) *(15–19)*. To target the crossed-primed T cells with costimulatory ligands, some groups have injected soluble forms of B7 molecules in combination with irradiated tumor cells *(20,21)*. Soluble B7.1-Ig and B7.2-Ig were equally effective in curing three murine tumors (MethA, P815, and MB49) *(21)*, and they also significantly increased the survival of mice implanted with the poorly immunogenic tumor, B16/F10 *(21)*. The combination of B7.1-Ig and chemotherapy was more effective than either therapy alone *(20)*. The inherent problem with using molecules that target CD28 on T cells to enhance costimulation is the ability of these molecules to also target the negative regulator CTLA-4, which could potentially decrease T-cell function. Current strategies in tumor immunotherapy have blocked CTLA-4 interaction with CD80/86 via an anti-CTLA-4 antibody, and two sections of this chapter are devoted to the biology of CTLA-4 function and enhancing T-cell function through CTLA-4 blockade.

Other members of the B7 family that have been implicated at the effector T-cell stage include B7RP-1, B7RP-2, and B7-DC (eliciting positive T-cell signals) and PDL-1/PDL-2, which are negative regulators of T-cell activation and function. B7RP-1(B7h), which is expressed on activated B cells, macrophages, and non-immune tissues, is a type 1 transmembrane protein with 20% aa identity to CD80 *(22,23)*. The ligand for B7RP-1, known as ICOS *(23,24)*, is a 50-60-K_d dimer that shares 19% aa identity to CD28. ICOS is expressed primarily on activated CD4+ and CD8+ T-cells *(23)*. ICOS and B7RP-1 are a unique receptor/ligand pair; ICOS does not bind B7 and B7RP-1 does not bind to CD28 *(23)*. A B7RP-1-Fc fusion protein can enhance proliferation of anti-CD3 stimulated T cells, but appears to be more important for effector T-cell responses than naïve T-cell stimulation *(24–26)*. Transfection of the immunogenic tumor Sa1N with B7RP-1 resulted in rejection of the tumors within 20 d of subcutaneous (sc) administration, while the parental tumor was not rejected *(27)*. A similar effect was also observed with the plasmacytoma, J558, transfected with B7RP-1 *(28)*. Antibody depletion studies showed that rejection of B7RP-1 tumors was dependent on CD8, but not CD4 T cells.

Members of the TNF-receptor family that play a significant role in T-cell costimulation include 4-1BB, CD27, and OX40 *(5)*. 4-1BB (CD137) is expressed on activated CD4 and CD8 T cells as well as natural killer (NK), dendritic, and endothelial cells *(5,29–31)*. Long-term survival of CD8+ T cells *(32)* and cytotoxic T lymphocyte (CTL) generation *(33,34)* is greatly enhanced upon ligation of 4-1BB in vivo. The 4-1BB ligand (a tumor necrosis factor [TNF] homolog) is expressed on the surface of activated APC *(35)*, and is a costimulatory ligand that is necessary for the optimal development of Ag-specific CD8 memory T cells following viral exposure *(36)*. Engagement of 4-1BB with an antibody in tumor-bearing hosts causes significant tumor regression, and can lead to protective immunity in several tumor models *(37)*. Engagement of 4-1BB acts synergistically in combination with CD28 signaling to reject poorly immunogenic tumors *(38)*. In addition, transfection of CD80 and CD86 were not sufficient to induce a potent immune response to the B-cell lymphoma A20 in the absence of 4-1BBL expressed on the tumor *(39)*. Therefore, it appears that 4-1BB bioactivity can be augmented through CD28 signaling, and combining these two signals in tumor-bearing hosts synergizes to enhance antitumor immunity.

CD27 is expressed on NK cells and B cells as well as naive CD4 and CD8 T cells *(40)*. The TNF-/TNF-R pair CD70/CD27 will costimulate the priming of the naive T cell, as determined by proliferation and cytokine production *(41–43)*. Engagement of CD27 also enhances NK cell function *(44)*. CD27-

knockout mice showed that CD27 signaling plays an important role in CD4+ and CD8+ T-cell expansion, survival, and lymphocyte homing during a primary and secondary immune response *(45)*. The ligand for CD27 (CD70) *(46)* is transiently expressed on T and B cells upon engagement of the antigen receptor *(47,48)*. Two reports have demonstrated that expression of CD70 on tumors cells leads to enhanced tumor immunity and tumor rejection *(49,50)*. Although the CD27/CD70-mediated rejection of tumor was primarily mediated by NK cells, the antitumor augmentation led to increased CD8 T-cell cytotoxicity against the parental tumor cell line *(49)*.

2. BIOLOGIC FUNCTION OF OX40 (CD134)

OX40 has a unique pattern of expression—it is for the most part restricted to lymphoid tissue *(51)*, and is mainly expressed on activated CD4+ T cells *(52)*. The OX40 ligand (OX40L) is transiently expressed and found on activated APC such as B cells, macrophage/microglia, DC, and endothelial cells *(53–57)*. OX40 expression on recently activated naïve T cells peaks within 24–48 h after TCR engagement by peptide Ag in the context of MHC class II and returns to baseline levels 120 h later *(58)*. Effector T cells upregulate OX40 expression more rapidly than naïve T cells, expressing OX40 within 4 h after Ag stimulation *(58)*. Transient expression of OX40 is observed both in vitro and in vivo (58, 59). OX40+ T cells are found preferentially at sites of inflammation and OX40 is not normally expressed on peripheral T cells *(60)*. In both autoimmunity and tumor models, sorting for OX40+ T cells enriched for the recently stimulated auto- or tumor Ag-specific T cells *(61–63)*. Therefore, OX40 represents a convenient target by which the function of Ag-specific T-cell responses can be modulated in various disease models, even without prior knowledge of the specific Ag(s) involved *(60)*. In essence, manipulation of OX40+ T cells in vivo targets the ongoing "endogenous" immune responses, but ignores the remainder of the peripheral T-cell repertoire. OX40+ T cells have been detected at the inflammatory site in several human autoimmune diseases *(60)* and in the following human cancers: melanoma, breast, colon, head and neck, and most recently, prostate cancer *(60,64,65)*. Therefore, manipulation of OX40 in patients with a variety of diseases could have a wide range of clinical benefits.

Engagement of OX40 causes a potent costimulatory response that can lead to enhanced effector T-cell function both in vitro and in vivo *(63,66,67)*. The control point for OX40-specific costimulation appears to be at the level of OX40L expression during an ongoing immune response in vivo. Evidence supporting this theory is drawn from two separate transgenic mouse models that overexpress the OX40L. When immunized with Ag, the OX40L transgenic mice had greatly enhanced Ag recall responses when compared to nontransgenic control mice *(68,69)*. Addition of an agonist OX40 antibody (Ab)

Table 1
Analysis of Ova-Specific T Cells 62 d Postimmunization

Treatment[a]	*Spleen Cells*[b]	*LN*[b]
No OVA	2.62 ± 0.91	1.76 ± 0.17
OVA/IgG	3.21 ± 1.54	1.26 ± 0.59
OVA/anti-OX40	39.63 ± 20.25	7.63 ± 4.67
OVA/LPS/IgG	5.24 ± 0.19	1.88 ± 0.11
OVA/LPS/anti-OX40	191.85 ± 30.92	12.06 ± 2.23

[a]On d 1, 3.6×10^6 DO11.10 T cells were injected into thymectomized Balb/c recipients. Five groups were organized and injected as described in Table 1 using 500 mg of anti-OX40 or rat IgG and 40 mg of LPS. On d 62 after the initial OVA injection, the LN and spleen T cells were isolated. Cells were counted, stained with anti-CD4 and KJ1-26 Abs, and analyzed by flow cytometry. These data represent mean numbers ± SEM from one representative experiment of two involving three mice per group.

[b]Number of CD4 KJ1-26+ (Ova-specific) T cells $\times 10^4$

or soluble OX40L:Ig fusion protein during primary immunization can also enhance ongoing immune responses that were similar to the transgenic mice previously described. Mice injected with reagents designed to engage OX40 during an inflammatory response show increased effector T-cell cytokine production, increased Ag-specific antibody production, increased memory T-cell generation, and the ability to overcome peripheral tolerance *(58,67,70–72)*. The majority of OX40-induced effects on the immune system can be attributed to enhanced CD4+ T-cell function, although a few studies show that CD8 T cells can be directly augmented by OX40 engagement *(73)*. An example of the potent proinflammatory capability of OX40 engagement in vivo is shown in Table 1, in which TCR transgenic T cells were transferred into naïve hosts and stimulated with Ag in the presence or absence of anti-OX40. These particular TCR transgenic T cells (D011.10 model) are specific for ovalbumin (ova) and can be monitered with the anti-T cell-receptor clonotypic Ab, KJ1-26 *(74)*. Table 1 demonstrates that the number of Ag-specific T cells that survived 60 d postimmunization was increased by the addition of anti-OX40 during the immunization protocol and the addition of a "danger" signal lipopolysaccharide (LPS) enhanced the effect *(72)*. Table 1 also suggests that engagement of OX40 inhibits activation-induced cell death in vivo, which ultimately leads to increased memory T-cell development.

Engagement of OX40 has also been shown to break peripheral T-cell tolerance both in vivo and in vitro *(70)*. If T cells are presented with Ag in the context of MHC without "proper" costimulation, they are rendered unresponsive/tolerant upon subsequent encounter with Ag *(75,76)*. This unresponsiveness can be visualized in hosts that have encountered Ag in a non-inflammatory

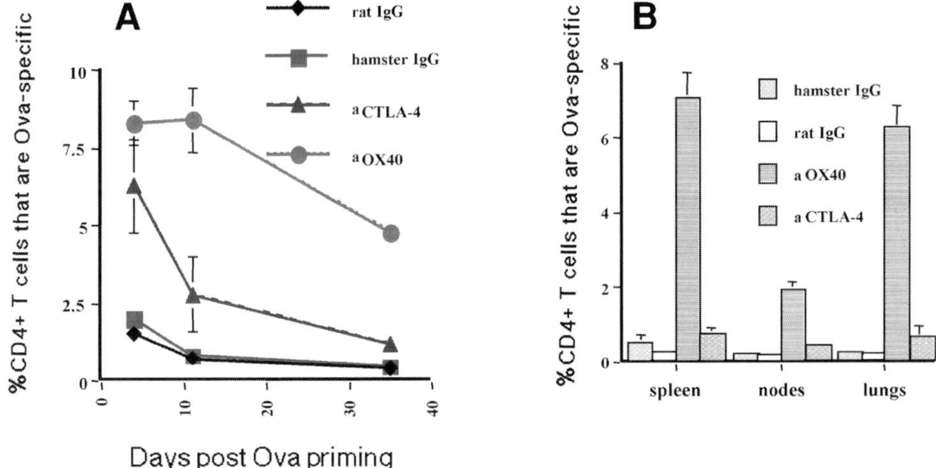

Fig. 2. Anti-OX40 has a more pronounced effect than anti-CTLA-4 on CD4+ T-cell survival. One × 10^6 KJ1-26+ CD4+ spleen cells from D011.10 mice were transferred (iv) into naïve Balb/c recipients. Three days later (d 0), mice were injected subcutaneously with 500 μg of ova in saline and either 50 μg of anti-OX40, 100 μg of anti-CTLA-4, or the appropriate IgG control. **(A)** Mice were bled via the tail vein on the day indicated, and the blood was analyzed by flow cytometry for the presence of ova-specific KJ1-26+ CD4+ T-cells. **(B)** The percentage of ova-specific KJ1-26+ CD4+ T cells in the spleen, lymph nodes, and lungs at d 43 in mice. The mean of five mice/group (no LPS) ± one standard error is shown.

environment, such as intravenous (iv) administration of high doses of peptide in saline or when Ag(s) are expressed on peripheral tissues *(74)*. Engagement of OX40 during the induction of anergy can prevent T-cell tolerance, while signaling through OX40 can also break an existing state of tolerance in the CD4+ T-cell compartment *(70)*. Several studies have shown that tumor Ag-specific T cells isolated from tumor-bearing hosts are tolerant to Ag restimulation *(77,78)*. Therefore, it is possible that engagement of OX40 in tumor-bearing hosts can break peripheral T-cell tolerance, leading to productive immune responses that are ultimately responsible for T-cell-mediated tumor regression. Another mechanism that has been described to limit tolerant T-cell responses is the blockade of CTLA-4 signaling in vivo during an ongoing immune response. Both OX40 engagement and CTLA-4 blockade exhibit enhanced antitumor responses in tumor-bearing mice; therefore, we performed a direct comparison of their abilities to accentuate CD4 T-cell responses in the D011.10 model. Figure 2 shows that both immune-accentuating Abs administered during the early stages of Ag-priming were able to increase the numbers of Ag-specific CD4+ T cells early in the peripheral blood. However, only OX40 treatment increased the survival of long-lasting memory T cells *(67)*. The combination of anti-OX40 engagement and CTLA-4 blockade was no better than anti-OX40 alone at generating or maintaining long-term memory T cells (data not shown). Therefore, it appears that engagement of OX40 during Ag priming in vivo may be more efficient than CTLA-4 blockade in achieving long-lasting CD4 T-cell memory.

3. ENHANCING ANTITUMOR IMMUNITY THROUGH OX40 ENGAGEMENT IN VIVO

OX40 is expressed on both tumor-infiltrating lymphocytes (TIL) and on tumor-draining lymph-node T cells, and this expression has allowed for targeted immunotherapy in tumor-bearing mice with specific designs to enhance antitumor immunity *(60)*. A tumor model was developed to test whether engagement of OX40 in tumor-bearing mice would lead to increased antitumor immunity. Figure 3 shows that OX40 engagement in vivo increased the survival of mice that received a lethal inoculum of sc tumor (MCA 303). Mice were treated on d 3 and d 7 post-tumor inoculation with 100 μg of the OX40 ligand : Ig (OX40L : Ig) fusion protein, a control fusion protein DR3 : Ig (another TNF-R family member) that does not bind OX40, or saline. It was necessary to sacrifice saline-treated mice and mice treated with DR3 : Ig at approximately a similar time because of progressive tumor growth. In contrast, all the mice that received OX40L : Ig experienced delayed tumor growth, and 60% remained tumor-free for >70 d *(63)* (Fig. 3). The OX40L : Ig-treated mice that survived the initial tumor challenge shown in Fig. 2 were shown to be immune to rechallenge with the same MCA 303 tumor-cell line, suggesting that these surviving mice had functional T-cell memory to the immunizing tumor *(63)*. Subsequently, it was shown that a monoclonal antibody (MAb) specific for OX40 had similar antitumor efficacy to the OX40L : Ig fusion protein *(63)*. Most of the evidence in the literature has implicated CD8 T cells as the ultimate effector that destroys tumor cells, but some recent studies suggest that CD4 memory T cells are critical in the maintenance of tumor-free mice in the battle against metastatic disease *(79)*. Because reagents that bind OX40 primarily target CD4 T cells, we hypothesized that the CD4 memory T cells may have been accentuated in the OX40-treated mice. To test this hypothesis, we performed adoptive transfers from the spleens of mice that had been cured through OX40 ligation into naïve recipients. Prior to the adoptive transfer, CD8 T cells were depleted from the spleens, and the mice receiving the "memory CD4 T cells" were challenged with the original inoculating tumor. All the mice that received the CD8-depleted spleen cells were able to resist the tumor challenge, and control mice that received CD8-depleted spleen cells from naïve mice succumbed to the tumor challenge. The data suggest that OX40 ligation during the initial tumor challenge increased the numbers of CD4 memory T cells, and those tumor-specific T cells were able to confer therapeutic antitumor immunity to naïve hosts.

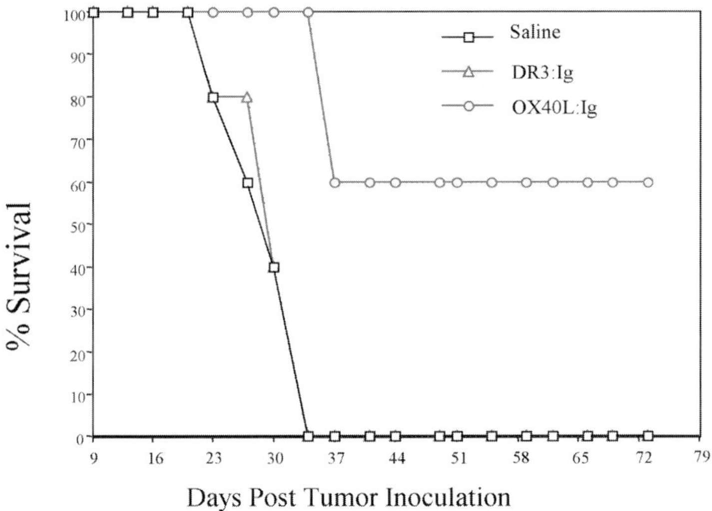

Fig. 3. Therapeutic antitumor immunity after engagement of OX40 in vivo. Mice were inoculated with a lethal sc dose of MCA 303 sarcoma and injected with OX40L : Ig, DR3 : Ig (a control TNF-R family member), or the same volume of intraperitoneal saline on d 3 and 7 post-inoculation (five mice per group). The mice were then followed for evidence of tumor growth, and were sacrificed if their tumor reached 200 mm^2.

Although the data implicate OX40 as helpful target in the immune battle against cancer, they also suggest that a strong backbone of tumor-specific CD4 memory T cells is important in order to initiate and maintain antitumor immunity *(63,79)*.

Engagement of OX40 increases cancer-free survival in a number of tumor models, including sarcomas (MCA 203, 205, 303), glioma (GL261), melamoma (F10), mammary cancer (4T1 and SM1), and colon cancer (CT-26). Although most of the benefits were described in sc tumor models, anti-OX40 treatment has also shown an increased survival benefit when mice were inoculated intracranially with tumors *(80)*. The role of T-cell subsets in the OX40-mediated antitumor response was evaluated in the intracranial tumor model (GL261). Mice were inoculated intracranially with the GL261 glioma and CD4 or CD8 T cells were depleted 3 d prior to OX40 engagment in vivo. The results showed that both CD4 and CD8 T cells were essential for the OX40-mediated antitumor response *(80)*. Since the GL261 is MHC class-II negative, we theorize that the termimal effector immune population responsible for tumor-cell killing was most likely CD8+ T cells. The T-cell depletion studies suggest that OX40 engagement could have boosted the helper function of CD4+ tumor-reactive T cells, which in turn may have boosted the antitumor activity of the CD8+ T cells. Since both CD4 and CD8 TIL express OX40, an alternative explanation is that anti-OX40 directly stimulated both CD4 and CD8 T cells to enhance antitumor immunity.

Adoptive immunotherapy can also be enhanced by treatment with anti-OX40 in both lung and brain metastases tumor models *(81)*. The anti-OX40 therapy showed tumor-antigen specificity in an MCA 205/207 sarcoma "criss-cross" experiment *(81)*. MCA 205-specific T cells had no therapeutic effect upon anti-OX40 administration on MCA 207 lung metastases, and vice versa. Anti-OX40 was only effective when MCA 205-specific T cells were transferred into mice bearing MCA 205 lung metastases (the same was true for MCA 207). The data suggest that OX40-mediated tumor therapy directly targets and enhances tumor Ag-specific T cells. Treatment with IL-2 or anti-OX40 showed similar levels of enhancement in the adoptive immunotherapy setting in the lung metastases model. However, anti-OX40 enhancement of adoptive immunotherapy in a brain metastases model was far superior to in vivo administration of IL-2 *(81)*. These data show that anti-OX40 can enhance tumor Ag-specific T-cell function in both brain and lung metastases models, and suggests that OX40-specific immunotherapy may be able to replace IL-2 injections in the future because of the toxicity associated with IL-2 in cancer patients *(82)*.

Other new and promising agents associated with immune-therapy for enhancing tumor regression in cancer-bearing hosts include granulocyte-macrophage colony-stimulating factor (GM-CSF) secreting tumor vaccines *(83)*, engagement of 4-1BB *(37)*, or blockade of CTLA-4 during tumor priming *(84,85)*. Most likely, the combination of efficient tumor-specific immune priming in conjunction with OX40 engagement will prove to be the most effective use of OX40-specific reagents in the future. The next two sections are devoted to the immune-enhancing properties of blocking CTLA-4 and how that strategy has been used in tumor models to increase antitumor immunity.

4. OVERVIEW OF CTLA-4 BIOLOGY: EXPRESSION AND FUNCTION

Upon activation, T cells express a second receptor for B7 (CD80 and 86) known as CTL antigen 4 (CTLA-4, CD152). Originally, it was proposed that CTLA-4 either had a redundant costimulatory function for T-cell activation *(86)* or exerted apoptotic effects *(87)*. However, the generation of MAbs directed against epitopes critical for B7 binding revealed a different function for CTLA-4 *(3,88–90)*. When used in soluble form, these antibodies enhanced T-cell activation both in vitro and in vivo. More striking was the effect of these antibodies when immobilized on plastic surfaces, where they could crosslink and engage CTLA-4 signaling. In such studies, it was demonstrated that CTLA-4 ligation inhibited T-cell responses. This inhibitory effect manifests itself through the inhibition of IL-2 production, loss of proliferation via blockade of cell-cycle progression, and decreased cytokine production *(91)*.

Although it is generally accepted that CTLA-4 delivers an inhibitory signal during T-cell activation, it is unclear how this occurs. CTLA-4 may serve to terminate ongoing T-cell responses, or alternatively, it may serve to set a threshold for the initiation of activation of T-cell responses *(92)*. One mechanism by which CTLA-4 may exert its inhibitory effects is by tightly regulated expression at the immunological synapse. CTLA-4 appears to be stored in intracellular vesicles, and activation stimulates export to the cell surface *(93,94)*. However, only low levels of CTLA-4 protein are detected on the extracellular surface *(95)*. The low level of CTLA-4 expression may be compensated for by the significantly higher affinity that CTLA-4 has for CD80/86 as compared to CD28 *(96)*. Accordingly, at low levels of CD80/86 expression, CTLA-4 may "outcompete" CD28 and inhibitory signals may prevail. However, an emerging story suggests that lower-affinity TCR ligands may not successfully deliver CTLA-4 to the immunologic synapse *(92)*. This may prevent CTLA-4 from regulating T cells with low avidity for MHC/peptide interactions.

The critical biologic role of CTLA-4 is underscored by the phenotype of *ctla-4*-deficient mice *(97,98)*. These mice exhibit a severe lymphoproliferative disorder that is characterized by chronic T-cell activation, infiltration into many non-lymphoid tissues, and lethality by 6 wk of age. The severity of this phenotype is lessened when mice are backcrossed onto a TCR transgenic background or when the T-cell repertoire is rendered chimeric via a single TCR (through a bone-marrow transplant with TCR transgenic bone marrow) *(99–101)*. These findings indicate that in the absence of CTLA-4, T cells have a reduced threshold for activation and may be chronically activated. These observations also support other findings that demonstrate a key role for CTLA-4 in regulation of autoimmune disease.

Because of the lethality of the phenotype of *ctla-4*-deficient mice, most studies that have characterized the role of CTLA-4 in the immune response have relied on antibodies directed against CTLA-4 that block the interaction with CD80 and/or CD86. In vitro, these antibodies can be used to crosslink CTLA-4 and deliver an inhibitory signal. However, these antibodies function to block antibodies in vivo and enhance T-cell responses. Such reagents have been used to demonstrate that CTLA-4 can regulate adaptive responses to infectious agents such as *Leishmania major (102)*, *Mycobacterium bovis (103)*, human immunodeficiency virus (HIV) *(104)*, and *Cryptococcus neoformans (105)*. Other studies have demonstrated a role for CTLA-4 in restricting autoimmune disease progression. CTLA-4 blockade was sufficient to reveal and exacerbate type I diabetic responses in both susceptible NOD and resistant Balb/c strains *(106–108)*. In addition, a role for CTLA-4 in regulating autoimmune responses in the central nervous system (CNS) was demonstrated using Experimental Autoimmune Encephalomyelitis, a murine model for multiple sclerosis *(109–112)*. In these studies, CTLA-4 was shown to regulate autopathogenicity in both susceptible and resistant strains. As a whole, the studies that use a reagent to remove CTLA-4-mediated inhibition all demonstrate that CTLA-4 is a key regulator of T-cell responses in both infectious and autoimmune disease.

A role for CTLA-4 in regulating tolerance has also been described. It was initially suggested that *ctla-4*-deficient mice exhibited signs of autoimmune disease. However, little evidence exists for tissue antigen-specific autoimmune disease in these mice. Rather, the pathogenicity may be caused by diffuse ischemia and necrosis as a result of lymphocytosis. Many studies have examined the role of CTLA-4 in tolerance induction *(113–115)*. All of these studies indicate that tolerance induction can be thwarted by blocking CTLA-4: CD80/86 interactions. However, in most of these studies, delivery of tolerizing antigen comes in the form of exogenous antigen sensitization. Thus, it is unclear whether CTLA-4 blockade truly interrupts the tolerization process or whether CTLA-4 blockade acts on recent thymic emigrants that were not fully tolerized in the periphery. Alternatively, CTLA-4 blockade may boost third-party responses that provide help "in trans" during the tolerization process. A more controversial role for CTLA-4 in tolerance to tumor antigens exists, and is discussed further in the following section.

5. THE ROLE OF CTLA-4 IN ANTITUMOR RESPONSES: ACCENTUATING VIA CTLA-4 BLOCKADE

Two studies have examined the role of CTLA-4 in tumor tolerance. Both used models in which tumors that expressed surrogate tumor antigens were implanted into mice. Tumor antigen-specific T cells derived from TCR-transgenic mice were adoptively transferred into tumor-bearing mice. In one study, Levitsky and colleagues demonstrated that although CTLA-4 blockade enhanced early T-cell responses to mice challenged with a class II-restricted tumor antigen-expressing tumor, long-term tolerance was not prevented *(116)*. In contrast, Shrikant et al. reported that CTLA-4 blockade following tumor challenge can prevent tolerance to a class I-restricted antigen in a CD4+ T cell- and IL-2-dependent mechanism *(117)*. These two studies differed in the use of different antigens expressed by various tumors recognized by different T-cell subsets, and thus, further studies will be required to clarify these opposing findings.

Several studies have exploited the fact that recently activated T cells express CTLA-4, and have demonstrated a role for CTLA-4 in suppressing antitumor responses (Table 2). Originally, Leach and colleagues reported that CTLA-4 blockade accelerates regression of a B7+ tumor, and could also promote regression of unmodified tumors *(118)*. Tumor immunity was dependent on CD8+ T cells, and conferred long-lasting protection to rechallenge. These findings

Table 2
Effects of CTLA-4 Blockade on Different Tumor Models

Tumor Model	*Tumor Type*	*αCTLA-4*	*Combination**
EL4	Thymoma	+/–	ND
SAI/N	Fibrosarcoma	+	ND
51BLim 10	Colorectal carcinoma	+	ND
RENCA	Renal carcinoma	+	ND
K1735	Melanoma	+/–	ND
TRAMPC	Prostatic carcinoma	+	ND
SM1	Mammary carcinoma	–	GM*
B16/BL6	Melanoma	–	GM*
MOPC-315	Plasmacytoma	–	Mel*
RLÔ1	Leukemia	–	CD40*
TRAMP	Primary prostatic carcinoma	–	GM*

ND, not determined; +, full rejection (>80%); +/–, partial rejection (40–80%); –, low rejection (<40%); *, Combination of α-CTLA-4 with GM-CSF-expressing vaccine (GM), melphalan (Mel), or α-CD40 (CD40 resulted in therapeutic tumor immunity)

were subsequently extended using tumors of other tissue origins in transplantable tumor models *(119,120)*. However, the success of this approach was restricted to immunogenic tumors. Thus, tumors with little or no inherent immunogenicity were refractory to CTLA-4 blockade. This approach was also applied to a model of minimal residual disease, and was successful in eliminating metastases in both lymphoid and non-lymphoid compartments *(121)*.

One tumor in which CTLA-4 blockade had no effect was the murine melanoma, B16. Interestingly, the combination of CTLA-4 blockade and a B16 cell-based vaccine expressing GM-CSF was sufficient to protect against rechallenge *(122)* and to treat recently established melanoma tumors as well as pulmonary metastases *(123)*. In the B16 model, only CD8+ T cells and NK cells were required for the therapeutic activity of anti-CTLA-4. Somewhat surprisingly, depletion of CD4+ cells actually enhanced tumor immunity. More striking was the observation that in this melanoma model, immunity to the B16 tumors was also accompanied by immune destruction of normal melanocytes. This manifests itself as a vitiligo-like depigmentation of the hairs, and is reminiscent of the vitiligo observed in melanoma patients undergoing immunotherapy *(124,125)*. More importantly, this indicated that the immune response is at least in part directed against normal tissue antigens and not solely tumor-specific antigens, as the vitiligo-like depigmentation was only observed in mice treated with anti-CTLA-4. This finding also suggests that the power of CTLA-4 blockade, in the context of a cell-based vaccine that expresses both tissue-specific antigens and pro-inflammatory signals (GM-CSF), is sufficient to overcome tolerance to the pigmentation antigens and elicit an autoimmune response.

A similar approach was also applied to a primary murine model of prostate cancer *(84)*. The Transgenic Adenocarcinoma of the Mouse Prostate (TRAMP) model consists of mice that bear the SV40 T antigen under the transcriptional regulation of the rat probasin promoter, an androgen-regulated promoter that directs expression to the prostatic basolateral epithelium *(126)*. TRAMP mice develop prostatic tumors with 100% penetrance, and disease progression is comparable to that found in man. To test the efficacy of CTLA-4 blockade in a primary tumor model, TRAMP mice with early neoplastic lesions were vaccinated with a TRAMP-derived prostate cancer-cell vaccine and treated with anti-CTLA-4. This approach reduced both primary tumor incidence and tumor grade. The antitumor effect of CTLA-4 blockade was dependent on an exogenous source of antigen from the cell-based vaccine. Provision of GM-CSF in the vaccine appeared to offer some additional protection, but this did not significantly differ from those animals treated with the unmodified cell-based vaccine. The most prominent histological finding in this study was the accumulation of inflammatory cells in the interductal spaces of prostates of TRAMP mice treated with GM-CSF-expressing vaccine in combination with anti-CTLA-4, suggestive of autoimmune prostatitis. A similar vaccination approach applied to wild-type mice also resulted in prostatitis, suggesting that like the B16 model, immune-reactivity was in part directed against normal tissue antigens. The ability of this combinatorial approach to elicit a response against a tumor model in which the entire organ is undergoing transformation provided the translational support for the initiation of a clinical trial to test CTLA-4 blockade in human cancers.

CTLA-4 blockade has also been combined with other cancer therapies, both immune- and non-immune-mediated. The synergy between CTLA-4 blockade and GM-CSF-secreting tumor-cell vaccination suggests that activation of APC by GM-CSF can potentiate the effectiveness of anti-CTLA-4. It was also reported that in vivo activation of host APCs via the CD40-CD40 ligand pathway can synergize with CTLA-4 blockade to induce tumor cell-specific CTL activity *(127)*. In this study, the researcher combined anti-CD40 with anti-CTLA-4 administration, which resulted in marked increases in antigen-specific CTL activity following liposomal delivery of tumor-specific peptides. Moreover, responses raised by vaccination with liposomal tumor Ags and co-administration of anti-CD40 and anti-CTLA-4 were sufficient to extend the survival of mice challenged with the RL1 lymphoma. Another approach to increase the efficacy of CTLA-4 blockade as an antitumor therapy included its use in combination with low-dose chemotherapy. Low-dose melphalan administration followed immediately by CTLA-4 blockade was shown to cause enhanced tumor regression and improve survival of mice bearing recently established sc tumors *(128)*. It was suggested that CTLA-4 blockade may enhance the effectiveness of suboptimal melphalan therapy that was previously demonstrated to promote a shift toward a T_H1 environment, thus favoring the generation of potent tumor-specific CD8+ T cells. However, subsequent studies by the same group demonstrated that melphalan may upregulate B7 expression on some solid tumors *(129)*.

6. SUMMARY

In conclusion, the field of T-cell costimulation has merged with the field of tumor immunology, and has created some promise in helping T cells to eradicate tumors and keeping hosts tumor-free by accentuating long-lasting immunity ("memory"). This chapter describes a number of T-cell costimulatory targets that have shown therapeutic promise in the field of tumor immunology, and focuses on blockade of CTLA-4 and OX40 engagement as two of the most promising targets. Although accentuating the immune system during Ag priming in basic immunology models through costimulatory ligands and/or antibodies appears to enhance immunity, it is an arduous task to enhance antitumor immunity in a cancer-bearing host. The tumor environment can be extremely immune-suppressive, and reversing this suppression may actually require a combination of costimulatory molecules working together to aggressively achieve potent antitumor immunity. In the coming years, clinical trials with cancer patients will be performed to evaluate the efficacy of the individual costimulatory pathways. Future clinical trials are likely to incorporate the knowledge of these individual trials to determine the most effective costimulatory pathways to be used in combination with cytokines and/or chemotherapeutics in patients with cancer.

REFERENCES

1. Dubey C, Croft M, Swain SL. Costimulatory requirements of naive CD4+ T cells. ICAM-1 or B7-1 can costimulate naive CD4 T cell activation but both are required for optimum response. *J Immunol* 1995;155:45–57.
2. Chambers CA, Krummel MF, Boitel B, et al. The role of CTLA-4 in the regulation and initiation of T-cell responses. *Immunol Rev* 1996;153:27–46.
3. Krummel MF, Allison JP. CD28 and CTLA-4 have opposing effects on the response of T cells to stimulation. *J Exp Med* 1995;182:459–466.
4. Walunas T, Bakker CY, Bluestone JA. CTLA-4 ligation blocks CD28-dependent T cell activation. *J Exp Med* 1996;183:2541–2550.
5. Watts TH, DeBenedette MA. T cell co-stimulatory molecules other than CD28. *Curr Opin Immunol* 1999;11:286–293.
6. Weinberg AD, Vella AT, Croft M. OX-40: life beyond the effector T cell stage. *Semin Immunol* 1998;10:471–480.
7. Freedman AS, Freeman G, Horowitz JC, Daley J, Nadler LM. B7, a B-cell-restricted antigen that identifies preactivated B cells. *J Immunol* 1987;139:3260–3267.

8. Freeman GJ, Borriello F, Hodes RJ, et al. Murine B7-2, an alternative CTLA-4 counter-receptor that costimulates T cell proliferation and interleukin-2 production. *J Exp Med* 1993;178:2185–2192.
9. Freeman GJ, Borriello F, Hodes RJ, et al. Uncovering of functional alternative CTLA-4 counter-receptor in B7-deficient mice. *Science* 1993;262:907–909.
10. Baskar S, Ostrand-Rosenberg S, Nabavi N, Nadler LM, Freeman GJ, Glimcher LH. Constitutive expression of B7 restores immunogenicity of tumor cells expressing truncated major histocompatibility complex II molecules. *Proc Natl Acad Sci USA* 1993; 90:5687–5690.
11. Chen L, Ashe S, Brady WA, et al. Costimulation of anti-tumor immunity by the B7 counterrecptor for the T lymphocyte molecules CD28 and CTLA-4. *Cell* 1992;71:1093–1102.
12. Chen L, McGowan P, Ashe S, et al. Tumor immunogenicity determines the effect of B7 costimulation on T cell-mediated tumor immunity. *J Exp Med* 1994;179:523–532.
13. Townsend S, Allison JP. Tumor rejection after direct costimulation of CD8+ T cells by B7-transfected melanoma cells. *Science* 1993;259:368–370.
14. Townsend SE, Su FW, Atherton JM, Allison JP. Specificity and longevity of anti-tumor immune responses induced by B7-transfected tumors. *Cancer Res* 1994;54:6477–6483.
15. Bevan MJ. Cross-priming for a secondary cytotoxic response to minor H antigens with H-2 congenic cells which do not cross-react in the cytotoxic assay. *J Exp Med* 1976; 143:1283–1288.
16. Bevan MJ. Minor H antigens introduced on H-2 different stimulating cells cross-react at the cytotoxic T cell level during in vivo priming. *J Immunol* 1976;117:2233–2238.
17. Carbone FR, Kurts C, Bennett SR, Miller JF, Heath WR. Cross-presentation: a general mechanism for CTL immunity and tolerance. *Immunol Today* 1998;19:368–373.
18. Huang AYC, Golumbek P, Ahmadzedeh M, Jaffee E, Pardoll D, Levitsky H. Role of bone-marrow derived cells in presenting MHC Class I-restricted tumor antigens. *Science* 1994; 264:961–965.
19. Jeannin P, Renno T, Goetsch L, et al. Omp A targets dendritic cells, induces their maturation and delivers antigen into the MHC class I presentation pathway. *Nat Immunol* 2000; 1:502–509.
20. Runyon K, Lee K, Zuberek K, Collins M, Leonard JP, Dunussi-Joannopoulos K. The combination of chemotherapy and systemic immunotherapy with soluble B7-immunoglobulin G leads to cure of murine leukemia and lymphoma and demonstration of tumor-specific memory responses. *Blood* 2001;97:2420–2426.
21. Sturmhoefel K, Lee K, Gray GS, et al. Potent activity of soluble B7-IgG fusion proteins in therapy of established tumors and as vaccine adjuvant. *Cancer Res* 1999;59:4964–4972.
22. Swallow MM, Wallin JJ, Sha WC. B7h, a novel costimulatory homolog of B7.1 and B7.2, is induced by TNFalpha. *Immunity* 1999;11:423–432.
23. Yoshinaga SK, Whoriskey JS, Khare SD, et al. T-cell co-stimulation through B7RP-1 and ICOS. *Nature* 1999;402:827–832.
24. Hutloff A, Dittrich AM, Beier KC, et al. ICOS is an inducible T-cell co-stimulator structurally and functionally related to CD28. *Nature* 1999;397:263–266.
25. Coyle AJ, Lehar S, Lloyd C, et al. The CD28-related molecule ICOS is required for effective T cell-dependent immune responses. *Immunity* 2000;13:95–105.
26. McAdam AJ, Chang TT, Lumelsky AE, et al. Mouse inducible costimulatory molecule (ICOS) expression is enhanced by CD28 costimulation and regulates differentiation of CD4+ T cells. *J Immunol* 2000;165:5035–5040.
27. Wallin JJ, Liang L, Bakardjiev A, Sha WC. Enhancement of CD8+ T cell responses by ICOS/B7h costimulation. *J Immunol* 2001;167:132–139.
28. Liu X, Bai XF, Wen J, et al. B7H costimulates clonal expansion of, and cognate destruction of tumor cells by, CD8(+) T lymphocytes in vivo. *J Exp Med* 2001;194:1339–1348.

29. Pauly S, Broll K, Wittmann M, Giegerich G, Schwarz H. CD137 is expressed by follicular dendritic cells and costimulates B lymphocyte activation in germinal centers. *J Leukoc Biol* 2002;72:35–42.
30. Broll K, Richter G, Pauly S, Hofstaedter F, Schwarz H. CD137 expression in tumor vessel walls. High correlation with malignant tumors. *Am J Clin Pathol* 2001;115:543–549.
31. Wilcox RA, Tamada K, Strome SE, Chen L. Signaling through NK cell-associated CD137 promotes both helper function for CD8+ cytolytic T cells and responsiveness to IL-2 but not cytolytic activity. *J Immunol* 2002;169:4230–4236.
32. Takahashi C, Mittler RS, Vella AT. Cutting edge: 4-1BB is a bona fide CD8 T cell survival signal. *J Immunol* 1999;162:5037–5040.
33. DeBenedette MA, Chu NR, Pollok KE, et al. Role of 4-1BB ligand in costimulation of T lymphocyte growth and its upregulation on M12 B lymphomas by cAMP. *J Exp Med* 1995;181:985–992.
34. Hurtado JC, Kim SH, Pollok KE, Lee ZH, Kwon BS. Potential role of 4-1BB in T cell activation. Comparison with the costimulatory molecule CD28. *J Immunol* 1995;155: 3360–3367.
35. Alderson MR, Smith CA, Tough TW, et al. Molecular and biological characterization of human 4-1BB and its ligand. *Eur J Immunol* 1994;24:2219–2227.
36. Wen T, Bukczynski J, Watts TH. 4-1BB ligand-mediated costimulation of human T cells induces CD4 and CD8 T cell expansion, cytokine production, and the development of cytolytic effector function. *J Immunol* 2002;168:4897–4906.
37. Melero I, Shuford WW, Newby SA, et al. Monoclonal antibodies against the 4-1BB T-cell activation molecule eradicate established tumors. *Nat Med* 1997;3:682–685.
38. Melero I, Johnston JV, Shufford WW, Mittler RS, Chen L. NK1.1 cells express 4-1BB (CDw137) costimulatory molecule and are required for tumor immunity elicited by anti-4-1BB monoclonal antibodies. *Cell Immunol* 1998;190:167–172.
39. Guinn BA, DeBenedette MA, Watts TH, Berinstein NL. 4-1BBL cooperates with B7-1 and B7-2 in converting a B cell lymphoma cell line into a long-lasting antitumor vaccine. *J Immunol* 1999;162:5003–5010.
40. Hintzen RQ, de Jong R, Lens SM, Brouwer M, Baars P, van Lier RA. Regulation of CD27 expression on subsets of mature T-lymphocytes. *J Immunol* 1993;151:2426–2435.
41. Gravestein LA, Nieland JD, Kruisbeek AM, Borst J. Novel mAbs reveal potent co-stimulatory activity of murine CD27. *Int Immunol* 1995;7:551–557.
42. Hintzen RQ, Lens SM, Lammers K, Kuiper H, Beckmann MP, van Lier RA. Engagement of CD27 with its ligand CD70 provides a second signal for T cell activation. *J Immunol* 1995;154:2612–2623.
43. Kobata T, Jacquot S, Kozlowski S, Agematsu K, Schlossman SF, Morimoto C. CD27-CD70 interactions regulate B-cell activation by T cells. *Proc Natl Acad Sci USA* 1995;92: 11,249–11,253.
44. Yang FC, Agematsu K, Nakazawa T, et al. CD27/CD70 interaction directly induces natural killer cell killing activity. *Immunology* 1996;88:289–293.
45. Hendriks J, Gravestein LA, Tesselaar K, van Lier RA, Schumacher TN, Borst J. CD27 is required for generation and long-term maintenance of T cell immunity. *Nat Immunol* 2000; 1:433–440.
46. Hintzen RQ, Lens SM, Beckmann MP, Goodwin RG, Lynch D, van Lier RAW. Characterization of the human CD27 ligand, a novel member of the TNF gene family. *J Immunol* 1994;152:1762–1773.
47. Lens SM, Tesselaar K, van Oers MH, van Lier RA. Control of lymphocyte function through CD27-CD70 interactions. *Semin Immunol* 1998;10:491–499.
48. Oshima H, Nakano H, Nohara C, et al. Characterization of murine CD70 by molecular cloning and mAb. *Int Immunol* 1998;10:517–526.

49. Kelly JM, Darcy PK, Markby JL, et al. Induction of tumor-specific T cell memory by NK cell-mediated tumor rejection. *Nat Immunol* 2002;3:83–90.
50. Lorenz MG, Kantor JA, Schlom J, Hodge JW. Anti-tumor immunity elicited by a recombinant vaccinia virus expressing CD70 (CD27L). *Hum Gene Ther* 1999;10:1095–1103.
51. Baum PR, Gayle RB, 3rd, Ramsdell F, et al. Molecular characterization of murine and human OX40/OX40 ligand systems: identification of a human OX40 ligand as the HTLV-1-regulated protein gp34. *EMBO J* 1994;13:3992–4001.
52. Paterson DJ, Jefferies WA, Green JR, et al. Antigens of activated rat T lymphocytes including a molecule of 50,000 Mr detected only on CD4 positive T blasts. *Mol Immunol* 1987; 24:1281–1290.
53. Ohshima Y, Tanaka Y, Tozawa H, Takahashi Y, Maliszewski C, Delespesse G. Expression and function of OX40 ligand on human dendritic cells. *J Immunol* 1997;159:3838–3848.
54. Stuber E, Neurath M, Calderhead D, Fell HP, Strober W. Cross-linking of OX40 ligand, a member of the TNF/NGF cytokine family, induces proliferation and differentiation in murine splenic B cells. *Immunity* 1995;2:507–521.
55. Weinberg AD, Wegmann KW, Funatake C, Whitham RH. Blocking OX-40/OX-40 ligand interaction in vitro and in vivo leads to decreased T cell function and amelioration of experimental allergic encephalomyelitis. *J Immunol* 1999;162:1818–1826.
56. Imura A, Hori T, Imada K, et al. The human OX40/gp34 system directly mediates adhesion of activated T cells to vascular endothelial cells. *J Exp Med* 1996;183:2185–2195.
57. Kunitomi A, Hori T, Imura A, Uchiyama T. Vascular endothelial cells provide T cells with costimulatory signals via the OX40/gp34 system. *J Leukoc Biol* 2000;68:111–118.
58. Gramaglia I, Weinberg AD, Lemon M, Croft M. Ox-40 ligand: a potent costimulatory molecule for sustaining primary CD4 T cell responses. *J Immunol* 1998;161:6510–6517.
59. Weinberg AD, Wallin JJ, Jones RE, et al. Target organ-specific up-regulation of the MRC OX-40 marker and selective production of Th1 lymphokine mRNA by encephalitogenic T helper cells isolated from the spinal cord of rats with experimental autoimmune enciphalomyelitis. *J Immunol* 1994;152:4712–4721.
60. Weinberg AD. OX40: targeted immunotherapy—implications for tempering autoimmunity and enhancing vaccines. *Trends in Immunology* 2002;23:102–109.
61. Buenafe AC, Weinberg AD, Culbertson NE, Vandenbark AA, Offner H. V beta CDR3 motifs associated with BP recognition are enriched in OX-40+ spinal cord T cells of Lewis rats with EAE. *J Neurosci Res* 1996;44:562–567.
62. Weinberg AD, Bourdette DN, Sullivan TJ, et al. Selective depletion of myelin-reactive T cells with the anti-OX-40 antibody ameliorates autoimmune encephalomyelitis. *Nat Med* 1996;2:183–189.
63. Weinberg AD, Rivera MM, Prell R, et al. Engagement of the OX-40 receptor in vivo enhances antitumor immunity. *J Immunol* 2000;164:2160–2169.
64. Ramstad T, Lawnicki L, Vetto J, Weinberg A. Immunohistochemical analysis of primary breast tumors and tumor-draining lymph nodes by means of the T-cell costimulatory molecule OX-40. *Am J Surg* 2000;179:400–406.
65. Vetto JT, Lum S, Morris A, et al. Presence of the T-cell activation marker OX-40 on tumor infiltrating lymphocytes and draining lymph node cells from patients with melanoma and head and neck cancers. *Am J Surg* 1997;174:258–265.
66. Kaleeba JA, Offner H, Vandenbark AA, Lublinski A, Weinberg AD. The OX-40 receptor provides a potent co-stimulatory signal capable of inducing encephalitogenicity in myelin-specific CD4+ T cells. *Int Immunol* 1998;10:453–461.
67. Evans DE, Prell RA, Thalhofer CJ, Hurwitz AA, Weinberg AD. Engagement of OX40 enhances antigen-specific CD4(+) T cell mobilization/memory development and humoral immunity: comparison of alphaOX-40 with alphaCTLA-4. *J Immunol* 2001;167:6804–6811.

68. Brocker T, Gulbranson-Judge A, Flynn S, Riedinger M, Raykundalia C, Lane P. CD4 T cell traffic control: in vivo evidence that ligation of OX40 on CD4 T cells by OX40-ligand expressed on dendritic cells leads to the accumulation of CD4 T cells in B follicles. *Eur J Immunol* 1999;29:1610–1616.
69. Murata K, Nose M, Ndhlovu LC, Sato T, Sugamura K, Ishii N. Constitutive OX40/OX40 ligand interaction induces autoimmune-like diseases. *J Immunol* 2002;169:4628–4636.
70. Bansal-Pakala P, Gebre-Hiwot Jember A, Croft M. Signaling through OX40 (CD134) breaks peripheral T-cell tolerance. *Nat Med* 2001;7:907–912.
71. Gramaglia I, Jember A, Pippig SD, Weinberg AD, Killeen N, Croft M. The OX40 costimulatory receptor determines the development of CD4 memory by regulating primary clonal expansion. *J Immunol* 2000;165:3043–3050.
72. Maxwell JR, Weinberg A, Prell RA, Vella AT. Danger and OX40 receptor signaling synergize to enhance memory T cell survival by inhibiting peripheral deletion. *J Immunol* 2000; 164:107–112.
73. Wang HC, Klein JR. Multiple levels of activation of murine CD8(+) intraepithelial lymphocytes defined by OX40 (CD134) expression: effects on cell-mediated cytotoxicity, IFN-gamma, and IL-10 regulation. *J Immunol* 2001;167:6717–6723.
74. Kearney ER, Pape KA, Loh DY, Jenkins MK. Visualization of peptide-specific T cell immunity and peripheral tolerance induction in vivo. *Immunity* 1994;1:327–339.
75. Harding FA, McArthur JG, Gross JA, Raulet DH, Allison JP. CD28-mediated signalling co-stimulates murine T cells and prevents induction of anergy in T-cell clones. *Nature* 1992; 356:607–609.
76. Croft M, Joseph SB, Miner KT. Partial activation of naive CD4 T cells and tolerance induction in response to peptide presented by resting B cells. *J Immunol* 1997;159:3257–3265.
77. Sotomayor EM, Borrello I, Tubb E, et al. Conversion of tumor-specific CD4+ T-cell tolerance to T-cell priming through in vivo ligation of CD40. *Nat Med* 1999;5:780–787.
78. Staveley-O'Carroll K, Sotomayor E, Montgomery J, et al. Induction of antigen-specific T cell anergy: An early event in the course of tumor progression. *Proc Natl Acad Sci USA* 1998;95:1178–1183.
79. Hu HM, Winter H, Urba WJ, Fox BA. Divergent roles for CD4+ T cells in the priming and effector/memory phases of adoptive immunotherapy. *J Immunol* 2000;165:4246–4253.
80. Kjaergaard J, Tanaka J, Kim JA, Rothchild K, Weinberg A, Shu S. Therapeutic efficacy of OX-40 receptor antibody depends on tumor immunogenicity and anatomic site of tumor growth. *Cancer Res* 2000;60:5514–5521.
81. Kjaergaard J, Peng L, Cohen PA, Drazba JA, Weinberg AD, Shu S. Augmentation vs. Inhibition: Effects of conjunctional OX40R mAb and IL-2 treatment on adoptive immunotherapy of advanced tumor. *J Immunol* 2001;167:6669.
82. Siegel JP, Puri RK. Interleukin-2 toxicity. *J Clin Oncol* 1991;9:694–704.
83. Hurwitz AA, Yu TF, Leach DR, Allison JP. CTLA-4 blockade synergizes with tumor-derived granulocyte-macrophage colony-stimulating factor for treatment of an experimental mammary carcinoma. *Proc Natl Acad Sci USA* 1998;95:10,067–10,071.
84. Hurwitz AA, Foster BA, Kwon ED, et al. Combination immunotherapy of primary prostate cancer in a transgenic mouse model using CTLA-4 blockade. *Cancer Res* 2000;60: 2444–2448.
85. Kwon ED, Hurwitz AA, Foster BA, et al. Manipulation of T cell costimulatory and inhibitory signals for immunotherapy of prostate cancer. *Proc Natl Acad Sci USA* 1997;94:8099–8103.
86. Linsley PS, Greene JL, Tan P, et al. Coexpression and functional cooperation of CTLA-4 and CD28 on activated T lymphocytes. *J Exp Med* 1992;176:1595–1604.
87. Gribben JG, Freeman GJ, Boussiotis VA, et al. CTLA4 mediates antigen-specific apoptosis of human T cells. *Proc Natl Acad Sci USA* 1995;92:811–815.

88. Krummel MF, Allison JP. CTLA-4 engagement inhibits IL-2 accumulation and cell cycle progression upon activation of resting T cells. *J Exp Med* 1996;183:2533–2540.
89. Walunas TL, Bakker CY, Bluestone JA. CTLA-4 ligation blocks CD28-dependent T cell activation. *J Exp Med* 1996;183:2541–2550.
90. Walunas TL, Lenschow DJ, Bakker CY, et al. CTLA-4 can function as a negative regulator of T cell activation. *Immunity* 1994; 1:405–413.
91. Chambers CA, Kuhns MS, Egen JG, Allison JP. CTLA-4-mediated inhibition in regulation of T cell responses: mechanisms and manipulation in tumor immunotherapy. *Annu Rev Immunol* 2001;19:565–594.
92. Egen JG, Allison JP. Cytotoxic T lymphocyte antigen-4 accumulation in the immunological synapse is regulated by TCR signal strength. *Immunity* 2002;16:23–35.
93. Chuang E, Alegre ML, Duckett CS, Noel PJ, Vander Heiden MG, Thompson CB. Interaction of CTLA-4 with the clathrin-associated protein AP50 results in ligand-independent endocytosis that limits cell surface expression. *J Immunol* 1997;159: 144–151.
94. Zhang Y, Allison JP. Interaction of CTLA-4 with AP50, a clathrin-coated pit adaptor protein. *Proc Natl Acad Sci USA* 1997;94:9273–9278.
95. Linsley PS, Bradshaw J, Greene J, Peach R, Bennett KL, Mittler RS. Intracellular trafficking of CTLA-4 and focal localization towards sites of TCR engagement. *Immunity* 1996;4:535–543.
96. Linsley PS, Greene JL, Brady W, Bajorath J, Ledbetter JA, Peach R. Human B7-1 (CD80) and B7-2 (CD86) bind with similar avidities but distinct kinetics to CD28 and CTLA-4 receptors. *Immunity* 1994;1:793–801.
97. Chambers CA, Cado D, Truong T, Allison JP. Thymocyte development is normal in CTLA-4-deficient mice. *Proc Natl Acad Sci USA* 1997;94:9296–9301.
98. Waterhouse P, Penninger JM, Timms E, et al. Lymphoproliferative disorders with early lethality in mice deficient in CTLA-4. *Science* 1995;270:985–988.
99. Bachmann MF, Kohler G, Ecabert B, Mak TW, Kopf M. Cutting edge: lymphoproliferative disease in the absence of CTLA-4 is not T cell autonomous. *J Immunol* 1999; 163:1128–1131.
100. Chambers CA, Kuhns MS, Allison JP. Cytotoxic T lymphocyte antigen-4 (CTLA-4) regulates primary and secondary peptide-specific CD4(+) T cell responses. *Proc Natl Acad Sci USA* 1999;96:8603–8608.
101. Chambers CA, Sullivan TJ, Truong T, Allison JP. Secondary but not primary T cell responses are enhanced in CTLA-4-deficient CD8+ T cells. *Eur J Immunol* 1998;28: 3137–3143.
102. Murphy ML, Cotterell SE, Gorak PM, Engwerda CR, Kaye PM. Blockade of CTLA-4 enhances host resistance to the intracellular pathogen, Leishmania donovani. *J Immunol* 1998;161:4153–4160.
103. Kirman J, McCoy K, Hook S, et al. CTLA-4 blockade enhances the immune response induced by mycobacterial infection but does not lead to increased protection. *Infect Immun* 1999;67:3786–3792.
104. Riley JL, Schlienger K, Blair PJ, et al. Modulation of susceptibility to HIV-1 infection by the cytotoxic T lymphocyte antigen 4 costimulatory molecule. *J Exp Med* 2000;191: 1987–1997.
105. McGaha T, Murphy JW. CTLA-4 down-regulates the protective anticryptococcal cell-mediated immune response. *Infect Immun* 2000;68:4624–4630.
106. Luhder F, Hoglund P, Allison JP, Benoist C, Mathis D. Cytotoxic T lymphocyte-associated antigen 4 (CTLA-4) regulates the unfolding of autoimmune diabetes. *J Exp Med* 1998;187:427–432.

107. Piganelli JD, Poulin M, Martin T, Allison JP, Haskins K. Cytotoxic T lymphocyte antigen 4 (CD152) regulates self-reactive T cells in BALB/c but not in the autoimmune NOD mouse. *J Autoimmun* 2000;14:123–131.
108. Salomon B, Lenschow DJ, Rhee L, et al. B7/CD28 costimulation is essential for the homeostasis of the CD4+CD25+ immunoregulatory T cells that control autoimmune diabetes. *Immunity* 2000;12:431–440.
109. Hurwitz AA, Sullivan TJ, Krummel MF, Sobel RA, Allison JP. Specific blockade of CTLA-4/B7 interactions results in exacerbated clinical and histologic disease in an actively-induced model of experiemntal allergic encephalomyelitis. *J Neuroimmunol* 1997; 73:57–62.
110. Hurwitz AA, Sullivan TJ, Sobel RA, Allison JP. Cytotoxic T lymphocyte antigen-4 (CTLA-4) limits the expansion of encephalitogenic T cells in experimental autoimmune encephalomyelitis (EAE)-resistant BALB/c mice. *Proc Natl Acad Sci USA* 2002;99: 3013–3017.
111. Karandikar NJ, Vanderlugt CL, Walunas TL, Miler SD, J.A. B. CTLA-4: A negative regulator of autoimmune disease. *J Exp Med* 1996;184:783–788.
112. Perrin PJ, Maldonado JH, Davis TA, June CH, Racke MK. CTLA-4 blockade enhances clinical disease and cytokine production during experimental allergic encephalomyelitis. *J Immunol* 1996;157:1333–1336.
113. Perez VL, Van Parijs L, Biuckians A, Zheng XX, Strom TB, Abbas AK. Induction of peripheral T cell tolerance in vivo requires CTLA-4 engagement. *Immunity* 1997;6: 411–417.
114. Ratts RB, Arredondo LR, Bittner P, Perrin PJ, Lovett-Racke AE, Racke MK. The role of CTLA-4 in tolerance induction and antigen administration cell differentiation in experimental autoimmune encephalomyelitis: i.v. antigen administration. *Int Immunol* 1999; 11:1889–1896.
115. Samoilova EB, Horton JL, Zhang H, Khoury SJ, Weiner HL, Chen Y. CTLA-4 is required for the induction of high dose oral tolerance. *Int Immunol* 1998;10:491–498.
116. Sotomayor EM, Borrello I, Tubb E, Allison JP, Levitsky HI. In vivo blockade of CTLA-4 enhances the priming of responsive T cells but fails to prevent the induction of tumor antigen-specific tolerance. *Proc Natl Acad Sci USA* 1999;96:11,476–11,481.
117. Shrikant P, Khoruts A, Mescher MF. CTLA-4 blockade reverses CD8+ T cell tolerance to tumor by a CD4+ T cell- and IL-2-dependent mechanism. *Immunity* 1999;11:483–493.
118. Leach DR, Krummel MF, Allison JP. Enhancement of antitumor immunity by CTLA-4 blockade. *Science* 1996;271:1734–1736.
119. Kwon ED, Hurwitz AA, Foster BA, et al. Manipulation of T cell costimulatory and inhibitory signals for immunotherapy of prostate cancer. *Proc Natl Acad Sci USA* 1997; 94:8099–8103.
120. Yang YF, Zou JP, Mu J, et al. Enhanced induction of antitumor T-cell responses by cytotoxic T lymphocyte-associated molecule-4 blockade: the effect is manifested only at the restricted tumor-bearing stages. *Cancer Res* 1997;57:4036–4041.
121. Kwon ED, Foster BA, Hurwitz AA, et al. Elimination of residual metastatic prostate cancer after surgery and adjunctive cytotoxic T lymphocyte-associated antigen 4 (CTLA-4) blockade immunotherapy. *Proc Natl Acad Sci USA* 1999;96:15,074–15,079.
122. van Elsas A, Sutmuller RP, Hurwitz AA, et al. Elucidating the autoimmune and antitumor effector mechanisms of a treatment based on cytotoxic T lymphocyte antigen-4 blockade in combination with a B16 melanoma vaccine: comparison of prophylaxis and therapy. *J Exp Med* 2001;194:481–489.
123. van Elsas A, Hurwitz AA, Allison JP. Combination immunotherapy of B16 melanoma using anti-cytotoxic T lymphocyte-associated antigen 4 (CTLA-4) and granulocyte/macrophage

colony-stimulating factor (GM-CSF)-producing vaccines induces rejection of subcutaneous and metastatic tumors accompanied by autoimmune depigmentation. *J Exp Med* 1999;190:355–366.

124. Dudley ME, Wunderlich JR, Robbins PF, et al. Cancer regression and autoimmunity in patients after clonal repopulation with antitumor lymphocytes. *Science* 2002;298:850–854.
125. Rosenberg SA, White DE. Vitiligo in patients with melanoma: normal tissue antigens can be targets for cancer immunotherapy. *J Immunother Emphasis Tumor Immunol* 1996; 19:81–84.
126. Greenberg NM, DeMayo F, Finegold MJ, et al. Prostate cancer in a transgenic mouse. *Proc Natl Acad Sci USA* 1995;92:3439–3443.
127. Ito D, Ogasawara K, Iwabuchi K, Inuyama Y, Onoe K. Induction of CTL responses by simultaneous administration of liposomal peptide vaccine with anti-CD40 and anti-CTLA-4 mAb. *J Immunol* 2000;164:1230–1235.
128. Mokyr MB, Kalinichenko T, Gorelik L, Bluestone JA. Realization of the therapeutic potential of CTLA-4 blockade in low-dose chemotherapy-treated tumor-bearing mice. *Cancer Res* 1998;58:5301–5304.
129. Sojka DK, Donepudi M, Bluestone JA, Mokyr MB. Melphalan and other anticancer modalities Up-regulate B7-1 gene expression in tumor cells. *J Immunol* 2000;164:6230–6236.

11 Optimizing T-Cell Adoptive Immunotherapy to Overcome Tumor Evasion

Peter A. Cohen, MD, Gregory E. Plautz, MD, James H. Finke, PhD, and Suyu Shu, PhD

CONTENTS

1. INTRODUCTION

The normal immune system has the capacity to develop tolerant relationships with strongly antigenic environments, including the placenta and the bacteria-laden large intestine *(1–3)*. Such chronic tolerance is as important to the immune system as its capacity to destroy pathogens, since it is essential that the host does not reject a growing fetus or loops of bowel that house commensual bacteria. A vast array of physiological immunosuppressive factors, including interleukin (IL)-10, transforming growth factor-β (TGF-β), and cyclic adenosine 5′ monophosphate (cAMP)-elevating prostaglandins, contribute to the induction and maintenance of such tolerance, and are variously produced by T lymphocytes themselves and/or by ambient host cells such as macrophages *(4–12)*.

From: *Current Clinical Oncology: Cancer Immunotherapy at the Crossroads: How Tumors Evade Immunity and What Can Be Done*
Edited by: J. H. Finke and R. M. Bukowski

Tumors, whether benign or malignant, represent the pathologic subversion of physiological tolerance. If human papillomavirus (HPV)-containing warts can routinely avoid rejection, what are the realistic prospects for far less antigenic tumors to be rejected, given the inherent potential of all tumors to mimic physiologic secretion of immunosuppressive factors? How can the immune system distinguish a solid tumor from placenta, if the cytokine environment within the tumor itself is indistinguishable? Thus, it has been proposed that solid tumors pose a formidable immunosuppressive "barrier" to T-cell-mediated tumor rejection, epitomized by the observation that within the same mouse host an allogeneic tumor challenge continues to grow before, during, and after the successful rejection of a crossreactive allograft of normal skin *(13)*.

Despite the unquestioned validity of such observations, adoptive immunotherapy (AIT) with appropriately activated effector T cells (T_E) can already overcome this barrier in aggressive mouse tumor models *(14,15)*. Furthermore, markedly improved therapeutic outcomes in a recent NCI melanoma AIT trial confirm that this barrier can also be surmounted in the clinical setting *(16)*. The strategy that is currently most successful in mouse models relies on the following three observations:

1. In its most effective form, AIT employs "stand alone" doses of optimally activated T_E to cure advanced solid tumors without co-administration of adjunct biologics such as IL-2.
2. Adequate T_E dosing and optimum T_E activation are essential to successful therapy, and these are largely determined by culture conditions after T_E are extracorporealized.
3. At the present time, adjunct sublethal irradiation or chemotherapy remains necessary prior to T_E reinfusion to facilitate rejection of extrapulmonary tumor burdens *(14,15)*.

Although it may ultimately be possible to achieve similar T_E expansion and activation in vivo through vaccine maneuvers, it must be emphasized that recent culture improvements (notably anti-CD3 stimulation) were directly responsible for revealing the superior activation state in which T_E can reject advanced tumors *(14,15,17–19)*. That activation state is probably never achieved naturally within the tumor-bearing host, and may only be achieved transiently following most vaccine maneuvers *(20–24)*. Furthermore, current evidence favors blunting of T_E activation as the primary mechanism by which tumors escape the immune system, rather than a failure of T-cell sensitization. Growth of even weakly immunogenic tumors is accompanied by sensitization and prolonged proliferation of tumor-specific pre-effector T cells within tumor-draining lymph nodes (TDLN) *(25,26)*. Such sensitized T cells naturally redistribute, not only to distant lymphoid organs such as the spleen, but even into the tumor bed, where they are known as tumor-infiltrating lymphocytes (TIL) *(23,24,27–29)*.

Despite such T-cell sensitization and redistribution, spontaneous tumor rejection is seldom observed in these mouse models. In fact, as already noted, hosts can competently mediate rejection of normal tissue allografts while challenges of alloantigen-expressing tumor continue to grow progressively *(13)*.

This failure of tumor rejection despite efficient T-cell sensitization may best be explained by a regional blunting of the effector response, much as the placenta is spared in otherwise immunocompetent mothers. This blunting is most likely the result of immunosuppression and/or tepid immunostimulation within the tumor environment, causing the local effector response to subside into a tolerant state with elements of split anergy *(20–24)*. Although this usually constitutes the end of any effective antitumor response, many tumor-specific T_E may persist indefinitely within the host, and even intratumorally, in this hypoactivated state. Such persistence is dramatically demonstrated by the ability to culture-activate gigantic numbers of tumor-specific TIL ($>10^{11}$) even from the long-standing, progressively enlarging tumor nodules of melanoma patients *(16,30–32)*.

The persistence of sensitized T_E in the tumor host therefore provides a natural resource from which to generate T cell-based immunotherapy. Thanks to recent advances in mouse tumor studies and in clinical trials, for the first time, strong evidence now exists that the efficacy of tumor-specific T_E is not limited to microscopic disease or to minute tumor burdens. Furthermore, there is no evidence that any anatomic location in the host constitutes a true sanctuary site for tumor cells to escape immunological recognition. To the contrary, investigations in aggressive mouse tumor models have proven beyond any doubt that optimally activated T_E given as AIT can achieve rejection of advanced, widely disseminated tumors, including established brain tumors *(14,15,19,33)*.

This chapter addresses the evidence that points to blunting of the effector response as a primary avenue of tumor escape (Subheadings 2.1. and 2.2.), as well as recent clinical evidence that potent T_E persist during such blunting, even in patients with long-standing tumors (Subheading 2.2.). Subheading 3 reviews we reviews elements of T-cell function, already achievable ex vivo, that can overcome such tumor evasion, and explains how adjunct chemotherapy/radiation therapy is currently necessary to modulate such curative therapy.

2. TUMOR ESCAPE FROM REJECTION IS TYPICALLY ASSOCIATED WITH BLUNTING OR FATIGUE OF THE EFFECTOR T-CELL (T_E) RESPONSE

2.1. Mouse Models

Current evidence strongly indicates that T-cell sensitization to tumor-associated antigen (TAA) often occurs regardless of whether a therapeutic effector T-cell response ensues. Most typically, sensitization occurs at a site removed from the tumor bed itself, namely TDLN. In fact, extirpation experiments have demonstrated that the tumor bed itself must only be present for 3 d to enable T-cell sensitization, whereas TDLN must remain undisturbed for almost 2 wk to propagate complete resistance to subsequent tumor challenges. Such data support the importance of a transient event at the tumor site, followed by a sustained event at the TDLN, after which sensitized T cells disseminate more widely in the host *(27)*.

That transient event within the tumor bed often appears to be processing of tumor-associated antigens (Ag) by transiting host antigen-presenting cells (APC), which subsequently transport the Ag to TDLN. T-cell sensitization within TDLN occurs regardless of whether tumor cells themselves actually metastasize to the lymph nodes. Experiments conducted by several groups confirm the capacity of host APC to "cross-present" tumor Ag both to CD4+ and to CD8+ T cells *(14,15,19,33)*. Dendritic cells (DC) are the host APC that are best equipped physiologically to accomplish the multiple migrations necessary in this sequence of events *(14,15,19,34,35)*.

Within the TDLN, proliferative expansion of antitumor T cells proceeds in the shadow of the growing upstream tumor. Somewhat surprisingly, more rapidly growing tumor burdens appear to hasten and even enhance the phase of T_E sensitization and proliferative expansion within TDLN, possibly because of a more robust delivery of tumor Ag to the TDLN by DC *(25,26)*. In fact, challenges with growing tumor are more effectively sensitizing than challenges with irradiated (non-growing) tumor cells. Current evidence suggests that proliferation of the CD8+ component in TDLN is often contingent to activation of the CD4+ subset *(25,26)*. This is consistent with several studies that have demonstrated that CD4+ T cells can "condition" DC through CD40-CD40L or other interactions to promote CD8+ T-cell sensitization *(36–39)*. Nonetheless, at least a subset of CD8+ T cells is helper-independent, and is effectively sensitized to tumor Ag even in CD4-knockout animals *(19)*.

Although a persistent tumor burden is permissive and even stimulatory for T-cell sensitization, it also typically inhibits subsequent mounting of the effector response. At least some of the time, such effector inhibition is not systemic, but rather confined to the end target—e.g., the tumor bed. As demonstrated by Wick et al., concomitant challenges of normal skin allografts that are antigenically crossreactive with a tumor can still be rejected, confirming the host's enduring capacity for an undiminished effector response *(13)*. Therefore, it is not surprising that upstream tumor progression does not prevent sensitized T cells from redistributing to extranodal locations, even including the tumor bed itself. In weakly immunogenic mouse-tumor models, sensitized T cells can be retrieved from both TDLN and the growing tumor bed, despite the absence of a therapeutically evident antitumor response *(28,29,40)*. Similarly, the ability to culture-activate tumor-specific T cells (TIL) from the long-standing nodules of melanoma patients demonstrates that even tumor progression does not preclude T-cell sensitization, redistribution in the host, and long-term accumulation within tumor beds *(16)*.

The ability of a growing tumor to evade immune rejection through effector fatigue was elegantly demonstrated by Speiser et al. in a rat model of spontaneous insulinoma development *(20)*. Mice were rendered transgenic for the the tumor-promoting SV40 virus TAg expressed under control of the rat insulin promoter (RIP). Resultant "spontaneous" insulinomas were rendered more antigenic by crossing these rats with rats that were transgenic for a strongly antigenic virus glycoprotein (LCMV-GP) also under RIP control. Finally, these rats were crossed with rats that were transgenic for a T-cell receptor (TCR) enabling major histocompatibility complex (MHC) class I-restricted recognition of an LCMV-GP-derived peptide. The latter rats spontaneously developed insulinomas expressing LCMV-GP, but also possessed CD8+ T cells capable of recognizing tumor-expressing LCMV-GP. These rats displayed no spontaneous tumor rejection, but did display transient partial tumor regressions following vaccine challenges with intact LCMV virus. Such vaccination acutely increased the anti-LCMV cytolytic activity of CD8+ T cells, but this activity subsided with recurrent tumor progression. Remarkably, repeated vaccinations again resulted in transient tumor regressions and cytolytic reactivation of anti-LCMV CD8+ T cells, indicating that tumor escape did not involve apoptotic elimination of the anti-LCMV CD8+ T-cell repertoire. Furthermore, the insulinomas continued to express LCMV-GP at each recurrence, demonstrating that tumor escape was not accomplished through deleted expression of LCMV-GP. Anti-LCMV CD8+ T cells remained in evidence during subsequent tumor progressions, but not in a cytolytically activated state *(20)*.

These studies clearly demonstrated that expression of a strong viral Ag by established tumors was itself insufficient to stimulate a sustained and strongly activated effector T-cell response. Although the mechanism of effector fatigue remained unclear, transiently effective activations or reactivations of the effector response could readily be accomplished by presenting the Ag more potently and repetitively in the form of virus infection *(20)*.

Similar studies from Shrikant, Deeths et al. have elegantly monitored the sequence of events that occur when naïve CD8+ T cells are first exposed to an intraperitoneal tumor challenge *(22–24)*. CD8+ T cells from OT1 transgenic mice express TCR that recognize an MHC class I-restricted ovalbumin (OVA) peptide, and enable recognition of syngeneic EL-4 lymphoma transfected to express OVA (EL-4-OVA). Such T cells are Thy 1.2^{pos}, enabling precise monitoring of their fate when they are adoptively transferred into otherwise syngeneic Thy 1.1^{pos} hosts. One day after adoptive transfer of naïve OT1 CD8+ T cells, recipient mice were challenged intraperitoneally with EL-4-OVA or parent EL-4.

The adoptively transferred naïve OT1 CD8+ T cells transiently accumulated at the intraperitoneal site of tumor, increased in numbers, and controlled tumor growth if the challenge was EL4-OVA, but not parent EL-4. Such T-cell activation included conversion from a naïve to a memory ($CD44^{pos}$) phenotype. However, this activation did not result in a sustained antitumor response. Rather, the OT1 CD8+ T cells that were activated within the peritoneum spontaneously migrated away from the tumor challenge to remote lymphoid locations, resulting in unfettered tumor progression. When migrated OT1 CD8+ T cells were later recovered from host spleen, they retained their capacity to specifically lyse EL4-OVA targets, but had lost their capacity to spontaneously proliferate when exposed to OVA peptide. This was deemed split anergy, or antigen-induced nonresponsiveness (AINR) *(23)*.

Subsequent studies demonstrated that elements of this AINR reflected a normal T-cell response to Ag encounter *(22)*. Naïve CD8+ T cells undergoing primary TCR-stimulation and co-stimulation in vitro displayed transient IL-2 production, IFN-γ production and acquisition of lytic activity against the appropriate targets. However, after several days of further culture, proliferation ceased, resulting in CD8+ T cells that could be restimulated at Ag encounter to produce IFN-γ or lyse targets, but not to produce IL-2. Addition of exogenous rIL-2 could be used to overcome such split anergy and reinduce proliferation, after which the CD8+ T cells could again transiently produce IL-2 and proliferate upon TCR restimulation, even without additional costimulation *(22)*. In vivo data suggested that following an initial transient burst of IL-2 production by CD8+ T cells, CD4+ T cells may normally be required to provide IL-2 to "reverse" split anergy and free CD8+ T cells for more sustained autocrine activation with reduced signaling requirements *(24)*. Nonetheless, similar "split anergy" has also been observed in CD4+ T cells, suggesting a more complicated phenomenon than simple "helper dependence" *(22)*.

In summary, these mouse studies graphically illustrate the challenge of sustaining an effective antitumor response even when initial activation is brisk and effective, as a result of physiological fatigue or pathological blunting of the effector response.

2.2. Clinical Studies

A similar phenomenon consistent with regional T_E fatigue has been identified in vaccinated melanoma patients by Kammula et al. *(21)*. HLA-tetramer and real-time PCR analyses revealed that melanoma patients challenged with relevant antigenic peptides transiently developed an enrichment of Ag-specific CD8+ T cells within tumor nodules, and that such T cells produced interferon (IFN)-γ within the tumor bed as a transient response to the vaccination. Despite this unequivocal demonstration of vaccine-linked intratumoral T_E activation, no objective nodule regressions were observed in this study, indicating a failure in the effector response's magnitude or sustenance parallel to that repeatedly observed by Speiser et al. *(20)*.

Common to these studies is a persistence of tumor-specific T_E in the host, even in the absence of a therapeutically effective antitumor response. As shown by Speiser et al., later reactivation of such T_E can result in undiminished therapeutic effects, suggesting that no therapeutic potential has been lost between initial T-cell sensitization and the later breaking of exhaustion, AINR, or tolerance. However, the reality may be considerably more complex in cancer patients, in whom tumors can exist for many years before immunotherapy is considered. Even if there are persistent hypoactivated antitumor T cells in cancer patients, are they truly representative of the originally sensitized T-cell repertoire? Since T-cell apoptosis is a frequently observed and chronic event within tumors *(41–43)*, a selection process may theoretically occur in which there is clonal deletion of higher-affinity antitumor T_E, leaving only T_E with a considerably reduced therapeutic potential. This dismal possibility seemed consistent with the historically disappointing outcome of clinical trials in which melanoma patients were reinfused with immense numbers of autologous in vitro expanded TIL *(16,30–32)*.

Fortunately, a recent TIL clinical trial at the National Cancer Institute strongly suggests that the previous therapeutic deficiencies of TIL were the result of suboptimal culture activation, rather than to tumor-induced deletion of the potent T_E subset. Dramatic and sometimes sustained body-wide objective tumor regressions were recently observed in 6 of the first 13 melanoma patients who received a modified preparation of autologous TIL and conjunctional rIL-2 following nonmyeloablative chemotherapy *(16)*. Ongoing objective responses (>15–24 mo) have occurred in patients who previously failed other immunotherapy and chemotherapy regimens, and in several instances, transferred TIL were found in peripheral blood of patients for many months following transfer *(16)*.

This improved clinical outcome was predicated on two modifications to the Surgery Branch's previous strategy. Patients received chemotherapy consisting of high-dose cyclophosphamide (120 mg/kg) and fludarabine instead of lower doses of cyclophosphamide alone (25 mg/kg). Nonetheless, the newer chemotherapy regimen recently proved ineffective when melanoma patients received traditionally cultured TIL, or hyperexpanded autologous T-cell clones with high avidity to melanoma cells *(16,31,32)*. Instead, the current trial's success hinged on a distinctive culture modification in which TIL were conventionally established from each patient, screened for strong in vitro antitumor reactivity, and then, for the first time, further hyperexpanded by anti-CD3/IL-2 activation prior to adoptive transfer *(16)*. This highlights the pivotal role of T-cell culture conditions on therapeutic outcome, since the procedures for TIL derivation, adoptive transfer, and IL-2 administration were unchanged from previous NCI TIL trials.

This Surgery Branch report is probably the first compelling clinical demonstration that AIT can play a significant role in the treatment of human cancer. Furthermore, it validates the continuing importance of the weakly and poorly immunogenic mouse tumor models which have proven to be predictive in the development, understanding, and troubleshooting of AIT. Ongoing preclinical studies in these same tumor models corroborate the current clinical success at the Surgery Branch, and also point to the likelihood of continued clinical advances as the mechanism of successful AIT is better understood, and reliable culture techniques for surmounting tumor evasion are further optimized. These topics are discussed in the following section.

3. ELEMENTS OF T-CELL FUNCTION REQUIRED FOR SUCCESSFUL AIT OF ADVANCED TUMORS (TABLE 1)

3.1. Tumor-Sensitized T_E Are Confined to the Freely Trafficking L-Selectin^{low} Subset

Within tumor-bearing hosts, sensitized pre-effectors are concentrated within the T-cell subset of TDLN with downregulated L-selectin expression *(17)*. Concentration of pre-effectors within the L-selectin^{low} subset also follows vaccination maneuvers *(44)*. Following ex vivo activation with anti-CD3 or bacterial superantigen, this subpopulation constitutes a stand-alone and renewable effector population *(17,19)*. Because of their enhanced capacity to peripheralize and redistribute into tumor deposits *(45,46)*, such L-selectin^{low} T_E appear to be analogous to the L-selectin^{low} "memory effector" T cells recently described in non-tumor studies *(47–49)*.

For mouse TDLN, isolation of the L-selectin^{low} T-cell component prior to culture results in marked enrichment of effector activity. Only TDLN T cells that have downregulated L-selectin expression prior to extracorporealization, and which remain L-selectin^{low} during culture, constitute tumor-specific T_E *(17–19)*. Such stably low L-selectin expression is also consistent with "memory effector" function *(47,49)*. In contrast, although the great majority of T cells in TDLN are L-selectin^{high} at harvest, this L-selectin^{high} subset makes no positive contribution to AIT, although it largely downregulates L-selectin expression during culture *(17,18,33)*. It is thus likely that TDLN do not contain tumor-specific L-selectin^{high} "central memory" T cells at this juncture *(47)*.

Although L-selectin downregulation is strongly associated with the capacity of antitumor T_E to redistribute into tumor deposits, this appears to be a general property of all L-selectin^{low} T cells, including L-selectin^{low} normal splenocytes and even L-selectin downregulated suppressor T cells *(33,45,46)*. Therefore, ini-

Table 1
Principles of Successful Adoptive T-Cell Immunotherapy to Overcome Tumor Evasion

1. Tumor-sensitized pre-effector T cells are concentrated within the small subset of T cells with L-selectin^{low} expression. Spontaneous reversion to an L-selectin^{high} state has not yet been demonstrated, consistent with "memory effector" function.
2. Curative tumor rejection depends completely on the dose and activation status of L-selectin^{low} effector T cells (T_E).
3. Since culture conditions determine T_E dose and activation status, culture itself largely dictates therapeutic outcome.
4. T_E preparations with identical Vβ repertoires and similar avidity vary widely in therapeutic outcome, suggesting that successful culture-activation modifies other aspects of T_E function, such as resistance to apoptosis.
5. Adoptively transferred L-selectin^{low} T_E migrate successfully into tumor deposits at all tested anatomic locations, and proliferate intratumorally upon exposure to relevant tumor Ag.
6. The CD4+ and CD8+ subsets of L-selectin^{low} T_E are synergistic therapeutically, but can each be administered successfully as "stand alone" therapy, even without adjuncts such as rIL-2.
7. L-selectin^{low} T_E adoptive therapy can be therapeutically subverted by co-administration of tumor-induced suppressor T cells (T_S). Depending on their activation status, such T_S may be L-selectin^{high} or L-selectin^{low}.
8. Adjunct immunosensitizing sublethal irradiation, or more clinically appropriate chemotherapy, is currently necessary for successful adoptive therapy of established extrapulmonary tumors. Intratumoral T_E proliferation is heightened by such sublethal irradiation.

tial entry into tumors is probably a random event for circulating L-selectin^{low} T cells, with long-term retention and proliferation of only those L-selectin^{low} T cells that recognize relevant Ag within the tumor bed *(14,15)*.

Consistent with their capacity to migrate into tumors at all tested anatomic locations, optimally culture-activated L-selectin^{low} T_E are able to mediate curative rejection of advanced established tumors at all tested locations, including pulmonary, intracranial, hepatic, and subcutaneous (sc) challenges *(14,15,19)*. This contrasts with earlier T-cell preparations ("in vitro sensitized" T cells and TIL) prepared from identical TDLN, which were, for example, totally ineffective against experimental sc tumors, regardless of the T-cell dose, with or without conjunctional IL-2 *(14,15)*. At present, it is unknown whether the therapeutic deficiencies of such earlier preparations were the result of disparate T_E lineage, or disparate culture activation (e.g., a lack of anti-CD3 stimulation).

3.2. AIT With L-Selectin^{low} T_E is Highly Dose-Dependent

One striking and consistent observation in all AIT experiments is that threshold doses of L-selectin^{low} T_E must be adoptively transferred to achieve curative rejection of established tumors *(14,15,17–19)*. These doses differ for individual tumor models, and even a halving of the T_E dose can result in complete therapeutic failure. The particular "impact" that the threshold T_E dose must achieve is unknown. Knockout studies have demonstrated that this impact is not IFN-γ secretion *(50)*, and it is not linked to very high initial accumulation of T_E within the tumor bed, since established mouse sc tumors have a notoriously low initial T_E accumulation (logs-fold less than pulmonary or intracranial tumors), yet rejection is still observed *(33,45)*. Although the mechanistic basis of this "threshold" effect is unknown, it is evident that meeting this threshold by adoptively transferring putatively effective doses of culture-activated T_E is a much more straightforward method than providing it through vaccine maneuvers.

3.3. Variable Efficacy of Conjunctional Treatments

Because the capacity of adoptively transferred L-selectin^{low} T_E to mediate curative tumor rejection is highly dose-dependent, it is important to consider the capacity of conjunctional treatments to compensate for subtherapeutic T_E doses. Although rIL-2 is often administered as an AIT adjunct, its therapeutic significance in this context has not been established in randomized clinical trials. Its original testing was predicated on observations that classically derived mouse TIL lacked any therapeutic effect in the absence of rIL-2 co-administration *(28,29)*.

Since therapeutically superior L-selectin^{low} T_E display no such absolute dependence upon conjunctional rIL-2 in mouse models, we recently compared the effects of conjunctional treatments upon AIT, using "therapeutic" or "subtherapeutic" doses of L-selectin^{low} T_E. For the treatment of advanced (10-d established) pulmonary metastases, co-administration of either rIL-2 or the costimulatory ligand OX-40R MAb enhanced the therapeutic effect of suboptimal doses of L-selectin^{low} T_E. For advanced (10-d) intracranial tumors, OX-40R MAb was similarly enhancing, but conjunctional IL-2 was non-enhancing, and also impeded AIT by otherwise curative doses of L-selectin^{low} T_E *(51)*. rIL-2's therapeutic blockade was associated with inhibition of T_E trafficking into intracranial tumors *(51)*. Similarly, Shrikant et al. have described undesirable pro-apoptotic effects of adjunct rIL-2 during AIT of malignant ascites *(52)*.

Importantly, adjunct IL-2 and OX-40R MAb had no significant impact (enhancement or inhibition) upon the treatment of established 10d hepatic metastases by L-selectin^{low} T_E. In this virtually pre-terminal treatment model, untreated mice survive only 1 wk past the day of therapy. Despite this strikingly brief therapeutic window of opportunity, and the uselessness of conjunctional treatments, adoptive transfer of "stand-alone," adequately dosed L-selectin^{low} T_E still proved to be curative (manuscript in preparation).

These data clearly demonstrate that the impact of adjunct treatments upon AIT is vulnerable to major anatomic variances. Although modifying schedules of adjunct biologic factors may address certain undesirable or paradoxical effects, the use of such adjuncts is simply unnecessary when adequate doses of L-selectin^{low} T_E are administered.

3.4. Passenger Suppressor T Cells (T_S) Can Cause Effector T-Cell Blockade

As a purely pragmatic consideration, elimination of the non-therapeutic L-selectin^{high} subset at the beginning of culture markedly reduces the numbers of T cells that must be propagated and adoptively transferred, and reduces consumption of culture medium and growth-stimulatory factors. However, these practical incentives have become a near mandate now that it has been determined that the L-selectin^{high} subset can also be a source of therapeutically ruinous passenger T_S *(33)*. In contrast to previously characterized T_S that primarily inhibit the afferent limb of the immune response (e.g., CD4+CD25+ T_S) *(53)*, L-selectin^{high} passenger T_S exert effector blockade. This poses an ultimate liability to successful AIT, since culture-activated L-selectin^{low} T_E remain fully vulnerable to L-selectin^{high} T_S, even when afferent blockade is no longer a factor *(33)*.

Tumor-induced L-selectin^{high} T_S appear in TDLN between d 9 and 12 following tumor challenge. They can be isolated, anti-CD3-activated, and co-transferred with either d 9 or d 12 L-selectin^{low} T_E to prevent tumor rejection. These T_S are predominantly CD8+, but CD4+ participation has not been ruled out *(33)*.

By purging L-selectin^{high} cells prior to culture, freshly harvested d 12 TDLN can readily be divested of passenger T_S. This is only transiently available as a purging technique, since T_S downregulate L-selectin expression during culture-activation. L-selectin downregulated T_S are currently indistinguishable from L-selectin^{low} T_E, showing equivalent expression patterns for CD25, CD28, CTLA4 and CD44 *(33)*. L-selectin downregulated T_S also resemble L-selectin^{low} T_E in their superior ability to traffick into tumor beds, providing favorable stoichiometrics for effector blockade *(33)*.

Separately anti-CD3-activated L-selectin^{high} T cells from d 12 TDLN can already inhibit tumor-specific IFN-γ production by L-selectin^{low} T_E prior to adoptive transfer. In contrast, when such T_S are anti-CD3-activated as a component of unfractionated d 12 TDLN T cells, they remain functionally silent until adoptive transfer, at which time they prevent tumor rejection. A significant element of T_S activation therefore normally occurs following re-infusion.

In mouse models, AIT of established sc tumors is particularly vulnerable to L-selectin^{high} T_S, corresponding to the relatively low initial accumulation of even L-selectin^{low} T_E at this experimental challenge site. Remarkably, mice that have been triply challenged with sc, pulmonary, and intracranial tumors can be cured by adoptive transfer of purified L-selectin^{low} T_E or unfractionated T cells from d 9 TDLN, but develop mixed responses and ultimately treatment failure when treated with unfractionated T cells from d 12 TDLN, because of the latter's T_S content.

Many features augur the clinical significance of this T_S phenomenon. Historically, adoptive transfer of culture-activated T_E to melanoma patients has typically resulted in nonsustained and/or mixed responses at best, with no demonstrable survival advantage *(30)*. Even in the recent, generally more promising NCI Surgery Branch trial, this has remained a problem for the majority of treated patients *(16)*. Such disappointing clinical outcomes have occurred despite in vitro evidence that many and sometimes all patients received tumor-specific T cells capable of T1-type cytokine production and direct tumor lysis *(54)*. The therapeutic discrepancy between in vitro and in vivo performance has traditionally been attributed to a trafficking failure of cultured T cells, although such a trafficking defect has never been validated by clinical studies *(55–57)*.

Mouse studies display remarkable reasonance with this clinical performance discrepancy: when unfractionated T cells from d 12 TDLN are employed as AIT, mixed tumor responses and ultimate treatment failure is observed, despite the T cells' strong capacity in vitro for tumor-specific IFN-γ production prior to infusion, and their excellent subsequent trafficking proficiency in vivo.

3.5. Relative Roles of CD4+ and CD8+ L-Selectin^{low} T_E Subsets

Knockout mice studies have confirmed that CD8+ L-selectin^{low} antitumor T_E can be sensitized in the absence of CD4+ T cells, and vice versa *(19)*. Since each subset is also therapeutically active against tumors as "stand alone" adoptive therapy without IL-2 co-administration, it is apparent that L-selectin^{low} CD8+ T_E constitute "helper-independent" T cells *(14,18,45,58)*.

It is apparent that L-selectin^{low} CD4+ and CD8+ T_E also have significant functional differences, beginning with different practical requirements for recognizing tumor Ag. The CD8+ subset produces IFN-γ and granulocyte-macrophage colony-stimulating factor (GM-CSF) when exposed either to relevant MHC class I-expressing tumor targets or tumor-associated macrophages (TAM); in contrast, L-selectin^{low} CD4+ T_E fail to react with relevant, MHC Class II^{neg} tumor, but produce IFN-γ when exposed to relevant TAM *(19)*. The ability to interact directly with MHC Class I^{pos}/II^{neg} tumor cells may confer a therapeutic advantage to L-selectin^{low} CD8+ T_E by facilitating direct perforin-mediated tumor-cell lysis in addition to indirect mechanisms of tumor rejection *(59)*.

Despite the capacity of either subset for "stand alone" therapy, it is also evident that they are not simply interchangeable as adoptive therapy, but rather play distinctive and complementary roles. For example, adoptively transferred L-selectin^{low} CD4+ T_E have proven to be relatively more potent on a cell-number basis for eradicating 3-d sc tumors, whereas L-selectin^{low} CD8+ T_E have proven to be more effective against 10-d pulmonary metastases *(19)*. Although the therapeutic efficacy of purified L-selectin^{low} CD8+ T_E varies strongly in proportion to observed accumulation efficiencies at these sites (pulmonary tumors > intracranial tumors >> sc tumors) *(19,45)*, the therapeutic efficacy of purified L-selectin^{low} CD4+ T_E appears to be largely independent of such trafficking variances. This may reflect the superior abilities of L-selectin^{low} CD4+ T_E to proliferate intratumorally, provide APC conditioning, and/or gradually recruit additional host-effector elements, including CD8+ T_E *(60–65)*. Nonetheless, purified L-selectin^{low} CD8+ T_E display greater efficacy than purified L-selectin^{low} CD4+ T_E in eradicating advanced (d 10) pulmonary tumors, even without co-administration of exogenous rIL-2, and are essential for achieving rapid rejection of sc tumors *(19)*. It has not been determined whether the latter reflects the L-selectin^{low} CD8+ T cell's superior capacity to interact directly with MHC Class I^{pos}/Class II^{neg} tumor cells.

Given the relative insensitivity of L-selectin^{low} CD4+ T cells to trafficking variances and the rapid effector impact of L-selectin^{low} CD8+ T cells even against advanced tumors, it is not surprising that these subsets are often therapeutically superior and even synergistic when administered together, despite their respective capacities for "stand alone" therapy when administered at threshold doses.

3.6. Therapeutic Potency of T_E Is Ultimately Dictated by Culture Conditions

Recent studies have confirmed that extended culture does not diminish the *per cell* therapeutic potency of L-selectin^{low} T_E, yet provides opportunities for numeric expansion that can provide T_E doses well above the therapeutic "threshold" (*66*; manuscripts in preparation). Although extended culture *per se* does not detectably impact therapeutic potency, certain culture modifications, including substitution of mouse serum (MS) for fetal calf serum (FCS) *(67)* have proven to have a profoundly enhancing impact on mouse T_E. Despite the therapeutic superiority of T_E following culture in MS compared to FCS, intracellular cytokine assays at the end of culture demonstrate an similar frequency of tumor-specific T_E with a virtually identical TCR-Vβ-chain repertoire. Furthermore, higher avidity is not evident in the T_E cultured in MS. The major, consistently observed in vitro distinction between L-selectin^{low} T_E prepared in MS vs FCS is the former's superior resistance to apoptosis when restimulated with anti-CD3 or with whole-cell tumor digests (manuscript in preparation).

Such data demonstrate that culture itself largely dictates therapeutic outcome, even in the absence of affinity divergences or avidity modulations. It is now proving feasible to identify culture modifications that not only generate therapeutic doses of L-selectin^{low} T_E, but also proactively confer potent therapeutic characteristics. Ironically, such data indicate that the already impressive therapeutic potential of L-selectin^{low} T_E had been considerably underestimated when they were prepared exclusively in FCS.

3.7. Adjunct Irradiation or Chemotherapy Is Currently Essential to Successful AIT

With the exception of pulmonary metastases, for which T_E trafficking is exceptionally robust, effective AIT has consistently required the adjunct administration of either sublethal radiation therapy (RT) or chemotherapy prior to T-cell adoptive transfer *(68,69)*. This is as true for high-performance L-selectin^{low} T_E as it is for less potent T-cell preparations. Adjunct RT or chemotherapy enables adoptively transferred, "stand-alone" doses of L-selectin^{low} T_E to reject advanced poorly immunogenic tumors (intracranial, sc, and intrahepatic), and is also required for rejection of early tumors at certain anatomic locations (e.g., sc and intracranial) *(14,15,50)*.

Experiments performed in the mid-1980s demonstrated that adjunct sublethal total body irradiation (TBI, 500R) could potentiate AIT of MCA-105 even when TBI was applied prior to tumor inoculation, 5 d prior to adoptive transfer *(70)*. This indicated that a host alteration rather than a direct antitumor effect was vital to the observed potentiation. Although it was initially theorized that this host alteration was ablation of suppressor T cells, this was not validated in subsequent mechanistic studies that addressed this possibility *(69)*.

The recent melanoma AIT trial at the NCI Surgery Branch incorporated high-dose chemotherapy as part of its regimen *(16)*, and that trial's early success will undoubtedly inspire the continued use of adjunct chemotherapy, even in the absence of a sure mechanistic rationale. Clarifying the therapeutic mechanisms of adjunct RT/chemotherapy remains essential to develop less toxic, but equally effective alternatives. Although chemotherapy is clinically more acceptable than RT, mechanistic studies in mice are more readily accomplished with RT, because regional and total body RT can be compared. We recently defined several unique effects of adjunct RT upon individual elements of T-cell function:

1. Although adjunct RT itself has no discernible impact upon the trafficking of adoptively transferred L-selectin^{low} T_E into tumor deposits, it potentiates proliferation of adoptively transferred, fluorescently tagged (CFSE-labeled) T_E. Tumor-specific proliferation within the tumor bed is especially potentiated, suggesting that adjunct RT enhances intratumoral Ag presentation or costimulation by an unidentified mechanism *(71)*.

2. Adjunct RT reduces the performance demands upon T_E to achieve tumor rejection. In non-irradiated hosts, we and others have demonstrated that rejection of early pulmonary tumors requires adoptively transferred T_E to produce IFN-γ. In contrast, in irradiated hosts, T_E, or host-cell production of IFN-γ has proved to be completely unnecessary to tumor rejection, regardless of the site of tumor implantation (e.g., pulmonary, sc, or intracranial) *(50)*. This observation was subsequently corroborated by other investigators *(72)*.

Administration of high-dose (100 mg/kg) cyclophosphamide several hours prior to adoptive therapy has proven to be equally as effective as TBI to enable adoptively transferred L-selectin^{low} T_E to cure a variety of tumor models *(69)*. Despite blood–brain barrier concerns, TBI or cyclophosphamide given on the same day as T_E enabled cure of both MCA-105 and MCA-205 tumors, whether established sc or intracranially (manuscript in preparation). These studies suggest that "same day" adjunct RT or chemotherapy may have broad therapeutic applicability, and single-agent "high-dose" cyclophosphamide is clinically preferable to TBI.

Because evidence strongly suggests that the immunosensitizing effect of these adjuncts reflects host modulation rather than a direct antitumor effect, better elucidation of their mechanism(s) of action is very likely to reveal less toxic treatment alternatives.

4. CONCLUSION

Despite the strongly evident capacity of established solid tumors to resist recognition and rejection by naturally sensitized T cells, extracorporealization of those T_E affords the opportunity to remedy dosing and activation issues that are critical to successful AIT. The immunosuppressive "barrier" posed by established solid tumors is insufficient to prevent curative AIT when T_E are optimally activated and adjunct chemotherapy or RT is provided. Because adjunct chemotherapy is clinically acceptable, there are no insurmountable barriers to successful AIT in cancer patients.

REFERENCES

1. Wojtowicz-Praga S. Reversal of tumor-induced immunosuppression: a new approach to cancer therapy. *J Immunother* 1997;20(3):165–177.
2. Gabrilovich D, Ishida T, Oyama T, Ran S, Kravtsov V, Nadaf S, et al. Vascular endothelial growth factor inhibits the development of dendritic cells and dramatically affects the differentiation of multiple hematopoietic lineages in vivo. *Blood* 1998;92(11):4150–4166.
3. Kavanaugh DY, Carbone DP. Immunologic dysfunction in cancer. *Hematol Oncol Clin N Am* 1996;10(4):927–951.
4. Kullberg MC, Ward JM, Gorelick PL, Caspar P, Hieny S, Cheever A, et al. Helicobacter hepaticus triggers colitis in specific-pathogen-free interleukin-10 (IL-10)-deficient mice

through an IL-12- and gamma interferon-dependent mechanism. *Infect Immun* 1998; 66(11):5157–5166.

5. Davidson NJ, Hudak SA, Lesley RE, Menon S, Leach MW, Rennick DM. IL-12, but not IFN-gamma, plays a major role in sustaining the chronic phase of colitis in IL-10-deficient mice. *J Immunol* 1998;161(6):3143–3149.
6. Reuter BK, Asfaha S, Buret A, Sharkey KA, Wallace JL. Exacerbation of inflammation-associated colonic injury in rat through inhibition of cyclooxygenase-2. *J Clin Investig* 1996;98(9):2076–2085.
7. Lane JS, Todd KE, Lewis MP, Gloor B, Ashley SW, Reber HA, et al. Interleukin-10 reduces the systemic inflammatory response in a murine model of intestinal ischemia/reperfusion. *Surgery* 1997;122(2):288–294.
8. Strober W, Kelsall B, Fuss I, Marth T, Ludviksson B, Ehrhardt R, et al. Reciprocal IFN-gamma and TGF-beta responses regulate the occurrence of mucosal inflammation. *Immunol Today* 1997;18(2):61–64.
9. Powrie F, Carlino J, Leach MW, Mauze S, Coffman RL. A critical role for transforming growth factor-beta but not interleukin 4 in the suppression of T helper type 1-mediated colitis by CD45RB(low) CD4+ T cells. *J Exp Med* 1996;183(6):2669–2674.
10. Giladi E, Raz E, Karmeli F, Okon E, Rachmilewitz D. Transforming growth factor-beta gene therapy ameliorates experimental colitis in rats. *Eur J Gastroenterol Hepatol* 1995; 7(4):341–347.
11. Seo N, Hayakawa S, Takigawa M, Tokura Y. Interleukin-10 expressed at early tumour sites induces subsequent generation of CD4(+) T-regulatory cells and systemic collapse of anti-tumour immunity. *Immunology* 2001;103(4):449–457.
12. Nakamura K, Kitani A, Strober W. Cell contact-dependent immunosuppression by CD4(+) CD25(+) regulatory T cells is mediated by cell surface-bound transforming growth factor beta. *J Exp Med* 2001;194(5):629–644.
13. Wick M, Dubey P, Koeppen H, Siegel CT, Fields PE, Chen L, et al. Antigenic cancer cells grow progressively in immune hosts without evidence for T cell exhaustion or systemic anergy. *J Exp Med* 1997;186(2):229–238.
14. Cohen PA, Peng L, Plautz GE, Kim KK, Weng DE, Shu S. CD4+ T Cells in Adoptive Immunotherapy and the Indirect Mechanism of Tumor Rejection. *Crit Rev Immunol* 2000; 20(1):17–56.
15. Cohen PA, Peng L, Kjaergaard J, Plautz GE, Finke JH, Koski GK, et al. T-cell adoptive therapy of tumors: mechanisms of improved therapeutic performance. *Crit Rev Immunol* 2001;21(1–3):215–248.
16. Dudley ME, Wunderlich JR, Robbins PF, Yang JC, Hwu P, Schwartzentruber DJ, et al. Cancer regression and autoimmunity in patients after clonal repopulation with antitumor lymphocytes. *Science* 2002;298(5594):850–854.
17. Kagamu H, Touhalisky JE, Plautz GE, Krauss JC, Shu S. Isolation based on L-selectin expression of immune effector T cells derived from tumor-draining lymph nodes. *Cancer Res* 1996;56(19):4338–4342.
18. Kagamu H, Shu S. Purification of L-selectin(low) cells promotes the generation of highly potent CD4 antitumor effector T lymphocytes. *J Immunol* 1998;160(7): 3444–3452.
19. Peng L, Kjaergaard J, Weng DE, Plautz GE, Shu S, Cohen PA. Helper-independent CD8+/CD62L low T Cells with broad anti-tumor efficacy are naturally sensitized during tumor progression. *J Immunol* 2000;165:5738–5749.
20. Speiser DE, Miranda R, Zakarian A, Bachmann MF, McKall-Faienza K, Odermatt B, et al. Self antigens expressed by solid tumors Do not efficiently stimulate naive or activated T cells: implications for immunotherapy. *J Exp Med* 1997;186(5):645–653.

21. Kammula US, Lee K-H, Riker AI, Wang E, Ohnmacht GA, Rosenberg SA, et al. Functional analysis of antigen-specific T lymphocytes by serial measurement of gene expression in peripheral blood mononuclear cells and tumor specimens. *J Immunol* 1999;163(12):6867–6875.
22. Deeths MJ, Kedl RM, Mescher MF. CD8+ T cells become nonresponsive (anergic) following activation in the presence of costimulation. *J Immunol* 1999;163(1):102–110.
23. Shrikant P, Mescher MF. Control of syngeneic tumor growth by activation of CD8+ T cells: efficacy is limited by migration away from the site and induction of nonresponsiveness. *J Immunol* 1999;162(5):2858–2866.
24. Shrikant P, Khoruts A, Mescher MF. CTLA-4 blockade reverses CD8+ T cell tolerance to tumor by a CD4+ T cell- and IL-2-dependent mechanism. *Immunity* 1999;11(4):483–493.
25. Marzo AL, Kinnear BF, Lake RA, Frelinger JJ, Collins EJ, Robinson BW, et al. Tumor-specific CD4+ T cells have a major "post-licensing" role in CTL mediated anti-tumor immunity. *J Immunol* 2000; 165(11):6047–6055.
26. Marzo AL, Lake RA, Lo D, Sherman L, McWilliam A, Nelson D, et al. Tumor antigens are constitutively presented in the draining lymph nodes. *J Immunol* 1999;162(10):5838–5845.
27. Stephenson KR, Perry-Lalley D, Griffith KD, Shu S, Chang AE. Development of antitumor reactivity in regional draining lymph nodes from tumor-immunized and tumor-bearing murine hosts. *Surgery* 1989;105(4):523–528.
28. Rosenberg SA, Spiess P, Lafreniere R. A new approach to the adoptive immunotherapy of cancer with tumor-infiltrating lymphocytes. *Science* 1986;233(4770):1318–1321.
29. Barth RJ, Jr., Mule JJ, Asher AL, Sanda MG, Rosenberg SA. Identification of unique murine tumor associated antigens by tumor infiltrating lymphocytes using tumor specific secretion of interferon-gamma and tumor necrosis factor. *J Immunol Methods* 1991;140: 269–279.
30. Rosenberg SA, Yannelli JR, Yang JC, Topalian SL, Schwartzentruber DJ, Weber JS, et al. Treatment of patients with metastatic melanoma with autologous tumor-infiltrating lymphocytes and interleukin2. *J Natl Cancer Inst* 1994;86:1159–1166.
31. Dudley ME, Wunderlich JR, Yang JC, Hwu P, Schwartzentruber DJ, Topalian SL, et al. A phase I study of nonmyeloablative chemotherapy and adoptive transfer of autologous tumor antigen-specific T lymphocytes in patients with metastatic melanoma. *J Immunother* 2002; 25(3):243–251.
32. Dudley ME, Wunderlich J, Nishimura MI, Yu D, Yang JC, Topalian SL, et al. Adoptive transfer of cloned melanoma-reactive T lymphocytes for the treatment of patients with metastatic melanoma. *J Immunother* 2001;24(4):363–373.
33. Peng L, Kjaergaard J, Plautz GE, Awad M, Drazba JA, Shu S, et al. Tumor-induced Lselectin^{high} suppressor T cells mediate potent effector T cell blockade and cause failure of otherwise curative adoptive immunotherapy. *J Immunol* 2002;169:4811–4821.
34. Cruz PD, Bergstresser PR. Antigen processing and presentation by epidermal Langerhans cells, induction of immunity or unresponsiveness. *Dermatol Clin* 1990;8:633–646.
35. Girolomoni G, Simon JC, Bergstresser PR, Cruz PD. Freshly isolated spleen dendritic cells and epidermal Langerhans cells undergo similar phenotypic and functional changes during short term culture. *J Immunol* 1990;145:2820–2826.
36. Caux C, Massacrier C, Vanbervliet B, Dubois B, Van Kooten C, Durand I, et al. Activation of human dendritic cells through CD40 cross-linking. *J Exp Med* 1994;180: 1263–1272.
37. Toes REM, Schoenberger SP, van der Voort EIH, Offringa R, Melief CJM. CD40-CD40Ligand interactions and their role in cytotoxic T lymphocyte priming and anti-tumor immunity. *Semin Immunol* 1998;10(6):443–448.
38. Ridge JP, Di Rosa F, Matzinger P. A conditioned dendritic cell can be a temporal bridge between a CD4+ T-helper and a T-killer cell. *Nature* 1998;393(6684):474–478.

39. Lu Z, Yuan L, Zhou X, Sotomayor E, Levitsky HI, Pardoll DM. CD40-independent pathways of T cell help for priming of CD8(+) cytotoxic T lymphocytes. *J Exp Med* 2000; 191(3):541–550 2000; 191(3):541–550.
40. Chou T, Chang AE, Shu SY. Generation of therapeutic T lymphocytes from tumor-bearing mice by in vitro sensitization. Culture requirements and characterization of immunologic specificity. *J Immunol* 1988;140(7):2453–2461.
41. Uzzo RG, Rayman P, Kolenko V, Clark PE, Bloom T, Ward AM, et al. Mechanisms of apoptosis in T cells from patients with renal cell carcinoma. *Clin Cancer Res* 1999;5: 1219–1229.
42. Gastman BR, Johnson DE, Whiteside TL, Rabinowich H. Tumor-induced apoptosis of T lymphocytes: elucidation of intracellular apoptotic events. *Blood* 2000 Mar 15;95(6):2015–2023 2000; 95(6):2015–2023.
43. Whiteside TL. Immune cells in the tumor microenvironment. Mechanisms responsible for functional and signaling defects. *Adv Exp Med Biol* 1998;451:167–171.
44. Tanaka H, Yoshizawa H, Yamaguchi Y, Ito K, Kagamu H, Suzuki E, et al. Successful doptive immunotherapy of murine poorly immunogenic tumor with specific effector cells generated from gene-modified tumor-primed lymph node cells. *J Immunol* 1999; 162(6):3574–3582.
45. Kjaergaard J, Shu S. Tumor infiltration by adoptively transferred T cells is independent of immunologic specificity but requires down-regulation of L-selectin expression. *J Immunol* 1999;163:751–759.
46. Mukai S, Kjaergaard J, Shu S, Plautz GE. Infiltration of tumors by systemically transferred tumor-reactive T lymphocytes is required for antitumor efficacy. *Cancer Res* 1999; 59(20):5245–5249.
47. Sallusto F, Lenig D, Forster R, Lipp M, Lanzavecchia A. Two subsets of memory T lymphocytes with distinct homing potentials and effector functions. *Nature* 1999;401(6754): 708–712.
48. Tussey L, Speller S, Gallimore A, Vessey R. Functionally distinct CD8+ memory T cell subsets in persistent EBV infection are differentiated by migratory receptor expression. *Eur J Immunol* 2000;30(7):1823–1829.
49. Masopust D, Vezys V, Marzo AL, Lefrancois L. Preferential localization of effector memory cells in nonlymphoid tissue. *Science* 2001;291(5512):2413–2417.
50. Peng L, Krauss JC, Plautz GE, Mukai S, Shu S, Cohen PA. T cell-mediated tumor rejection displays diverse dependence upon perforin and IFN-gamma mechanisms that cannot be predicted from in vitro T cell characteristics. *J Immunol* 2000;165(12):7116–7124.
51. Kjaergaard J, Peng L, Cohen PA, Drazba JA, Weinberg AD, Shu S. Augmentation vs. inhibition: effects of conjunctional OX-40 receptor monoclonal antibody and IL-2 treatment on adoptive immunotherapy of advanced tumor. *J Immunol* 2001;167:6669–6677.
52. Shrikant P, Mescher MF. Opposing effects of IL-2 in tumor immunotherapy: promoting CD8 T cell growth and inducing apoptosis. *J Immunol* 2002;169(4):1753–1759.
53. Tanaka H, Tanaka J, Kjaergaard J, Shu S. Depletion of CD4+CD25+ regulatory cells aguments the generation of specific immune T cells in tumor-draining lymph nodes. *J Immunother* 2002;25:207–217.
54. Schwartzentruber DJ, Hom SS, Dadmarz R, White DE, Yannelli JR, Steinberg SM, et al. In vitro predictors of therapeutic response in melanoma patients receiving tumor-infiltrating lymphocytes and interleukin-2. *J Clin Oncol* 1994;12(7):1475–1483.
55. Pockaj BA, Sherry RM, Wei JP, Yannelli JR, Carter CS, Leitman SF, et al. Localization of 111indium-labeled tumor infiltrating lymphocytes to tumor in patients receiving adoptive immunotherapy. Augmentation with cyclophosphamide and correlation with response. *Cancer* 1994;73(6):1731–1737.

56. Yee C, Gilbert MJ, Riddell SR, Brichard VG, Fefer A, Thompson JA, et al. Isolation of tyrosinase-specific CD8+ and CD4+ T cell clones from the peripheral blood of melanoma patients following in vitro stimulation with recombinant vaccinia virus. *J Immunol* 1996;157(9): 4079–4086.
57. Yee C, Thompson JA, Byrd D, Riddell SR, Roche P, Celis E, et al. Adoptive T cell therapy using antigen-specific CD8+ T cell clones for the treatment of patients with metastatic melanoma: in vivo persistence, migration, and antitumor effect of transferred T cells. *Proc Natl Acad Sci USA* 2002;99(25):16,168–16,173.
58. Mukai S, Kagamu H, Shu S, Plautz GE. Critical role of CD11a (LFA-1) in therapeutic efficacy of systemically transferred antitumor effector T cells. *Cell Immunol* 1999;192: 122–132.
59. Peng L, Krauss JC, Plautz GE, Mukai S, Shu S, Cohen PA. T-cell mediated rejection of established tumors displays a varied requirement for perforin and IFN-gamma expression which is not predicted by in vitro lytic capacity. *J Immunol* 2000;165:7116–7124.
60. Ridge JP, Di Rosa F, Matzinger P. A conditioned dendritic cell can be a temporal bridge between a CD4+ T-helper and a T-killer cell. *Nature* 1998;393(6684):474–478.
61. Surman DR, Dudley ME, Overwijk WW, Restifo NP. CD4+ T cell control of CD8+ T cell reactivity to a model tumor antigen. *J Immunol* 2000;164:562–565.
62. Thivolet C, Bendelac A, Bedossa P, Bach JF, Carnaud C. CD8+ T cell homing to the pancreas in the nonobese diabetic mouse is CD4+ T cell-dependent. *J Immunol* 1991; 146(1):85–88.
63. Miki S, Ksander B, Streilein JW. Studies on the minimum requirements for in vitro "cure" of tumor cells by cytotoxic T lymphocytes. *Reg Immunol* 1992;4(6):352–362.
64. Ksander BR, Acevedo J, Streilein JW. Local T helper cell signals by lymphocytes infiltrating intraocular tumors. *J Immunol* 1992;148(6):1955–1963.
65. Bando Y, Ksander BR, Streilein JW. Characterization of specific T helper cell activity in mice bearing alloantigenic tumors in the anterior chamber of the eye. *Eur J Immunol* 1991; 21(8):1923–1931.
66. Wang LX, Chen BG, Plautz GE. Adoptive immunotherapy of advanced tumors with CD62 L-selectin(low) tumor-sensitized T lymphocytes following ex vivo hyperexpansion. *J Immunol* 2002;169(6):3314–3320.
67. Cohen PA, Fowler DJ, Kim H, White RL, Czerniecki BJ, Carter C, et al. Propagation of murine and human T cells with defined antigen specificity and function. In: Ciba Foundation Symposium No 187: Vaccines against virally induced cancers (Frazer I, Chadwick D, Marsh J, eds.), Wiley & Sons Ltd, Chichester, 1994, pp. 179–193.
68. Plautz GE, Inoue M, Shu S. Defining the synergistic effects of irradiation and T-cell immunotherapy for murine intracranial tumors. *Cell Immunol* 1996;171(2):277–284.
69. Peng L, Shu S, Krauss JC. Treatment of subcutaneous tumor with adoptively transferred T cells. *Cell Immunol* 1997;178(1):24–32.
70. Chang AE, Shu S, Chou T, Lafreniere R, Rosenberg SA. Differences in the effects of host suppression on the adoptive immunotherapy of subcutaneous and visceral tumors. *Cancer Res* 1986;46(7):3426–3430.
71. Kjaergaard J, Peng L, Cohen PA, Shu S. Therapeutic efficacy of adoptive immunotherapy is predicated on in vivo antigen-specific proliferation of donor T cells. *Clin Immunol* 2003;108(1):8–20.
72. Winter H, Hu HM, McClain K, Urba WJ, Fox BA. Immunotherapy of melanoma: a dichotomy in the requirement for IFN-gamma in vaccine-induced antitumor immunity versus adoptive immunotherapy. *J Immunol* 2001;166(12):7370–7380.

12 Tumor Resistance to Apoptosis

Mechanisms of Evasion and Implications for Radiation and Chemotherapeutic Strategies

Robert G. Uzzo, MD, *Paul Cairns,* PhD,
Nickolai Dulin, PhD, *Eric M. Horwitz,* MD,
Alan Pollack, MD, PhD,
and Vladimir Kolenko, MD, PhD

CONTENTS

1. MOLECULAR MECHANISMS OF APOPTOSIS IN CANCER CELLS

Anticancer therapeutic regimens such as chemo-, radiation-, and immunotherapy may trigger tumor-cell death through the induction of apoptosis. Alterations in the apoptotic pathways may determine tumor resistance to current therapeutic strategies. An understanding of the molecular mechanisms involved in the regulation of apoptosis and how tumor cells evade apoptotic death may provide insight into the processes of carcinogenesis and the pro-

From: *Current Clinical Oncology: Cancer Immunotherapy at the Crossroads: How Tumors Evade Immunity and What Can Be Done*
Edited by: J. H. Finke and R. M. Bukowski © Humana Press Inc., Totowa, NJ

gression of various malignancies, making it possible to use more rational approaches to antitumor therapy.

Apoptosis is a specific process that causes programmed cell death by activating evolutionarily conserved intracellular pathways. Apoptotic cell death is characterized by a series of unique biochemical and morphological events such as cleavage of multiple proteins, phosphatidyl serine exposure, cell shrinkage, and condensation and fragmentation of chromatin. Apoptosis can be initiated through two alternative pathways: death receptors located on a cell surface (the extrinsic pathway) or mitochondrial mechanisms (the intrinsic pathway) (Fig. 1). The first pathway involves ligand-induced activation of death receptors such as CD95/APO-1/Fas, tumor necrosis factor (TNF)-R1, DR4 (TRAIL-R1), and DR5 (TRAIL-R2), which leads to receptor trimerization and recruitment of adaptor proteins to the intracellular death domain followed by proteolytic activation of procaspase-8 *(1–3)*. Activated caspase-8 cleaves various proteins including procaspase-3, which results in its activation and development of the apoptotic process *(2,4)*. Interestingly, activation of the cell-death receptor may occur in the absence of the corresponding ligand. CD95L-independent oligomerization of CD95 receptor by cytotoxic drugs or ultraviolet (UV) irradiation is sufficient to activate downstream caspases *(5–7)*. The relative contribution of death receptor vs mitochondrial pathways may depend on the dose and kinetics of a particular stress agent, and may also reflect the existence of two different cell types with respect to CD95 signaling. Type I cells undergo CD95-mediated apoptosis without the involvement of mitochondria, whereas type II cells require the release of cytochrome c from mitochondria in order for CD95 to perform its apoptotic effect *(8,9)*. Tumorigenic disruptions in the death-receptor pathway occur less frequently than in the intrinsic pathway. Nevertheless, tumor cells are often resistant to death-receptor-mediated apoptosis, and various alterations in CD95, TNF, and TRAIL receptors signaling do occur in human malignancies.

Chemotherapy and irradiation can directly activate the mitochondrial pathway (Fig. 1). The principal role of mitochondria in the regulation of the intrinsic cell-death pathway has only recently being recognized when experiments identified direct involvement of cytochrome c in the initiation of caspase activation *(10)*. Mitochondria are induced to release cytochrome c in response to most anticancer drugs and other stress agents, either by the opening of channels in the outer membrane or because of the mitochondria swelling and rupture that occurs following permeability-transition pore opening *(2,11,12)*. The release of cytochrome c into the cytosol results in activation of the caspase adaptor Apaf-1 and procaspase-9 *(13,14)*. Caspase-9 in turn activates other caspases, including caspase-3 and caspase-8 *(2,15)*. Mitochondrial-membrane permeabilization is regulated by the opposing action of pro- and anti-apoptotic Bcl-2 family members. The pro-apoptotic Bcl-2 proteins (Bak and Bax) can be

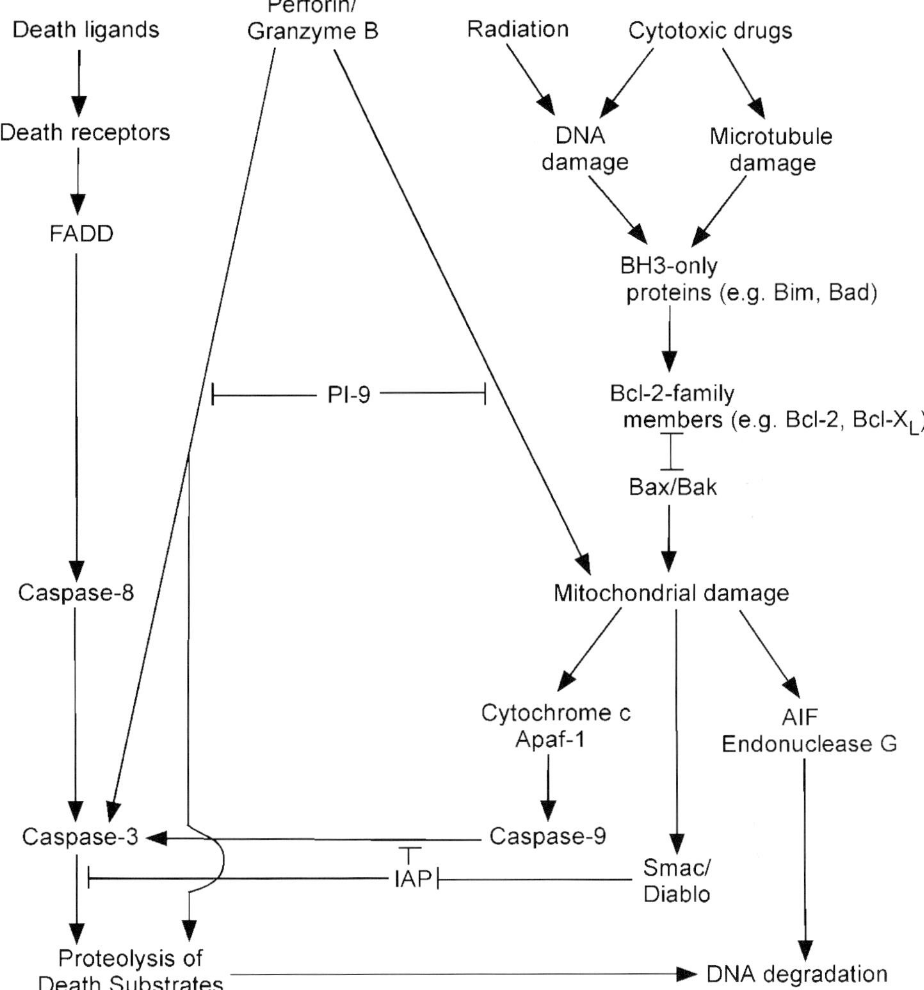

Fig. 1. A schematic diagram showing some of the known components of the extrinsic and intrinsic apoptotic pathways.

activated directly following interaction with Bid, another member of this family. Alternatively, binding of the other pro-apoptotic proteins (Noxa, Puma, Bad, and Bim) to anti-apoptotic Bcl-2 family proteins (Bcl-2 and Bcl-X_L) results in the activation of Bax and Bak *(16–19)*. Whether Bcl-2 proteins control mitochondrial membrane permeability by directly forming pores in the outer membrane or by regulating the opening and closing of permeability transition pores remains unclear *(16,20)*.

Activation of mitochondria-mediated apoptosis represents a major antitumor response of the *p53* molecule. One of the mechanisms for *p53* to induce mitochondria-mediated cell death events is to activate pro-apoptotic Bcl-2 family members that are directly involved in the initiation of mitochondria-induced apoptosis, such as Noxa, PUMA, and Bax. All these proteins have been shown to be direct targets in *p53*-mediated apoptosis *(21)*. *p53* also represses anti-apoptotic Bcl-2 proteins (Bcl-2 and Bcl-X_L) and inhibitor of apoptosis protein (IAPs) *(16,22–24)*.

Both extrinsic and intrinsic pathways converge on the activation of caspase family members organized in a branched proteolytic cascade *(25)*. Active caspases cleave numerous intracellular substrates that activate or deactivate them, leading to various nuclear and cytoplasmic alterations and culminating in DNA fragmentation and cell death. Members of the caspase family have long been considered indispensable executioners of programmed cell death (PCD). However, recent studies demonstrate that apoptosis can occur in the complete absence of functional caspase activity. Like classic apoptosis, caspase-independent PCD is often dependent on activation of non-caspase proteases such as the calpains, cathepsins B, D, and L, and granzymes A and B *(26–29)*. These proteases often cooperate with caspases in classic apoptosis, and can also induce PCD accompanied by morphological changes typical for apoptosis in a caspase-independent mode *(26,28–30)*. Other proteases that have been associated with PCD include the recently identified serine protease Omi (also known as HtrA2), which can induce apoptosis in both a caspase-dependent and -independent manner *(31,32)* and apoptotic protease 24 (AP24) *(33,34)*. AP24 was capable of triggering internucleosomal DNA fragmentation in isolated nuclei and mediating DNA fragmentation in leukemia cells in response to TNF, ultraviolet (UV) light, and various chemotherapeutic agents *(33,34)*. Apoptosis-like PCD can also be induced by apoptosis-inducing factor (AIF) *(35)* and endonuclease G *(36,37)*, which are released from mitochondria upon death stimuli and do not require prior processing by caspases for their DNase activity.

2. CHEMOTHERAPY AND CANCER-CELL RESISTANCE TO APOPTOSIS

The resistance of cancer cells to multiple chemotherapeutic agents poses a major problem in the successful treatment of various malignancies. Failure to activate the apoptotic program represents an important mechanism of tumor drug resistance. Therefore, the increasing interest in apoptosis has been driven by the expectation that a better understanding of the molecular pathways that control cell death will enable us to overcome tumor drug resistance. There is strong evidence that the sensitivity of various tumor types to current therapeutic methods critically depends on the expression and activation of multiple

Table 1
Genetic Alterations Associated With Apoptosis Resistance in Cancer Cells

Protein	*Role in Drug Resistance*	*References*
CD95/Fas	Downregulated and mutated in lymphoid and solid tumors	*146*
Caspase family members	Deficient in the expression or activation of in many types of tumor including breast cancer, neuroblastoma, and renal cell carcinoma	*45–47*
Bcl-2	Elevated in many tumors. Inhibits drug-induced apoptosis	*2,57*
Bcl-X_L	Determines drug resistance in several tumor types, including multiple myeloma	*56,89*
Bak	Decreased expression in some tumors, including gastric and colorectal cancers. Involved in mitochondrial membrane damage	*147*
Bax	Decreased expression in some tumors. Involved in mitochondrial membrane damage	*57,58*
p53	Mutated in many types of cancer. *p53*$^{-/-}$ cells are resistant to drug-induced apoptosis	*141,148*
IAPs	Overexpressed in cancer. Downregulation of XIAP induces apoptosis in chemoresistant tumors.	*149,150*
NF-κB	Induces drug-resistance in many tumors. Activates expression of anti-apoptotic Bcl-2and IAP family members	*2,151*
Apaf-1	Mutated in melanoma and leukemia-cell lines. Apaf$^{-/-}$ cells are drug-resistant	*152*

apoptosis-regulatory proteins. Tumors may overcome sensitivity to apoptotic stimuli by selective defects in the intracellular signaling proteins and caspases that are central to apoptotic pathways (Table 1). These defects may provide a selective advantage for transformed cells, thereby rendering them resistant to various forms of chemotherapy, which depend on the induction of apoptosis in tumor cells.

Many lines of evidence obtained over the last several years reveal an overlap between chemosensitivity of tumor cells and activation of the CD95 system *(38–40)*. In chemosensitive Hodgkin's lymphoma, Ewing's sarcoma, colon carcinoma, and small-cell lung cancer (SCLC) cells, induction of CD95, CD95 ligand (CD95L), and caspase activity were identified upon treatment with doxorubicin *(38)*. CD95-resistant and doxorubicin-resistant leukemia and neuroblastoma cells display cross-resistance to apoptotic modes of cell death *(41)*. Resistant cells did not exhibit different drug uptake or drug efflux in comparison to drug-sensitive cells, suggesting that non-multidrug-resistant mechanisms are involved *(41)*. Drug-resistant cells also fail to upregulate CD95L, and display complete loss or reduced expression of CD95 *(41,42)*. However, other studies have disputed this hypothesis, based largely on the inability of exogenously added anti-Fas/FasL reagents to attenuate drug-induced apoptosis in their studies. These data suggest that most anticancer drugs can trigger apoptosis in the absence of the functional CD95 pathway via alternative death pathways *(7,43,44)*.

Tumor-cell variants that are deficient in the expression or activation of caspase family members have a significant survival advantage when exposed to various death stimuli. For example, MCF-7 breast-cancer cells are deficient in the caspase-3 expression, which determines their resistance to many chemotherapeutic agents. Reconstitution of caspase-3 renders these cells sensitive to etoposide and doxorubicin *(45)*. In neuroblastoma, the gene for caspase-8 is frequently inactivated, making caspase 8-null neuroblastoma cells resistant to doxorubicin-mediated apoptosis. This defect may be corrected by programmed expression of the enzyme *(46)*. Similarly, resistance to apoptosis in renal cell carcinoma (RCC) lines is correlated with almost complete loss of caspase-3 expression and variable downregulation of caspases-7, -8, and -10 *(47)*.

The functions of caspases are modulated by a set of proteins known as IAP. Expression of the IAP family protein survivin was found in most human tumors, but not in normal cells *(48,49)*. In neuroblastoma, survivin expression correlates with more aggressive and unfavorable disease *(50)*. Expression of a nonphosphorylated mutant of survivin in a melanoma xenograft tumor model suppressed tumor growth and reduced intraperitoneal tumor dissemination *(51,52)*. Another IAP family member, ML-IAP, is expressed at high levels in melanoma-cell lines, but not in primary melanocytes. Melanoma cells that express ML-IAP are significantly more resistant to drug-induced apoptosis than cells that lack ML-IAP *(53)*.

Anticancer drugs can activate the mitochondrial pathway without involvement of upstream caspases. The finding that mitochondrial alterations represent an irreversible step in the cellular death process has significant implications for the further development of antineoplastic agents. Cytotoxic agents that are capable of triggering mitochondrial changes directly may overcome drug-resistance of tumor cells that results from the deficient expression or activation of caspase family members. This has been documented in experiments with caspase-deficient renal carcinoma cells. These cells were almost completely resistant to apoptosis in response to the intracellular zinc chelator, *N,N,N′N′*,-

tetrakis (2-pyridylmethyl) ethylenediamine (TPEN), although TPEN treatment resulted in a significant increase in the number of necrotic cells in culture *(47)*.

The coexistence of both caspase-dependent and -independent pathways has been demonstrated in non-small-cell lung carcinoma (NSCLC) cells. NSCLC cells are cross-resistant to a broad spectrum of apoptotic stimuli, including receptor stimulation, cytotoxic drugs and gamma-radiation. In contrast to irradiation and chemotherapeutic agents, staurosporine induced mitochondrial dysfunction in NSCLC cells, followed by release of cytochrome c, translocation of AIF into the nuclei, activation of apical and effector caspases, and morphological changes that were specific for apoptosis. Thus, in NSCLC cells, in which the caspase-dependent pathway is less efficient, the triggering of an AIF-mediated caspase-independent mechanism circumvents the resistance of these cells to cytotoxic treatment *(54)*.

Members of the bcl-2 family represent attractive targets for gene therapy because the failure of antitumor agents to induce cell death in target cells may be the result of the altered expression of these proteins in malignant cells. Anti-apoptotic Bcl-2 and Bcl-X_L proteins have been implicated as key elements of drug resistance in multiple myeloma *(55,56)* and chronic lymphocytic leukemia *(57)*, whereas mutation or deletion of the pro-apoptotic bax gene is associated with resistance to chemotherapy in patients with colon cancer *(58)*. Drug resistance in SCLC was paralleled by strong upregulation of Bcl-2, which diminished apoptosis by inhibiting the loss of the mitochondrial transmembrane potential and the release of cytochrome c *(59)*. Excessive expression of anti-apoptotic proteins can make tumor cells extremely resistant to diverse cytotoxic insults, including γ-irradiation and cytotoxic drugs, since Bcl-2 and Bcl-X_L proteins protect cells from both caspase-dependent and -independent death *(12,60)*. The downregulation of Bcl-X_L in prostate cancer DU-145 cells has led to their resistance to cytotoxic agents, including docetaxel, mitoxantrone, etoposide, vinblastine, and carboplatin *(59)*. Reduction of Bcl-2 level using anti-sense treatment or intracellular expression of anti-Bcl-2 antibody renders tumor cells susceptible to drug-induced cell death *(55,61)*. In this respect, encouraging results were obtained in experiments with expression of oncogenically mutate *ras* gene in human glioma and gastric cancer-cell lines *(62)*. Oncogenic Ras-induced cell death occurred in the absence of caspase activation, and was not inhibited by the overexpression of Bcl-2 protein *(62)*. Considering these results, it appears that gene therapy may ultimately become a successful component in the treatment of drug-resistant tumors.

One of key elements controlling apoptosis induction in cancer cells is the *p53* molecule. Disruption of *p53* function frequently occurs in human cancers, and is associated with an unfavorable prognosis. Loss of *p53* expression or specific *p53* mutations have been linked to primary chemoresistance and early relapse in breast, leukemia, testicular, and Wilms cancers *(63)*. Mutant *p53* is also associated with prostate-cancer resistance to cytotoxic agents. Re-introduction of wild-type *p53* into *p53* null tumor cells re-establish their chemosensitivity *(64)*. Wild-type *p53* is also known to repress a number of cellular promoters that may be important for an apoptotic response, cell-cycle control, and other important biological functions. For example, expression of the anti-apoptotic Bcl-2 is suppressed by wild-type *p53 (65)*. Therefore, loss of this repression by *p53* mutation or inactivation may lead to an upregulation of Bcl-2 expression and an impaired apoptotic response to chemotherapeutic agents. However, certain tumors that possess either mutation or deletion of the *p53* gene are still capable of undergoing apoptosis, such as breast or gastric cancer cells upon exposure to taxol *(66,67)*.

Multiple studies have established the role of genes controlled by the NF-κB transcription factor in malignant transformation *(68)* and progression of cancer to hormone-independent growth *(69–73)*. Overexpression of anti-apoptotic proteins controlled by NF-κB family members has been implicated as a key element of drug resistance in a wide variety of tumors *(55–57)*. Constitutive activation of NF-κB in androgen-independent prostate-cancer cells explains the observation that these cells are remarkably resistant to therapeutic agents operating through the induction of apoptosis *(74)*. Many studies have documented that the inhibition of NF-κB activity enhances the apoptotic effect of a variety of death inducers *(75–77)*, whereas pretreatment of cells with NF-κB inducers confers resistance against apoptosis *(78,79)*. Inhibition of NF-κB activity enhances TNF-related apoptosis-inducing ligand (TRAIL)-mediated apoptosis in malignant cells *(80)*, and activation of NF-κB has the opposite effect *(81)*. Inhibition of NF-κB also sensitizes previously insensitive cancer cells to TNF-α *(82,83)* and chemotherapy *(84)*. Downregulation of the NF-κB regulated anti-apoptotic protein Bcl-X_L restores sensitivity to apoptosis in androgen-independent PC-3 and DU-145 cell lines *(85–87)*.

Considering the importance of apoptosis as a potential outcome of tumor-cell response to chemotherapeutic regimens, further studies are needed to identify the contribution of individual components of the complex apoptotic pathways in the sensitivity to anti-cancer therapy. These may include novel proteomic approaches, analysis of gene-expression profiles and functional in vitro and in vivo studies of malignant cells from patients who are undergoing cancer therapy.

3. RADIOTHERAPY AND CANCER-CELL RESISTANCE TO APOPTOSIS

The genetic composition of cells and their sensitivity to radiation-induced apoptosis are equally critical as in chemotherapy-induced apoptosis. It appears that cells that are resistant to the induction of apoptosis in response to chemotherapeutic agents are also resistant to radiotherapy. It has been demonstrated that tumors with a high apoptotic index prior to the initiation of radiotherapy are more sensitive to the cytotoxic effects of the radiation, and that these patients have a significantly longer survival *(88,89)*.

Pathways leading to apoptosis are rather complex, and it is unlikely that resistance of tumor cells to radiotherapy can be ascribed to a single component. Ionizing radiation can act as a response-enhancing agent for CD95-mediated cell death. This complementation exists for a wide range of tumor cells. Therefore, stimulation of antitumor immunity at the completion of radiotherapy might be beneficial for inducing apoptosis through the CD95/CD95L system *(90)*. However, a block in intracellular signaling can prevent CD95-mediated apoptosis, even in cells that express a high level of CD95 *(91)*. A number of reports have indicated that ionizing radiation triggers activation of the caspase cascade in susceptible tumor cells. The mechanism by which radiation activates caspases is unclear, although it has been reported that radiation acts on cellular membranes to generate the apoptosis-inducing molecule ceramide *(92)*. Indeed, radiation resistance in prostate-cancer cells was reversed by generation of ceramide via activation of the enzyme ceramide synthase *(93)*. Ionizing irradiation also triggers the activation of caspase-8 *(94,95)* and caspase-9 *(90,96)*. Thus, the lack of functional caspase activity in tumor cells can be responsible, at least in part, for tumor resistance to radiation therapy. Paradoxically, androgen deprivation reduces radiosensitivity of androgen-dependent prostate-cancer cells, possibly by triggering cell-cycle delay, which results in a reduction of post-mitotic apoptosis *(97)*.

Activation of the transcription factor NF-κB is part of the immediate early response of tissues to ionizing irradiation. There is increasing evidence to support a central role for NF-κB regulation in cellular intrinsic radiation sensitivity and apoptosis after exposure to ionizing radiation *(98–100)*. Expression of a mutant IκB inhibited NF-κB and sensitized head and neck squamous cell carcinoma (HNSCC) to radiation *(101)*. Inhibition of NF-κB activation also increased radiation-induced apoptosis and enhanced radiosensitivity in colorectal cancer cells, both in vitro and in vivo *(100)*. However, inhibition of NF-κB activity in the PC-3 prostate cancer and HD-MyZ Hodgkin's lymphoma cells failed to alter their intrinsic radiosensitivity *(102)*. NF-κB exerts its protective effect by upregulating expression of numerous genes with known anti-apoptotic activity. Indeed, excessive expression of NF-κB controlled anti-apoptotic proteins can make tumor cells extremely resistant to diverse cytotoxic insults, including irradiation, since such proteins protect cells from both caspase-dependent and -independent death *(12,60)*. A significant association between the bcl-2 and bax status of the tumors and histopathologic subtypes and grades has been noted in patients with epithelial ovarian carcinoma *(103)*. Controversially, in patients with advanced esophageal squamous cell carcinoma who underwent chemotherapy and/or radiation therapy after surgery, Bax and Bcl-X_L expression was not related to clinical outcome *(104)*.

Although *p53* protein plays an important role in the regulation of radio-and chemosensitivity in many tumors, the role of *p53* in the combined management of tumors that harbor mutations in the *p53* gene has not been fully defined. Many researchers have attempted to link *p53* mutation and spontaneous apoptosis to the effectiveness of radiochemotherapy and with prognosis in several malignancies. Recent studies revealed that *p53* status has a significant impact on radiation sensitivity of pancreatic tumors. Tumor cells carrying wild-type *p53* are significantly more radiosensitive than mutant cell lines. When radiation therapy and 5-fluorouracil were combined, this led only to an additive effect in wild-type cell lines and to a synergistic effect in mutant cell lines *(105)*. The induction of wild-type *p53* potentiated the cytotoxicity of both irradiation and 5-fluorouracil in colorectal cancer cells *(106)*. A high level of spontaneous apoptosis induced by overexpression of bax may increase the sensitivity of radiochemotherapy, resulting in a good prognosis. *p53* mutation may lead to resistance against radiochemotherapy, resulting in a poor prognosis *(107)*. *p53* status in pretreatment biopsies also strongly predicted long-term biochemical control after radiation therapy in favorable-to-intermediate-risk prostate-cancer patients, suggesting that abnormal *p53* status may favor surgical management, aggressive dose escalation, or *p53*-targeted therapy *(108)*.

4. IMMUNOTHERAPY AND CANCER-CELL RESISTANCE TO APOPTOSIS

The antitumor effect of cytotoxic T lymphocytes (CTL) is executed through at least two distinct mechanisms. The first pathway depends on crosslinking of CD95 on target cells by CD95L expressed on a surface of CTL. As discussed previously, target cell death mediated through the CD95/CD95L pathway is entirely caspase-dependent. During the process of malignant transformation, multiple defects along the CD95 signaling complex may provide cells with a selective advantage that renders them insensitive to CD95-mediated death signals. The second pathway involves exocytosis of preformed granules that act as lytic effectors and initiate target-cell death. This mechanism requires the pore-forming protein perforin (PFN), which is inserted into the target-cell membrane and facilitates entry and release from endosomal compartments of the serine proteases, granzymes (Gr), capable of processing caspases and initiating apoptosis (*109*; Fig. 1).

Loss of CD95 expression on tumor cells may contribute to immune evasion. The expression of CD95 was found to be reduced in hepatocellular carcinoma, melanoma, and other tumors *(110–112)*. CD95 gene mutations have been demonstrated in myeloma and adult T cell leukemia *(113,114)*. Recent data suggest that de novo expression of the CD95L in tumors may result in the elimination of CD95 positive antitumor lymphocytes *(115)*.

An expression of soluble receptors that act as decoys for death ligands by tumor cells may represent a potential mechanism to escape immune destruction. High serum levels of soluble CD95 are associated with a poor prognosis in melanoma *(116,117)*. Secretion of soluble CD95 found in RCC was suggested to contribute to the resistance of this tumor to CD95-mediated apoptosis *(118)*. Expression of another CD95L-binding decoy receptor 3 (DcR3) is increased in several lung and colon carcinomas, glioma cell lines, and glioblastomas *(119–121)*. Ectopic expression of DcR3 in glioma model resulted in decreased immune-cell infiltration in vivo *(121)*.

Recent studies with caspase inhibitors suggest the presence of non-apoptotic caspase-independent pathways when target-cell death is induced by CTL granule exocytosis *(122,123)*. Caspase inhibitors can effectively block tumor-cell death induced by the cytotoxic drugs camphotecin and cisplatin, but fail to inhibit lysis of cells induced by the granule exocytosis *(122)*. Caspase-deficient human RCCs were resistant to apoptosis induced by GrB/PFN; however, despite this endogenous defect, the addition of PFN and GrB was capable of triggering non-apoptotic necrotic death in these cells *(124)*. These data demonstrate that CTL may overcome tumor resistance to apoptotic modes of cell death via GrB-mediated cellular necrosis. Thus, the ability of cytotoxic lymphocyte granules to bypass the requirement for caspases in the death pathway may guarantee killing of tumor cells with a caspase pathway that is incomplete or under strict endogenous control.

Tumor cells can still resist CTL-mediated killing through interference with the perforin/GrB pathway. This escape mechanism involves expression of the serine protease inhibitor PI-9/SPI-6, which inactivates GrB. Expression of PI-9 was observed in a variety of human and murine tumors, and determined the resistance of tumor cells to CTL-mediated killing both in vitro and in vivo *(125)*. Tumor cells may also evade immune destruction by causing apoptotic death in immune cells *(126,127)*.

Interestingly, the exposure of macrophages to necrotic tumor cells causes pronounced stimulation of macrophage antitumor activity, and exposure to apoptotic tumor cells results in impairment of macrophage-mediated tumor defenses and may even support tumor-cell growth *(128)*. Therefore, treatment modalities aimed at inducing tumor-cell necrosis rather than apoptosis may result in final eradication of tumors via nonspecific activation of the immune system.

5. NEW APPROACHES TO OVERCOMING APOPTOSIS RESISTANCE IN CANCER CELLS

The heterogeneity of cancer cells with respect to their sensitivity to various stress agents emphasizes the need for the activation of additional death pathways in the therapeutic control of cancer-cell death. Recent studies have provided new agents that may circumvent defects in apoptotic pathways found in tumors. One such agent is the death ligand TRAIL, a member of the TNF family. TRAIL cytotoxic activity was found to be relatively selective to the human tumor-cell lines with a minor effect on the normal cells. TRAIL implements antitumor activity without causing toxicity, as shown by studies with several xenograft models *(129)*. Chemotherapy and radiation sensitized resistant cells to TRAIL-mediated apoptosis, both in vitro and in vivo *(130,131)*. The pro-apoptotic mitochondrial protein SMAC/DIABLO was also shown to sensitize malignant cells to TRAIL-mediated apoptosis. Expression of a cytosolic Smac/DIABLO allowed TRAIL to bypass Bcl-X_L inhibition of death receptor-induced apoptosis. In addition, SMAC/DIABLO may be used as a selective agent to downregulate IAP family members in melanoma cells *(132)*.

Molecules that inhibit activation of NF-κB have been the focus of much attention as potential anticancer agents. NF-κB activation is regulated by phosphorylation of IkappaB inhibitor molecules that are subsequently targeted for degradation by the ubiquitin-proteasome pathway. PS-341 is a specific and selective inhibitor of the proteasome that inhibits NF-κB activation and enhances cytotoxic effects of chemotherapy in vitro and in vivo. An 84% reduction in initial tumor volume was obtained in colorectal cancer xenografts that received radiation and PS-341 *(100)*. The drug is well-tolerated, has few adverse side effects, and may be beneficial in combination therapies with reduced doses of chemotherapeutic agents *(16,133)*.

Anti-sense approaches to decrease expression of anti-apoptotic genes including Bcl-2, Ras, XIAP, and Mdm2 are in various stages of preclinical and clinical studies *(16,134–139)*. Experiments, both in vitro and in vivo, have demonstrated the potential feasibility of such approaches.

The importance of *p53* in the regulation of apoptosis, growth arrest, genomic stability, cell senescence, and differentiation makes it an attractive target for pharmacological intervention. Reintroduction of wild-type *p53* into tumor cells suppresses tumor growth and potentiates the cytotoxicity of DNA-damaging drugs *(106,140,141)*. Intratumoral injection with *p53*-expressing adenovirus (Ad-*p53*) in combination with cisplatin is well-tolerated *(142)*.

Other promising therapeutic agents include small-molecule inhibitors of PI-3 kinase/Akt *(143)* and farnysyltransferases needed for the activity of *ras* *(144)*. These compounds induce apoptosis both in vitro and in vivo, are relatively nontoxic to normal cells, and have been shown to mediate tumor regression in mice *(16)*. Interesting results were also obtained with small peptides composed of two functional domains. The "homing" domain was designed to guide the peptide to targeted cells and allow its internalization. The "pro-apoptotic" domain was designed to be nontoxic outside cells, but toxic when internalized into targeted cells by the disruption of mitochondrial membranes. In mice, these peptides displayed antitumor activity, but no apparent toxicity *(145)*.

6. CONCLUSION

The resistance of tumor cells to anticancer therapies may result from a failure to activate apoptotic pathways in response to drug treatment. A better understanding of the molecular mechanisms of cell death in response to chemo-, radio-, and immunotherapeutic strategies will help to avoid ineffective treatment regimens and provide a molecular basis for the new therapeutic modalities targeting apoptosis-resistant forms of cancer. Finally, an understanding of such mechanisms may reveal potential targets for one of the most promising approaches to cancer treatment—gene therapy.

REFERENCES

1. Igney FH, Krammer PH. Death and anti-death: tumour resistance to apoptosis. *Nat Rev Cancer* 2002;2:277–288.
2. Herr I, Debatin KM. Cellular stress response and apoptosis in cancer therapy. *Blood* 2001; 98:2603–2614.
3. Green DR. Apoptotic pathways: paper wraps stone blunts scissors. *Cell* 2000;102:1–4.
4. Krammer PH. CD95's deadly mission in the immune system. *Nature* 2000;407:789–795.
5. Rehemtulla A, Hamilton CA, Chinnaiyan AM, Dixit VM. Ultraviolet radiation-induced apoptosis is mediated by activation of CD-95 (Fas/APO-1). *J Biol Chem* 1997; 272:25,783–25,786.
6. Aragane Y, Kulms D, Metze D, Wilkes G, Poppelmann B, Luger TA, et al. Ultraviolet light induces apoptosis via direct activation of CD95 (Fas/APO-1) independently of its ligand CD95L. *J Cell Biol* 1998;140:171–182.
7. Micheau O, Solary E, Hammann A, Dimanche-Boitrel MT. Fas ligand-independent, FADD-mediated activation of the Fas death pathway by anticancer drugs. *J Biol Chem* 1999; 274:7987–7992.
8. Roy S, Nicholson DW. Cross-talk in cell death signaling. *J Exp Med* 2000;192:21–26.
9. Fulda S, Meyer E, Friesen C, Susin SA, Kroemer G, Debatin KM. Cell type specific involvement of death receptor and mitochondrial pathways in drug-induced apoptosis. *Oncogene* 2001;20:1063–1075.
10. Liu X, Kim CN, Yang J, Jemmerson R, Wang X. Induction of apoptotic program in cell-free extracts: requirement for dATP and cytochrome c. *Cell* 1996;86:147–157.
11. Kroemer G, Reed JC. Mitochondrial control of cell death. *Nat Med* 2000;16:513–519.
12. Reed JC. Mechanisms of apoptosis avoidance in cancer. *Curr Opin Oncol* 1999;11:68–75.
13. Zou H, Li Y, Liu X, Wang X. An APAF-1.cytochrome c multimeric complex is a functional apoptosome that activates procaspase-9. *J Biol Chem* 1999;274:11,549–11,556.
14. Wang X. The expanding role of mitochondria in apoptosis. *Genes Dev* 2001;15:2922–2933.
15. Rodriguez J, Lazebnik Y. Caspase-9 and APAF-1 form an active holoenzyme. *Genes Dev* 1999;13:3179–3184.

16. Johnstone RW, Ruefli AA, Lowe SW. Apoptosis: a link between cancer genetics and chemotherapy. *Cell* 2002;108:153–164.
17. Huang DC, Strasser A. BH3-Only proteins-essential initiators of apoptotic cell death. *Cell* 2000;103:839–842.
18. Nakano K, Vousden KH. PUMA, a novel proapoptotic gene, is induced by p53. *Mol Cell* 2001;7:683–694.
19. Oda E, Ohki R, Murasawa H, Nemoto J, Shibue T, Yamashita T, et al. Noxa, a BH3-only member of the Bcl-2 family and candidate mediator of p53-induced apoptosis. *Science* 2000;288:1053–1058.
20. Martinou JC, Green DR. Breaking the mitochondrial barrier. *Nat Rev Mol Cell Biol* 2001;2:63–67.
21. Wu X, Deng Y. Bax and BH3-domain-only proteins in p53-mediated apoptosis. *Front Biosci* 2002;7:d151–d156.
22. Wu Y, Mehew JW, Heckman CA, Arcinas M, Boxer LM. Negative regulation of bcl-2 expression by p53 in hematopoietic cells. *Oncogene* 2001;20:240–251.
23. Ryan KM, Phillips AC, Vousden KH. Regulation and function of the p53 tumor suppressor protein. *Curr Opin Cell Biol* 2001;13:332–337.
24. Hoffman WH, Biade S, Zilfou JT, Chen J, Murphy M. Transcriptional repression of the anti-apoptotic survivin gene by wild type p53. *J Biol Chem* 2002;277:3247–3257.
25. Hirata H, Takahashi A, Kobayashi S, Yonehara S, Sawai H, Okazaki T, et al. Caspases are activated in a branched protease cascade and control distinct downstream processes in Fas-induced apoptosis. *J Exp Med* 1998;187:587–600.
26. Johnson DE. Noncaspase proteases in apoptosis. *Leukemia* 2000;14:1695–1703.
27. Kitanaka C, Kuchino Y. Caspase-independent programmed cell death with necrotic morphology. *Cell Death Differ* 1999;6:508–515.
28. Leist M, Jaattela M. Four deaths and a funeral: from caspases to alternative mechanisms. *Nat Rev Mol Cell Biol* 2001;2:589–598.
29. Mathiasen IS, Jaattela M. Triggering caspase-independent cell death to combat cancer. *Trends Mol Med* 2002;8:212–220.
30. Wang KK. Calpain and caspase: can you tell the difference? *Trends Neurosci* 2000;23: 20–26.
31. Wolf BB, Green DR. Apoptosis: letting slip the dogs of war. *Curr Biol* 2002;12: R177–R179.
32. Hegde R, Srinivasula SM, Zhang Z, Wassell R, Mukattash R, Cilenti L, et al. Identification of Omi/HtrA2 as a mitochondrial apoptotic serine protease that disrupts inhibitor of apoptosis protein-caspase interaction. *J Biol Chem* 2002;277:432–438.
33. Wright SC, Schellenberger U, Wang H, Wang Y, Kinder DH. Chemotherapeutic drug activation of the AP24 protease in apoptosis: requirement for caspase 3-like-proteases. *Biochem Biophys Res Commun* 1998;245:797–803.
34. Wright SC, Schellenberger U, Wang H, Kinder DH, Talhouk JW, Larrick, JW. Activation of CPP32-like proteases is not sufficient to trigger apoptosis: inhibition of apoptosis by agents that suppress activation of AP24, but not CPP32-like activity. *J Exp Med* 1997; 186:1107–1117.
35. Susin SA, Lorenzo, HK, Zamzami N, Marzo I, Snow BE, Brothers GM, et al. Molecular characterization of mitochondrial apoptosis-inducing factor. *Nature* 1999;397:441–446.
36. Parrish J, Li L, Klotz K, Ledwich D, Wang X, Xue D. Mitochondrial endonuclease G is important for apoptosis in C. elegans. *Nature* 2001;412:90–94.
37. Li LY, Luo X, Wang X. Endonuclease G is an apoptotic DNase when released from mitochondria. *Nature* 2001;412:95–99.
38. Fulda S, Los M, Friesen C, Debatin KM. Chemosensitivity of solid tumor cells in vitro is related to activation of the CD95 system. *Int J Cancer* 1998;76:105–114.

39. Los M, Herr I, Friesen C, Fulda S, Schulze-Osthoff K, Debatin KM. Cross-resistance of CD95- and drug-induced apoptosis as a consequence of deficient activation of caspases (ICE/Ced-3 proteases). *Blood* 1997;90:3118–3129.
40. Friesen C, Fulda S, Debatin KM. Cytotoxic drugs and the CD95 pathway. *Leukemia* 1999; 13:1854–1858.
41. Friesen C, Fulda S, Debatin KM. Deficient activation of the CD95 (APO-1/Fas) system in drug-resistant cells. *Leukemia* 1997;11:1833–1841.
42. Martinez-Lorenzo MJ, Gamen S, Etxeberria J, Lasierra P, Larrad L, Pineiro A, et al. Resistance to apoptosis correlates with a highly proliferative phenotype and loss of Fas and CPP32 (caspase-3) expression in human leukemia cells. *Int J Cancer* 1998;75:473–481.
43. Wesselborg S, Engels IH, Rossmann E, Los M, Schulze-Osthoff K. Anticancer drugs induce caspase-8/FLICE activation and apoptosis in the absence of CD95 receptor/ligand interaction. *Blood* 1999;93:3053–3063.
44. Tolomeo M, Dusonchet L, Meli M, Grimaudo S, D′Alessandro N, Papoff G, et al. The CD95/CD95 ligand system is not the major effector in anticancer drug-mediated apoptosis. *Cell Death Differ* 1998;5:735–742.
45. Yang XH, Sladek TL, Liu X, Butler BR, Froelich CJ, Thor AD. Reconstitution of caspase 3 sensitizes MCF-7 breast cancer cells to doxorubicin- and etoposide-induced apoptosis. *Cancer Res* 2001;61:348–354.
46. Teitz T, Wei T, Valentine MB, Vanin EF, Grenet J, Valentine VA, et al. Caspase 8 is deleted or silenced preferentially in childhood neuroblastomas with amplification of MYCN. *Nat Med* 2000;6:529–535.
47. Kolenko V, Uzzo RG, Bukowski R, Bander NH, Novick AC, Hsi ED, et al. Dead or dying: necrosis versus apoptosis in caspase-deficient human renal cell carcinoma. *Cancer Res* 1999; 59:2838–2842.
48. Reed JC. The Survivin saga goes in vivo. *J Clin Investig* 2001;108:965–969.
49. Ambrosini G, Adida C, Altieri DC. A novel anti-apoptosis gene, survivin, expressed in cancer and lymphoma. *Nat Med* 1997;3:917–921.
50. Adida C, Berrebi D, Peuchmaur M, Reyes-Mugica M, Altieri DC. Anti-apoptosis gene, survivin, and prognosis of neuroblastoma. *Lancet* 1998;351:882–883.
51. Mesri M, Wall NR, Li J, Kim RW, Altieri DC. Cancer gene therapy using a survivin mutant adenovirus. *J Clin Investig* 2001;108:981–990.
52. Grossman D, Kim PJ, Schechner JS, Altieri DC. Inhibition of melanoma tumor growth in vivo by survivin targeting. *Proc Natl Acad Sci USA* 2001;98:635–640.
53. Vucic D, Stennicke HR, Pisabarro MT, Salvesen GS, Dixit VM. ML-IAP, a novel inhibitor of apoptosis that is preferentially expressed in human melanomas. *Curr Biol* 2000;10: 1359–1366.
54. Joseph B, Marchetti P, Formstecher P, Kroemer G, Lewensohn R, Zhivotovsky B. Mitochondrial dysfunction is an essential step for killing of non-small cell lung carcinomas resistant to conventional treatment. *Oncogene* 2002;21:65–77.
55. Bloem A, Lockhorst H. Bcl-2 antisense therapy in multiple myeloma. *Pathol Biol (Paris)* 1999;47:216–220.
56. Tu Y, Renner S, Xu F, Fleishman A, Taylor J, Weisz J, et al. BCL-X expression in multiple myeloma: possible indicator of chemoresistance. *Cancer Res* 1998;58:256–262.
57. McConkey DJ, Chandra J, Wright S, Plunkett W, McDonnell TJ, Reed JC, et al. Apoptosis sensitivity in chronic lymphocytic leukemia is determined by endogenous endonuclease content and relative expression of BCL-2 and BAX. *J Immunol* 1996; 156:2624–2630.
58. Rampino N, Yamamoto H, Ionov Y, Li Y, Sawai H, Reed JC, et al. Somatic frameshift mutations in the BAX gene in colon cancers of the microsatellite mutator phenotype. *Science* 1997;275:967–969.

59. Vilenchik M, Raffo AJ, Benimetskaya L, Shames D, Stein CA. Antisense RNA down-regulation of bcl-xL Expression in prostate cancer cells leads to diminished rates of cellular proliferation and resistance to cytotoxic chemotherapeutic agents. *Cancer Res* 2002;62:2175–2183.
60. Okuno S, Shimizu S, Ito T, Nomura M, Hamada E, Tsujimoto Y, et al. Bcl-2 prevents caspase-independent cell death. *J Biol Chem* 1998;273:34,272–34,277.
61. Piche A, Grim J, Rancourt C, Gomez-Navarro J, Reed JC, Curiel DT. Modulation of Bcl-2 protein levels by an intracellular anti-Bcl-2 single-chain antibody increases drug-induced cytotoxicity in the breast cancer cell line MCF-7. *Cancer Res* 1998;58:2134–2140.
62. Chi S, Kitanaka C, Noguchi K, Mochizuki T, Nagashima Y, Shirouzu M, et al. Oncogenic Ras triggers cell suicide through the activation of a caspase-independent cell death program in human cancer cells. *Oncogene* 1999;18:2281–2290.
63. Aas T, Borresen AL, Geisler S, Smith-Sorensen B, Johnsen H, Varhaug JE, et al. Specific P53 mutations are associated with de novo resistance to doxorubicin in breast cancer patients. *Nat Med* 1996;2:811–814.
64. Wallace-Brodeur RR, Lowe SW. Clinical implications of p53 mutations. *Cell Mol Life Sci* 1999;55:64–75.
65. Miyashita T, Krajewski S, Krajewska M, Wang HG, Lin HK, Liebermann DA, et al. Tumor suppressor p53 is a regulator of bcl-2 and bax gene expression in vitro and in vivo. *Oncogene* 1994;9:1799–1805.
66. Chang YF, Li LL, Wu CW, Liu TY, Lui WY, P′Eng FK, et al. Paclitaxel-induced apoptosis in human gastric carcinoma cell lines. *Cancer*1996;77:14–18.
67. Strobel T, Swanson L, Korsmeyer S, Cannistra SA. BAX enhances paclitaxel-induced apoptosis through a p53-independent pathway. *Proc Natl Acad Sci USA* 1996;93: 14,094–14,099.
68. Hsu TC, Nair R, Tulsian P, Camalier CE, Hegamyer GA, Young MR, et al. Transformation nonresponsive cells owe their resistance to lack of p65/nuclear factor-kappaB activation. *Cancer Res* 2001;61:4160–4168.
69. Nakshatri H, Bhat-Nakshatri P, Martin DA, Goulet RJ, Jr., Sledge GW, Jr. Constitutive activation of NF-kappaB during progression of breast cancer to hormone-independent growth. *Mol Cell Biol* 1997;17:3629–3639.
70. Palayoor ST, Youmell MY, Calderwood SK, Coleman CN, Price BD. Constitutive activation of IkappaB kinase alpha and NF-kappaB in prostate cancer cells is inhibited by ibuprofen. *Oncogene* 1999;18:7389–7394.
71. Supakar PC, Jung MH, Song CS, Chatterjee B, Roy AK. Nuclear factor kappa B functions as a negative regulator for the rat androgen receptor gene and NF-kappa B activity increases during the age-dependent desensitization of the liver. *J Biol Chem* 1995;270:837–842.
72. Mizokami A, Gotoh A, Yamada H, Keller ET, Matsumoto T. Tumor necrosis factor-alpha represses androgen sensitivity in the LNCaP prostate cancer cell line. *J Urol* 2000; 164:800–805.
73. Nakajima Y, DelliPizzi A, Mallouh C, Ferreri NR. Effect of tumor necrosis factor-alpha and interferon-gamma on the growth of human prostate cancer cell lines. *Urol Res* 1995; 23:205–210.
74. Howell SB. Resistance to apoptosis in prostate cancer cells. *Mol Urol* 2000;4:225–229; discussion 231.
75. Wang CY, Mayo MW, Baldwin AS, Jr. TNF- and cancer therapy-induced apoptosis: potentiation by inhibition of NF-kappaB. *Science* 1996;274:784–787.
76. Van Antwerp DJ, Martin SJ, Kafri T, Green DR, Verma IM. Suppression of TNF-alpha-induced apoptosis by NF-kappaB. *Science* 1996;274:787–789.
77. Beg AA, Baltimore D. An essential role for NF-kappaB in preventing TNF-alpha-induced cell death. *Science* 1996;274:782–784.

78. Kothny-Wilkes G, Kulms D, Poppelmann B, Luger TA, Kubin M, Schwarz T. Interleukin-1 protects transformed keratinocytes from tumor necrosis factor-related apoptosis-inducing ligand. *J Biol Chem* 1998;273:29,247–29,253.
79. Hess S, Gottfried E, Smola H, Grunwald U, Schuchmann M, Engelmann H. CD40 induces resistance to TNF-mediated apoptosis in a fibroblast cell line. *Eur J Immunol* 1998; 28:3594–3604.
80. Keane MM, Rubinstein Y, Cuello M, Ettenberg SA, Banerjee P, Nau MM, et al. Inhibition of NF-kappaB activity enhances TRAIL mediated apoptosis in breast cancer cell lines. *Breast Cancer Res Treat* 2000;64:211–219.
81. Oya M, Ohtsubo M, Takayanagi A, Tachibana M, Shimizu N, Murai M. Constitutive activation of nuclear factor-kappaB prevents TRAIL-induced apoptosis in renal cancer cells. *Oncogene* 2001;20:3888–3896.
82. Sumitomo M, Tachibana M, Nakashima J, Murai M, Miyajima A, Kimura F, et al. An essential role for nuclear factor kappa B in preventing TNF-alpha-induced cell death in prostate cancer cells. *J Urol* 1999;161:674–679.
83. Muenchen HJ, Lin DL, Walsh MA, Keller ET, Pienta KJ. Tumor necrosis factor-alpha-induced apoptosis in prostate cancer cells through inhibition of nuclear factor-kappaB by an IkappaBalpha "super-repressor". *Clin Cancer Res* 2000;6:1969–1977.
84. Baldwin AS. Control of oncogenesis and cancer therapy resistance by the transcription factor NF-kappaB. *J Clin Investig* 2001;107:241–246.
85. Marcelli M, Marani M, Li X, Sturgis L, Haidacher SJ, Trial JA, et al. Heterogeneous apoptotic responses of prostate cancer cell lines identify an association between sensitivity to staurosporine-induced apoptosis, expression of Bcl-2 family members, and caspase activation. *Prostate* 2000;42:260–273.
86. Li X, Marani M, Mannucci R, Kinsey B, Andriani F, Nicoletti I, et al. Overexpression of BCL-X(L) underlies the molecular basis for resistance to staurosporine-induced apoptosis in PC-3 cells. *Cancer Res* 2001;61:1699–1706.
87. Shirahama T, Sakakura C, Sweeney EA, Ozawa M, Takemoto M, Nishiyama K, et al. Sphingosine induces apoptosis in androgen-independent human prostatic carcinoma DU-145 cells by suppression of bcl-X(L) gene expression. *FEBS Lett* 1997;407:97–100.
88. Dewey WC, Ling CC, Meyn RE. Radiation-induced apoptosis: relevance to radiotherapy. *Int J Radiat Oncol Biol Phys* 1995;33:781–796.
89. Bold RJ, Termuhlen PM, McConkey DJ. Apoptosis, cancer and cancer therapy. *Surg Oncol* 1997;6:133–142.
90. Sheard MA. Ionizing radiation as a response-enhancing agent for CD95-mediated apoptosis. *Int J Cancer* 2001;96:213–220.
91. Owen-Schaub LB, Radinsky R, Kruzel E, Berry K, Yonehara S. Anti-Fas on non-hematopoietic tumors: levels of Fas/APO-1 and bcl-2 are not predictive of biological esponsiveness. *Cancer Res* 1994;54:1580–1586.
92. Haimovitz-Friedman A, Kan CC, Ehleiter D, Persaud RS, McLoughlin M, Fuks Z, et al. Ionizing radiation acts on cellular membranes to generate ceramide and initiate apoptosis. *J Exp Med* 1994;180:525–535.
93. Garzotto M, Haimovitz-Friedman A, Liao WC, White-Jones M, Huryk R, Heston WD, et al. Reversal of radiation resistance in LNCaP cells by targeting apoptosis through ceramide synthase. *Cancer Res* 1999;59:5194–5201.
94. Belka C, Marini P, Lepple-Wienhues A, Budach W, Jekle A, Los M, et al. The tyrosine kinase lck is required for CD95-independent caspase-8 activation and apoptosis in response to ionizing radiation. *Oncogene* 1999;18:4983–4992.
95. Belka C, Rudner J, Wesselborg S, Stepczynska A, Marini P, Lepple-Wienhues A, et al. Differential role of caspase-8 and BID activation during radiation- and CD95-induced apoptosis. *Oncogene* 2000;19:1181–1190.

96. Yoshida H, Kong YY, Yoshida R, Elia AJ, Hakem A, Hakem R, et al. Apaf1 is required for mitochondrial pathways of apoptosis and brain development. *Cell* 1998;94:739–750.
97. Garzotto M. Combined androgen deprivation with radiotherapy for prostate cancer: does it make sense? *Mol Urol* 2000;4: 209–213; discussion 215.
98. Gewirtz DA. Growth arrest and cell death in the breast tumor cell in response to ionizing radiation and chemotherapeutic agents which induce DNA damage. *Breast Cancer Res Treat* 2000;62:223–235.
99. Jung M, Dritschilo A. NF-kappa B signaling pathway as a target for human tumor radiosensitization. *Semin Radiat Oncol* 2001;11:346–351.
100. Russo SM, Tepper JE, Baldwin AS, Jr., Liu R, Adams J, Elliott P, et al. Enhancement of radiosensitivity by proteasome inhibition: implications for a role of NF-kappaB. *Int J Radiat Oncol Biol Phys* 2001;50:183–193.
101. Kato T, Duffey DC, Ondrey FG, Dong G, Chen Z, Cook JA, et al. Cisplatin and radiation sensitivity in human head and neck squamous carcinomas are independently modulated by glutathione and transcription factor NF-kappaB. *Head Neck* 2000;22:748–759.
102. Pajonk F, Pajonk K, McBride WH. Inhibition of NF-kappaB, clonogenicity, and radiosensitivity of human cancer cells. *J Natl Cancer Inst* 1999;91:1956–1960.
103. Skirnisdottir I, Sorbe B, Seidal T. P53, bcl-2, and bax: their relationship and effect on prognosis in early stage epithelial ovarian carcinoma. *Int J Gynecol Cancer* 2001;11: 147–158.
104. Natsugoe S, Matsumoto M, Okumura H, Nakashima S, Sakamoto F, Sakita H, et al. Bax and Bcl-X(L) expression are not related to prognosis in patients with advanced esophageal squamous cell carcinoma. *Cancer Lett* 2001;174:91–97.
105. Mohiuddin M, Chendil D, Dey S, Alcock RA, Regine W, Ahmed MM. Influence of p53 status on radiation and 5-flourouracil synergy in pancreatic cancer cells. *Anticancer Res* 2002;22:825–830.
106. Yang B, Eshleman JR, Berger NA, Markowitz SD. Wild-type p53 protein potentiates cytotoxicity of therapeutic agents in human colon cancer cells. *Clin Cancer Res* 1996; 2:1649–1657.
107. Bandoh N, Hayashi T, Kishibe K, Takahara M, Imada M, Nonaka S, et al. Prognostic value of p53 mutations, bax, and spontaneous apoptosis in maxillary sinus squamous cell carcinoma. *Cancer* 2002;94:1968–1980.
108. Ritter MA, Gilchrist KW, Voytovich M, Chappell RJ, Verhoven BM. The role of p53 in radiation therapy outcomes for favorable-to-intermediate-risk prostate cancer. *Int J Radiat Oncol Biol Phys* 2002;53:574–580.
109. Pinkoski MJ, Hobman M, Heibein JA, Tomaselli K, Li F, Seth P, et al. Entry and trafficking of granzyme B in target cells during granzyme B-perforin-mediated apoptosis. *Blood* 1998;92:1044–1054.
110. Volkmann M, Schiff JH, Hajjar Y, Otto G, Stilgenbauer F, Fiehn W, et al. Loss of CD95 expression is linked to most but not all p53 mutants in European hepatocellular carcinoma. *J Mol Med* 2001;79:594–600.
111. Strand S, Hofmann WJ, Hug H, Muller M, Otto G, Strand D, et al. Lymphocyte apoptosis induced by CD95 (APO-1/Fas) ligand-expressing tumor cells—a mechanism of immune evasion? *Nat Med* 1996;2:1361–1366.
112. Leithauser F, Dhein J, Mechtersheimer G, Koretz K, Bruderlein S, Henne C, et al. Constitutive and induced expression of APO-1, a new member of the nerve growth factor/tumor necrosis factor receptor superfamily, in normal and neoplastic cells. *Lab Investig* 1993;69:415–429.
113. Landowski TH, Qu N, Buyuksal I, Painter JS, Dalton WS. Mutations in the Fas antigen in patients with multiple myeloma. *Blood* 1997;90:4266–4270.

114. Maeda T, Yamada Y, Moriuchi R, Sugahara K, Tsuruda K, Joh T, et al. Fas gene mutation in the progression of adult T cell leukemia. *J Exp Med* 1999;189:1063–1071.
115. Strand S, Galle PR. Immune evasion by tumours: involvement of the CD95 (APO-1/Fas) system and its clinical implications. *Mol Med Today* 1998;4:63–68.
116. Midis GP, Shen Y, Owen-Schaub LB. Elevated soluble Fas (sFas) levels in non-hematopoietic human malignancy. *Cancer Res* 1996;56:3870–3874.
117. Ugurel S, Rappl G, Tilgen W, Reinhold U. Increased soluble CD95 (sFas/CD95) serum level correlates with poor prognosis in melanoma patients. *Clin Cancer Res* 2001; 7:1282–1286.
118. Gerharz CD, Ramp U, Dejosez M, Mahotka C, Czarnotta B, Bretschneider U, et al. Resistance to CD95 (APO-1/Fas)-mediated apoptosis in human renal cell carcinomas: an important factor for evasion from negative growth control. *Lab Investig* 1999; 79:1521–1534.
119. Yu KY, Kwon B, Ni J, Zhai Y, Ebner R, Kwon BS. A newly identified member of tumor necrosis factor receptor superfamily (TR6) suppresses LIGHT-mediated apoptosis. *J Biol Chem* 1999;274:13,733–13,736.
120. Pitti RM, Marsters SA, Lawrence DA, Roy M, Kischkel FC, Dowd P, et al. Genomic amplification of a decoy receptor for Fas ligand in lung and colon cancer. *Nature* 1998;396:699–703.
121. Roth W, Isenmann S, Nakamura M, Platten M, Wick W, Kleihues P, et al. Soluble decoy receptor 3 is expressed by malignant gliomas and suppresses CD95 ligand-induced apoptosis and chemotaxis. *Cancer Res* 2001;61:2759–2765.
122. Sarin A, Williams MS, Alexander-Miller MA, Berzofsky JA, Zacharchuk CM, Henkart PA. Target cell lysis by CTL granule exocytosis is independent of ICE/Ced-3 family proteases. *Immunity* 1997;6:209–215.
123. Beresford PJ, Xia Z, Greenberg AH, Lieberman J. Granzyme A loading induces rapid cytolysis and a novel form of DNA damage independently of caspase activation. *Immunity* 1999; 10:585–594.
124. Uzzo RG, Kolenko V, Froelich CJ, Tannenbaum C, Molto L, Novick AC, et al. The T cell death knell: immune-mediated tumor death in renal cell carcinoma. *Clin Cancer Res* 2001;7:3276–3281.
125. Medema JP, de Jong J, Peltenburg LT, Verdegaal EM, Gorter A, Bres SA, et al. Blockade of the granzyme B/perforin pathway through overexpression of the serine protease inhibitor PI-9/SPI-6 constitutes a mechanism for immune escape by tumors. *Proc Natl Acad Sci USA* 2001;98:11,515–11,520.
126. Uzzo RG, Rayman P, Kolenko V, Clark PE, Bloom T, Ward AM, et al. Mechanisms of apoptosis in T cells from patients with renal cell carcinoma. *Clin Cancer Res* 1999; 5:1219–1229.
127. Pirtskhalaishvili G, Shurin GV, Gambotto A, Esche C, Wahl M, Yurkovetsky ZR, et al. Transduction of dendritic cells with Bcl-xL increases their resistance to prostate cancer-induced apoptosis and antitumor effect in mice. *J Immunol* 2000;165:1956–1964.
128. Reiter I, Krammer B, Schwamberger G. Cutting edge: differential effect of apoptotic versus necrotic tumor cells on macrophage antitumor activities. *J Immunol* 1999;163: 1730–1732.
129. Srivastava RK. TRAIL/Apo-2L: mechanisms and clinical applications in cancer. *Neoplasia* 2001;3:535–546.
130. Chinnaiyan AM, Prasad U, Shankar S, Hamstra DA, Shanaiah M, Chenevert TL, et al. Combined effect of tumor necrosis factor-related apoptosis-inducing ligand and ionizing radiation in breast cancer therapy. *Proc Natl Acad Sci USA* 2000;97: 1754–1759.

131. Keane MM, Ettenberg SA, Nau MM, Russell EK, Lipkowitz S. Chemotherapy augments TRAIL-induced apoptosis in breast cell lines. *Cancer Res* 1999;59:734–741.
132. Srinivasula SM, Datta P, Fan XJ, Fernandes-Alnemri T, Huang Z, Alnemri ES. Molecular determinants of the caspase-promoting activity of Smac/DIABLO and its role in the death receptor pathway. *J Biol Chem* 2000;275:36,152–36,157.
133. Adams J. Proteasome inhibition in cancer: development of PS-341. *Semin Oncol* 2001; 28:613–619.
134. Tamm I, Dorken B, Hartmann G. Antisense therapy in oncology: new hope for an old idea? *Lancet* 2001;358:489–497.
135. Sasaki H, Sheng Y, Kotsuji F, Tsang BK. Down-regulation of X-linked inhibitor of apoptosis protein induces apoptosis in chemoresistant human ovarian cancer cells. *Cancer Res* 2000;60:5659–5666.
136. Cunningham CC, Holmlund JT, Geary RS, Kwoh TJ, Dorr A, Johnston JF, et al. Phase I trial of H-ras antisense oligonucleotide ISIS 2503 administered as a continuous intravenous infusion in patients with advanced carcinoma. *Cancer* 2001;92:1265–1271.
137. Jansen B, Wacheck V, Heere-Ress E, Schlagbauer-Wadl H, Hoeller C, Lucas T, et al. Chemosensitisation of malignant melanoma by BCL2 antisense therapy. *Lancet* 2000; 356:1728–1733.
138. Morse MA. Technology evaluation: ISIS-2503, Isis Pharmaceuticals. *Curr Opin Mol Ther* 2001;3:589–594.
139. Kausch I, Bohle A. Antisense oligonucleotide therapy for urologic tumors. *Curr Urol Rep* 2003;4:60–69.
140. Blagosklonny MV, el-Deiry WS. In vitro evaluation of a p53-expressing adenovirus as an anti-cancer drug. *Int J Cancer* 1996;67:386–392.
141. Blagosklonny MV. P53: an ubiquitous target of anticancer drugs. *Int J Cancer* 2002; 98:161–166.
142. Nemunaitis J, Swisher SG, Timmons T, Connors D, Mack M, Doerksen L, et al. Adenovirus-mediated p53 gene transfer in sequence with cisplatin to tumors of patients with non-small-cell lung cancer. *J Clin Oncol* 2000;18:609–622.
143. Ng SSW, Tsao MS, Chow S, Hedley DW. Inhibition of phosphatidylinositide 3-kinase enhances gemcitabine-induced apoptosis in human pancreatic cancer cells. *Cancer Res* 2000;60:5451–5455.
144. Omer CA, Chen Z, Diehl RE, Conner MW, Chen HY, Trumbauer ME, et al. Mouse mammary tumor virus-Ki-rasB transgenic mice develop mammary carcinomas that can be growth-inhibited by a farnesyl: protein transferase inhibitor. *Cancer Res* 2000; 60:2680–2688.
145. Ellerby HM, Arap W, Ellerby LM, Kain R, Andrusiak R, Rio GD, et al. Anti-cancer activity of targeted pro-apoptotic peptides. *Nat Med* 1999;5:1032–1038.
146. Poulaki V, Mitsiades CS, Mitsiades N. The role of Fas and FasL as mediators of anticancer chemotherapy. *Drug Resist Updat* 2001;4:233–242.
147. Kondo S, Shinomura Y, Miyazaki Y, Kiyohara T, Tsutsui S, Kitamura S, et al. Mutations of the bak gene in human gastric and colorectal cancers. *Cancer Res* 2000;60:4328–4330.
148. Vogelstein B, Lane D, Levine AJ. Surfing the p53 network. *Nature* 2000;408:307–310.
149. LaCasse EC, Baird S, Korneluk RG, MacKenzie AE. The inhibitors of apoptosis (IAPs) and their emerging role in cancer. *Oncogene* 1998;17:3247–3259.
150. Holcik M, Gibson H, Korneluk RG. XIAP: apoptotic brake and promising therapeutic target. *Apoptosis* 2001;6:253–261.
151. Bours V, Bentires-Alj M, Hellin AC, Viatour P, Robe P, Delhalle S, et al. Nuclear factor-kappa B, cancer, and apoptosis. *Biochem Pharmacol* 2000;60:1085–1089.
152. Soengas MS, Capodieci P, Polsky D, Mora J, Esteller M, Opitz-Araya X, et al. Inactivation of the apoptosis effector Apaf-1 in malignant melanoma. *Nature* 2001;409:207–211.

II Clinical Relevance of Immune Evasion

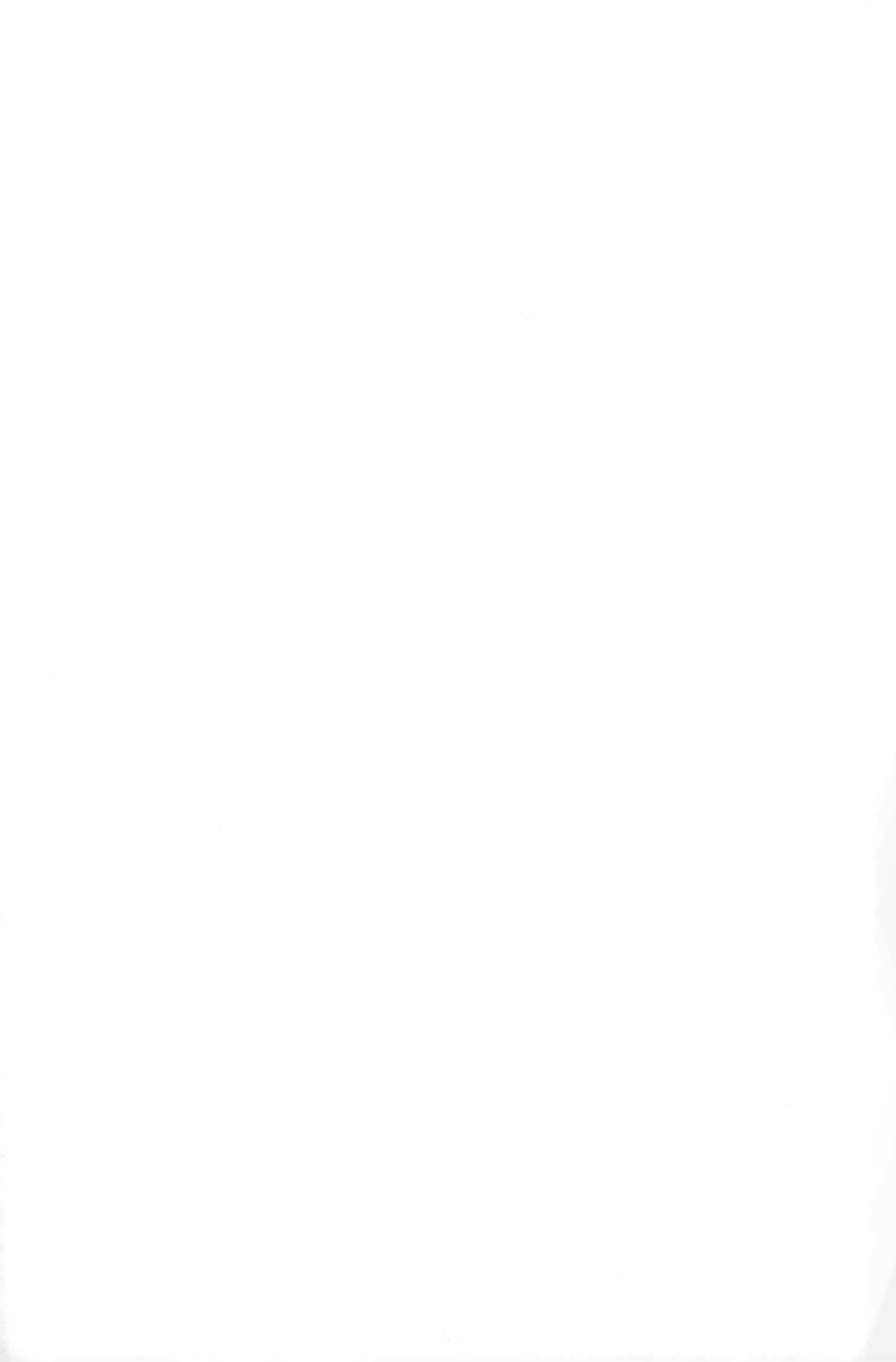

13 The Development and Reversal of T-Cell Tolerance in Cancer Patients Receiving Peptide-Based Vaccines

Ena Wang, MD
and Francesco M. Marincola, MD

CONTENTS

1. INTRODUCTION

A key question that has remained unanswered in the field of tumor immunology is whether the observed tumor-specific immune responses are intrinsically insufficient to induce cancer rejection or—although adequate for this task—are most often counteracted by an evolving disease that is capable of escaping them through continuous phenotypic changes. A combination of the two is probably at the basis of the relatively rare observation of tumor regression in response to immune manipulation. However, in this chapter, we emphasize the importance that the latter possibility may have in influencing the success of most anticancer immunization strategies. We also discuss strategies that may help to

From: *Current Clinical Oncology: Cancer Immunotherapy at the Crossroads: How Tumors Evade Immunity and What Can Be Done*
Edited by: J. H. Finke and R. M. Bukowski

understand this complex phenomenon, with the ultimate goal of identifying the true algorithm that modulates the immune rejection of cancer.

During the last decade, impressive advances have been made in the understanding of the biology of tumor host interactions in humans. A highly significant breakthrough was the molecular characterization of tumor antigens (TA) recognized by the cellular and/or the humoral arm of the immune response *(1–3)*. This information led to the preparation of clinical trials designed for the active specific immunization of patients with cancer with single or polyepitope vaccines from one or several TA *(1,4)*. This strategy is deemed feasible because most lineage-specific and tumor-specific TA are non-mutated molecules with an expression that is shared by a wide variety of tumors and a large number of patients *(5)*. Although only marginally successful in clinical terms, immunization with TA has facilitated the understanding of the immunological response to vaccines by limiting the analysis to one or few human leukocyte antigen (HLA) allele/epitope combination(s), allowing direct analysis of epitope-specific circulating T cells ex vivo as well as the phenotypic changes occurring in tumor-cell changes in response to immunization *(6)*.

The implementation of an immunization protocol and respective monitoring of immunological parameters, together with changes in tumor-cell phenotypes, has been more productive in raising new questions than in answering old ones *(7)*. Such questions encompass biological phenomena related to immune responsiveness and tolerance toward self molecules, as well as a broader appreciation for the genetic instability of the neoplastic process and its heterogeneity among different individuals and within the same individual during a period of time. These variations may in turn be responsible for the immune-escape of cancer cells from recognition by a competent immune system *(8)*.

There is no question that a dialogue is naturally established between cells of the innate and adaptive immune system and cancer. The most striking evidence is the ease with which tumor-infiltrating lymphocytes (TIL) that are capable of specifically recognizing and killing tumor cells can be expanded from tumor deposits *(9)*. This observation suggests that within the tumor microenvironment, tools are available for the recruitment from the systemic circulation of T cells that are specific for TA expressed by tumor cells or antigen-presenting cells (APC) that have taken up remnants of the death tumor cell. Intriguingly, the identification of TA-specific TIL occurs in tumor deposits that are nevertheless happily growing, suggesting that the naturally occurring immune response is, for reasons that remain unclear, insufficient to complete its effector function. The paradoxical observation of the pacific co-existence of tumor cells and their killers could be explained partly by the fact that the strong cytotoxic activity of TIL against tumor cells is observed after their in vitro expansion in the presence of cytokines associated with powerful T-cell activation and proliferation properties such as interleukin-2 (IL-2). Thus, it is likely that this in vitro potency of TIL represents an exaggeration of the immune reactivity in vivo at the tumor site, where naturally cytokines are not constitutionally expressed in large amounts *(8)*.

Supporting this hypothesis is the observation that systemic IL-2 administration, as a single agent or in combination with the adoptive transfer of TIL, can induce complete regression of metastatic cancer *(10,11)*. In addition, the adoptive transfer of TIL combined with IL-2 appeared to increase the rate of cancer regressions compared to IL-2 alone. Although it remains unclear how IL-2 works when given in pharmacological doses, these observations corroborate the hypothesis that a second stimulus is necessary to complement the naturally ongoing immune response for a successful induction of immunologically mediated cancer rejection. We have recently followed changes in the transcriptional profile of melanoma metastases sequentially biopsied before and during systemic IL-2 administration *(12)*. Surprisingly, IL-2 had no direct effect on T-cell migration to the tumor site or on their activation or proliferation. Instead, IL-2 affected T-cell function indirectly through powerful activation of innate immunity mechanisms centered on activation of APC with secondary release of potent chemokines and of natural killer (NK) cell activity. These findings corroborate the concept that the activity of TIL observed in vitro is not representative of the in vivo situation in which the tumor microenvironment is not capable of providing—in natural conditions—the signaling necessary for the maintenance of a brisk immune response, and additional stimuli must be provided. Thus, it is possible that tumor-cell co-existence with competent immune cells within the tumor microenvironment is a default occurrence, and potent stimuli must be delivered in the target tissue to overcome this indolent relationship.

A cornerstone in the understanding of tumor/host interactions was the identification of the first TA recognized by T-cells through the characterization of the immune reactivity of a T-cell clone expanded from circulating lymphocytes of a long-term cancer survivor *(13)*. Following this identification, a large number of TA have been identified in association with various tumor types to the point that a comprehensive list of TA and related epitopes is readily available. However, for the purpose of this discussion, several TA can be categorized into conceptually similar subsets according to their genetic origin and tissue distribution *(6,14)*. An important clinical conclusion that can be drawn from a survey of the TA thus far identified is that a significant number of these are expressed by a relatively broad range of tumor types and by a large percentage of patients within each type of tumor. This is particularly true for the cancer/testis antigens *(3)*, whose expression in normal tissues is restricted to testes, and for the tumor differentiation antigens *(15)*, which represent remnants of the cellular lineage of origin of a cancer of a particular histology. One practical implication of these findings is that many of the TA identified could serve as immunogens to implement specific immunotherapy in large patient populations.

The identification of TA has allowed a detailed analysis of the immune reactivity toward them in natural conditions or in response to immunologic manipulation. Surprisingly, non-tumor-bearing individuals naturally demonstrate acquired cellular immune responses against TA *(16,17)*, although to a lesser extent than cancer-bearing individuals *(16,18–20)*. As a corollary to this observation, it became obvious that although individuals may be capable of mounting systemic immune responses toward TA, these are not sufficient in themselves to prevent tumor occurrence and progression. At the same time, these observations raised the hope that increasing the intensity of naturally occurring immune responses against cancer with TA-specific immunization could improve the survival of patients with cancer. Several clinical trials have been conducted to test this hypothesis *(21–31)*. The global impression yielded confidence that most immunization strategies are effective in inducing systemic tumor-specific T-cell responses, but with few exceptions *(29–31)*, the extent of the observed immune response is not correlated in the clinical outcome.

An interesting point that can be drawn from a review of these early studies is that the combination of IL-2 and immunization appears to yield response rates at higher frequency than could be expected with the administration of either IL-2 or the vaccine alone *(27)*. This point is far from established, since no randomized study has been performed to demonstrate the effectiveness of this combination. However, based on these preliminary observations and ongoing clinical experience, it is reasonable to assume as a working hypothesis that the combination of immunization with nonspecific immune stimulation may be beneficial. Paradoxically, the higher frequency of clinical responsiveness observed with the IL-2/vaccine combination is associated with a decreased ability to identify circulating immunization-induced TA-specific T cells. Some researchers have suggested that the disappearance of TA-reactive T cells caused by IL-2 administration could be the result of a surge of CTL migration toward the extravascular space—and more specifically, the tumor microenvironment—in response to the increased vascular permeability caused by IL-2 *(27,32)*. However, in a recent study, we failed to identify such evidence of migration, as the frequency of various T-cell markers did not change during IL-2 therapy *(12)*. Another line of evidence suggests that IL-2 is not directly responsible for the migration of T cells at the tumor site. We serially followed the gene expression of various cytokines in melanoma metastases undergoing therapy by obtaining fine-needle aspirates (FNA) before and after treatment. When patients received TA-specific immunization in the absence of systemic IL-2 therapy, we observed increased expression of IFN-γ in post-treatment FNA that correlated with enhanced systemic immune reactivity *(33)*. In addition, increased IFN-γ transcript was correlated to levels of expression of the TA targeted by the immunization, and was associated with an increased frequency of TA-specific T cells, as demonstrated by tetrameric HLA/peptide (tHLA)-complexes phenotyping. When patients received the same immunization schedule in combination with IL-2 administration, we could not document systemic enhancement of TA-specific immune reactivity. This finding also correlated with a lack of localization of T cells at the tumor site, as we did not observe increased in IFN-γ levels in tumor deposits following treatment or an increased number of tHLA-staining CD8+ T cells. Thus, the addition of IL-2 to immunization does not seem to enhance response rates by directly facilitating the migration of T cells to the tumor site, but rather works through different mechanisms.

Thus, the reason(s) why cancer treatments based on active-specific immunization are sporadically successful remain(s) elusive. In addition, the reason(s) that general immune stimulants such as IL-2 exert antitumor effects in vivo remain(s) unknown, mostly because little is known about their actual mechanism of action within the tumor microenvironment. Because the ultimate goal of anticancer vaccines to induce tumor regression has remained elusive and dissociates from the achievement of immune sensitization, two types of logical explanations have been raised. On the one side, it may be postulated that the observed immune responses to vaccination are in quantitative or qualitative terms insufficient to achieve a threshold required for tumor clearance. An alternative—and not exclusive—hypothesis suggests that the immune response elicited by immunization are of an optimal nature, and tumor regression may not occur because within the tumor microenvironment, a variety of factors may modulate the sensitivity of tumor cells to the effects of immunization.

IL-2 may fit in both models by being responsible for the enhancement of the immune response in the former and for overcoming the tumor resistance to immune cells in the latter by indirectly promoting the migration and activation of TA-specific T cells at the tumor site or further activating T cells that are already localized at the tumor site. In addition, IL-2 can overturn immunosuppressive signals in the tumor microenvironment or induce tumor death through a nonspecific outburst of cytokine production. We favor the second hypothesis based on our direct ex vivo observations of changes in the genetic profile of melanoma metastases in patients who are undergoing systemic IL-2 therapy *(12)*.

The study of the mechanism of action of IL-2 as an adjuvant to tumor vaccines may have implications beyond the biology of this cytokine, and may be seen as a model for understanding the complex algorithm governing tumor rejection by the immune system. The field of human tumor immunology is a hybrid that combines two different disciplines. One is the study of human immunology that encompasses the understanding of recognition of self and/or non-self molecules in the context of human polymorphism. The second field that we believe has been somewhat neglected in the past is the appreciation of the extreme heterogeneity and instability of cancer *(34)*. Thus, as some researchers are aggressively pursuing the optimization of T-cell stimulation in vivo with the purpose of inducing immune responses of intensity sufficient to eradicate a conceptually constant target, others search for reasons why, given comparable immune responses, different tumors may respond differently. Indeed, various tumors may differ in their sensitivity to immune recognition, or may modulate the immune response through paracrine secretion of immune-regulatory substances. Possibly, systemic treatments such as IL-2 administration may work not only by increasing the intensity of the immune response, but also by inducing a tumor microenvironment that is conducive to the recruitment and maintenance of such a response by overcoming tolerogenic signals released by tumor cells. We believe that at this crossroad, more resources should be used in an attempt to identify the reason(s) for the capriciousness of immune-mediated cancer rejection by analysis of tumor/host interactions directly within the tumor microenvironment. This may lead to the identification of the parameters that truly regulate tumor rejection by the innate and/or adaptive immune response, and may consequently identify molecular targets that are likely to achieve this purpose. Therefore, we will discuss both models in this chapter.

2. THE FAILURE OF IMMUNIZATION TRIALS AS A RESULT OF QUANTITATIVELY OR QUALITATIVELY INADEQUATE IMMUNE RESPONSES

Various assays have been described that can estimate the intensity of cellular immune reactivity toward a given epitope, and a recent workshop sponsored by the Society of Biological Therapy has summarized the pros and cons of most of them *(35)*. Originally, vaccine-induced immune responses had been demonstrated and characterized using parallel in vitro sensitization (IVS) of leukapheresis products obtained from patients before and at various time-points during immunization *(22)*. Although IVS provided the first conclusive evidence that TA-specific immunization could elicit enhancement of systemic anticancer immune responses, it was criticized because it provided non-quantitative information, since the expansion of vaccine-specific T cells was performed under arbitrary conditions such as, the selection of antigen and cytokine concentration used for the assay. Thus, assays that could document the extent of the immune response to immunization ex vivo have gradually taken over IVS.

The ELISPOT assay has enjoyed notable popularity because of its simplicity, accuracy, and sensitivity *(36,37)*. This assay consists in the enumeration of T-cell colonies spotted on a semi-solid surface producing IFN-γ, or another cytokine, in response to a cognate stimulus. Similar assay have been described that include immune phenotyping of TA-reactive T cells through the detection of specific surface or intracellular cytokine expression by fluorescence-activated cell sorting (FACS) analysis *(38–40)*. Because of the dependency on cytokine secretion, "functional" assays may underestimate the actual frequency of vaccine-induced T-cell precursors by missing T cells with a threshold for cytokine expression/proliferation above the stimulus applied by the assay *(41)*. Thus, other assays have been proposed that may more directly enumerate the frequency of epitope-specific T cells, such as tetrameric HLA/epitope complexes (tHLA) *(42)*. Indeed, measurements by these assays reveal CTL precursor frequencies that are considerably higher than those suggested by ELISPOT, limiting dilution analysis, or intracellular FACS analysis *(41,43)*. Levels of tumor-reactive T cells reached up to 5% of the circulating CD8+ T-cell population, yet no correlation was noted between their number in individual patients and treatment efficacy *(43,44)*. Conceptually, this makes sense, considering the heterogeneity of tumor cells in different individuals that could be differentially sensitive to a particularly intensity of immune recognition *(6)*. The lack of a relationship between immune and clinical response may be related to the fact that enumeration of vaccine-specific T cells has been predominantly performed on blood samples obtained several weeks (generally 3–4 wk) after treatment. This timing of sampling may not reflect the peak of activity of the T cells in response to the immunogen. Thus, it is possible that this discrepancy may reflect the survival rate or extravascular distribution of vaccine-induced T cells rather than a discrepancy between their frequency and effectiveness at the time of treatment. No information is presenbly available about the short-term kinetics of immune responses to immunization and during combined treatment with systemic cytokine administration. This information may be critical if future studies are to confirm the usefulness of this combined approach *(27)*. Evidence based on the comparison of various vaccination strategies suggests that vaccination protocols that are most effective in inducing immune responses are associated with a higher rate of clinical responses, suggesting that a general correlation may exist between immune and clinical response if patient heterogeneity is mitigated by random distribution of tumor phenotypes among random patient populations *(27)*.

It is possible that the frequency of TA-specific T cells induced by vaccination may not reach a numerical threshold that is sufficient to initiate and sustain an effective rejection of cancer. At present, no information is available about the frequency of circulating T cells required to achieve a particular effect on a target tissue. However, it is clear that a much higher frequency of epitope-specific T cells than those noted after TA-specific immunization have been observed in the context of some, but not all, acute and chronic viral infections, and in the context of autoimmune diseases *(41,45–48)*. Our recent studies suggest that prolonged vaccination schedules may progressively increase the frequency of TA-specific circulating T cells by broadening the recruitment of T cells bearing diverse and non-overlapping T-cell receptor (TCR) repertoires *(49)*. These results were similar to those reported by Dietrich et al. *(50)*, who also provided evidence against the usage of highly restricted TCR-repertoire utilization in response to a self-differentiation TA. We also noted that the schedule of administration had marked effects on the number of vaccine-specific T cells induced, and closer vaccine administrations appeared to be most effective *(49)*.

The blunted status of activation of tumor-specific T cells may be the cause of their ineffectiveness *(51)*. TA-specific T cells may be incapable of releasing IFN-γ or being cytoxic upon encountering relevant tumor-cell targets. This hypothesis cannot be generalized because it is based on a single patient observation *(51)* and has not been confirmed by other investigators. A recent analysis of PBMC from patients with melanoma identified TA-specific T cells with an effector/memory phenotype capable of IFN-γ release ex vivo upon cognate stimulation *(40)*. Functional differences in cytokine expression by various subsets of TA-specific lymphocytes in tumor-bearing patients may merely reflect various functional subsets of naïve/memory/effector T cells *(52)* (Fig. 1). Dunbar et al. have shown that different subsets of TA-specific T cells can be identified in melanoma patients *(53)*. In the context of human T-cell lymphotropic virus type I infection, symptoms of myelopathy were associated with a high frequency of CD45RA-CD27-effector cells expressing perforin and demonstrating cytolytic function *(48)*. A dissociation between cytokine secretion and cytolytic function upon cognate stimulation has been observed in other human viral models *(54)* and in the context of TA-specific vaccination *(23)*. Thus, the observed increase in TA-specific, IFN-γ secreting T cells following immunization may give the misleading impression of the presence of the circulation of powerful effector cells.

As previously discussed, active specific immunization alone is rarely associated with clinical responses. The best results seem to be observed when the immunogen is delivered in combination with adjuvants such as APC *(24,25)* or immune-stimulatory cytokines *(27,55)*. However, the effectiveness of APC has

---

Fig. 1. *(facing page)* Steps supposedly required for immunization-induced tumor regression. Immunogens may have varying potency in relation to their stability and solubility, the patient's histotype and the milieu in which they are delivered (e.g., chemical adjuvants, cytokines, APC). The induction of an effective local response matures APC that migrate to draining lymph nodes (LND) to present antigen to naïve/memory T cells (locoregional response). Upon antigen-exposure, T cells enter the circulation (systemic response), where various factors may influence their effectiveness, including their frequency, status of differentiation, and/or activation. Some T cells can localize in peripheral tissues to exert effector function (peripheral response). Upon T-cell receptor/epitope engagement, cytotoxicity occurs. T cells also may release cytokines such as interferons (IFN), tumor necrosis factor (TNF), granulocyte-macrophage colony-stimulating factor (GM-CSF) and interleukin-2 (IL-2), with potent inflammatory properties capable of sustaining the ongoing or stimulating a novel immune response. In some circumstances, this could be facilitated by a conducive tumor microenvironment pre-conditioned by cytokines that are constitutively produced by a tumor or infiltrating normal cells. A deficient clinical response could be caused by loss of antigen expression or presentation by tumor cells, or production of immunosuppressive factors.

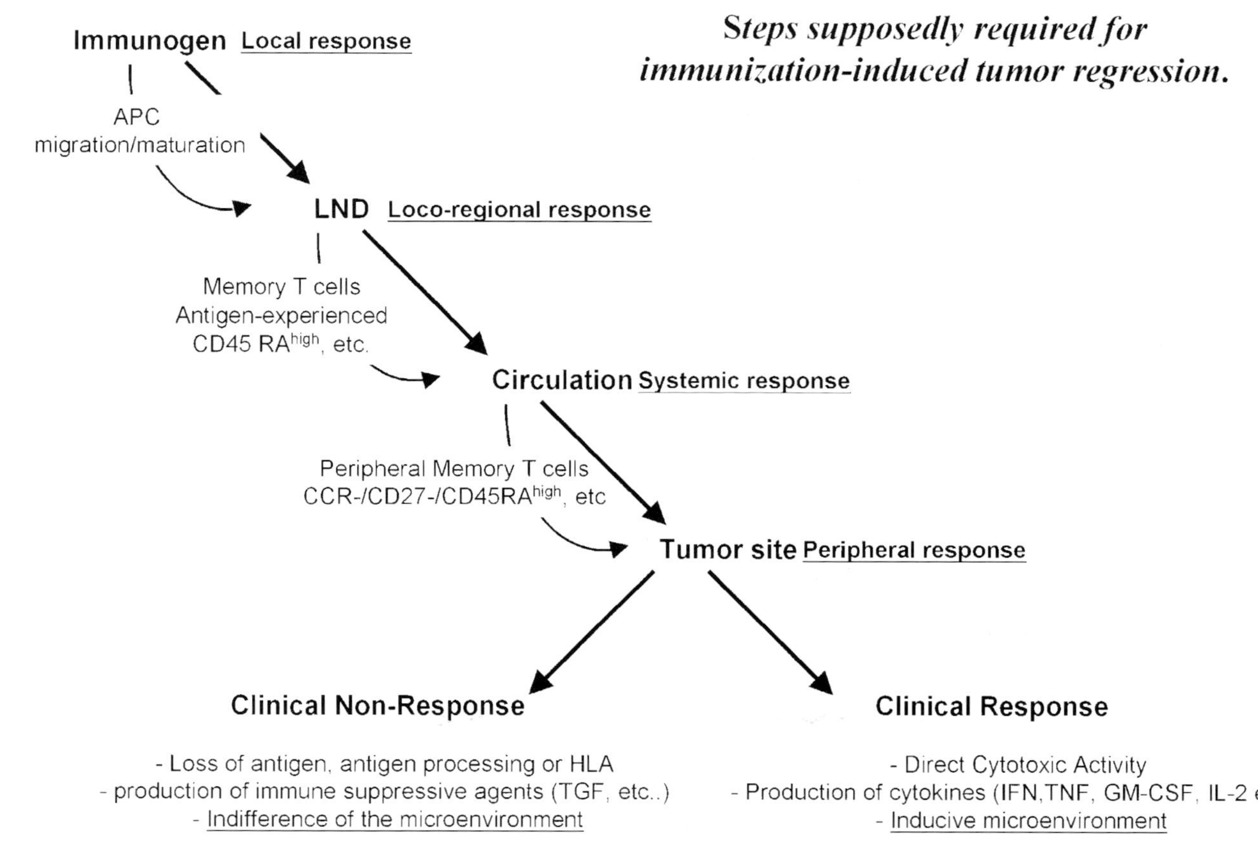
Steps supposedly required for immunization-induced tumor regression.
Immunogen Local response
APC
migration/maturation
LND Loco-regional response
Memory T cells
Antigen-experienced
CD45 RAhigh, etc.
Circulation Systemic response
Peripheral Memory T cells
CCR-/CD27-/CD45RAhigh, etc
Tumor site Peripheral response
Clinical Non-Response
- Loss of antigen, antigen processing or HLA
- production of immune suppressive agents (TGF, etc..)
- Indifference of the microenvironment
Clinical Response
- Direct Cytotoxic Activity
- Production of cytokines (IFN,TNF, GM-CSF, IL-2 etc..)
- Inducive microenvironment

not been confirmed by other investigators *(56,57)*. The combination of systemic immune stimulation with cytokines with immunization also appears to offer an additional benefit over immunization alone. In particular, anticancer vaccines in association with IL-2 *(27)* or granulocyte-macrophage colony-stimulating factor (GM-CSF) *(55)* can dramatically increase the frequency of clinical responses compared with historical controls *(58)*. At present, it is unclear whether these results represent a true additional benefit of the combination. A randomized multi-institutional clinical protocol for the treatment of HLA-A*0201 patients with metastatic melanoma that is currently in progress may help to answer this question by randomizing patients between an arm offering systemic high-dose IL-2 and a second arm receiving the combination IL-2 and an HLA-A*0201-associated gp100-derived epitope.

Based on the working hypothesis that the combination of immunization and IL-2 therapy may synergistically enhance immune rejection, we have been interested in investigating the mechanism of action of IL-2 when systemically administered at high doses *(12)*. It has been suggested that the anticancer effects of IL-2 are mediated through its ability to expand and activate in vivo CTL of the NK and T-cell subsets *(59)*. However, it has become quite apparent that IL-2 at the more than physiologic doses in which it is systemically administered has effects beyond the simple activation of cells carrying the IL-2 receptor *(32,60)*. In a recent study *(12)*, we compared early changes in transcriptional profiles of circulating mononuclear cells with those that occur within the microenvironment of melanoma metastases following systemic IL-2 administration. The results suggested that the immediate effect of IL-2 administration on the tumor microenvironment is transcriptional activation of genes predominantly associated with monocytic cell function, and minimal effects were noted on migration, activation, and proliferation of T cells. However, production of chemokines and markers of adhesion and migration within a few hours of IL-2 administration may be responsible for a secondary recruitment of immune cells to the tumor site at a later time-point. The results of this study suggest that IL-2 administration induces inflammation at the tumor site with three predominant secondary effects: i) activation of antigen-presenting monocytes; ii) a massive production of chemoattractants that may recruit other immune cells to the tumor site including MIG and PARC, specific for T cells; and iii) activation of lytic mechanisms attributable to monocytes (Calgranulin, Grancalcin) and NK cells (NKG5, NK4).

Another question that remains to be resolved is whether TA-specific T cells reach the tumor site, and whether this is a requirement for their effector function. Pockaj et al. *(61)*, in a conceptually similar study, observed that the localization at tumor site of adoptively transferred ^{111}Indium-labeled TIL was required for tumor regression. By analogy, vaccine-elicited T cells may not effectively reach the tissue, where they are supposed to exert their effector function, and this may limit their efficacy. For instance, we noted a functional dissociation between systemic and intra-tumoral immune reactivity following vaccination *(62)*. Vaccine-elicited T cells could be readily expanded in circulating lymphocytes, but could not be identified among TIL expanded from a simultaneously obtained FNA biopsy *(63)*. This discrepancy may be best explained by the loss of the TA targeted by the vaccination by the cancer cells during treatment. Others have reported similar findings, as summarized in a recent review by Yee et al. *(64)*. When tumor variant cases are excluded, localization of CD8+ T cells within tumors may occur, as reported in the context of vaccination with MAGE-3 *(25)*, MART-1 *(30,65)*, and gp100 *(33,65)* peptides. Yet, the localization does not correlate with tumor regression. In a recent study, we noted that IFN-γ messenger RNA expression is increased after vaccination in melanoma metastases that did not respond to treatment, and this increase is associated with expression of the TA targeted by the vaccination, suggesting that the lack of responsiveness is unlikely to be the result of an antigen-unresponsive state or to a lack of target TA expression *(33)*. In addition, since all the lesions studied expressed the relevant HLA class I antigen, lack of HLA expression could also be excluded in this cohort of patients as the cause for treatment failure. Overall, our studies and others suggest that vaccine-induced immune responses can localize within the tumor microenvironment, and that such localization is not sufficient in most cases to induce clinical regression of tumors.

3. IS THE TUMOR MICROENVIRONMENT A POTENT MODULATOR OF THE IMMUNE RESPONSE IN THE TARGET ORGAN?

Most studies have monitored the effect of TA-directed immunization in humans on circulating lymphocytes because of the easy access to patient's blood. Although this strategy documents whether a locally administered immunogen may induce a systemic effect, it does not mention whether the immunogenic wave induced by the vaccine fades before or as its reaches the target tissue. Thus, we emphasize the importance of complementing the analysis of systemic immune responses with the study of changes within the tumor microenvironment induced by the immunization and associated treatments. This is not easily achievable, for several reasons. Solid tumors cannot be sampled as easily and repeatedly as blood. Therefore, the kinetics of the immune response to vaccination and the natural history of tumor phenotypes evolving with time and/or in response to therapy cannot be readily appreciated. Indeed, in the past, studies involving the tumor microenvironment have largely relied on excisional biopsies that yield a large quantity of material to study, but do not allow for serial sampling of the same lesions or for the prospective documentation of its natural and/or treatment-induced history. Thus, morphological studies based on excisional biopsies infer their relevance to the clinical setting on the assumption that any lesion excised from a given patient is prognostic of the behavior of those left *in situ*. However, because of its inherited genetic instability *(34)*, cancer is a disease that is not likely to satisfy this presumption. Although in the context of early-stage cancer, genetic profiling has suggested that primary lesions do not significantly differ from their locoregional metastases or seem to significantly vary in time *(66)*, in the context of advanced melanoma, our studies and others have found that specific biological markers may vary significantly among synchronous lesions and/or within the same lesions in a short observation period *(62,67,68)*. Tumor cells can lose expression of TA and/or the HLA alleles associated with their presentation *(6,67,69–72)*, and the kinetics of expression of TA may provide an explanation for the paradoxical co-existence of cancer cells in the tumor-competent host *(6)* as loss or downregulation of epitopes on the surface of cancer sells occurs in association with TA-specific immunization *(67,70–72)*, and it might explain tumor survival *(73)*. Thus, analysis of individual lesions frozen into a specific time-point of a disease process that is continuously in evolution may not adequately address the evolving nature of tumor–host interactions.

In addition to yielding a stationary aspect of an evolving pathophysiology, excisional biopsies allow only limited analysis of functional parameters through the semi-quantitative analysis of protein expression in fixed tissues. Expansion and growth of cells in cultures has been utilized extensively to attempt to link extensive functional characterization of a pathological situation to the physiologic state of the same disease in vivo, but it may not be accurately representative *(74)*. Thus, until now, very limited information could be obtained by directly studying the tumor microenvironment both in temporal and functional terms.

We have proposed that dynamic analyses of host–tumor adaptation to immunotherapy could be most successfully performed by correlating T-cell induction, activation, trafficking, and survival at the tumor site with the simultaneously occurring genetic or immune-mediated alterations of tumor cells within a given lesion that could be easily accessed by repeated FNA *(64,75)*. Although this strategy may not be readily applicable to all clinical situations, the principles learned from some human tumor models, such as subcutaneous (sc) melanoma metastases or basal cell carcinoma, may exemplify a broader range of tumor–host interactions that occur in the context of other cancers.

Epitope-specific vaccination is well-suited to the purpose of studying the dynamics of tumor–host interactions because it restricts the number of variables to be analysis in effector and target cells to a single epitope–HLA allele combination. Despite this simplification, several other variable remain unexplored that are unrelated to the direct relationship between the specificity of the immune reaction elicited by the vaccine and the present of relevant target molecules on the surface of cancer cells. Indeed, several other factors that are independent of the specific TCR–HLA–epitope complex interaction may influence the effector function of T cells. We have previously attempted a categorization of such variables according to broad conceptual families *(6)*. Direct cell-to-cell interactions that may increase or decrease the effector function of T cells on their targets (e.g., adhesion molecule enhancement of cytolytic function, FAS/FAS ligand, HLA allele interaction with inhibitory receptors on T cells) may play a prominent role in modulating cellular immune function. In addition, a wealth of secreted factors may be produced by tumor cells or normal cells that infiltrate them with potent chemotactic, inflammatory, and angio-regulatory effects *(6)*. The list of such factors and the complexity of their interaction is likely to rapidly increase in the next few years as a result of high-throughput technology, which has become recently available and allows for a global view of the pathophysiology of a given disease by identifying their extended gene-expression profiles *(76)* or by directly estimating the density of candidate molecules in various tissues *(74,77)*.

Thus, we advocate a strategy in which the kinetics of expression of relevant marker molecules could be tested at different time-points within the same metastasis by the use of serial FNA *(62,75)*. With this approach, we observed a rapid decrease in TA expression in response to vaccination that preceded tumor disappearance, and no changes were noted in non-regressing lesions *(68)*. These observations suggested that when successful, vaccination triggers a broad inflammatory reaction that can lead to tumor destruction despite immune selection. More importantly, these findings suggest that a lack of clinical response is associated with minimal changes in the tumor microenvironment rather than the selection of tumor-cell variants by an overwhelming immune response. Loss of TA or HLA molecules may still play a later role in the metastatic process by allowing TA-deprived cells that have survived the short-term effects of treatment to grow and reconstitute new lesions *(62)*. However, this line of research suggests that the tumor microenvironment is usually insensitive to the immune changes associated with vaccination, and emphasizes the importance of the studies that address the kinetic nature of tumor–host interactions.

The validation of an RNA amplification method that maintains the proportional expression of various genes *(78,79)* has recently allowed the utilization of material obtained from FNA for global transcript analysis studies. With this strategy, the molecular profile of various disease states could be temporally followed, with minimal disturbance of their microenvironment *(75)*. Thus, we have started a prospective collection of FNA samples from lesions of patients in the process of undergoing various forms of immunotherapy. The lesions are then followed for their clinical behavior so that a direct correlation can be made between their natural and/or treatment-induced history and their genetic profile.

4. WHAT CAN BE DONE TO ESCAPE ESCAPE MECHANISMS

We believe that the limited success of immunologic approaches to the treatment of advanced cancer is related to limitations in their design resulting from a lack of understanding of the biology of tumorhost interactions in humans. The last decade, although prolific in identifying molecular mechanisms that could individually be responsible for the modulation of tumor growth in an immune-competent host, has raised more questions than answers without solving several fundamental puzzles related to this field. Although attention to the identification of candidate molecules expressed by tumor cells that could be targets of T-cell killing has yielded a large number of alternate immunogens for immunization, little progress has been made in attempting to understand why ongoing immunizations are not achieving the desired clinical effect. Some studies have suggested that the primary reason for tumor escape from immunization is the ability of tumor cells to elude the effects of vaccination by losing or downregulating the expression of molecules on their surface targeted by the immunization. For this reason, these investigators recommend vaccines that are broad in immunogenic potential, which could immunize across the HLA polymorphism spectrum through presentation of different peptide sequences derived from multiple antigens or even whole-tumor-cell preparations *(80,81)*. With this strategy, loss of individual HLA allele and/or TA expression would have a lower impact than when a single epitope/HLA allele combination is targeted. Others believe that the reason that anticancer vaccines are not effective should be sought in the fine-tuning of the immunization effects on the functional phenotype of T cells *(23,40,52)*. Subtypes of effector and memory CD8+ T cells may predict the outcome of therapy in the future (Fig. 1).

We do not disagree with either of these hypotheses. However, we would like to introduce another possibility—that the primary reason for failure of immunotherapy in the majority of patients may be related to the inherent biologic characteristics of individual tumors. Fundamental questions must be answered in this regard before rational therapies can be designed. For instance, is it really necessary to individualize immunological treatments to the extent pursued by present immunization strategies? More fundamentally, are the mechanisms that lead to tumor rejection similar in all tumor types, independent of their histology or their site of occurrence? In addition, is the mechanism leading to tumor rejection similar for all treatments that modulate the host immune system, or does the specificity of each treatment play a uniquely significant role? Finally, is immunologically mediated tumor rejection a phenomenon with overlapping biological characteristics with autoimmune and infectious disease, and if so, to what extent? Should we look more closely at experiences from these other clinical aspects of immunology to further our insight of cancer immune biology and its relationship with the host? We believe that the answer to these questions are presently buried within the tissues targeted by our therapies—in our case, the tumor microenvironment—and thus, our efforts should be aimed at the implementation of the study of these sites as a complement to the study of systemic individual responses to immunization.

REFERENCES

1. Boon T, Coulie PG, Van den Eynde B. Tumor antigens recognized by T cells. *Immunol Today* 1997;18(6):267–268.
2. Rosenberg SA. Cancer vaccines based on the identification of genes encoding cancer regression antigens. *Immunol Today* 1997;18(4):175–182.
3. Old LJ, Chen YT. New paths in human cancer serology. *J Exp Med* 1998;187(8):1163–1167.
4. Rosenberg SA, Kawakami Y, Robbins PF, Wang R. Identification of the genes encoding cancer antigens: implications for cancer immunotherapy. *Adv Cancer Res* 1996;70: 145–77:145–177.
5. Renkvist N, Castelli C, Robbins PF, Parmiani G. A listing of human tumor antigens recognized by T cells. *Cancer Immunol Immunother* 2001;50(1):3–15.
6. Marincola FM, Jaffe EM, Hicklin DJ, Ferrone S. Escape of human solid tumors from T cell recognition: molecular mechanisms and functional significance. *Adv Immunol* 2000;74:181–273.
7. Sznol M, Marincola FM (2000) Principles of immune monitoring in cancer vaccine trials. In: Principles and Practice of the Biologic Therapy of Cancer (Rosenberg SA, ed.), Lippincott Williams & Wilkins, Philadelphia, PA, pp. 617–631.
8. Marincola FM (2000) Mechanisms of immune escape and immune tolerance. In: *Principles and Practice of the Biologic Therapy of Cancer* (Rosenberg SA, ed.), Lippincott Williams & Wilkins, Philadelphia, PA, pp. 601–617.
9. Wolfel T, Klehmann E, Muller C, Schutt KH, Meyer zum Buschenfelde KH, Knuth A. Lysis of human melanoma cells by autologous cytolytic T cell clones. Identification of human histocompatibility leukocyte antigen A2 as a restriction element for three different antigens. *J Exp Med* 1989;170:797–810.
10. Parkinson DR, Abrams JS, Wiernik PH, Rayner AA, Margolin KA, Van Echo DA, et al. Interleukin-2 therapy in patients with metastatic malignant melanoma: a phase II study. *J Clin Oncol* 1990;8:1650–1656.
11. Rosenberg SA, Packard BS, Aebersold PM, Solomon D, Topalian SL, Toy ST, et al. Use of tumor-infiltrating lymphocytes and interleukin-2 in the immunotherapy of patients with metastatic melanoma. A preliminary report. *N Engl J Med* 1988;319:1676–1680.
12. Panelli MC, Wang E, Phan G, Puhlman M, Miller L, Ohnmacht GA, et al. Genetic profiling of peripharal mononuclear cells and melanoma metastases in response to systemic interleukin-2 administration. *Genome Biol* 2002;3(7): RESEARCH0035.
13. van der Bruggen P, Traversari C, Chomez P, Lurquin C, De Plaen E, Van den Eynde B, et al. A gene encoding an antigen recognized by cytolytic T lymphocytes on a human melanoma. *Science* 1991;254:1643–1647.
14. Jager D, Jager E, Knuth A. Vaccination for malignant melanoma: recent developments. *Oncology* 2001;60(1):1–7.
15. Kawakami Y, Rosenberg SA. Immunobiology of human melanoma antigens MART-1 and gp100 and their use for immuno-gene therapy. *Int Rev Immunol* 1997;14(2–3):173–192.
16. Marincola FM, Rivoltini L, Salgaller ML, Player M, Rosenberg SA. Differential anti-MART-1/MelanA CTL activity in peripheral blood of HLA-A2 melanoma patients in comparison to healthy donors: evidence for in vivo priming by tumor cells. *J Immunother* 1996;19(4):266–277.

17. Pittet MJ, Valmori D, Dumbar PR, Speiser DE, Lienard D, Lejeune F, et al. High frequencies of naive Melan-A/MART-1-specific CD8(+) T cells in a large proportion of human histocompatibility leukocyte antigen (HLA)-A2 individuals. *J Exp Med* 1999; 190(5):705–715.
18. Coulie PG, Somville M, Lehmann F, Hainaut P, Brasseur F, Devos R, et al. Precursor frequency analysis of human cytolytic T lymphocytes directed against autologous melanoma cells. *Int J Cancer* 1992;50:289–297.
19. D'Souza S, Rimoldi D, Lienard D, Lejeune F, Cerottini JC, Romero P. Circulating Melan-A/Mart-1 specific cytolytic T lymphocyte precursors in HLA-A2+ melanoma patients have a memory phenotype. *Int J Cancer* 1998;78(6):699–706.
20. Letsch A, Keilholz U, Schadendorf D, Nagorsen D, Schmittel A, Thiel E et al. High frequencies of circulating melanoma-reactive T cells in patients with advanced melanoma. *Int J Cancer* 2000;87(5):659–664.
21. Marchand M, van Baren N, Weynants P, Brichard V, Dreno B, Tessier MH, et al. Tumor regressions observed in patients with metastatic melanoma treated with an antigenic peptide encoded by gene MAGE-3 and presented by HLA-A1. *Int J Cancer* 1999;80(2): 219–230.
22. Cormier JN, Salgaller ML, Prevette T, Barracchini KC, Rivoltini L, Restifo NP, et al. Enhancement of cellular immunity in melanoma patients immunized with a peptide from MART-1/Melan A [see comments]. *Cancer J Sci Am* 1997;3(1):37–44.
23. Pittet MJ, Speiser DE, Lienard D, Valmori D, Guillaume P, Dutoit V, et al. Expansion and functional maturation of human tumor antigen-specific CD8+ T cells after vaccination with antigenic peptide. *Clin Cancer Res* 2001;7(3):796s–803s.
24. Nestle FO, Alijagic S, Gilliet M, Sun Y, Grabbe S, Dummer R, et al. Vaccination of melanoma patients with peptide- or tumor lysate-pulsed dendritic cells. *Nat Med* 1998;4(3): 328–332.
25. Thurner B, Haendle I, Roder C, Dieckmann D, Keikavoussi P, Jonuleit H, et al. Vaccination with MAGE-3A1 peptide-pulsed mature, monocyte-derived dendritic cells expands specific cytotoxic T cells and induces regression of some metastases in advanced stage IV melanoma. *J Exp Med* 1999;190(11):1669–1678.
26. Scheibenbogen C, Schmittel A, Keilholz U, Allgauer T, Hofmann U, Max R, et al. Phase 2 trial of vaccination with tyrosinase peptides and granulocyte-macrophage colony-stimulating factor in patients with metastatic melanoma. *J Immunother* 2000;23(2):275–281.
27. Rosenberg SA, Yang JC, Schwartzentruber D, Hwu P, Marincola FM, Topalian SL, et al. Immunologic and therapeutic evaluation of a synthetic tumor associated peptide vaccine for the treatment of patients with metastatic melanoma. *Nat Med* 98 A.D.;4(3):321–327.
28. Laforet M, Froelich N, Parissiadis A, Bausinger H, Pfeiffer B, Tongio MM. An intronic mutation responsible for a low level of expression of an HLA-A*24 allele. *Tissue Antigens* 1997;50(4):340–346.
29. Jager E, Gnjatic S, Nagata Y, Stockert E, Jager D, Karbach J, et al. Induction of primary NY-ESO-1 immunity: CD8+ T lymphocyte and antibody responses in peptide-vaccinated patients with NY-ESO-1+ cancers. *Proc Natl Acad Sci USA* 2000;97(22):12198–12203.
30. Jager E, Maeurer MJ, Hohn H, Karbach J, Jager D, Zidianakis Z, et al. Clonal expansion of Melan A-specific cytotoxic T lymphocytes in a melanoma patient responding to continued immunization with melanoma-associated peptides. *Int J Cancer* 2000;86(4):538–547.
31. Wang F, Bade E, Kuniyoshi C, Spears L, Jeffery G, Marthy V, et al. Phase I trial of a MART-1 peptide vaccine with incomplete Freund's adjuvant for resected high-risk melanoma. *Clin Cancer Res* 1999;5(10):2756–2765.
32. Cotran RS, Pober JS, Gimbrone MA, Jr., Springer TA, Wiebke EA, Gaspari AA, et al. Endothelial activation during interleukin 2 immunotherapy. A possible mechanism for the vascular leak syndrome. *J Immunol* 1988;140:1883–1888.

33. Kammula US, Lee K-H, Riker A, Wang E, Ohnmacht GA, Rosenberg SA, et al. Functional analysis of antigen-specific T lymphocytes by serial measurement of gene expression in peripheral blood mononuclear cells and tumor specimens. *J Immunol* 1999;163:6867–6879.
34. Lengauer C, Kinzler KW, Vogelstein B. Genetic instabilities in human cancers. *Nature* 1998;396(6712):643–649.
35. Keilholz U, Weber J, Finke J, Gabrilovich D, Kast WM, Disis N, et al. Immunologic monitoring of cancer vaccine therapy: results of a Workshop sponsored by the Society of Biological Therapy. *J Immunother* 2002;25(2):97–138.
36. Scheibenbogen C, Lee KH, Stevanovic S, Witzens M, Willhauck M, Waldmann V, et al. Analysis of the T cell response to tumor and viral peptide antigens by an IFNgamma-ELISPOT assay. *Int J Cancer* 1997;71(6):932–936.
37. Pass HA, Schwarz SL, Wunderlich JR, Rosenberg SA. Immunization of patients with melanoma peptide vaccines: immunologic assessment using the ELISPOT assay [see comments]. *Cancer J Sci Am* 1998;4(5):316–323.
38. Papa P, Hussell T, Openshaw PJ. Flow cytometric measurement of intracellular cytokines. *J Immunol Methods* 2000;243(1–2):107–124.
39. Asemissen AM, Nargosen D, Keilholz U, Letsch A, Schmittel A, Thiel E, et al. Flw cytometric determination of intracellular or secreted IFNgamma for the quantitation of antigen reactive T cells. *J Immunol Methods* 2001;251(1–2):101–108.
40. Pittet MJ, Zippelius A, Speiser DE, Assenmacher M, Guillaume P, Valmori D, et al. Ex vivo IFN-γ secretion by circulating CD8 T lymphocytes: implications of a novel approach for T cell monitoring in infectious and malignant diseases. *J Immunol* 2001;166:7634–7640.
41. Tan LC, Gudgeon N, Annels NE, Hansasuta P, O'Callaghan CA, Rowland-Jones S, et al. A re-evaluation of the frequency of CD8(+) T cells specific for EBV in healthy virus carriers. *J Immunol* 1999;162(3):1827–1835.
42. Altman JD, Moss PH, Goulder PR, Barouch DH, McHeyzer-Williams MG, Bell JI, et al. Phenotypic analysis of antigen-specific T lymphocytes [published erratum appears in Science 1998 Jun 19;280(5371):1821]. *Science* 1996;274(5284):94–96.
43. Nielsen M-B, Monsurro′ V, Miguelse S, Wang E, Perez-Diez A, Lee K-H, et al. Status of activation of circulating vaccine-elicited CD8+ T cells. *J Immunol* 2000;165(4):2287–2296.
44. Lee K-H, Wang E, Nielsen M-B, Wunderlich J, Migueles S., Connors M, et al. Increased vaccine-specific T cell frequency after peptide-based vaccination correlates with increased susceptibility to in vitro stimulation but does not lead to tumor regression. *J Immunol* 1999;163:6292–6300.
45. Ogg GS, Jin X, Bonhoeffer S, Dunbar PR, Nowak MA, Monard S, et al. Quantitation of HIV-1-specific cytotoxic T lymphocytes and plasma load of viral RNA. *Science* 1998; 279(5359):2103–2106.
46. Gray CM, Lawrence J, Schapiro JM, Altman JD, Winters MA, Crompton M, et al. Frequency of class I HLA-restricted anti-HIV CD8(+) T cells in individuals receiving highly active antiretroviral therapy (HAART). *J Immunol* 1999;162(3):1780–1788.
47. Bieganowska K, Hollsberg P, Buckle GJ, Lim DG, Greten TF, Schneck J, et al. Direct analysis of viral-specific CD8(+) T cells with soluble HLA-A2/Tax 11-19 tetramer complexes in patients with human T cell lymphotropic virus-associated myelopathy. *J Immunol* 1999;162(3):1765–1771.
48. Nagai M, Kubota R, Greten TF, Schneck JP, Leist TP, Jacobson S. Increased activated human T cell lymphotropic virus type I (HTLV-I) Tax11-19-specific memory and effector CD8+ cells in patients with HLTV-I-associated myelopathy/tropical spastic paraparesis: correlation with HTLV-I provirus load. *J Infect Dis* 2001;183:197–205.
49. Monsurro V, Nielsen M-B, Perez-Diez A, Dudley ME, Wang E, Rosenberg SA, et al. Kinetics of TCR use in response to repeated epitope-specific immunization. *J Immunol* 2001; 166:5817–5825.

50. Dietrich PY, Walker PR, Quiquerez AL, Perrin G, Dutoit V, Lienard D, et al. Melanoma patients respond to a cytotoxic T lymphocyte-defined self-peptide with diverse and nonoverlapping T-cell receptor repertoires. *Cancer Res* 2001;61(5):2047–2054.
51. Lee PP, Yee C, Savage PA, Fong L, Brockstedt D, Weber JS, et al. Characterization of circulating T cells specific for tumor-associated antigens in melanoma patients. *Nat Med* 1999;5(6):677–685.
52. Sallusto F, Lenig D, Forster R, Lipp M, Lanzavecchia A. Two subsets of memory T lymphocytes with distinct homing potentials and effector functions. *Nature* 1999; 401(6754):659–660.
53. Dunbar PR, Smith CL, Chao D, Salio M, Shepherd DM, Mirza F, et al. A shift in the phenotype of MelanA-specific CTL identifies melanoma patients with an active tumor-specific immune response. *J Immunol* 2000;165(11):6644–6652.
54. Appay V, Nixon DF, Donahoe SM, Gillespie GM, Dong T, King A, et al. HIV-specific CD8(+) T cells produce antiviral cytokines but are impaired in cytolytic function. *J Exp Med* 2000;192(1):63–75.
55. Jager E, Ringhoffer M, Dienes HP, Arand M, Karbach J, Jager D, et al. Granulocyte-macrophage-colony-stimulating factor enhances immune responses to melanoma-associated peptides in vivo. *Int J Cancer* 1996;67(1):54–62.
56. Panelli MC, Wunderlich J, Jeffries J, Wang E, Mixon A, Rosenberg SA, et al. Phase I study in patients with metastatic melanoma of immunization with dendritic cells presenting epitopes derived from the melanoma associated antigens MART-1 and gp100. *J Immunother* 1999;23(4):487–498.
57. Lau R, Wang F, Jeffery G, Marty V, Kuniyoshi J, Bade E, et al. Phase I trial of intravenous peptide-pulsed dendritic cells in patients with metastatic melanoma. *J Immunother* 2001;24(1):66–78.
58. Rosenberg SA, Yang JC, Topalian SL, Schwartzentruber DJ, Weber JS, Parkinson DR, et al. Treatment of 283 consecutive patients with metastatic melanoma or renal cell cancer using high-dose bolus interleukin 2 [see comments]. *JAMA* 1994;271:907–913.
59. Margolin KA. Interleukin-2 in the treatment of renal cancer. *Semin Oncol* 2000;27(2):194–203.
60. Kasid A, Director EP, Rosenberg SA. Induction of endogenous cytokine-mRNA in circulating peripheral blood mononuclear cells by IL-2 administration to cancer patients. *J Immunol* 1989;143:736–739.
61. Pockaj BA, Sherry RM, Wei JP, Yannelli JR, Carter CS, Leitman SF, et al. Localization of 111indium-labeled tumor infiltrating lymphocytes to tumor in patients receiving adoptive immunotherapy. Augmentation with cyclophosphamide and correlation with response. *Cancer* 1994;73:1731–1737.
62. Lee K-H, Panelli MC, Kim CJ, Riker A, Roden M, Fetsch PA, et al. Functional dissociation between local and systemic immune response following peptide vaccination. *J Immunol* 1998;161:4183–4194.
63. Panelli MC, Bettinotti MP, Lally K, Li Y, Ohnmacht GA, Robbins PA, et al. Identification of a tumor infiltrating lymphocyte recognizing MAGE-12 in a melanoma metastasis with decreased expression of melanoma differentiation antigens. *J Immunol* 2000;164: 4382–4392.
64. Yee C, Riddell SR, Greenberg PD. In vivo tracking of tumor-specific T cells. *Curr Opin Immunol* 2001;13:141–146.
65. Panelli MC, Riker A, Kammula US, Lee K-H, Wang E, Rosenberg SA, et al. Expansion of Tumor/T cell pairs from Fine Needle Aspirates (FNA) of Melanoma Metastases. *J Immunol* 2000;164(1):495–504.
66. Perou CM, Sertle T, Eisen MB, van de Rijn M, Jeffrey SS, Rees CA, et al. Molecular portraits of human breast tumorurs. *Nature* 2000;406:747–752.

67. Jager E, Ringhoffer M, Altmannsberger M, Arand M, Karbach J, Jager D, et al. Immunoselection in vivo: independent loss of MHC class I and melanocyte differentiation antigen expression in metastatic melanoma. *Int J Cancer* 1997;71(2):142–147.
68. Ohnmacht GA, Wang E, Mocellin S, Abati A, Filie A, Fetsch PA, et al. Short term kinetics of tumor antigen expression in response to vaccination. *J Immunol* 2001;167:1809–1820.
69. Ferrone S, Marincola FM. Loss of HLA class I antigens by melanoma cells: molecular mechanisms, functional significance and clinical relevance. *Immunol Today* 1995;16:487–494.
70. Cormier JN, Hijazi YM, Abati A, Fetsch P, Bettinotti M, Steinberg SM, et al. Heterogeneous expression of melanoma-associated antigens (MAA) and HLA-A2 in metastatic melanoma in vivo. *Int J Cancer* 1998;75:517–524.
71 Scheibenbogen C, Weyers I, Ruiter D, Willhauck M, Bittinger A, Keilholz U. Expression of gp100 in melanoma metastases resected before or after treatment with IFN alpha and IL-2. *J Immunother* 1996;19(5):375–380.
72. Riker A, Kammula US, Panelli MC, Wang E, Abati A, Fetsch P, et al. Immune selection following antigen specific immunotherapy of melanoma. *Surgery* 1999;126(2):112–120.
73. Anichini A, Molla A, Mortarini R, Tragni G, Bersani I, Di Nicola M, et al. An expanded peripheral T cell population to a cytotoxic T lymphocyte (CTL)-defined, melanocyte-specific antigen in metastatic melanoma patients impacts on generation of peptide-specific CTLs but does not overcome tumor escape from immune surveillance in metastatic lesions. *J Exp Med* 1999;190(5):651–667.
74. Page MJ, Amess B, Townsend RR, Parekh RB, Herath A, Brunsten L, et al. Proteomic definition of normal human luminal and myoepithelial breast cells purified from reduction mammoplasties. *Proc Natl Acad Sci USA* 1999;96(22):12,589–12,594.
75. Wang E, Marincola FM. A natural history of melanoma: serial gene expression analysis. *Immunol Today* 2000;21(12):619–623.
76. Brown PO, Botstein D. Exploring the new world of the genome with DNA microarrays. *Nat Genet* 1999;21:33–37.
77. Paweletz CP, Charboneau L, Bichsel VE, Simone NL, Chen T, Gillespie JW, et al. Reverse phase protein microarrays which capture disease progression show activation of pre-survival pathways at the cancer invasion front. *Oncogene* 2001;20:1981–1989.
78. Wang E, Miller L, Ohnmacht GA, Liu E, Marincola FM. High fidelity mRNA amplification for gene profiling using cDNA microarrays. *Nat Biotechnol* 2000;17(4):457–459.
79. Feldman AL, Costouros NG, Wang E, Qian M, Marincola FM, Alexander HR, et al. Advantages of mRNA amplification for microarray analysis. *Biotechniques* 2002;33(4):906–914.
80. Mitchell MS. Perspective on allogeneic melanoma lysates in active specific immunotherapy. *Semin Oncol* 1998;25(6):623–635.
81. Bystryn JC, Zaleniuch-Jacquotte A, Oratz R, Shapiro RL, Harris MN, Roses DF. Double-blind trial of polyvalent, shed-antigen, melanoma vaccine. *Clin Cancer Res* 2001;7(7): 1882–1887.

14 Altered Signaling in T Lymphocytes of Patients With Cancer

A Biomarker of Prognosis?

Theresa L. Whiteside, PhD

Contents

1. INTRODUCTION

The role of the host immune system in cancer development and progression has been debated for most of the last century. On the one hand, the concept of immune surveillance advanced the notion that the immune system protected the host from insults by infectious agents and played a significant role in elimination of abnormal cells. On the other hand, evidence indicating that cancer developed and progressed in subjects with a normally functioning immune system argued against immune-mediated control of cancer progression. Early experiments with transplantable tumors in syngeneic mice showed that it was possible to successfully immunize animals against tumors and that immune protection was mediated by lymphocytes *(1,2)*. Later on, it became clear that transfer of T lymphocytes, antibodies, or cytokines to tumor-bearing hosts was often successful in the control of tumor growth in animals *(3,4)*, but frequently failed in man *(5)*. By then, the field of tumor immunology had evolved, and principles of tumor immunity had been established. The central role played by T-lymphocyte subsets in tumor control has now been widely accepted, although it remained unclear why T cells were unable to exercise this control successfully in cases of tumor progression and metastasis. Although it has been recognized that the host is not ignorant of the developing tumor, the scientific

From: *Current Clinical Oncology: Cancer Immunotherapy at the Crossroads: How Tumors Evade Immunity and What Can Be Done*
Edited by: J. H. Finke and R. M. Bukowski

community was reluctant to accept evidence that tumors are able to manipulate and subvert the host immune system. The last few years have witnessed a change in this respect, which was largely brought about by frequent difficulties with achieving therapeutic effects with cancer vaccines, even when highly sophisticated therapeutic strategies were used in "immunologically responsive" cancers, such as melanoma *(6,7)*. The question of why T cells in tumor-bearing hosts are unable to prevent or interfere with tumor growth, although they apparently can control invading pathogens, remains one of the key issues in tumor immunology today. Clearly, tumor-specific T cells are present in the circulation of patients with cancer, as demonstrated by using tetramers or ELISPOT assays *(8,9)*. It may be expected that these T cells would be able to effectively eliminate the tumor or arrest its metastases. One possible answer to this dilemma may be that tumor antigen-specific T lymphocytes, although present, may not be able to exercise their functions in the tumor microenvironment or, more broadly, in the host bearing the tumor. The goal of this chapter is to review evidence in support of this possibility and to show that T lymphocytes in tumor-bearing human hosts are functionally compromised and thus unable to successfully complete the fundamental molecular pathway that leads to their activation upon the encounter with a cognate antigen.

1.1. Characteristics of T Lymphocytes in the Blood and Tumor Tissues of Patients With Cancer

Phenotypic and functional studies of T lymphocytes at the tumor site and in the peripheral circulation of patients with cancer have revealed that in many respects, these cells are different from their counterparts in normal subjects *(10,11)*. As reviewed elsewhere in this volume (e.g., Chapters 1 and 2) tumor-infiltrating lymphocytes (TIL) are functionally impaired despite the fact that they have an activation phenotype—e.g., express the activation surface markers usually associated with functional effector cells *(10)*. The loss or decrease of functional attributes by TIL has been extensively evaluated and ascribed to a variety of different mechanisms related to or mediated by the tumor *(12,13)*. In marked contrast, activated T cells that infiltrate inflammatory non-cancerous lesions are largely able to function normally. Thus, the conclusion that the tumor subverts TIL functions can be reached. We have also observed that TIL in human solid tumors contain variable proportions of T cells with fragmented DNA (e.g., TUNEL + TIL) *(12)*. Thus, it appeared that TIL undergo apoptosis *in situ*, which might be related to expression of FasL, and perhaps other death-related molecules on the surface of tumor cells *(14)*. Immunostaining performed on sections of tumor biopsies indicated that FasL+ tumors were infiltrated by Fas+ TIL, and that many showed evidence of apoptosis *(13–15)*. These observations have led to a proposal that tumors "counterattack" and eliminate TIL *(16)*.

Earlier studies in our laboratory and others showed that circulating T cells in patients with cancer were also functionally impaired, and that they shared some of the characteristics ascribed to TIL *(10,17)*. For instance, we have reported that apoptosis of lymphocytes in subjects with cancer is not limited to the tumor microenvironment, but is also detectable in circulating peripheral-blood lymphocytes (PBLs) *(17,18)*. These newer data strongly suggested that the immunosuppressive effects of the tumor extend beyond its microenvironment. To test this hypothesis, we searched for evidence to support a direct association between T-cell dysfunction and the apoptosis seen in TIL and autologous PBL by comparing TIL with PBL obtained from 28 patients with oral carcinoma *(15)*. The comparison showed that functional impairments (e.g., low expression of the T-cell receptor (TCR)-associated ζ chain and low proliferation in response to anti-CD3 Ab) were concomitantly present in TIL and PBL, and that low ζ expression correlated with increased proportions of apoptotic T cells in paired TIL and PBL populations *(15)*. Thus, a link was established between signaling abnormalities in T cells and spontaneous apoptosis of circulating lymphocytes seen in patients with cancer. This study also confirmed that low expression of the ζ chain, depressed immune function, and apoptosis of T cells correlated with high levels of FasL expression on the tumor *(15)*.

The significant associations observed between immune abnormalities and apoptosis in TIL and PBL suggested to us that lymphocytes are re-circulating or turning over more rapidly in patients with cancer than in normal controls. A recently completed evaluation of absolute lymphocyte counts in a large cohort of more than 90 patients with head and neck cancer (HNC) showed that some CD3+ and CD4+ T cells, but not CD8+ T cells, were significantly decreased in these patients compared to normal age-matched controls *(19)*. This result appears to be in conflict with our other studies, which show that spontaneous apoptosis in the peripheral compartment selectively targets CD8+ effector T-cell subsets *(17,18)*. However, the explanation is that the rate of turnover might be different for CD4+ and CD8+ T-cell subsets, as formally shown for patients with acquired immunodeficiency syndrome (AIDS) *(20)*. If CD8+ T cells are selectively driven into the apoptotic pathway, their turnover is expected to be rapid, and their swift ingress from the bone-marrow stores may be able to maintain homeostasis and account for the normal CD8+ T-cell number. This appears to be true for most patients we studied, except for those few with a strikingly low CD8+ T-cell count in the circulation (unpublished data, I. Kuss and T.L. Whiteside). Although the clinical significance of this finding is currently under investigation, it is reasonable to suggest that rapid turnover of T cells in patients with cancer exists, and that it is driven by excessive apoptosis of these T cells *(18)*.

The second suggestion that can be made based on our studies is that in patients with cancer, TIL and PBL have several features in common, including the sensitivity to apoptosis and the presence of signaling defects, which result in a depressed functional potential of T lymphocytes. These features distinguish T cells of patients with cancer from their normal counterparts in the circulation of age-matched controls without cancer.

1.2. The TCR-Associated Signaling Complex

The TCR-associated ζ chain is responsible for transduction of signals delivered via the receptor, and therefore, its expression is essential for activation of T cells *(21)*. TCR is a complex of several molecules that cooperate in the process of recognition and binding of the peptide presented by the MHC on the antigen-presenting cell (APC).

It has been determined that there are six phosphorylation sites or ITAMs (immune receptor tyrosine-based activation motifs) on each of the two ζ chains in the TCR (*see* Fig. 1). The effective TCR signal induces ordered successive phosphorylation of all six ITAMs. Interactions of correctly assembled TCRs on the cell surface with the APC present a cognate MHC-peptide complex that triggers the receptors. The process of T-cell triggering is self-limited, and downregulation of triggered TCR involves a loss of ζ protein. The mechanisms responsible for this loss are unclear, although internalization and lysosomal degradation of TCR chains, including the ζ chain, have been observed in experiments involving human T-cell clones that are specific for tetanus toxoid peptides *(22)*. The T cells then replace the internalized receptors on the cell surface and interact again with the immunogenic peptide. However, lysosomal degradation may not be the only mechanism of cellular degradation of ζ, as discussed here. Nevertheless, it is important to note that chronic antigenic stimulation via TCR may lead to prolonged or even permanent downregulation of ζ expression and to partial or complete T-cell anergy. Low or absent ζ chain expression in circulating lymphocytes is not confined to patients with cancer; it has been also documented in chronic infections such as leprosy and AIDS *(23,24)*, as well as autoimmune diseases associated with circulating immune complexes, such as systemic lupus erythematosus (SLE) *(25)*.

The crucial importance of ζ in T-cell signaling via TCR underscores the attention attracted by the first report on the low expression of this molecule as well as *p56* ^{lck} and *p59* ^{fyn} in splenocytes of mice bearing established tumors *(26,27)*. The implication of this finding was that the TCR complex in lymphocytes of tumor-bearing animals had been altered, and thus was unable to signal with optimal efficiency. Indeed, splenocytes of these mice had depressed effector-cell functions as compared to animals without tumors *(26)*. Subsequently, similarly low expression of ζ was observed in TIL and circulating T lymphocytes of patients with various cancers *(28–32)*. However, considerable variation in the expression of TCR-associated proteins was being reported, ranging from their absence in the lymphocytes of some patients with cancer to normal levels of

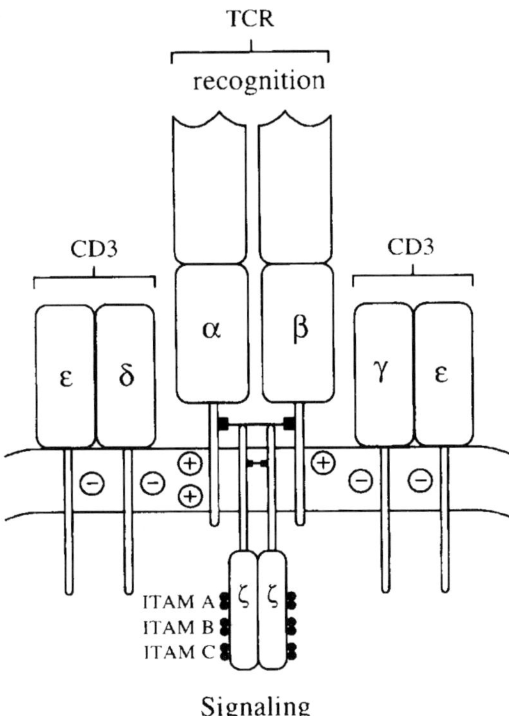

Fig. 1. Schematic representation of TCR expressed on the surface of T lymphocytes. Note that the ζ chain homodimer is a signaling component of the complex. A single ζ chain contains three ITAMS, each incorporating two phosphotyrosines. Upon full T-cell activation, all six tyrosines become phosphorylated. (Reproduced from *Immunology for Surgeons*, Andrew P. Zbar, Pierre J. Guillou, Kirby I. Bland, Konstantinos N. Syrigos [eds.], Springer-Verlag, London, 2002.)

expression in others. More consistently, TIL were found to express less ζ than PBL-T, and this was interpreted as evidence that signaling abnormalities were induced in T cells by the tumor, and therefore, were more pronounced at the tumor site than in the peripheral circulation. A survey of tumor-bearing mouse strains failed to detect decreases in the expression of ζ using Western blots *(33)*. One report suggests that low or absent expression of ζ in PBL-T may be an artifact induced by granulocyte- or monocyte-derived proteases released during tissue or blood processing *(34)* generated skepticism about decreased ζ expression in tumor-bearing hosts and its biologic significance.

1.3. Measurements of ζ Chain Expression in Lymphocytes

One of the reasons for variabiation in the results for ζ expression in TIL or PBL-T of patients with cancer or other diseases was the methodology used for

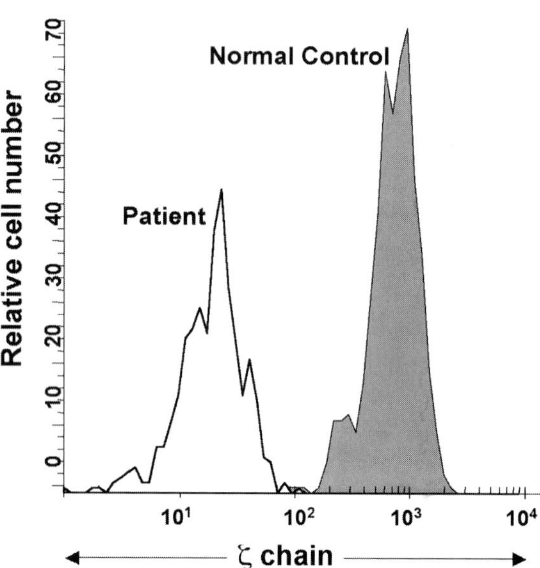

Fig. 2. A representative flow cytometry histogram, showing MFI of the ζ chain in effector T cells of a patient and a normal control. The gate was set on CD8+CD45RO–CD27– effector T cells. Note the substantial decrease of ζ MFI in the patient's T cells. (Reproduced from ref. *61*.)

its detection. The prevailing use of Western blots—which are not quantitative or sensitive—and the fact that ζ was decreased rather than completely absent in most cases contributed to difficulties in the interpretation of ζ expression in T cells of patient with cancer. It was not until quantitative flow cytometry was applied to the analysis of TCR and ζ that a more consistent picture began to emerge. Staining for ζ expression requires cell permeabilization; however, and it is important to ensure that the procedure is performed under optimized conditions, with normal T cells serving as the control. Scoring lymphocytes for ζ expression by mean fluorescence intensity (MFI) provides a quantitative measurement in suspensions of cells. The analysis is performed after setting the lymphocyte gate (FCS/SCC) and backgating to CD3+, CD4+, or CD8+ populations in order to determine their MFI. As shown in Fig. 2, the MFI of each patient's T cells can be measured in this way relative to that of normal control tested in parallel. By establishing a normal range of ζ expression in T lymphocytes obtained from healthy donors, it is possible to determine the deviation of patients' T cells from this range. In addition to MFI, the percentage of ζ-negative cells in the gate can be determined based on the cutoff level established by using the MFI value for an isotype control. The use of fluorescent beads (e.g., Quantum 27 beads) as a standard allows for even more precise quantification of the ζ chain in appropriately stained lymphocyte populations.

In tissues, ζ expression in T lymphocytes is measured by immunocytochemistry, using cryosections of tumor biopsies embedded in ornithine carbamyl transferase (OCT) medium. We have also used paraffin specimens, but only after determining that anti-ζ antibodies are able to bind to the denatured ζ protein. In tumor tissue sections, staining intensity for ζ is graded as either reduced or normal relative to staining of T lymphocytes that infiltrate the adjacent non-tumor tissue or of T lymphocytes that are present in normal tissues used as controls. To avoid bias in interpretation, it is best to use an optical device to measure staining intensity, or to have more than one investigator perform the evaluation and use the mean score.

The use of quantitative flow cytometry facilitated the ζ chain analysis in T cells and highlighted its deficient expression in T cells of patients with cancer, including those with melanoma and ovarian, prostate, and oral as well as renal cell carcinomas (RCCs) *(28,29,32,35–37)*. Usually, the lowest ζ expression was seen in TIL and tumor-associated lymphocytes (TAL), in lymphocytes isolated from tumor-involved lymph nodes and in PBL-T obtained from patients with advanced metastatic disease *(38)*. Analysis of ζ expression by immunohistochemistry in cryosections of human tumors confirmed that this abnormality existed *in situ*, and thus could not result from release of enzymes during tissue processing *(39)*. In addition to low or absent ζ expression, that of the ε chain was often lower in T cells obtained from patients with cancer relative to PBL-T of normal donors *(39)*. In our experience, the loss of ζ expression was generally greater than that of CD3ε, and it was always greater in TIL or TAL than in the paired PBL-T *(38,39)*. Furthermore, this decrease in expression of the components of the TCR complex seemed to correlate with functional dysfunctions of the isolated T cells, including proliferation, cytotoxicity, or cytokine production *(38–40)*.

Most of the available data on ζ expression in T cells of patients with cancer have been obtained in cross-sectional studies that examined either PBL or TIL in cohorts of patients with a particular type of cancer and compared the phenotype and/or functions to those of PBL obtained from normal donors. Few studies have attempted to directly compare features of TIL with those of autologous PBL *(41)*. Yet, if the presence of the tumor contributes in some way to dysfunction of T cells, then a gradient of functional impairments extending from TIL to PBL in individual patients with cancer should be demonstrable. Therefore, we examined the ζ-chain expression, ability to proliferate ex vivo, and the frequency of apoptosis in paired TIL and PBL obtained from a cohort of 28 patients with oral cancer *(15)*. The results clearly showed that such a gradient exists, reinforcing the conclusion that the presence of the tumor has significant inhibitory effects on functions of the immune cells, and that these

Table 1
Expression of the ζ Chain in Paired TIL and PBL of Patients With Oral Carcinoma[a]

		TIL - ζ		
		Reduced	*Normal*	*Total*
PBL – ζ	Reduced	8	4	12
	Normal	1	15	16
	Total	9	19	28

[a]The data indicate the numbers of patients. Expression of ζ in paired TIL and PBL-T was determined by immunohistochemistry. Reduction of ζ expression in both TIL and PBL is significant at $p = 0.0012$.

effects are both local and systemic. As shown in Table 1, reduced expression of ζ in TIL was observed in 9 of 28 patients (32%), and in PBL in 12 of 28 (43%) of the patients. Concordant reduction of ζ in paired TIL and PBL was seen in 8 of 28 (29%) of the patients (p < 0.0012). Thus, ζ expression was reduced in only a subset of patients with oral cancer, but when present, the defect in signaling was usually detectable in both TIL and PBL *(15)*. The subset of 12 patients with low ζ expression in PBL was also found to have depressed proliferative responses to anti-CD3 Ab ($p < 0.0012$). Similarly, responses to anti-CD3 Ab of PBL-T obtained from patients whose TIL had low ζ expression were also significantly depressed, as would be predicted from a significant correlation established between concomitant low ζ expression in TIL and PBL. If TIL expressed normal levels of ζ, responses of PBL to anti-CD3 Ab were equal to those of normal T cells *(15)*. Interestingly, as shown in Table 2, we observed a significant correlation in both TIL and PBL between reduced expression of ζ in CD3+ cells and apoptosis ($p = 0.0015$ and $p = 0.0019$, respectively). This significant association between decreased ζ expression in autologous TIL and PBL and spontaneous apoptosis was not surprising, as it was consistent with the evidence reported by us earlier that ζ-chain degradation could be a manifestation of apoptosis.

1.4. Mechanisms Responsible for ζ-Chain Alterations in Cancer

In aggregate, our studies of TIL and PBL obtained from patients with various tumors showed that decreased expression of ζ in T cells was associated with significant functional defects, as manifested by reduced or absent Ca++ flux, decreased tyrosine kinase activity after TCR crosslinking with anti-CD3 Abs, an altered cytokine profile in TAL and TIL that reflected a significant decrease in IL-2 and IFN-γ (type 1 cytokines) at the RNA and protein levels, and by a increased propensity for spontaneous apoptosis (reviewed in ref. *38*). We

Table 2
Associations Between Apoptosis and ζ Expression in PBL and TIL of Patients With Oral Carcinoma[a]

		ζ Expression in PBL		
		Reduced	*Normal*	*Total*
PBL apoptosis	<5%	14	3	17
	≥5%	2	9	11
	Total	16	12	28
		ζ Expression in TIL		
		Reduced	*Normal*	*Total*
TIL apoptosis	None	13	1	14
	Present	5	8	13
	Total	18	9	27

[a]ζ expression in PBL or TIL was measured by immunocytochemical staining and apoptosis by TUNEL staining. Significant associations were observed between reduced ζ expression and apoptosis in PBL ($p = 0.0015$) and in TIL ($p < 0.0019$).

considered the possibility that the tumor induced signaling aberrations in T lymphocytes, because co-incubation of cultured or freshly isolated tumor cells with normal allogeneic or semi-allogeneic PBL-T resulted in a substantial reduction of ζ expression in T cells *(37,39)*. Furthermore, in vitro activated T lymphocytes were found to be highly susceptible to tumor-induced down-regulation of ζ expression. Pre-incubation of T cells with inhibitors of lysosomal or proteasomal peptidase activity prevented degradation of the ζ chain in these lymphocytes upon co-incubation with tumor cells. The results suggested that the tumor induced activation of intracellular peptidases in T cells, leading to enzyme-mediated protein cleavage, which included ζ *(38)*. This interpretation appeared to support findings indicating the presence of normal levels of mRNA for the ζ chain observed in our studies and others in TIL and TAL *(39,42)*. It was also consistent with the possibility that post-translational modifications in signaling molecules are present in these cells. Similar modifications could be induced in normal T cells co-incubated with the tumor *(43)*.

The tumor may contribute to ζ downregulation by secretion of soluble factors, as exemplified by the ζ inhibitory protein (ZIP) recently purified from ascites of women with ovarian carcinoma by Taylor et al. *(42)*. This 14-K_d protein selectively suppressed TCRζ without affecting *lck* or ZAP-70 in normal T cells by interfering with ζ-specific mRNA synthesis. The presence of this inhibitory factor in the sera of women with ovarian carcinoma was associated with a loss of ζ and diminished functional responses of T cells. However, the identity of the factor remains a mystery, as it has only been partially sequenced to date.

In addition to secreting factors that are capable of a direct inhibition of ζ production, the growing tumor is a source of multiple antigens, which are being processed and presented to T cells. Perhaps the simplest explanation for ζ downregulation in T-cells of patients with cancer is the state of chronic antigenic stimulation, which develops as a result of tumor progression. It has been shown that ex vivo T-cell activation by a specific antigen results in a rapid downregulation of CD3ε and ζ, which is followed by a restoration of these molecules on the cell surface in the course of a normal response *(22,44)*. However, when the stimulus is chronic—e.g., TCR is repeatedly triggered by an antigen or antigen-Ab complexes, a long-lasting depression or absence of ζ expression may be a result of its lysosomal degradation, which is not followed by sufficiently rapid recycling to ensure its re-expression. It has been shown that an inhibitor of lysosomal degradation (folimycin) markedly reduces ζ downregulation *(22)*. Thus, it is possible that in diseases characterized by chronic antigenic stimulation—e.g., infections, autoimmune syndromes, and cancer—reduced expression of ζ reflects its extensive utilization and processing without a concomitant recycling of the protein to the cell surface. This process has been referred to as immune "exhaustion."

Another mechanism that has been implicated in downregulation of ζ expression is mediated by reactive oxygen intermediates (ROI) released by activated monocytes or granulocytes in the tumor microenvironment. Kiessling and colleagues reported that tumor-derived or in vitro activated macrophages induced a decrease in ζ expression accompanied by functional impairments in T cells during co-incubation, which was totally abrogated in the presence of catalase, a scavenger of H_2O_2 *(45)*. The mechanism involving activation of granulocytes and oxidative stress mediated by H_2O_2 produced by ganulocytes in the circulation of patients with advanced cancer was described by Schmielau and Finn *(46)*. The sera of these patients contained elevated levels of 8-isoprostane, a product of lipid peroxidation and a marker of oxidative stress *(46)*.

A mechanism that links ζ expression to the availability of L-arginine has been investigated by Ochoa's group *(47,48)*. Jurkat cells cultured in the absence of L-arginine show a selective decrease in ζ expression and decreased proliferation. The effects of L-arginine depletion are mediated at the post-transcriptional level, as it appears that a decreased ζ mRNA half-life is related to the de novo synthesis of a regulatory protein. The process is completely reversed by the restoration of L-arginine *(47)*. There are indications that in the tumor microenvironment, activated macrophages or myeloid suppressor cells (MSC) described in mice *(49)* consume L-arginine in the process of nitric oxide (NO) generation mediated by inducible nitric oxide synthase (iNOS). This molecular pathway bridges the earlier observations of macrophage activation by the tumor with a decrease of ζ in T cells.

The tumor can influence signaling of immune cells in another way. Our studies and others have described the presence of FasL on tumor cells in culture and *in situ (14,16,50)*. TIL at the tumor site and the activated Fas+ T cell co-incubated with tumor cells contain activated caspases and DNA breaks, as demonstrated using (TUNEL) or JAM assays *(39,51)*. We showed earlier that the pan-caspase inhibitors Z-VAD-FMK and Z-DEVD-FMK cause a complete inhibition of apoptosis in T lymphocytes co-incubated with human tumor cells *(14)*. Conversely, a human tumor-cell line genetically modified to secrete FasL-induced apoptosis in activated T cells during a short-term co-incubation *(14,51)*. These apoptotic T cells, or T lymphocytes induced to initiate the apoptotic pathway by Fas-crosslinking Ab (CH-11) in another series of experiments, were characterized by low or absent expression of ζ *(43)*. Thus, both *in situ* and ex vivo experiments indicated that ζ degradation is a part of apoptosis that occurs spontaneously or is induced via the Fas pathway, respectively. Subsequent computer-assisted analysis of the amino acid sequence of the ζ chain showed the presence of sites that were sensitive to cleavage by caspases 3 and 7, confirming that the ζ chain is a suitable substrate for caspase-mediated degradation *(52)*. The conclusion we have drawn from these data suggests that tumor-induced activation of caspases is at least partially responsible for low or absent expression of ζ in T lymphocytes that are present in the tumor.

In light of these findings, the question arises about the identity of the mechanism triggering the apoptotic pathway in T cells of patients with cancer. Although Fas/FasL interactions are clearly implicated, and there is considerable evidence to support this mechanism, as reviewed elsewhere *(50)*, it does not adequately explain the phenomenon of spontaneous apoptosis of T cells seen in the circulation of patients with cancer. Although the great majority of circulating T cells are Fas+, levels of sFasL are not elevated, but rather are decreased in the sera of these patients *(15,17)*. More recently, an explanation has been provided by the discovery that FasL-containing vesicles, which originate from the surface membrane of tumor cells, are present in the sera of patients with ovarian carcinoma, and are able to induce Fas-mediated apoptosis as well as ζ degradation in activated T cells *(53)*. Similar vesicles containing FasL that were able to trigger Fas-dependent apoptosis of lymphocytes were recently described as being produced by melanoma *(54)*. Thus, the receptor (Fas)-initiated /FasL pathway has gained relative importance as the mediator of apoptosis-mediated downregulation of ζ in lymphocytes in cancer patients.

It is important to note that ζ is the target of simian immunodeficiency virus (SIV) Nef, which binds to the ζ chain at two different sites on its cytoplasmic domain *(55)*. The direct interaction of between SIV Nef and TCR ζ leads to downmodulation of the TCR/CD3 complex and to reduced availability of CD3ε for crosslinking with anti-CD3 Ab to induce T-cell proliferation *(55)*. In addition, nef targets two peptides, which represent portions of the first and second of three ITAMs that are essential for signaling via the ζ chain *(55)*.

The fact that many different mechanisms are being proposed to account for low/absent ζ expression emphasizes the importance of this signaling molecule for the integrity of the immune system in host defense. It is very likely that most or all of these mentioned mechanisms operate in the tumor microenvironment. In order to be successful, the tumor must fool or disable the immune system. The redundant attack by several distinct mechanisms at the key signaling molecule responsible for T-cell and natural killer (NK)-cell functions may be one example of how the tumor orchestrates its escape from the immune system.

1.5. Prognostic Importance of the ζ-Chain Expression in Patients With Cancer

Considering the key role ζ plays in TCR signaling, it may be expected that biologic consequences of its low/absent expression are considerable, as reflected in depressed antitumor immunity, poorer prognosis, and shorter overall survival. To address this issue, we performed a retrospective study in which ζ expression was measured in TIL present in biopsies of oral carcinoma obtained from 138 patients who underwent curative surgery and for whom a follow-up of >5 yr was available *(56)*. Absent or low expression of ζ in TIL was detected in 32% of tumors, and was significantly associated with a high tumor stage (T3 or T4) as well as nodal involvement. In oral carcinoma patients with advanced disease, normal expression of ζ in TIL was predictive of significantly better 5-yr survival independent of other established prognostic parameters *(56)*. Thus, expression of ζ was identified as an independent prognostic marker in oral carcinoma. In a more recent study using the same biopsy material, we reported that the number of tumor-infiltrating DCs (TIDCs) is also a highly significant prognostic parameter in patients with oral carcinoma. The absence or paucity of DC was strongly linked to abnormalities in the ζ chain expression in TIL *(57)*. Low density of DC and low or absent expression of ζ in TIL correlated with each other and predicted the poorest survival and the greatest risk in this cohort of patients with oral carcinoma (Fig. 3). These findings strongly suggest that a link exists between ζ expression in T cells accumulating at the tumor site and tumor progression, and that ζ expression in TIL may serve as a biomarker of survival.

Although decreased ζ expression in PBL-T is frequently seen in cancer, as discussed previously, aberrations in ζ are not detected in all patients with cancer, and when present, may be measurable in only a subset of T cells. For this reason, low expression of ζ expression may be missed completely if a small number of patients is studied (*see* ref. *58*). In a study comparing the presence of local (TIL) vs systemic (PBL) signaling defects in lymphocytes of patients

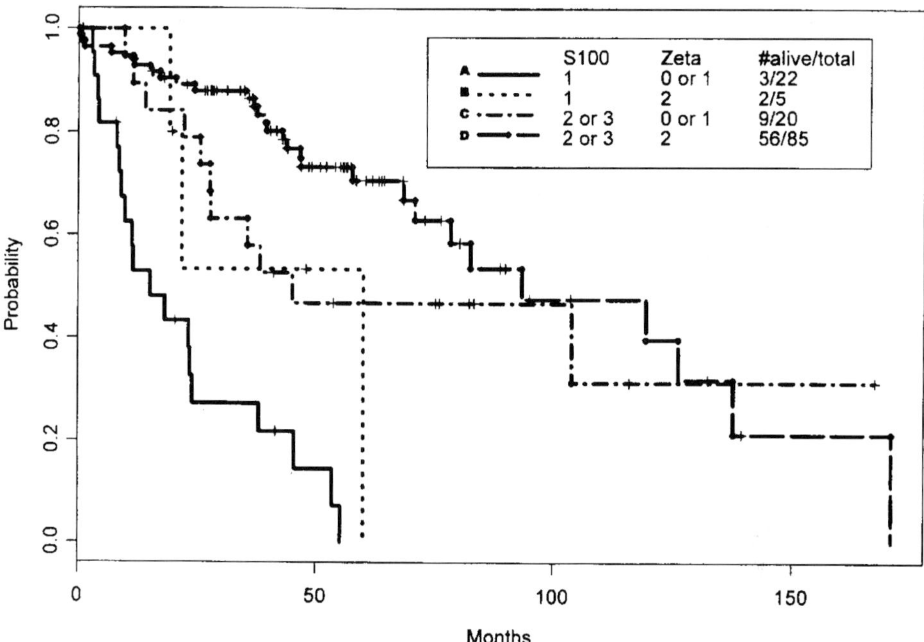

Fig. 3. Survival by S-100 status (S-100 is an antigen expressed on DC, and was used as a "marker" of DC) and ζ (Zeta) expression in TILs ($p = 1 \times 10^{-11}$). The numbers of TIL are described as follows: 1, low numbers of S-100-positive DCs; 2, intermediate numbers of S-100-positive DCs; and 3, high numbers of S-100-positive DCs. TILs are described as follows: 1, lymphocytes with no or low ζ expression; and 2, lymphocytes with normal ζ-chain expression. (Reproduced from ref. *57*.)

with oral carcinoma, we observed that low ζ occurred in a subset of patients, including some that did not have advanced disease *(15)*. Thus, it is important to determine the significance of local vs systemic defects in ζ expression for patients with cancer. It is possible that patients with concomitant local and systemic T-cell dysfunction have a poorer prognosis than those with only local immune dysfunction. Also, the presence of such defects in early stages of disease or in patients with recurrent disease *(36)* may be a poor prognostic sign. Although speculative, these considerations suggest that the presence and degree of immune dysfunction in TIL and PBL may reflect the aggressiveness of the tumor and its ability to induce immune suppression. Low ζ expression in PBL-T has been shown to have significance in regard to survival and prognosis in patients with cancer. Thus, Zea and colleagues observed a marked decrease in ζ expression in PBL-T of 19/44 (43%) patients with metastatic melanoma *(35)*. Importantly, overall survival of melanoma patients with low ζ expression in PBL-T was found to be significantly shorter than that of melanoma patients with normal ζ expression in circulating T cells *(35)*.

In a study including 22 women with cervical carcinoma, 23 with cervical intraepithelial neoplasias (CIN) and 21 normal controls, Kiessling and colleagues observed significant decreases in ζ expression in PBL-T obtained from both patient cohorts relative to controls *(59)*. This signaling impairment also correlated with significantly decreased ability of lymphocytes to produce TNF-α in response to TCR crosslinking by anti-CD3 Ab *(59)*. Furthermore, these aberrations were greater in women with cancer than those with CIN, an indication that they may be related to disease progression *(59)*. The data suggest that both the downregulation of ζ expression and cytokine production become impaired early in the disease progression. The implication of these findings is that ζ expression may be a biomarker of disease progression in those patients who exhibit immune abnormalities early in disease.

Our own cross-sectional studies of patients with HNC indicated that in patients who underwent curative surgery and had no evidence of disease (NED) at the time of blood collection, ζ expression in PBL-T was significantly decreased ($p < 0.0001$) relative to that measured in age- and sex-matched normal controls tested in the same assays as the patients *(36)*. Among these patients, those who had developed new primary tumors or recurrence of the primary disease since surgery had significantly lower ζ than patients who remained NED status. Also, patients with more aggressive types of carcinoma, such as oral carcinoma—which has a poor prognosis compared to laryngeal carcinoma—had markedly depressed ζ in PBL-T *(36)*. Again, these observations suggest that low ζ in PBL-T in patients with HNC may be a marker of aggressive disease with poor prognosis.

In our laboratory, which is strongly committed to the study of apoptosis of PBL-T in cancer, we have repeatedly linked ζ aberrations in T cells to apoptosis in patients with HNC and melanoma *(17,18)*. Our studies indicate that spontaneous apoptosis of T-cell subsets is accompanied by downregulation of ζ and, not surprisingly, that both high apoptosis and low ζ in PBL-T accurately discriminate between patients with cancer and normal controls—although the discrimination between patients with active disease and those with NED has been more difficult to confirm and is under current investigation (ref *18*). Our preliminary observations of preferential apoptosis in CD8+ T cells in patients with cancer *(17)* are of great interest, and they suggest that ζ expression may also be lower in this lymphocyte subset. When ζ expression in T cells of a cohort of patients with prostate carcinoma studied in our laboratory was compared with that found in normal controls, both the percentage of ζ -negative cells and the MFI for ζ were significantly lower for CD3+ T cells of patients vs controls. However, CD4+ T cells unexpectedly showed reduced ζ expression, and CD8+ T cells did not *(60)*. Thus, the relationship between apoptosis and low or absent ζ expression is not straightforward, and requires further investigation. This is underscored by our recent observations that although the subset of CD8+ effector T cells (e.g., CD8+ CD45RO- CD27-) was significantly expanded in the circulation of patients with HNC relative to age-matched controls, these cells were found to have significantly decreased or absent ζ expression ($p < 0.0001$) compared with the same subset of CD8+ cells in controls *(61)*. Despite their expansion in the peripheral compartment, these effector cells had compromised signaling via TCR. Expression of the ζ chain was also found to be depressed in the naïve and memory subsets of CD8+ T cells in these patients *(61)*. The data suggest a complex picture of ζ downregulation in T-cell subsets of patients with cancer, possibly mediated by more than one mechanism, as discussed previously, and certainly are worthy of further examination.

1.6. ζ-chain Expression in Monitoring of Clinical Trials

Preliminary studies suggest that ζ may also be a marker of response to biologic therapy. Using samples of lymphocytes collected immediately before the start of a phase II trial for patients with ovarian carcinoma treated with intraperitoneal interleukin-2 (IL-2), we measured ζ expression in circulating T cells *(62)*. Of 19 patients with ovarian carcinoma who received intraperitoneal IL-2, 9 clinical responders to therapy had normal ζ expression in circulating T cells prior to therapy, yet in 10 non-responders to IL-2, ζ expression was significantly decreased *(62)*. This observation reinforces our initial belief that in patients with cancer, ζ may be a marker of immune competence in individuals most likely to respond favorably to biotherapy, and it emphasizes the need for further studies that will explore this intriguing possibility.

A related question concerns the restoration of ζ expression in circulating T cells following immunopotentiating therapies. Normalization in the level of ζ expression in melanoma TIL cultured in the presence of 1000 IU of IL-2 for 48h has been observed in our laboratory *(63)*. Although this normalization may represent selection in the culture of T cells that are not yet in the apoptotic pathway and thus are able to respond to IL-2 rather than "restoration" of ζ, in vivo effects of IL-2 in patients with cancer suggest that this cytokine can modulate ζ expression. In patients with metastatic melanoma who participated in a multi-institutional phase II study of the combination therapy with IL-2 and histamine dihydrochloride, ζ expression increased significantly in circulating lymphocytes of patients who completed at least two cycles of therapy *(64)*. Also, patients with stable disease following this therapy had a significantly higher percentage of ζ+ CD56+ NK cells than patients with progressive disease *(64)*. These results suggest that modulation of ζ expression may be a correlate of increased immunologic activity of effector cells (T and NK) and, by extension, of an improved clinical status. Others have reported that nonspecific immunotherapy with cytokines or adoptively transferred autologous lymphocytes plus IL-2 results in a recovery of ζ-chain expression in PBL-T of some of the treated patients with cancer *(65–67)*. In contrast, Farace and colleagues, who studied ζ expression in PBL-T obtained from patients with advanced cancers, including RCC, HNC, hepatic colon metastases, and others, reported no evidence for the upregulation of ζ after IL-2 therapy *(68)*. Again, these conflicting results indicate a need for further examination of in vivo effects of IL-2 or other cytokines on ζ expression in the T cells of patients with cancer.

To investigate the possibility that active, specific immunotherapy can normalize ζ-chain expression in the T cells of patients with prostate cancer and lead to improved T-cell functions, we studied a cohort of patients who had received PSA-based vaccines *(60)*. We have previously shown that the administration of a PSA-based vaccine resulted in the generation of PSA-reactive T cells in this cohort of patients, who had surgically incurable prostate cancer *(69)*. We evaluated lymphocytes that were obtained from the same patients prior to and after vaccination, to determine changes in ζ-chain expression in conjunction with monitoring the frequency of prostate-specific antigen (PSA)-reactive T cells in the peripheral circulation and cytokine profiles of the T cells. Our results indicate that in some of these patients, PSA-based vaccination resulted in the restoration of impaired ζ-chain expression and generation of PSA-reactive circulating T cells *(69)*. Figure 4 shows treatment-related changes in ζ expression in T cells of all the patients on this study. After the PSA vaccine, recovery of ζ was observed in 50% of the patients. In this study, no significant correlations could be established between ζ-chain expression before or after therapy and delayed-type hypersensitivity (DTH) responses to PSA or an increase in the frequency of PSA-reactive T cells after therapy and progression-free survival *(69)*. Nevertheless, some interesting insights were obtained. Three patients showed significant upregulation of ζ expression, as well as a substantial increase in PSA-reactive T cells after therapy. All three had strong positive DTH to PSA prior to therapy. The only patient who had a documented partial response to the vaccine was in this subgroup. However, the two patients with progressive disease had relatively normal ζ expression before and after therapy. Of the 15 patients with stable disease, there were eight with progression-free survival (PFS) >20 mo and seven with PFS <20 mo. In the former group, six of eight (75%) showed significant ζ upregulation after vaccination vs three of seven (42%) in the latter. This type of data suggest that ζ expression may have a relationship to clinical responses, and that larger prospective studies should be designed to determine the significance of ζ upregulation after cancer biotherapies.

2. CONCLUSIONS

The loss or decreased expression of the ζ chain in T cells of patients with cancer has been documented in many laboratories. Mechanisms that lead to this phenomenon seem to vary, and to be related to the presence of a tumor or its consequences. Newer, quantitative methods of ζ detection now permit more

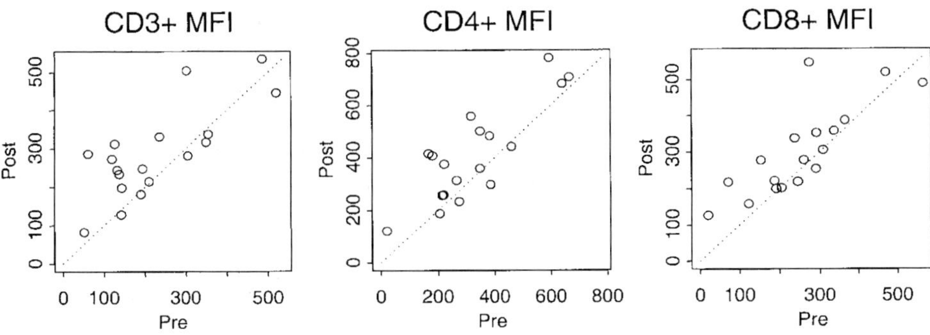

Fig. 4. Treatment-related changes in mean fluorescence intensity (MFI) for ζ chain in subsets of patients with prostate carcinoma treated with PSA-based vaccines. (Reproduced from ref. *60*.)

precise monitoring of changes in ζ expression in lymphocytes. There are indications that monitoring for ζ expression may be useful in the evaluation of immune competence of patients, and following changes in immunocompetence during therapies. Furthermore, ζ is emerging as a clinically relevant signaling molecule, because its expression may be related to prognosis and survival in patients with cancer. Thus far, only preliminary data have linked ζ expression to clinical assessments or prognosis. If ζ-chain expression in PBL-T—a marker of immune function—can be validated and then consistently used for patient monitoring, it may prove to be a promising criterion for stratifying patients for immunotherapy trials as well as a measure of disease progression, and ultimately of survival. Clearly, more work is needed before this signaling molecule can be considered to be a correlate of prognosis or of survival in patients with cancer.

REFERENCES

1. Foley, EJ. Antigenic properties of methylcholanthrene-induced tumors in mice of the strain of origin. *Cancer Res* 1953;13:835–841.
2. Prehn, RT, Main JM. Immunity to methylcholanthrene-induced sarcomas. *J Nat Cancer Inst* 1957;18:769–775.
3. Rosenberg SA, Spiess P, Lafreniere R. A new approach to the adoptive immunotherapy of cancer with tumor-infiltrating lymphocytes. *Science* 1986;233:1318–1321.
4. Yoshizawa H, Chang AE, Shu S. Specific adoptive immunotherapy mediated by tumor-draining lymph node cells sequentially activated with anti-CD3 and IL-2. *J Immunol* 1991; 147:729–737.
5. Rosenberg SA. Progress in human immunology and immunotherapy. *Nature* 2001; 411:380–384.
6. Lee KH, Wang E, Nielsen MB, et al. Increased vaccine-specific T-cell frequency after peptide-based vaccination correlates with increased susceptibility to in vitro stimulation but does not lead to tumor regression. *J Immunol* 1999;163:6292–6300.

7. Parmiani G, Castelli C, Dalerba P, Mortarini R, et al. Cancer immunotherapy with peptide-based vaccines: what have we achieved? Where are we going? *JNCI* 2002;94:805–818.
8. Hoffman TK, Donnenberg AD, Finkelstein SD, Donnenberg VS, Friebe-Hoffman F, Myers EN, et al. Frequencies of tetramer+ T cells specific for the wild-type sequence $p53_{264-272}$ peptide in the circulations of patients with head and neck cancer. *Cancer Res* 2002;62:3521–3529.
9. Letsch A, Keilholz U, Schadendorf D, et al. High frequencies of circulating melanoma-reactive CD8+ T cells in patients with advanced melanoma. *Int J Cancer* 2000;87: 659–664.
10. Whiteside TL (1993) *Tumor-Infiltrating Lymphocytes in Human Solid Tumors*. R.G. Landes, Austin, TX.
11. Whiteside TL, Parmiani G. Tumor-infiltrating lymphocytes: their phenotype, function and clinical use. *Cancer Immunol Immunother* 1994;39:15–21.
12. Whiteside, TL, Rabinowich H. The role of Fas/FasL in immunosuppression induced by human tumors. *Cancer Immunol Immunother* 1998;46:175–184.
13. Uzzo RG, Clark PE, Rayman P, et al. Alterations in NFκB activation in T lymphocytes of patients with renal cell carcinoma. *JNCI* 1999;91:718–721.
14. Gastman BR, Atarashi Y, Reichert TE, Saito T, Balkir L, Rabinowich H, et al. Fas ligand is expressed on human squamous cell carcinomas of the head and neck and it promotes apoptosis of T lymphocytes. *Cancer Res* 1999;59:5356–5364.
15. Reichert TE, Strauss L, Wagner EM, Gooding W, Whiteside TL. Signaling abnormalities and reduced proliferation of circulating and tumor-infiltrating lymphocytes in patients with oral carcinoma. *Clin Cancer Res* 2002;8:3137–3145.
16. O'Connell J, O'Sullivan GD, Collins, JK, et al. The Fas counterattack: Fas-mediated T cell killing by colon cancer cells expressing Fas ligand. *J Exp Med* 1996;184:1075–1082.
17. Hoffmann TK, Dworacki G, Meidenbauer N, Gooding W, Johnson JT, Whiteside TL. Spontaneous apoptosis of circulating T lymphocytes in patients with head and neck cancer and its clinical importance. *Clin Cancer Res* 2002;8:2553–2562.
18. Whiteside TL. Apoptosis of immune cells in the tumor microenvironment and peripheral circulation of patients with cancer: implications for immunotherapy. *Vaccine* 2002; 20:A46–A51.
19. Kuss I, Ferris RL, Gooding W, Whiteside TL. Lymphocyte subsets in patients with head and neck cancer. Submitted, 2003.
20. Hellerstein M, Hanley MB, Cesar D, Siler S, et al. Directly measured kinetics of circulating T lymphocytes in normal and HIV1-infected humans. *Nat Med* 1999;5:83–89.
21. Kersh EN, Shaw AS, Allen PM. Fidelity of T cell activation through multistep T cell receptor ζ phosphorylation. *Science* 1998;281:572–575.
22. Valitutti S, Muller S, Salio M, Lanzavecchia A. Degradation of T cell receptor (TCR)-CD3-ζ complexes after antigenic stimulation. *J Exp Med* 1997;185:1859–1864.
23. Stefanova I, Saville MW, Peters C, Cleghorn FR, Schwartz D, Venzon DF, et al. HIV infection-induced posttranslational modification of T cell signaling molecules associated with disease progression. *J Clin Investig* 1996;98:1290–1297.
24. Zea AH, Ochoa MT, Ghosh P, Longo DL, Alvord WG, Valderrama L, et al. Changes in expression of signal transduction proteins in T lymphocytes of patients with leprosy. *Infect Immun* 1998;66:499–504.
25. Liossis SN, Ding XZ, Dennis GJ, Tsokos GC. Altered pattern of TCR/CD3-mediated protein-tyrosylphosphorylation in T cells from patients with systemic lupus erythematosus. Deficient expression of the T cell receptor zeta chain. *J Clin Investig* 1998;101: 1448–1457.
26. Loeffler CM, Smyth MJ, Longo DL, Kopp WC, Harvery LK, Tribble HR, et al. Immunoregulation in cancer-bearing hosts. Down-regulation of gene expression and cytotoxic function in CD8+ T cells. *J Immunol* 1992;149:949–956.

27. Mizogushi H, O'Shea JJ, Longo DL, Loeffler CM, McVicar DW, Ochoa AC. Alteration in signal transduction molecules in T lymphocytes from tumor-bearing mice. *Science* 1992;258:1975–1978.
28. Lai P, Rabinowich H, Crowley-Nowick PA, Bell MC, Mantovani G, Whiteside TL. Alterations in expression and function of signal-transducing proteins in tumor-associated T and natural killer cells in patients with ovarian carcinoma. *Clin Cancer Res* 1996; 2:161–173.
29. Finke JH, Zea AH, Stanley J, Longo DL, Mizoguchi H, Tubbs RR, et al. Loss of T-cell receptor chain and p56^{lck} in T-cells infiltrating human renal cell carcinoma. *Cancer Res* 1993;53:5613–5616.
30. Nakagomi H, Petersson M, Magnusson I, Juhlin C, Matsuda M, Mellstedt H, et al. Decreased expression of the signal-transducing ζ chains in tumor-infiltrating T-cells and NK cells of patients with colorectal carcinoma. *Cancer Res* 1993;53:5610–5612.
31. Matsuda M, Petersson M, Lenke R, Taupin J-L, Magnusson I, Mellstedt H, et al. Alterations in the signal-transducing molecules of T cells and NK cells in colorectal tumor-infiltrating, gut mucosal and peripheral lymphocytes: correlation with the stage of the disease. *Int J Cancer* 1995;61:765–772.
32. Healy CG, Simons JW, Carducci MA, DeWeese TL, Bartkowski M, Tong KP, et al. Impaired expression and function of signal-transducing zeta chains in peripheral T cells and natural killer cells in patients with prostate cancer. *Cytometry* 1998;32:109–119.
33. Levey DL, Srivastava PK. T cells from late tumor-bearing mice express normal levels of p56^{lck}, p59^{fyn}, ZAP-70, and CD3ζ despite suppressed cytolytic activity. *J Exp Med* 1995;182:1029–1036.
34. Aoe T, Okamoto Y, Saito T. Activated macrophages induce structural abnormalities of the T cell receptor-CD3 complex. *J Exp Med* 1995;181:1881–1886.
35. Zea AH, Brendan CD, Longo DL, Alvord WG, Strobl SL, Mizoguchi H, et al. Alterations in T cell receptor and signal transduction molecules in melanoma patients. *Clin Cancer Res* 1995;1:1327–1335.
36. Kuss I, Saito T, Johnson JT, Whiteside TL. Clinical significance of decreased ζ chain expression in peripheral blood lymphocytes of patients with head and neck cancer. *Clin Cancer Res* 1999;5:329–334.
37. Rabinowich H, Reichert TE, Kashii Y, Bell MC, Whiteside TL. Lymphocyte apoptosis induced by Fas ligand-expressing ovarian carcinoma cells: implications for altered expression of TcR in tumor-associated lymphocytes. *J Clin Investig* 1988;101:2579–2588.
38. Whiteside TL. Signaling defects in T lymphocytes of patients with malignancy. Symposium-in-writing. *Cancer Immunol Immunother* 1999;48:346–352.
39. Reichert TE, Rabinowich H, Johnson JT, Whiteside TL. Immune cells in the tumor microenvironment: mechanisms responsible for signaling and functional defects. *J Immunother* 1998;21:295–306.
40. Rabinowich H, Suminami Y, Reichert TE, Crowley-Nowick P, Bell M, Edwards R, et al. Expression of cytokine genes or proteins and signaling molecules in lymphocytes associated with human ovarian carcinoma. *Int J Cancer* 1996;68:276–284.
41. Asselin-Paturel C, Echchakin H, Carayol G, Gay F, Opolon P, Grunenwald D, et al. Quantitative analysis of Th1, Th2 and TGF-β 1 cytokine expression in tumor, TIL and PBL of non-small lung cancer patients. *Int J Cancer* 1998;77:7–12.
42. Taylor DD, Bender DP, el-Taylor GEI, Stanson J, Whiteside, TL. Modulation of TcR/CD3-zeta chain expression by a circulating factor derived from ovarian cancer patients. *Br J Cancer* 2001;84:1624–1629.
43. Dworacki G, Meidenbauer N, Kuss I, Hoffmann TK, Gooding MS, Lotze M, et al. Decrease ζ chain expression and apoptosis in CD3+ peripheral blood T lymphocytes of patient with melanoma. *Clin Cancer Res* 2001;7:947–957.

44. Krishnan S, Warke VG, Nambiar MP, Wong HK, Tsokos GC, Farber DL. Generation and biochemical analysis of human effector CD4 T cells: alterations in tyrosine phosphorylation and loss of CD3 ζ expression. *Blood* 2001;15:3851–3859.
45. Kono K, Salazar-Onfray F, Petersson M, Hansson J, Masucci G, Wasserman K, et al. Hydrogen peroxide secreted by tumor-derived macrophages down-modulates signal-transducing ζ molecules and inhibits tumor-specific T cell- and natural killer cell-mediated cytoxicity. *Eur J Immunol* 1996;26:1308–1313.
46. Schmielau J, Finn OJ. Activated granulocytes and granulocyte-derived hydrogen peroxide are the underlying mechanism of suppression of T-cell function in advanced cancer patients. *Cancer Res* 2001;61:4756–4760.
47. Taheri F, Ochoa JB, Faghiri Z, Culotta K, Park HJ, Lan MS, et al. L-Arginine regulates the expression of the T-cell receptor zeta chain (CD3zeta) in Jurkat cells. *Clin Cancer Res* 2001;7:958s–965s.
48. Rodriguez PC, Zea AH, Culotta KS, Zabaleta J, Ochoa JB, Ochoa AC. Regulation of T cell receptor CD3zeta chain expression by L-arginine. *J Biol Chem* 2002;277: 21,123–21,129.
49. Mazzoni A, Bronte V, Visintin A, Spitzer JH, Apolloni E, Serafini P, et al. Myeloid suppressor lines inhibit T cell responses by an NO-dependent mechanism. *J Immunol* 2002;168:689–695.
50. Whiteside TL. Tumor-induced death of immune cells: its mechanisms and consequences. *Sem Cancer Biol* 2002;12:43–50.
51. Atarashi Y, Kanaya H, Whiteside TL. A modified JAM assay detects apoptosis induced in activated lymphocytes by FasL+ human adherent tumor cells. *J Immunol Methods* 1999;233:179–182.
52. Gastman BR, Johnson DE, Whiteside TL, Rabinowich J. Caspase-mediated degradation of TcR-ζ chain. *Cancer Res.* 1999;59:1422–1427.
53. Taylor DD, Gercel-Taylor C, Lyons KS, Stanson J, Whiteside TL. T-cell apoptosis and suppression of TcR/CD3-ζ by FasL-containing membrane vesicles shed from ovarian tumors. Submitted, 2002.
54. Andreola G, Rivoltini L, Castelli C, Huber V, et al. Induction of lymphocyte apoptosis by tumor cell secretion of FasL-bearing microvesicles. *J Exp Med* 2002;195:1303–1316.
55. Schaeffer TM, Bell I, Fallert BA, Reinhart TA. The T-cell receptor ζ contains two homologous domains with which similar immunodeficiency virus Nef interacts and mediates down-modulation. *J Virol* 2000;74:3273–3283.
56. Reichert TE, Day R, Wagner EM, Whiteside TL. Absent of low expression of the ζ chain in T cells at the tumor site correlates with poor survival in patients with oral carcinoma. *Cancer Res* 1998;58:5344–5347.
57. Reichert TE, Scheuer C, Day R, Wagner W, Whiteside TL. The number of intratumoral dendritic cells and ζ-chain expression in T cells as prognostic and survival biomarkers in patients with oral carcinoma. *Cancer* 2000;91:2136–2147.
58. Cardi G, Heaney JA, Schned AR, Phillips DM, Branda MT, Ernstoff MS. T-cell receptor ζ-chain expression on tumor-infiltrating lymphocytes from renal cell carcinoma. *Cancer Res* 1997;57:3517–3519.
59. Kono K, Ressing ME, Brandt RMP, Melief CJM, Potkul RK, Andersson B, et al. Decreased expression of signal-transducing ζ chain in peripheral T cells and natural killer cells in patients with cervical cancer. *Clin Cancer Res* 1996;2:1825–1828.
60. Meidenbauer N, Gooding W, Spliter L, Harris D, Whiteside TL. Recovery of ζ chain expression and changes in spontaneous IL-10 production after PSA-based vaccines in patients with prostate cancer. *Br J Cancer* 2002;86:168–178.
61. Kuss I, Donnenberg A, Gooding W, Whiteside TL. Effector CD8+CD45RO-CD27- T cells have signaling defects in patients with head and neck cancer. *Br J Cancer* 2003;88:223–230.

62. Kuss I, Rabinowich H, Gooding W, Edwards R, Whiteside TL. Expression of ζ in T cells prior to IL-2 therapy as a predictor of response and survival in patients with ovarian carcinoma. *Cancer Biother Radiopharm* 2002;17:631–640.
63. Rabinowich H, Banks M, Reichert TE, Logan TF, Kirkwood JM, Whiteside TL. Expression and activity of signaling molecules in T lymphocytes obtained from patients with metastatic melanoma before and after interleukin 2 therapy. *Clin Cancer Res* 1996;2: 1263–1272.
64. Whiteside TL, Gooding W, Elder E, Stover L, Glaspy J, McMasters K, et al. Immunomodulatory effects of combination therapy with histamine dihydrochloride and interleukin-2 during a phase II study in stage IV melanoma. Abstract. 17th Annual Scientific Meeting of the Society for Biological Therapy, La Jolla, CA, November, 2002.
65. Bukowski RM, Rayman P, Uzzo R, Bloom T, Sandstrom K, Peereboom D, et al. Signal transduction abnormalities in T lymphocytes from patients with advanced renal carcinoma: clinical relevance and effects of cytokine therapy. *Clin Cancer Res* 1998;4:2337–2347.
66. Gratama JW, Zea AH, Bolhuis RL, Ochoa AC. Restoration of expression of signal-transduction molecules in lymphocytes from patients with metastatic renal cell cancer after combination immunotherapy. *Cancer Immunol Immunother* 1999;48:263–269.
67. Tartour E, Latour S, Mathiot C, Thiounn N, Mosser V, Joyeux I, et al. Variable expression of CD3-ζ chain in tumor-infiltrating lymphocytes (TIL) derived from renal-cell carcinoma: relationship with TIL phenotype and function. *Int J Cancer* 1995;63:505–212.
68. Farace F, Angevin E, Vanderplancke J, Escudier B, Triebel F. The decreased expression of CD3 ζ chains in cancer patients is not reversed by IL-2 administration. *Int J Cancer* 1994;59:752–755.
69. Meidenbauer N, Harris DT, Spitler LE, Whiteside TL. Generation of PSA-reactive effector cells after vaccination with a PSA-based vaccine in patients with prostate cancer. *The Prostate* 2002;43:88–100.

15 Allogeneic Hematopoietic Blood-Cell Transplantation As Immunotherapy for Metastatic Renal Cell Carcinoma

Richard W. Childs, MD,
and Cristian A. Carvallo, MD

CONTENTS

1. INTRODUCTION

Once metastatic, the prognosis of patients with metastatic renal cell carcinoma (RCC) is extremely poor. Chemotherapy is usually ineffective, and radiotherapy is typically reserved for palliative purposes. Although most would

From: *Current Clinical Oncology: Cancer Immunotherapy at the Crossroads: How Tumors Evade Immunity and What Can Be Done*
Edited by: J. H. Finke and R. M. Bukowski © Humana Press Inc., Totowa, NJ

consider RCC to be an "immunoresponsive" solid tumor, the vast majority of patients treated with systemic immunomodulators fail to manifest a disease response. Nevertheless, kidney cancer remains one of the few solid tumors to manifest evidence of intrinsic vulnerability to immune attack. As a result, considerable efforts have been made to develop methods to direct the immune system against RCC, including treatment with cytokines (e.g., interleukin [IL]-2, IL-12, interferons), the adoptive infusion tumor-infiltrating lymphocytes (TIL) or lymphocytes activated by cytokines (lymphokine-activated killer cells [LAK]) and tumor vaccine-based approaches. More recently, investigators have begun to pursue an alternative immune-based strategy in patients who fail to respond to conventional cytokines—namely, immune enhancement via total immune replacement following "low-intensity" nonmyeloablative allogeneic stem-cell transplantation (NST). NST has recently been shown to produce potent immune-mediated antitumor responses against a variety of chemotherapy-refractory hematologic malignancies, and has been associated with lower morbidity and mortality rates than conventional "mega-dose" myeloablative regimens. Because RCC may be regulated by the immune system, testing allogeneic-based immunotherapy in this malignancy seemed logical. Pilot allogeneic transplant trials were initiated based on the hypothesis that graft-vs-tumor (GVT) effects, analogous to the graft-vs-leukemia (GVL) effect seen in hematological malignancies, might be generated against RCC following the transplantation of allogeneic lymphocytes from healthy human leukocyte antigen (HLA) matched siblings. The recent observation of regression of metastatic RCC following NST has provided proof of concept of the susceptibility of RCC to allogeneic immune attack. In this chapter, we discuss some of the intricacies of GVT and NST for cancer, and highlight the results of pilot trials that have applied allogeneic immunotherapy to patients with treatment-refractory metastatic kidney cancer.

2. THE FAILURE OF CONVENTIONAL CHEMOTHERAPY FOR TREATMENT OF RCC

Renal cell carcinoma remains a significant contributor to worldwide cancer mortality. In the United States, approx 30,000 new cases of RCC are diagnosed yearly *(1,2)*. At initial diagnosis, nearly 25% of patients with RCC will have metastatic disease, and an additional 25% will go on to develop metastatic disease despite apparent localized disease at time of therapy *(4)*. The long-term prognosis is abysmal once disease becomes metastatic with median survival of 1 yr or less and only a 1–2% survival at 5 yr *(5)*.

Conventional chemotherapy and radiotherapy for treatment of locally advanced and metastatic disease has been largely unsuccessful. Despite in vitro activity, Vinblastine and fluorouracil have response rates of 4% or less, and do not appear to provide a survival advantage *(6)*. Although responses to gemcitabine given alone or in combination with fluorouracil or cytokines have recently been described, complete responses have rarely been observed *(7,8)*. The failure of such cytotoxic therapy to improve survival has provided at least some of the motivation to explore alternative therapeutic approaches, including immunotherapy-based regimens for patients with metastatic RCC.

3. RATIONALE FOR IMMUNOTHERAPY

The peculiar natural history of RCC, with its occasional prolonged periods of stable disease, has perplexed investigators for decades. The first spontaneous regression of metastatic RCC after nephrectomy was first described in the late 1920s, and was attributed to an antibody-mediated immune response *(9)*. Since then, nearly 100 cases of spontaneous regression of metastatic RCC have been reported in the literature *(10)*. Evenson and Cole observed that RCC has the highest incidence of this phenomenon among all solid tumors *(11)*. The frequency of spontaneous regression is estimated to be 0.3% *(10–12)*, but in a randomized study comparing recombinant IFN-γ to placebo, a 6.6% objective response rate was noted in the placebo arm, suggesting a higher rate of spontaneous regression than had been previously reported *(13)*. The immune system has been hypothesized to be responsible for the disease regression observed in the absence of systemic treatment. The existence of spontaneous regression of metastatic tumors has been proposed to be one of the rationales for the utilization of immunologic approaches in the treatment of RCC.

The presence of TILs in kidney-cancer lesions that are lytic to tumor cells in vitro and the identification of tumor-associated antigens (TAA) on renal cancer cells all further support the notion that immune-based therapies for RCC are worthy of exploration *(14,15)*.

However, variables exist that significantly limit the ability to enhance autologous immunity against RCC. Indeed, recent observations suggest the presence of immune dysregulation and T-lymphocyte dysfunction in RCC patients. T-cell receptor (TCR) abnormalities, abnormal NF-κB activation, and enhanced apoptosis of T lymphocytes, both in peripheral blood and in the tumor, have been noted *(16–18)*. Allogeneic blood-cell transplantation thus could potentially provide a more potent immune system than the patient's own depressed immunity. However, even with complete immune replacement, tumors might still have mechanisms to avoid immune attack, including the induction of T-lymphocyte apoptosis mediated through the Fas/Fas-ligand-receptor system. Indeed, it was recently observed that RCC tumor cells expressing Fas-L could induce apoptosis in activated T cells from RCC patients *(18)*.

4. CYTOKINE THERAPY FOR METASTATIC RCC

Since the recognition of its immunologic responsiveness, immunotherapy for RCC has undergone a significant evolution since its inception more than two decades ago. The first attempts were aimed at reinforcing the immune system through the administration of cytokines such as IL-2, interferon-α (IFN-α), interferon-γ (IFN-γ), or various combinations with or without LAK or TIL.

IFN-α and IL-2 induce tumor regression in 10–15% of patients with metastatic disease. Responses appear to occur most frequently in patients with pulmonary metastasis and a good performance status *(19,20)*. Median response duration is 6–10 mo; however, durable complete responses have occasionally been seen *(20)*.

IL-2 remains the only US Food and Drug Administration-approved treatment for metastatic RCC. Controversy exists as to its best route of administration (high vs low dose), method of infusion (bolus vs continuous), and synergy with other cytokines such as IFN-α or LAK/TIL. A recent review of single-agent IL-2 administered to more than 1900 patients in a series of phase I and II clinical trials demonstrated an overall response rate of 15%, with complete responses in 3–5% of patients *(21,22)*.

Preclinical data suggested possible synergistic effects when IL-2 and IFN-α were combined *(23)*. A recent review of results of combination therapy from a series of phase I and II trials including more than 1400 patients demonstrated response rates of approx 20%, with complete responses in 5% of patients *(21)*. Negrier et al. published their results of the largest randomized trial comparing cytokine monotherapy vs combination therapy with IL-2 and IFN-α *(24)*. Although the overall response rates and event-free survival in patients who received combination therapy were statistically superior when compared to monotherapy with either agent, no improvement in survival was demonstrated.

It is clear from these studies that a subset of patients with metastatic RCC respond favorably to cytokine-based therapy. Unfortunately, the vast majority of patients with metastatic kidney cancer fail to benefit from conventional interferon/IL-2-based regimens. The poor results of the cytokine-based trials and the recent observation of disease responses seen following dendritic cell (DC)-based tumor vaccination strategies has provided at least some of the motivation for investigators to pursue new immune-based investigational approaches such as allogeneic transplantation *(21,25)*.

5. ALLOGENEIC TRANSPLANTATION: CONVENTIONAL "HIGH-DOSE" TREATMENT

Allogeneic bone-marrow transplantation offers many patients with chemotherapy-resistant leukemia the only chance for cure. More than 35 yr have passed since allogeneic stem-cell transplantation (SCT) was first applied as a treatment modality for cancer. Unfortunately, the toxicity associated with the procedure may at times be severe and even life-threatening. Despite a number of recent clinical advances, complications leading to mortality following fully myeloablative "high-dose" regimens remains in the range of 25–35%. It was previously believed that in order for an allogeneic transplant to be effective, "mega-dose" conditioning (chemotherapy with or without total body irradiation [TBI]) was required to eradicate all neoplastic cells. As a result of such intensive chemo/radiotherapy, the recipient's bone marrow and immune system are also eradicated. The allogeneic hematopoietic-cell allograft is infused intravenously following chemotherapy from a HLA-matched donor consisting of hematopoietic stem cells (typically procured from the donor's blood by an apheresis procedure following granulocyte-colony-stimulating factor [G-CSF]-mobilization). The allograft serves as a new source of bone-marrow stem cells, rescuing the patient from marrow aplasia and replacing the patient's immune system with donor natural killer (NK), B, and T cells that were eradicated by the conditioning regimen. Patients are usually placed on immunosuppressive agents such as cyclosporin (CSA) or tacrolimus for 6–12 mo following the procedure to prevent the engrafted donor immune cells from attacking normal host tissues such as the GI tract, liver, or skin, a process referred to as graft-vs-host disease (GVHD). GVHD ranges from mild and self-limiting to severe and life-threatening, and occurs in 15–50% of patients following the procedure. Toxicities directly related to the "mega-dose" conditioning regimen and acute GVHD are the major contributors to transplant-related morbidity and mortality (TRM) following conventional allogeneic transplant. Despite these limitations, myeloablative SCT has been shown to be capable of curing patients with a variety of relapsed hematological malignancies that would otherwise be uniformly fatal.

6. IMMUNE EFFECTS AGAINST CANCER FOLLOWING ALLOGENEIC TRANSPLANTATION

Although hypothesized from its inception, it was not until about 20 yr ago that investigators began to appreciate the anti-neoplastic effects that were generated by donor immune cells following allogeneic SCT. The observation that intensive conditioning regimens frequently failed to eradicate all leukemic cells in patients that were ultimately cured by SCT, and the association of a decreased risk of leukemia relapse in patients with a history of GVHD gave rise to the appreciation of the donor immune-mediated anti-malignancy effect known as GVL or the GVT effect. Evidence now exists that the GVL effect is the critical component required to cure hematological malignancies after an allotransplant *(26)* (Table 1). About 15 yr ago, it was demonstrated that donor

Table 1
Evidence to Support the Existence of a Donor Immune-Mediated GVT Effect Following Allogeneic Blood or Marrow Transplantation

Relapse rate lower after transplant in patients with acute and/or chronic GVHD
Relapse rate higher in patients receiving a transplant depleted of donor T cells
Relapse rate higher when syngeneic (identical) twin used as marrow donor
Remission of leukemia following DLI in patients with relapsed disease after transplantation

lymphocyte infusions in the absence of any cytoreductive chemotherapy could induce complete and durable remissions in patients with leukemia who relapsed after allogeneic bone-marrow transplantation *(27)*. Results such as these showing the GVT effect to be a potent and effective form of immunotherapy for hematologic malignancies *(28–31)* brought into question the need for toxic "high-dose" myeloablative conditioning regimens. Reduced-intensity conditioning regimens were subsequently tested as a less toxic alternative to the traditional myeloablative SCT *(32,33)*. These low-intensity or NST were designed to provide sufficient immunosuppression to allow engraftment of the donor immune system while minimizing toxicities associated with high-dose conditioning. NST relies on the GVT effect to eradicate cancer rather than dose-intensive conditioning agents. Clinical results utilizing NST in the treatment of hematologic malignancies have demonstrate that such regimens are generally well-tolerated, have a decreased incidence of TRM, and result in high levels of donor immune-system engraftment sufficient to achieve sustained remissions in some hematologic diseases *(34–38)*. Key principles related to NST are summarized in Table 2.

7. APPLYING ALLOGENEIC IMMUNOTHERAPY TO KIDNEY CANCER

The high risk of death associated with traditional myeloablative SCT has deterred investigators from applying this form of therapy to non-hematological malignancies. The lower risk of TRM associated with NST allotransplants now provides investigators with a method to more safely evaluate whether GVT effects may be generated against incurable solid tumors. Immunologic replacement with a healthy donor immune system following an allotransplant seems to be a potentially attractive approach, considering the observation of a systemic immunosuppressed state in patients with metastatic RCC *(39–41)*.

The transplant scheme currently used by the National Institutes of Health (NIH) to treat patients with cytokine-refractory RCC is shown in Fig. 1. Patients

Table 2
NST: Principles

Conditioning Regimen	
Lower intensity of conditioning compared to conventional myeloablative transplant	
Better toxicity profile	
Immunosuppression from conditioning will allow donor immune engraftment	
Mixed chimerism	
May induce tolerance to normal host tissues as well as tumor and prevent a GVT effect	
Withdrawal of cyclosporine or infusion of donor lymphocytes may covert to full donor chimerism	
Allogeneic (donor) T cells	
Capable of inducing immune responses against:	-Normal tissues (GVHD) -Recipient bone-marrow cells -Tumor cells (GVT)

receive a low-intensity conditioning regimen of cyclophosphamide (120 mg/kg) and fludarabine (125 mg/m^2) followed by the infusion of a G-CSF mobilized blood hematopoietic-cell allograft collected from an HLA-identical sibling that is transfused intravenously on transplant d 0. CSA and low-dose methotrexate are given in the post-transplant period to prevent acute GVHD. Peripheral blood is collected at multiple intervals after transplantation to determine, the percentage of donor engraftment in the T-lymphocyte and myeloid lineages, using a polymerase chain reaction (PCR)-based analysis of microsatellites that are polymorphic between the patient and donor. Patients with mixed T-cell chimerism (both patient and donor cells detectable) are tapered off CSA rapidly, and may receive transfusions of donor lymphocytes (DLI) in an attempt to enhance an immune effect. In contrast, patients with early full-donor T-cell chimerism are at higher risk of having acute GVHD, and are tapered off their CSA more slowly. The rate and degree of engraftment of the donor immune system varies among patients, and is facilitated by factors such as prior exposure to chemotherapy and the dose of CD34+ hematopoietic progenitor cells infused in the allograft *(42)*. Because many patients with metastatic RCC patients have not received pre-transplant chemotherapy, engraftment of the donor hematopoietic system is delayed compared to patients with hematologic malignancies who are undergoing the same procedure.

Although allogeneic SCT remains an investigational approach for the treatment of metastatic RCC, evidence for susceptibility of this tumor to a GVT effect has recently been described by several groups (*43–47*; Table 3).

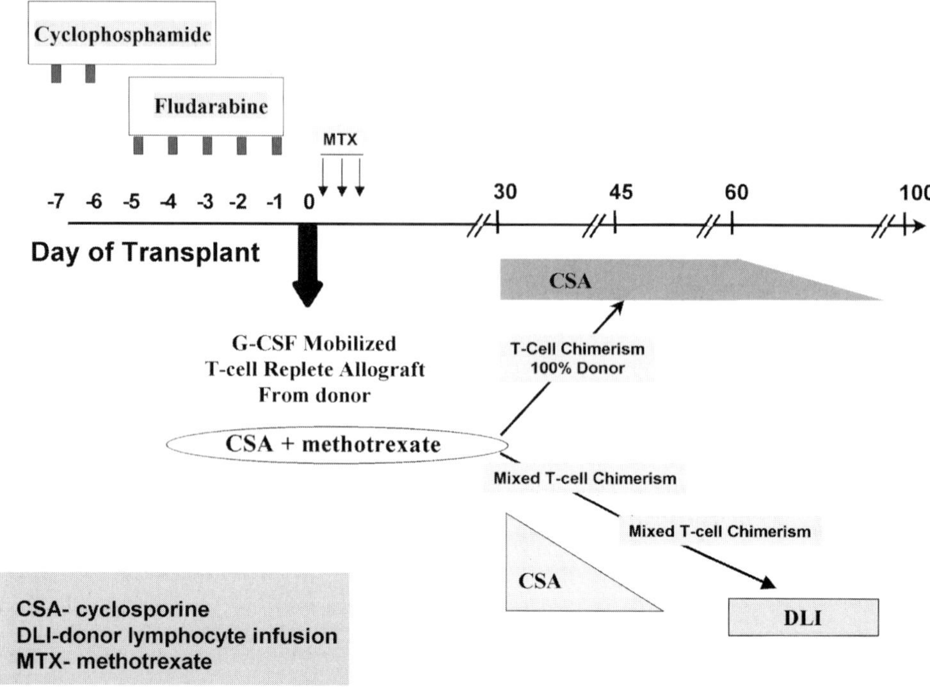

Fig. 1. The nonmyeloablative allogeneic blood SCT scheme currently utilized at the National Institutes of Health (NIH) to treat patients with cytokine-refractory RCC. Decisions regarding how rapidly CSA is tapered are dictated by the rate of donor T-cell engraftment and disease status.

Although results vary among transplant regimens, all have been reported to be well-tolerated.

Ten of the first 19 patients treated at the NIH with this approach had radiographic evidence of disease regression, including three complete responders and seven partial responses. Two patients died from complication of transplant-related events. More recently, a total of 58 patients have been treated, and 23 patients (40%) had radiographic evidence of disease regression consistent with a GVT effect. The first patient to achieve a complete response remains in remission 5 yr after transplantation. Although regression of metastasis has been observed in multiple locations, pulmonary responses have been observed most frequently (Fig. 2). Regression of metastatic disease typically does not occur until 4–8 mo following the transplant, and often follows tumor growth that occurred in the first few months following the procedure. As has been observed with hematological malignancies, regression of RCC may be delayed until T-cell chimerism

Table 3
Published Experience of Allogeneic Transplantation for Metastatic RCC

Investigator	*Conditioning regimens*	*GVHD prophylaxis*	*Other*
Childs et al. *(43)*	Cyclophosphamide 120 mg/kg Fludarabine 125 mg/m^2	Cyclosporine	Regression of RCC in 10/19 patients. High incidence of GVHD
Rini et al. *(44)*	Cyclophosphamide 2 g/m^2 Fludarabine 90 mg/m^2	FK 506 and MMF	4/9 engrafted patients had a GVT effect
Bregni et al. *(47)*	Thiotepa 10 mg/kg Fludarabine Cyclophosphamide	Cyclosporine + Methotrexate	Delayed disease regression observed in 4/7 treated patients
Pedrazzoli *(45)*	Cyclophosphamide 60 mg/kg Fludarabine 120 mg/m^2	Cyclosporine + Methotrexate	No responses in 7 patients. Patients had advanced disease and died early after transplant

has become predominantly donor and after CSA tapering. Furthermore, a prior history of acute GVHD has been favorably associated with achieving a disease response. Transplant-related events, as well as the engraftment kinetics and their relationship to clinical outcome in patients with RCC following cyclophosphamide/fludarabine-based conditioning, are shown in Fig. 3.

Rini and colleagues recently published their experience with NST in the treatment of metastatic RCC. Because of an unacceptably high rate of graft rejection (3/4 patients), their conditioning regimen was subsequently "dose-intensified." Overall, 4 of 9 patients (44%) who engrafted had radiographic evidence of a partial response. Acute and chronic GVHD occurred in two and six patients respectively, with a 30% incidence of transplant-related mortality.

Bregni and colleagues recently reported the results of their allogeneic transplant regimen, which used thiotepa, fludarabine, and cyclophosphamide with CSA and methotrexate for GVHD prophylaxis. Four of seven RCC patients had partial regression of metastatic disease. The regimen was reported to be well-tolerated, with a low incidence of acute GVHD *(47)*. Pedrazzoli and colleagues also recently published their experience of reduced-intensity transplantation in seven patients with cytokine-refractory RCC conditioned with 120 mg/m^2 of fludarabine and 60 mg/kg of cyclophosphamide *(45)*. Following treatment with

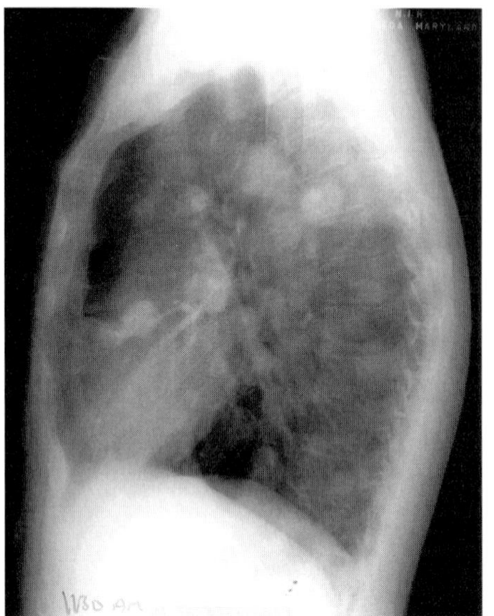
Pre-transplant chest X-RAY
RCC with extensive lung metastasis

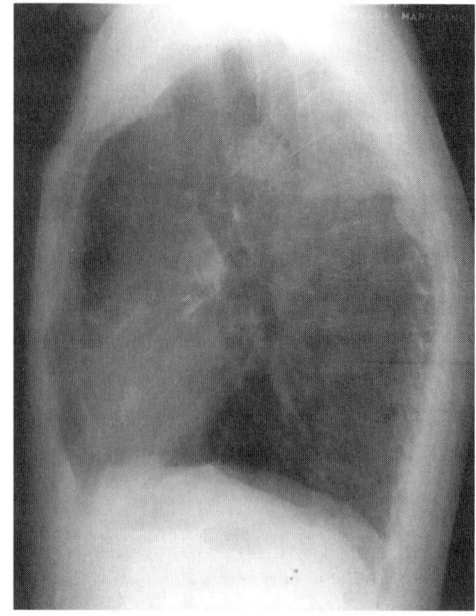
Complete regression of all lung metastasis
8 months after allogeneic transplantation

Fig. 2. Regression of multiple pulmonary metastases in a patient with IL-2-refractory RCC (clear-cell type) following a nonmyeloablative transplant.

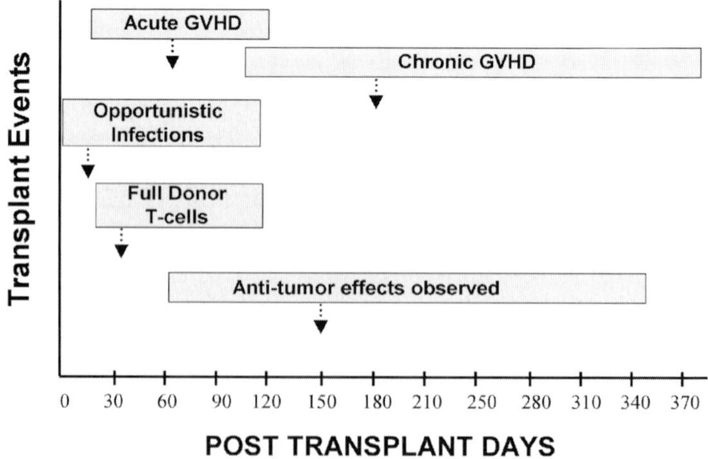

Fig. 3. Timeline of events observed after nonmyeloablative transplantation.

this regimen, they observed that complete donor chimerism was only achieved in patients with a history of more intensive prior chemotherapy treatment. None of their RCC patients achieved full-donor chimerism, and all seven died from rapid disease progression shortly after the transplant.

Table 4
Factors That Currently Limit Allogeneic Transplant for Patients With Metastatic RCC

Toxicity	*Incidence (%)*
Acute GVHD	40–60
Chronic GVHD	30–60
CMV reactivation	20–40
Graft rejection	5–10
Regimen-related morality	10–20

Responses not observed until months after the transplant. Patients with rapidly progressive unlikely to survive long enough to see benefit. Need for an HLA-matched sibling.

Table 5
Candidates for NST

Failed cytokine therapy
Progressive metastatic disease
Expected survival >6 mo
No CNS involvement
No hypercalcemia
HLA-compatible sibling

8. TOXICITY AND OTHER RISKS OF ALLOGENEIC IMMUNOTHERAPY

Although early evidence supports the susceptibility of RCC to allogeneic lymphocytes, transplant-related toxicity and other factors currently limit a broader application of this approach (Table 4). Although most patients can be expected to tolerate the conditioning regimen well, the risk of dying as a result of a transplant-related event runs in the range of 10–30%. Complications related to acute GVHD and infections are the two greatest contributors to TRM. Because some patients who receive IL-2 and IFN may achieve a durable complete response (albeit a low percentage), most investigators have reserved this procedure for patients with progressive metastatic disease who have failed conventional cytokine-based immunotherapy (Table 5). Also, given the substantial lag time of 4–8 mo between transplantation and the induction of a GVT effect, patients with rapidly progressing disease or poor performance status should be precluded from this form of therapy. When feasible, surgical debulking of the tumor in select patients may be used as a method to prolong survival to allow time for a GVT effect to occur.

Sound clinical judgment of the patient's prior clinical course, tumor-growth kinetics, and anticipated survival must be factored into the decision to treat patients with this form of therapy. Finally, in order to decrease the risk of fatal GVHD, most centers that investigate NST have required patients to have an HLA-matched sibling to serve as an allograft donor. This limits the application of this procedure to only 25–30% of patients with metastatic RCC. Whether NST can be performed safely and effectively in patients using HLA-matched unrelated donors is only now being investigated *(46)*.

9. MECHANISMS OF GVT RESPONSE TO ALLOGENEIC IMMUNOTHERAPY IN METASTATIC RCC

The observation that disease regression is associated with GVHD, is delayed in onset, and does not occur until CSA has been tapered in the setting of full donor T-cell chimerism strongly implicates the donor immune system as mediating tumor regression Recently, our studies and others have isolated cytotoxic CD8+ T-cell populations that kill RCC cells in vitro from the peripheral blood of patients obtained after transplant during periods of disease regression *(48–50)*. In vitro studies show that many of these T-cell populations kill patient tumor cells and patient hematopoietic cells, strongly implicating minor histocompatibility antigens—disparate between the patient and the donor—as a potential target for a GVT effect. However, disease regression observed in the absence of acute GVHD as well as the isolation of a number of donor T-cell clones with a tumor-restricted cytotoxicity pattern (expanded from a responding patient) also suggest that tumor-specific immune effects may be generated against RCC in some patients after allogeneic transplantation. It is also possible that RCC cells may be more susceptible to allogeneic NK cells than autologous NK cells as a result of mismatching between NK-cell killer Ig-like inhibitory receptors (KIR) and their inactivating ligands *(51)*. Further studies to delineate the exact cells that mediate GVT effects in RCC, as well as characterization of their target antigens, might lead to more efficacious regimens in the future that "tailor" the donor immune system to the patient's tumor.

10. CONCLUSION AND FUTURE DIRECTIONS

The low efficacy of chemotherapeutics, radiotherapy, and conventional cytokine-based immunotherapy has catalyzed enthusiasm for investigating NST as a novel form of immunotherapy in patients with metastatic RCC. The observation that cytokine-refractory metastatic RCC may sometimes regress following allogeneic transplantation has provided proof of concept that attests to the powerful nature of the GVT effect. Although toxicity remains a major limiting factor, early pilot trials have provided preliminary clinical data that clinically meaningful regression of a metastatic RCC may occur in some patients who follow this approach. Further advances in methods to prevent opportunistic infections and acute GVHD, as well as methods to target the allogeneic immune system to the tumor, will hopefully improve the safety and efficacy of this promising investigational therapy.

REFERENCES

1. Landis SH, Murray T, Bolden S, Wingo PA. Cancer statistics. *CA Cancer J Clin* 1999;49:8–31.
2. Chow WH, Devesa SS Warren JL, Fraumeni JFJ. Rising incidence of renal cell cancer in the United States. *JAMA* 1999;281:1628–1631.
3. Motzer RJ, Bander NH, Nanus DM. Renal cell carcinoma. *NEJM* 1996;335:856.
4. Lokich J, Harrison, JH. Renal cell carcinoma: natural history and chemotherapeutic experience. *J Urol* 1975;114–371.
5. Linehan WM, Shipley WU, Parkinson DR. (1993) Cancer of the kidney and ureter In *Cancer: Principles and Practice of Oncology,* fourth ed. (Devita VT Jr., ed.) JB Lippincott, Philadelphia, PA, 1993, pp.
6. Yagoda A, Petrylak D, Thompson S. Cytotoxic chemotherapy for advanced renal cell carcinoma *Urol Clin North Am* 1993;20:303–314.
7. Rini BI, Vogelzang NJ, Dumas MC, Wade JL 3rd, Taber DA, Stadler WM. Phase II trial of weekly intravenous gemcitabine with continuous infusion fluorouracil in patients with metastatic renal cell cancer. *J Clin Oncol* 2000;(12):2419–2426 .
8. Ryan CW, Vogelzang NJ, Stadler WM. A phase II trial of intravenous gemcitabine and 5-fluorouracil with subcutaneous interleukin-2 and interferon-alpha in patients with metastatic renal cell carcinoma. *Cancer* 2002;15;94(10):2602–2609.
9. Bumpus HC. The apparent disappearance of pulmonary metastasis in a case of hypernephroma following nephrectomy. *J Urol* 1928;20:185–191.
10. Fairlamb DJ. Spontaneous regression of metastatic renal cell cancer. *Cancer* 1981;47:2102–2106.
11. Evanson TC, Cole WH (1996) *Spontaneous Regression of Cancer*. WB Saunders, Philadelphia, PA, pp. 11–87.
12. Bloom HJG (1972) Renal cancer. In *Endocrine therapy of Malignant Disease*. WB Saunders, Philadelphia, PA, pp. 339–367.
13. Gleave ME, Elhilali M, Fredet Y, et al. Interferon gamma-1b compared with placebo in metastatic renal cell carcinoma. *N Engl J Med* 1998;338:1265–1271.
14. Finke JH, Rayman P, Hart L, et al. Characterization of TIL subsets from human renal cell carcinoma: specific reactivity defined by cytotoxicity, INF-γ secretion and proliferation. *J Immunother* 1994;15:91–104.
15. Gaugler B Brownvenstijn N, Vantomme V, et al. A new gene coding for an antigen recognized by autologous cytolytic T- Lymphocytes on human renal cell carcinoma. *Immunogenetics* 1996;44:323–330.
16. Finke JH, Zea AH, Stanley J, et al. Loss of T-cell receptor Zeta chain and p56lck in T-cells infiltrating human renal cell carcinoma. *Cancer Res* 1993;53:5613–5616.
17. Li X, Liu J, Park JK, et al. T cells from renal cell carcinoma patients exhibit an abnormal pattern of Kappa B-specific DNA binding activity: a preliminary report. *Cancer Res* 1994;54:5424–5429.
18. Uzzo RG, Rayman P, Bloom T. Mechanisms of apoptosis in T-cells from patients with renal cell carcinoma. *Clin Cancer Res* 1999;5:1219–1229.
19. Bukowski RM, Novick AC. Clinical practice guidelines: Renal cell carcinoma. *Cleve Clin J Med* 1997;64(Suppl 1):1–48.

20. Minisian LM, Motzer RJ, Gluck L, et al. Interferon alpha 2-a in advanced remal cell carcinoma: Treatment results and survival in 159 patients with long term follow-up. *J Clin Oncol* 1993;11:1368–1375.
21. Bukowski RM. Natural history and therapy of metastatic renal cell carcinoma: the role of interleukin-2. *Cancer* 1997;80:1198–1220.
22. Bukowski RM, Dutcher JP (2000) Low dose interleukin-2. In *Genitourinary Oncology* (Vogelzang NJ, Scardino PT, Shipley WW, eds), Lippincott Williams & Williams, Philadelphia, PA. pp. 218–233.
23. Chikkala NF, Lewis I, Ulchaker J, et al. Interactive effects of alpha-interferon A/D and interleukin-2 on murine lyphokine-activated killer activity: analysis at the effector and precursor level. *Cancer Res* 1990;50:1176–1182.
24. Negrier S, Escudier B, Lasser C, et al. Recombinant human interleukin-2, recombinant interferon-alpha-2a, or both in metastatic renal cell carcinoma. *N Engl J Med* 1998; 338:1272–1278.
25. Marten A, Flieger D, Renoth S, Weineck S, Albers P, Compes M, et al. Therapeutic vaccination against metastatic renal cell carcinoma by autologous dendritic cells: preclinical results and outcome of a first clinical phase I/II trial. *Cancer Immunol Immunother* 200251(11–12):637-644 .
26. Horowitz M, Gale RP, Sondel P, et al. Graft-versus-leukemia reactions after bone marrow transplantation. *Blood* 1991;78:2120–2130.
27. Kolb HJ, Mittermueller J, Clemm C, et al. Donor leukocyte transfusions for treatment of recurrent chronic myelogenous leukemia in marrow transplant patients. *Blood* 1990; 76:2462–2465
28. van Besien KW, de Lima M, Giralt SA, et al. Management of lymphoma recurrence after allogeneic transplantation: the relevance of graft-versus-lymphoma effect. *Bone Marrow Transplant* 1997;19:977–982.
29. Verdonck L, Lokhorst H, Dekker A, et al. Graft-versus-myeloma effect in 2 cases. *Lancet* 1996;347:800–801.
30. Eibl B, Schwaighofer H, Nachbaur D, et al. Evidence of a graft-versus-tumor effect in a patient treated with marrow ablative chemotherapy and allogeneic bone marrow transplantation for breast cancer. *Blood* 1996;88:1501–1508.
31. Ueno NT, Rondon G, Mirza NQ, et al. Allogeneic peripheral-blood progenitor-cell transplantation for poor-risk patients with metastatic breast cancer. *J Clin Oncol* 1998; 16:986–993.
32. Giralt S, Estey E, Albitar M, et al. Engraftment of allogeneic hematopoietic progenitor cells with purine analog-containing chemotherapy: harnessing graft-versus-leukemia without myeloablative therapy. *Blood* 1997;89:4531–4536.
33. Slavin S, Nagler A, Naparastak E, et al. Nonmyeloablative stem cell transplantation and cell therapy as an alternative to conventional bone marrow transplantation with lethal cytoreduction for the treatment of malignant and non malignant hematologic diseases. *Blood* 1998;91:756–763.
34. Khouri IF, Saliba RM, Giralt SA, Lee MS, Okoroji GJ, Hagemeister FB, et al. Nonablative allogeneic hematopoietic transplantation as adoptive immunotherapy for indolent lymphoma: low incidence of toxicity, acute graft-versus-host disease, and treatment-related mortality. *Blood* 2001;98(13):3595–3599.
35. Sykes M, Preffer F, McAfee S, et al. Mixed lymphohaemopoietic chimerism and graft-versus-lymphoma effects after non-myeloablative therapy and HLA mismatched bone-marrow transplantation. *Lancet* 1999;353:1755–1759.
36. Childs R, Clave E, Contentin N, et al. Engraftment kinetics after nonmyeloablative allogeneic peripheral blood stem cell transplantation: full donor T-cell chimerism preceded alloimmune responses. *Blood* 1999;94:3234–3241.

37. McSweeney PA, Niederwieser D, Shizuru JA, Sandmaier BM, Molina AJ, Maloney DG, et al. Hematopoietic cell transplantation in older patients with hematologic malignancies: replacing high-dose cytotoxic therapy with graft-versus-tumor effects. *Blood* 2001; 97(11):3390–3400.
38. Bornhauser M, Thiede C, Schuler U, et al. Dose-reduced conditioning for allogeneic blood stem cell transplantation: durable engraftment without antithymocyte globulin. *Bone Marrow Transplant* 2000;26(2):119–125.
39. Finke JH, Zea AH, Stanley J, et al. Loss of T-cell receptor zeta chain and p56lck in T-cells infiltrating human renal cell carcinoma. *Cancer Res* 1993;53:5613–5616.
40. Li X, Liu J, Park JK, et al. T cells from renal cell carcinoma patients exhibit an abnormal pattern of kappa B-specific DNA binding activity: a preliminary report. *Cancer Res* 1994; 54:5424–5429.
41. Uzzo RG, Rayman P, Bloom T. Mechanisms of apoptosis in T-cells from patients with renal cell carcinoma. *Clin Cancer Res* 1999;5:1219–1229.
42. Carvallo C, Kurlander R, Geller N, Griffith L, Linehan WM, Childs R. Prior chemotherapy facilitates donor engraftment following nonmyeloablative allogeneic stem cell transplantation. *Blood* 2002;100(11):620a.
43. Childs R, Chernoff A, Contentin N, et al. Regression of metastatic renal-cell carcinoma after nonmyeloablative allogeneic peripheral-blood stem-cell transplantation. *N Engl J Med* 2000;343:750–758.
44. Rini B, Zimmerman TM, Stadler W, et al. Allogeneic stem-cell transplantation of Renal Cell Cancer after nonmyeloablative chemotherapy: feasibility, engraftment, and clinical results. *J Clin Onc* 2002;20(8): 2017–2024.
45. Pedrazzoli P, Da Prada G, Giorgiani G, et al. Allogeneic blood stem cell transplantation after reduced intensity, preparative regimen—a pilot study in patients with refractory malignancies. *Cancer* 2002;94(9);2409–2416.
46. Appelbaum FR, Sandmaier B. Sensitivity of renal cell cancer to nonmyeloablative allogeneic hematopoietic cell transplantations: unusual or unusually important? *J Clin Oncol* 2002 20(8):1965–1967.
47. Bregni M, Dodero A, Peccatori J, et al. Nonmyeloablative conditioning followed by hematopoietic cell allografting and donor lymphocyte infusions for patients with metastatic renal and breast cancer. *Blood* 2002;99(11):4234–4236.
48. Mena O, Igarashi T, Srinivasan R, et al. Immunologic mechanisms involved in the graft versus tumor effect in renal cell carcinoma (RCC) following nonmyeloablative allogeneic peripheral blood stem cell transplantation. *Blood* 2001;98:356a.
49. Childs RW, Mena OJ, Tykodi S, Riddell S, Warren E. Minor histocompatibility antigens (mHa) are expressed on renal cell carcinoma (RCC) cells and are potential targets for a graft-vs-tumor effect (GVT) following allogeneic blood stem cell transplantation (SCT). *Proceedings of the American Society of Clinical Oncology* 2002;21:433a.
50. Warren EH, Tykodi SS, Murata M, et al. T-cell therapy targeting minor histocompatibility Ags for the treatment of leukemia and renal-cell carcinoma. *Cytotherapy* 2002: 4(5);441–442.
51. Igarashi T, Srinivasan R, Wynberg J, Takahashi Y, Becknel B, Caligiuri M, et al. Generation of allogeneic NK cells cytotoxic to melanoma and renal cell carcinoma based on killer immunoglobulin-like receptor (KIR)-ligand incompatibility. *Blood* 2002;100(11):620a.

16 Immune Defects in Patients Suffering From Non-Hodgkin's Lymphoma

Thomas Zander, MD, *Daniel Re*, MD,
Michael von Bergwelt-Baildon, MD, PhD,
Jürgen Wolf, MD,
and *Joachim L. Schultze*, MD

Contents

1. INTRODUCTION

Therapeutic efforts to activate the immune system as a treatment for cancer were started more than 100 yr ago *(1,2)*. However, the concept of immunosurveillance of cancer was only introduced in 1967 by Burnet *(3)*. The importance of immunosurveillance appears to be most obvious in malignancies of the immune system itself. In the first part of this chapter, we describe clinical examples that support this concept. First, the introduction of immunosuppressive agents and the spread of human immunodeficiency virus (HIV) gave rise to an increasing incidence of lymphoma in these patients, providing special insight into lymphomagenesis. Second, chronic stimulation of the immune

From: *Current Clinical Oncology: Cancer Immunotherapy at the Crossroads: How Tumors Evade Immunity and What Can Be Done*
Edited by: J. H. Finke and R. M. Bukowski © Humana Press Inc., Totowa, NJ

system, as present in chronic *Helicobacter pylori*-positive (HP) gastritis, is associated with an increased incidence of lymphoma development. In the second part of this chapter, we explore the specific interactions between lymphoma cells and the various cellular players of the immune system. An understanding of this interaction will lead to the third part of this chapter, in which we describe efforts made to manipulate the immune system in order to mount a clinically relevant antitumor immune response.

1.1. Suppression of the Immune System as a Risk Factor for Lymphoma Development: Findings in Organ Transplant Recipients and AIDS Patients

The extensive use of immunosuppressive agents—especially in the field of transplantation and for autoimmune diseases—and the spread of HIV has given rise to an increasing incidence of lymphoma in these immunosuppressed patients. In HIV patients, a 60–100-fold higher incidence of non-Hodgkin's lymphoma (NHL) has been observed, which increases dramatically as immune function declines *(4–6)*. Similarly, in patients with post-organ transplantation and subsequent immunosuppressive treatment, a 30–50-fold increase in lymphoma incidence has been documented *(7)*. Even in patients with rheumatoid arthritis or inflammatory bowl disease after low-dose immunosuppression *(8,9)* or patients with rare congenital immunodeficiencies (e.g., Ataxia teleangiectatica, Wiskott-Aldrich syndrome, common variable immunodeficiency) *(10)* an, increased risk of lymphoma development is apparent. Lymphomas that develop in these patients share some common features, as they tend to present in extranodal sites, are of B-cell origin, and are associated with the presence of Epstein-Barr virus (EBV). Whereas reduction of immunosuppressive agents prevents lymphoma development in organ-transplant patients *(7)*, the introduction of highly active antiretroviral therapy) (HAART) in the treatment of HIV was not followed by a strong reduction in lymphoma development, probably because of the additional pathogenetic effects of the virus itself *(11)*. One possible mechanism is chronic B-cell stimulation, which was shown to be a risk factor for lymphoma development in HIV patients *(12)*.

1.2. Chronic Immune Stimulation As a Risk Factor for Lymphoma Development: **Helicobacter pylori** *in MALT-Lymphoma*

Lymphoma arising from the mucosa-associated lymphoid tissue (MALT) comprises about 8% of NHL were first described in 1983. Several lines of evidence suggest a pathogenetic role of *Helicobacter pylori* in MALT-lymphoma. MALT lymphoma develops in the gastric mucosa, where lymphocytes are not normally present. Only the preceding *H. pylori* infection acquires the MALT. In the early stage MALT lymphoma, *H. pylori* can be found in nearly all specimens *(13)* with a decreasing incidence as the lymphoma evolves from chronic gastritis to high-grade lymphomas *(14)*. Pathologic findings further support the interaction between the immune system and the pathogen. Individual gastric glands are invaded by lymphoma cells that form lymphoepithelial lesions, and a plasma-cell differentiation as well as transformed B-cell blasts are found in the tumor, resembling germinal centers *(14)*. The individual B-cell clone that causes MALT lymphoma is regularly found in HP gastritis specimens several years before the lymphoma develops *(15)*. In vitro MALT lymphoma cells are stimulated by *H. pylori* specific T-cells in the presence of the pathogen. Finally, the eradication of HP by antibiotics results in regression of MALT lymphoma in up to 75% of cases *(13)*. These data support the hypothesis that HP may lead to a chronic antigenic stimulation of B cells during gastritis preceding MALT lymphoma, and that *H. pylori* may also provide the antigenic stimulus that sustains lymphoma growth. Nevertheless, many patients with HP gastritis do not develop lymphoma, and it is widely accepted that further transforming events play a role in gastric lymphoma—e.g., translocations involving Bcl-10 or cIAP2 have been described in MALT lymphoma, and may be involved in the transforming events *(16)*. Recently, HCV has been associated with the development of splenic lymphoma with villous lymphocytes by inducing chronic B-cell proliferation, finally resulting in B-cell lymphoma. Similar to MALT lymphoma, splenic lymphomas are also derived from the marginal zone of lymphatic follicles. Interestingly, a complete remission is obtained by eliminating hepatitis C virus (HCV) in these patients *(17)*.

1.3. Clinical Findings in Lymphoma-Bearing Patients Demonstrate the Immunosuppressive Action of the Malignant Cells

As studies have shown, a balanced immune system is crucial for the prevention of lymphoma development, but the lymphoma cells themselves have the ability to modulate the function of the immune system. Patients who suffer from multiple myeloma, for example, are typically at risk for bacterial infections *(18–20)*. Furthermore, they have a disturbed ability to mount primary antibody responses, and show an inadequate humoral response to secondary antigen challenge in the setting of vaccination against standard pathogens such as pneumococcus or influenza *(21,22)*. This impaired humoral immune response has been known for many years and is caused not by a lack of specific B cells, but by an extrinsic inhibition of antigen-specific B cells. This finding has been associated with an increased number of immunoregulatory CD5+ B cells, which can be found in the spleen even prior to clinical manifestation of the disease *(23,24)*. Pilarski and colleagues have shown that the number of specific B cells for recall antigens such as tetanus toxoid are not reduced in these patients, but the ability to secret antigen-specific antibodies or to differentiate into antibody-secreting B cells is severely impaired. This is further highlighted by the increased number of pre-B cells found in circulation of multiple myeloma patients and a decreased absolute number of B cells *(25)*.

An inhibitory influence of lymphoma cells on the immune system is also reflected by the detection of soluble immune-inhibitory factors in the serum of lymphoma patients. Interleukin (IL)-10, a cytokine known to inhibit Th1 responses, has been established as a prognostic factor in lymphoma patients *(26)*. Moreover, serum levels of transforming growth factor β (TGF-β) in lymphoma patients were shown to correlate with immunoparesis (determined by the amount of polyclonal immunoglobulins in the serum) in multiple myeloma *(27)*. Adhesion molecules such as soluble intracellular adhesion molecules (sICAM) are also shown to be elevated in lymphoma patients. It has been suggested that sICAM may bind to its receptor and inhibit binding of cells to the ICAM receptor, thereby inhibiting important functions of the immune system *(28)*.

2. VARIOUS BRANCHES OF THE IMMUNE SYSTEM AFFECTED IN LYMPHOMA PATIENTS

2.1. Impairment of the T-Cell Function

Several mechanisms responsible for the inability of tumor-infiltrating T cells (TIL) to eliminate lymphoma cells have been described, including ignorance, anergy/tolerance, and systemic immune inhibition (Fig. 1). It is most likely that all these mechanisms may interact and play a role at different time-points during lymphomagenesis and for different lymphoma subtypes. Ignorance is characterized by the presence of tumor antigen-specific T cells in vivo without immune activation, despite the presence of the particular tumor antigen. These specific T cells are naïve, and can easily be activated in vitro by optimal antigen presentation. Ignorance may be a particular mechanism of tolerance or may be seen independently. A classical definition of tolerance is the inability of the whole antigen-specific T-cell repertoire to mount an effective immune response to an antigenic challenge. In vivo tolerance is achieved by deletion of antigen-specific T cells (e.g., systemic tolerance) or induction of anergy (a mechanism of peripheral tolerance) in a specific T-cell clone. Downregulation of the entire immune system by the lymphoma is defined as immune inhibition *(29)*.

B-cell NHL are invaded by CD4+ and CD8+ T cells that are believed to have antitumor activity. CD4+ as well as CD8+ cells are mainly of memory type (80% CD45RO+), and are found with a CD4/CD8 ratio ranging between 0.17 and 13 *(30)*. Although about 13% of these T cells express the activation marker

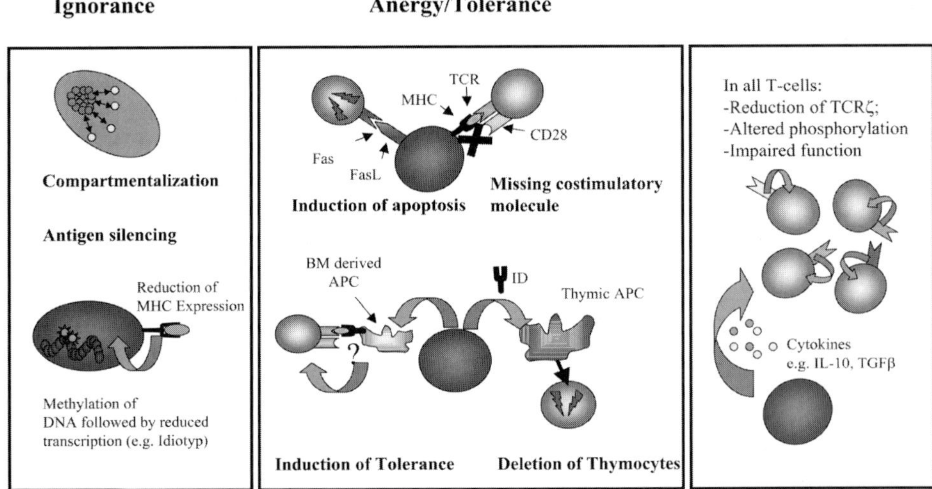

Fig. 1. Different mechanisms lead to an impaired T-cell antitumor response.

CD25 and 38% of the cells are HLA-DR positive *(31–33)*, tumor cells are not eliminated. Although these TIL recognize NHL cells in a major histocompatibility complex (MHC)-restricted manner *(34,35)* they show functional impairment in vitro *(36)*. Reduction of TCRζ expression observed in many tumors as well as in follicular lymphoma *(29)* and the hypophosphorylation of downstream kinases may explain this functional impairment *(37)*. Cytotoxicity of activated T cells is mediated by two systems: first, the release of perforin and granzymes, and second, the interaction of Fas with its ligand (FasL) *(38)*. T cells that infiltrate follicular lymphoma show no or a very weak expression of granzymeB and perforin *(29)*. Furthermore, B-cell lymphoma cells protect themselves against perforin and granzymeB-mediated apoptosis by expressing the serine protease inhibitor PI9 *(39)*. Fas ligand is expressed not only on tumor-infiltrating T cells, but also on the lymphoma cell itself, thereby inducing apoptosis of tumor-infiltrating T cells *(40,41)*.

Ignorance has been shown to be one reason for an impaired antitumor immune response in several tumor entities *(42–44)*. Antigen silencing has been described as a mechanism for ignorance. Using the murine lymphoma model EL4, it was demonstrated that despite the expression of several different CTL epitopes, only one epitope was recognized by T cells, and the other epitopes were silenced *(45)*. Reduced expression of the MHC is another possibility of antigen silencing *(46–49)*. For B-cell lymphoma, the idiotype can serve as tumor antigen, but is silenced in several entities by methylation of the promotor regions as yet another mechanism *(47,50)*. Compartmentalization within the secondary lymphoid organs has also been suggested as a possible mechanism of ignorance. For non-malignant B-cells, this tight regulation of B-cell trafficking has been clearly shown *(51–54)*. Further studies are needed to provide evidence for compartmentalization of lymphoma cells in vivo.

Tolerance in vivo against tumor antigens was demonstrated in several lymphoma models. In the spontaneous B cell lymphoma model of transgenic mice that express human HOX11 in B lymphocytes, Rosic-Kablar and colleagues demonstrated an antigen-specific tolerance of host T cells against lymphoma cells. Because the immune response against non-tumor-related antigens was not diminished, a general immune suppression was excluded *(55)*. The induction of this antigen-specific tolerance was shown to be an early event in the development of lymphoma *(56)*, and bone marrow-derived antigen-presenting cells (APC) play a key role in this process *(57)*. Reduction of costimulatory molecules is a key element in the induction of tolerance *(58–63)*. Induction of peripheral tolerance caused by T-cell deletion was directly demonstrated in a murine TCR-transgenic plasmocytoma model. Furthermore, deletion of T cells correlated with tumor burden *(64)*. This deletion of antigen-specific T cells may be mediated by Fas-FasL interactions between the tumor cells and T cells *(65)*, or centrally in the thymus by still unknown mechanisms *(66,67)*. Until recently, it was still unclear in the human whether an innate defect in the T-cell repertoire may account for an impaired tumor-specific immune response or whether the tumor itself inhibits the immune system. Assuming that the T-cell repertoire of monozygotic twins shows no major difference, we recently showed that inhibitory mechanisms during tumor growth—rather than a defective T-cell repertoire—are responsible for the impaired T-cell response in lymphoma *(68)*.

It is now well-documented that during the progression of disease, lymphoma induces a general immune suppression, which is phenotypically associated in T cells by downregulation of TCRζ (69) and functionally by a decreased response to recall antigens in vivo and in vitro. As shown in a murine plasmocytoma model, soluble factors account for general immune inhibition *(70)*. Cytokines such as TGF-β and IL-10, which are expressed by malignant B cells *(29,71,72)* and exert a direct or indirect suppressive effect on T cells *(73–76)*, may partially explain this immune inhibition.

Together, numerous mechanisms can contribute to the impaired host-immune response against lymphoma. In some lymphoma entities, tumor-infiltrating T cells even promote tumor growth. In MALT lymphoma malignant B cells grow in vitro only when stimulated by autologous tumor-infiltrating T cells. Interestingly, these T-cells are stimulated by *H. pylori*, the pathogen leading to MALT lymphoma *(77–78)*. An intense interaction of these mainly Th2 cells with the malignant B-cells in low-grade gastric MALT lymphoma via

CD40/CD40L, IL-4, and IL-10 was demonstrated to be responsible for the promotion of lymphoma growth *(79)*.

2.2. Impaired Humoral Immune Responses in Lymphoma Patients

Antibodies are an important part of the humoral immune response, and can in principle inhibit tumor growth via binding of complement (complement-mediated lysis) or via activation of natural killer (NK) cells or macrophages (antibody-dependent cell-mediated cytotoxicity). Furthermore, using the SEREX (serological analysis of autologous tumor antigens by recombinant cDNA cloning) method, natural antitumor antibodies have been detected in a variety of cancer patients including lymphoma patients *(80)*. However, the biological importance of these naturally occurring antibodies for protection against cancer is unclear. In contrast, humoral dysfunction secondary to lymphoma development is better understood. In chronic lymphocytic leukemia and multiple myeloma, hypogammaglobulinemia is associated with infectious complications in these patients. In particular, the quantitative loss of immunglobulin function, low mucosal IgM, and IgA and low-serum IgG subclasses may explain the occurrence of recurrent bacterial and herpesvirus infections *(81)*. In summary, impaired humoral dysfunction reflects a dysfunction of clonal and nonclonal B lymphocytes in lymphoma patients that is secondary to tumor progression.

2.3. Role of Professional APC in Antitumor Immunity

Although the role of APC in tumor-bearing hosts has not yet been extensively studied initial findings indicate an alteration in number and function: dendritic cells (DC) isolated from prostate cancer fail to show signs of increased recruitment and activation *(82)*. Similarly, DC in renal cell carcinoma display the same phenotype as DC from adjacent normal tissue and CD1a+ DC from transitional cell carcinoma show no signs of activation *(83)*. Gabrilovich showed that APC function of DC was reduced in breast cancer, yet patient T cells responded normally to mitogenic stimuli or DC from healthy donors *(84)*, and older studies indicate that DC frequencies correlate with prognosis *(85,86)*. Tumors secrete IL-10, TGF-β, and vascular endothelial growth factor (VEGF) that have been demonstrated to alter DC function *(87–88)*. The differentiation status of the DC also seems to be of importance since mature, murine blood-derived DC are impaired in their capacity to induce antitumor T-cell responses and marrow-derived DC are fully functional *(89)*. Few studies have investigated APC in lymphoma, and have focused mainly on morphology that demonstrate an altered network of follicular denritic cells (FDC) *(90–93)*. Ongoing efforts by our own group are currently addressing whether the function of such professional APC in lymphoma is altered.

2.4. Defects in the Innate Immune System: The Role of NK Cells in the Host Defense Against Lymphoma

In recent years, the role of several cell-surface receptors for the activation and inhibition of NK cell activity has been elucidated. The fate of NK-cell activity is ultimately regulated by the interaction of MHC class I and class I-like molecules on NK target cells and NK receptors such as killer-cell immunoglobulin-like receptors (KIR), C-type lectins, and natural cytotoxicity receptors (NCR). A number of other NK-cell (co)receptors such as CD40 ligand or CD69 are known, but the importance for NK-cell activity and the interaction with the previously mentioned receptors has not been described in detail *(94)*. In general, one of the major immunological functions of NK cells is to identify and destroy autologous cells that have altered or lost their self-MHC class-I molecules. It therefore may be theorized, that NK cells may play a role in host defense against MHC class-I-deficient tumor cells that are found, for example, in EBV-positive post-transplantation lymphoproliferative diseases. However, the precise role of NK cells in lymphoma is still not understood.

3. STRATEGIES TO OVERCOME IMMUNE DEFECTS IN LYMPHOMA PATIENTS AND ELICIT AN ANTITUMOR IMMUNE RESPONSE

3.1. Using the Potential of the Innate Immune System to Eliminate Lymphoma Cells

Evidence for the effectiveness of NK cells for treatment of malignancies has come from studies using ex vivo generated lymphokine-activated killer cells (LAK) or in vivo cytokine therapy (e.g., IL-2) to enhance autologous NK-cell activity *(95)*. Promising results from clinical phase III studies are mostly reported for renal cell carcinoma (RCC), but not for lymphoma patients. More recently it was demonstrated, that allogeneic NK cells exert a strong graft-vs-leukemia (GVL) effect in patients treated with HLA haplotype-mismatched hematopoietic stem cell transplantation for hematological malignancies *(96)*. In this study, alloreactive KIR-mismatched NK cells effectively killed malignant cells in acute and chronic myeloid leukemia but less effectively in acute lymphatic leukemia. In addition to showing a strong GVL effect, alloreactive KIR-mismatched NK cells also prevented the development of graft-vs-host disease (GVHD) in these patients. In a very recent mouse model, mice were protected from GVHD by the pre-transplant infusion of alloreactive NK cells and allowed subsequent transplantation of a higher amount of T cells, which in turn are known to exert an important antitumor effect themselves *(97)*. It is intriguing to speculate that in the near future new insights into the biology of NK cells will help to develop novel therapeutic strategies for the treatment of malignant disease, including lymphomas. Nevertheless, we ultimately must await the results of clinical trials testing activated NK-cell therapies in lymphoma patients in order to evaluate the postulated benefit of NK cell-based therapeutic strategies.

3.2. Exploiting the Antibody Specificity to Target Lymphoma Cells

The most advanced immunotherapy for B-cell lymphoma is the use of monoclonal antibodies (MAbs) targeting the CD20 cell-surface molecule of B cells. First attempts to use antibodies as a therapy for lymphoma were initiated in 1979 by Nadler *(98)*, demonstrating tumor-cell killing. Even patient-specific antibodies were administered, and lymphoma regression was demonstrated *(99)*. Further refinement of the antibodies by humanizing the constant regions lead to widely applicable MAbs such as the anti-CD20 antibody rituximab *(100)*. Several further antigens on B cell lymphomas were used as targets for antibodies. CD22, CD52w, and HLAII are examples that found their way into clinical application *(101–103)*. These MAbs are believed to induce tumor-cell killing via three different mechanisms: Complement-mediated cell death, antibody-dependent cellular cytotoxicity, and activation of apoptosis *(104)*. Further modification of MAbs were applied to increase lymphoma killing. Antibodies coupled to different radioactive nucleotides, such as Y90, I131, or Cu-67, were demonstrated to be safe and effective in the treatment of different lymphoma entities *(105–107)*.

3.3. Improved Antigen Presentation by Tumor Cells to Break Tolerance

Tumor cells have been demonstrated to present antigen poorly *(108)*. For successful T-cell induction, sufficient expression of adhesion, MHC, and costimulatory molecules is necessary. Among the costimulatory molecules, the B-7 family seems to be particularly important, since B7/CD28 interaction is necessary and sufficient to prevent anergy *(58–59)*. Several tumor models support the relevance of the B-7 pathway for the induction of antitumor immunity *(109–111)*. The majority of B-cell tumors express MHC class I and II, but fail to express B-7 family members, as well as important adhesion molecules *(112)*. Transfection of single key molecules, such as B7, would represent a rather limited strategy to overcome APC dysfunction in lymphoma. Simultaneous upregulation of several of these key molecules appears to be a more attractive goal. CD40 crosslinking is an important pathway involved in the activation of professional APC such as DC, for significant improvement of APC function *(113)*. CD40 is expressed by normal as well as malignant B cells. Ranheim and Kipps first demonstrated that CD40-activation of chronic lymphocytic leukemia (CLL) cells induces efficient presentation of antigen by the malignant B-CLL cells *(114)*. Similarly, expression of costimulatory and adhesion molecules and APC function of other B-cell tumors can be improved *(115–116)*. The potential clinical value of this approach was demonstrated by Wierda in a gene-therapy trial using CD40 ligand (CD40L [CD154])-transfected CLL cells *(117)*. As demonstrated by ELISPOT analysis and mixed lymphocyte reaction, B-CLL-specific T cells increased in frequency post-vaccination. Even more intriguing, a reduction of leukemia-cell counts as well as lymph-node size was observed, with no sign of induction of autoimmunity *(117)*.

3.4. Identification of Novel Lymphoma Antigens

Several potential targets for immunotherapy have been discovered in lymphoma (Table 1). The idiotype (Id) of the malignant B-cell clone represents a patient-specific tumor marker as well as a lymphoma-specific antigen *(118)*. Id is present on the cell surface, and Id-derived peptides have been shown to be presented in the context of MHC class I and II *(119–122)*. Id has therefore been targeted in vaccination approaches in mice and men *(123–125)*. Although this represents a highly targeted approach with little risk of autoimmunity and the potential for the induction of a significant immune response, clinical application will be limited because of technical difficulties and high costs. We have previously shown that framework-derived peptides can be used to induce tumor-specific immunity in B-cell malignacies *(126)*. These epitopes are shared by a subgroup of patients, and thus represent a less "customized" strategy. Nevertheless, they hardly meet the criteria of a broadly applicable vaccination approach, and a further search for tumor antigens that are shared by many patients, possibly beyond lymphoma, is warranted.

Although classical approaches focus on the dissection of pre-existing immune responses in cancer patients, novel strategies intend to use the vast information generated in the fields of proteomics and genomics to discover candidate tumor antigens that are ignored in cancer patients *(127–134)*. Using gene-expression profiling and reverse immunology, we have identified candidate epitopes from three potential tumor antigens in follicular lymphoma (von Bergwelt-Baildon, unpublished results). This strategy potentially circumvents the problem of boosting an apparently insufficient pre-existing antitumor immune response. Nevertheless, only extensive and well-monitored clinical trials will make it possible to determine the therapeutic potential of the candidate tumor antigens currently being studied (Table 1).

3.5 Targeting Effector and Helper Cells to the Lymphoma Site Through Chemokines

A major obstacle of any tumor-immunotherapy that specially uses adoptive-cell transfer is the recruitment of the effector and helper cells to the tumor site. Several attempts have been made to overcome this problem. In 1993, Luster and colleagues first used IP-10 (CXCL10)-transformed plasmocytoma cells in

Table 1
Different Antigens in Lymphoma May Serve as Targets for Antigen-Directed Immunotherapy

Target	*Antigen*	*Immune-induction*	*Entity*	*Reference*
Idiotype	Idiotype	DNA vaccine, cellular	Lymphoma, myeloma	*144*
	Idiotype	Adenoviral, cellular	A20 model	*145*
	Idiotype	Protein	NHL	*125*
Ig	Ig Framework	? cellular	B-NHL	*126*
TCR	TCR	DNA vaccine, cellular	T-cell lymphoma	*146*
Viral antigens	EBV	Adoptive transfer of T cells	PTLD	*147*
Mutated proto-oncogenes	*p53*			*148*
Products of chromosomal translocations	NPM/ALK	? cellular	Anablastic large-cell lymphoma	*149*
Specifically overexpressed genes	Sperm protein17	cellular	MM	*150*
	CD20	Antibody	Low grade NHL	*151,152,153*
			DLBCL	*154*
	CD52w	Antibody	CLL	*101*
	HLAII	Antibody	NHL	*102*
	CD22	Antibody	Low- and high-grade NHL	*103*
			NHL	
	B1	Antibody		*155*

Here we summarize some examples derived from different biological pathways. New antigens are expected by the use of proteomics and genomics.

a murine model. Tumor growth was clearly inhibited because of a strong immune response demonstrated by the infiltration of lymphocytes, neutrophils, and monocytes *(135)*. The role of the innate immune system in tumor rejection was highlighted by the study of Laning and colleagues, which described the antitumor activity of CCL1 in attracting only non-lymphocytes to the tumor site *(136)*. Many different chemokines were used to enhance tumor immunity *(137)*. Special attention was given to lymphotactin, which protected from established lymphoma, especially in combination with IL-2 *(138–139)*. The positive impact of inflammation at the tumor site further supports the important role of chemokines in attracting effector and helper cells to the tumor site *(140)*. Even the enhancement of tumor immunity by B7.1 transfection is partly the result of the chemotactic effect of chemokines such as MIP1α *(141)*. Apart from targeting effector cells to tumor sites efforts were made to target antigens to helper cells, which clearly enhanced tumor immunity *(142,143)*.

4. SUMMARY

A balanced immune system is crucial for the prevention of lymphoma development. This is demonstrated by the increasing incidence of lymphoma in patients with an impaired immune system—namely, organ transplant recipients, patients infected by HIV, and patients suffering from rare congenital immune defects. In those patients, an increase up to 100-fold in lymphoma incidence has been noted. Uncontrolled B-cell stimulation may be the underlying pathomechanism. This pathomechanism is also found in MALT lymphoma, in which the chronic infection with *H. pylori* is crucial for the lymphoma development.

Different members of the immune system interact with the lymphoma cells. Impairment of this interaction has been shown in various studies. Evidence for ignorance, as well as anergy/tolerance and systemic immune suppression, has been shown to prompt the interaction of T-cells with lymphoma cells. The humoral response is also alterated, which may explain the occurrence of recurrent bacterial and herpesvirus infections. The function of APC in the interaction with lymphoma cells has not been extensively studied, but an impaired network of follicular DC within the lymphoma has been demonstrated. An understanding of the intense interaction between the immune system and the lymphoma has allowed the development of different strategies to overcome the impaired immune system. The specificity of the antibody response was used to target lymphoma cells that already yield excellent clinical results. The recognition of lymphoma cells by the immune system was further enhanced by improving antigen presentation on the tumor cells itself, and by targeting the effector cells to the lymphoma site. In any case, new tumor antigens are needed for future therapeutic strategies.

REFERENCES

1. Coley WB. The treatment of malignant tumors by repeated inoculation of erysipelas: with a report of ten original cases. *Am J Med Sci* 1893;105:487–511.
2. Busch W. Aus der Sitzung der medicinischen Section vom 13 November 1867. *Berl Klin Wochenschr* 1867;5:137.
3. Burnet FM. Immunological aspects of malignant disease. *Lancet* 1967;1:1171–1174.
4. Rabkin CS, Biggar RJ, Baptiste MS, Abe T, Kohler BA, Nasca PC. Cancer incidence trends in women at high risk of human immunodeficiency virus (HIV) infection. *Int J Cancer* 1993; 55:208–212.
5. Munoz A, Schrager LK, Bacellar H, et al. Trends in the incidence of outcomes defining acquired immunodeficiency syndrome (AIDS) in the Multicenter AIDS Cohort Study: 1985-1991. *Am J Epidemiol* 1993;137:423–438.

6. Pluda JM, Venzon DJ, Tosato G, et al. Parameters affecting the development of non-Hodgkin's lymphoma in patients with severe human immunodeficiency virus infection receiving antiretroviral therapy. *J Clin Oncol* 1993;11:1099–1107.
7. Penn I. Post-transplant malignancy: the role of immunosuppression. *Drug Saf* 2000;23:101–113.
8. Kinlen LJ. Incidence of cancer in rheumatoid arthritis and other disorders after immunosuppressive treatment. *Am J Med* 1985;78:44–49.
9. Kamel OW. Iatrogenic lymphoproliferative disorders in non-transplantation settings. *Recent Results Cancer Res* 2002;159:19–26.
10. Elenitoba-Johnson KS, Jaffe ES. Lymphoproliferative disorders associated with congenital immunodeficiencies. *Semin Diagn Pathol* 1997;14:35–47.
11. Dal Maso L, Serraino D, Franceschi S. Epidemiology of AIDS-related tumours in developed and developing countries. *Eur J Cancer* 2001;37:1188–1201.
12. Grulich AE, Wan X, Law MG, et al. B-cell stimulation and prolonged immune deficiency are risk factors for non-Hodgkin's lymphoma in people with AIDS. *Aids* 2000;14: 133–140.
13. Wotherspoon AC, Ortiz-Hidalgo C, Falzon MR, Isaacson PG. Helicobacter pylori-associated gastritis and primary B-cell gastric lymphoma. *Lancet* 1991;338:1175–1176.
14. Doglioni C, Wotherspoon AC, Moschini A, de Boni M, Isaacson PG. High incidence of primary gastric lymphoma in northeastern Italy. *Lancet* 1992;339:834–835.
15. Zucca E, Bertoni F, Roggero E, et al. Molecular analysis of the progression from Helicobacter pylori- associated chronic gastritis to mucosa-associated lymphoid-tissue lymphoma of the stomach. *N Engl J Med* 1998;338:804–810.
16. Cavalli F, Isaacson PG, Gascoyne RD, Zucca E. MALT Lymphomas. *Hematology* (Am Soc Hematol Educ Program) 2001:241–258.
17. Hermine O, Lefrere F, Bronowicki JP, et al. Regression of splenic lymphoma with villous lymphocytes after treatment of hepatitis C virus infection. *N Engl J Med* 2002;347:89–94.
18. Chapel HM, Lee M, Hargreaves R, Pamphilon DH, Prentice AG. Randomised trial of intravenous immunoglobulin as prophylaxis against infection in plateau-phase multiple myeloma. The UK Group for Immunoglobulin Replacement Therapy in Multiple Myeloma. *Lancet* 1994;343:1059–1063.
19. Jacobson DR, Zolla-Pazner S. Immunosuppression and infection in multiple myeloma. *Semin Oncol* 1986;13:282–290.
20. Doughney KB, Williams DM, Penn RL. Multiple myeloma: infectious complications. *South Med J* 1988;81:855–858.
21. Birgens HS, Espersen F, Hertz JB, Pedersen FK, Drivsholm A. Antibody response to pneumococcal vaccination in patients with myelomatosis. *Scand J Haematol* 1983;30: 324–330.
22. Broder S, Muul L, Megson M, Waldmann TA. Abnormalities of immunoregulatory cells in immunodeficiency disease and cancer. *Prog Clin Biol Res* 1981;58:93–120.
23. MacKenzie MR, Paglieroni T, Caggiano V. CD5 positive immunoregulatory B cells in spleen populations from multiple myeloma patients. *Am J Hematol* 1991;37:163–166.
24. Paglieroni T, Caggiano V, MacKenzie M. Abnormalities in immune regulation precede the development of multiple myeloma. *Am J Hematol* 1992;40:51–55.
25. Pilarski LM, Mant MJ, Ruether BA, Belch A. Severe deficiency of B lymphocytes in peripheral blood from multiple myeloma patients. *J Clin Investig* 1984;74:1301–1306.
26. Cortes J, Kurzrock R. Interleukin-10 in non-Hodgkin's lymphoma. *Leuk Lymphoma* 1997;26:251–259.
27. Kyrtsonis MC, Repa C, Dedoussis GV, et al. Serum transforming growth factor-beta 1 is related to the degree of immunoparesis in patients with multiple myeloma. *Med Oncol* 1998; 15:124–128.

28. Christiansen I, Gidlof C, Kalkner KM, Hagberg H, Bennmarker H, Totterman T. Elevated serum levels of soluble ICAM-1 in non-Hodgkin's lymphomas correlate with tumour burden, disease activity and other prognostic markers. *Br J Haematol* 1996;92:639–646.
29. Schultze JL. Why do B cell lymphoma fail to elicit clinically sufficient T cell immune responses? *Leuk Lymphoma* 1999;32:223–236.
30. Xu Y, Kroft SH, McKenna RW, Aquino DB. Prognostic significance of tumour-infiltrating T lymphocytes and T-cell subsets in de novo diffuse large B-cell lymphoma: a multiparameter flow cytometry study. *Br J Haematol* 2001;112:945–949.
31. Diaz JI, Edinger MG, Stoler MH, Tubbs RR. Activated T-cell subsets in benign lymphoid hyperplasias and B-cell non-Hodgkin's lymphomas. *Am J Pathol* 1991;139:503–509.
32. Diaz JI, Edinger MG, Stoler M, Tubbs RR. Host tumor infiltrating lymphocytes in B cell non-Hodgkin's lymphomas. *Leuk Lymphoma* 1993;9:85–90.
33. Bonnefoix T, Claret E, Piccinni MP, Jacob MC, Zheng X, Sotto JJ. Detection, isolation and functional studies of CD25+ T cells in lymph nodes involved by B-cell non-Hodgkin's lymphomas. *Scand J Immunol* 1991;34:91–100.
34. Luna-Fineman S, Lee JE, Wesley PK, Clayberger C, Krensky AM. Human Cytotoxic T-Lymphocytes Specific for Autologous Follicular Lymphoma Recognize Immunoglobulin in a Major Histocompatibility Complex Restricted Fashion. *Cancer* 1992;70:2181–2186.
35. Schultze JL, Seamon MJ, Michalak S, Gribben JG, Nadler LM. Autologous tumor infiltrating T cells cytotoxic for follicular lymphoma cells can be expanded in vitro. *Blood* 1997;89: 3806–3816.
36. Bonnefoix T, Claret E, Piccinni MP, Jacob MC, Zheng XQ, Sotto JJ. Impaired clonogenic potential of CD25 positive T cells in lymph nodes involved by B cell non-Hodgkin's lymphomas. *Immunol Lett* 1991;27:135–139.
37. Wang Q, Stanley J, Kudoh S, et al. T cells infiltrating non-Hodgkin's B cell lymphomas show altered tyrosine phosphorylation pattern even though T cell receptor/CD3- associated kinases are present. *J Immunol* 1995;155:1382–1392.
38. Lowin B, Beermann F, Schmidt A, Tschopp J. A null mutation in the perforin gene impairs cytolytic T lymphocyte- and natural killer cell-mediated cytotoxicity. *Proc Natl Acad Sci USA* 1994;91:11,571–11,575.
39. Bladergroen BA, Meijer CJ, ten Berge RL, et al. Expression of the granzyme B inhibitor, protease inhibitor 9, by tumor cells in patients with non-Hodgkin and Hodgkin lymphoma: a novel protective mechanism for tumor cells to circumvent the immune system? *Blood* 2002;99:232–237.
40. Zeytun A, Hassuneh M, Nagarkatti M, Nagarkatti PS. Fas-Fas ligand-based interactions between tumor cells and tumor- specific cytotoxic T lymphocytes: a lethal two-way street. *Blood* 1997;90:1952–1959.
41. Ni X, Hazarika P, Zhang C, Talpur R, Duvic M. Fas ligand expression by neoplastic T lymphocytes mediates elimination of CD8+ cytotoxic T lymphocytes in mycosis fungoides: a potential mechanism of tumor immune escape? *Clin Cancer Res* 2001;7:2682–2692.
42. Wilcox RA, Flies DB, Zhu G, et al. Provision of antigen and CD137 signaling breaks immunological ignorance, promoting regression of poorly immunogenic tumors. *J Clin Investig* 2002;109:651–659.
43. Ochsenbein AF, Klenerman P, Karrer U, et al. Immune surveillance against a solid tumor fails because of immunological ignorance. *Proc Natl Acad Sci USA* 1999;96:2233–2238.
44. Wick M, Dubey P, Koeppen H, et al. Antigenic cancer cells grow progressively in immune hosts without evidence for T cell exhaustion or systemic anergy. *J Exp Med* 1997; 186:229–238.
45. Chen L, McGowan P, Ashe S, et al. Tumor immunogenicity determines the effect of B7 costimulation on T cell-mediated tumor immunity. *J Exp Med* 1994;179:523–532.

46. Ghosh N, Gyory I, Wright G, Wood J, Wright KL. Positive regulatory domain I binding factor 1 silences class II transactivator expression in multiple myeloma cells. *J Biol Chem* 2001;276:15,264–15,268.
47. Murphy SP, Holtz R, Lewandowski N, Tomasi TB, Fuji H. DNA Alkylating Agents Alleviate Silencing of Class II Transactivator Gene Expression in L1210 Lymphoma Cells. *J Immunol* 2002;169:3085–3093.
48. Seliger B, Harders C, Wollscheid U, Staege MS, Reske-Kunz AB, Huber C. Suppression of MHC class I antigens in oncogenic transformants: association with decreased recognition by cytotoxic T lymphocytes. *Exp Hematol* 1996;24:1275–1279.
49. Miller JF, Heath WR. Self-ignorance in the peripheral T-cell pool. *Immunol Rev* 1993; 133:131–150.
50. Malone CS, Miner MD, Doerr JR, et al. CmC(A/T)GG DNA methylation in mature B cell lymphoma gene silencing. *Proc Natl Acad Sci USA* 2001;98:10,404–10,409.
51. MacLennan IC, Gulbranson-Judge A, Toellner KM, et al. The changing preference of T and B cells for partners as T-dependent antibody responses develop. *Immunol Rev* 1997; 156:53–66.
52. Shokat KM, Goodnow CC. Antigen-induced B-cell death and elimination during germinal-centre immune responses. *Nature* 1995;375:334–338.
53. Rathmell JC, Cooke MP, Ho WY, et al. CD95 (Fas)-dependent elimination of self-reactive B cells upon interaction with CD4+ T cells. *Nature* 1995;376:181–184.
54. Cyster JG, Goodnow CC. Antigen-induced exclusion from follicles and anergy are separate and complementary processes that influence peripheral B cell fate. *Immunity* 1995;3:691–701.
55. Rosic-Kablar S, Chan K, Reis MD, Dube ID, Hough MR. Induction of tolerance to immunogenic tumor antigens associated with lymphomagenesis in HOX11 transgenic mice. *Proc Natl Acad Sci USA* 2000;97:13,300–13,305.
56. Staveley-O'Carroll K, Sotomayor E, Montgomery J, et al. Induction of antigen-specific T cell anergy: An early event in the course of tumor progression. *Proc Natl Acad Sci USA* 1998;95:1178–1183.
57. Sotomayor EM, Borrello I, Rattis FM, et al. Cross-presentation of tumor antigens by bone marrow-derived antigen- presenting cells is the dominant mechanism in the induction of T-cell tolerance during B-cell lymphoma progression. *Blood* 2001;98: 1070–1077.
58. Guinan EC, Gribben JG, Boussiotis VA, Freeman GJ, Nadler LM. Pivotal role of the B7:CD28 pathway in transplantation tolerance and tumor immunity. *Blood* 1994;84:3261–3282.
59. Schultze J, Nadler LM, Gribben JG. B7-mediated costimulation and the immune response. *Blood Rev* 1996;10:111–127.
60. Levitsky HI. Tumors derived from antigen presenting cells. *Semin Immunol* 1996;8:281–287.
61. Sotomayor EM, Borrello I, Levitsky HI. Tolerance and cancer: a critical issue in tumor immunology. *Crit Rev Oncog* 1996;7:433–456.
62. Schultze JL, Cardoso AA, Freeman GJ, et al. Follicular lymphomas can be induced to present alloantigen efficiently: a conceptual model to improve their tumor immunogenicity. *Proc Natl Acad Sci USA* 1995;92:8200–8204.
63. Dorfman DM, Schultze JL, Shahsafaei A, et al. In vivo expression of B7-1 and B7-2 on follicular lymphoma is not sufficient to induce significant T cell proferation but is sufficient to prevent T cell anergy in vitro. *Blood* 1997;90:4297–4306.
64. Bogen B. Peripheral T cell tolerance as a tumor escape mechanism: deletion of CD4+ T cells specific for a monoclonal immunoglobulin idiotype secreted by a plasmacytoma. *Eur J Immunol* 1996;26:2671–2679.

65. Ferrarini M, Consogno G, Rovere P, et al. Inhibition of caspases maintains the antineoplastic function of gammadelta T cells repeatedly challenged with lymphoma cells. *Cancer Res* 2001;61:3092–3095.
66. Lauritzsen GF, Hofgaard PO, Schenck K, Bogen B. Clonal deletion of thymocytes as a tumor escape mechanism. *Int J Cancer* 1998;78:216–222.
67. Bogen B, Dembic Z, Weiss S. Clonal deletion of specific thymocytes by an immunoglobulin idiotype. *EMBO J* 1993;12:357–363.
68. Gitelson E, Spaner D, Buckstein R, et al. T-cell analysis in identical twins reveals an impaired anti-follicular lymphoma immune response in the patient but not in the healthy twin. *Br J Haematol* 2002;116:122–127.
69. Massaia M, Attisano C, Beggiato E, Bianchi A, Pileri A. Correlation between disease activity and T-cell CD3 zeta chain expression in a B-cell lymphoma. *Br J Haematol* 1994;88:886–888.
70. Specht C, Bexten S, Kolsch E, Pauels HG. Prostaglandins, but not tumor-derived IL-10, shut down concomitant tumor-specific CTL responses during murine plasmacytoma progression. *Int J Cancer* 2001;91:705–712.
71. Otsuki T, Yamada O, Yata K, et al. Expression and production of interleukin 10 in human myeloma cell lines. *Br J Haematol* 2000;111:835–842.
72. Beaty RM, Rulli K, Bost KL, Pantginis J, Lenz J, Levy LS. High levels of IL-4 and IL-10 mRNA and low levels of IL-2, IL-9 and IFN- gamma mRNA in MuLV-induced lymphomas. *Virology* 1999;261:253–262.
73. Tada T, Ohzeki S, Utsumi K, et al. Transforming growth factor-beta-induced inhibition of T cell function. Susceptibility difference in T cells of various phenotypes and functions and its relevance to immunosuppression in the tumor-bearing state. *J Immunol* 1991;146:1077–1082.
74. Becker JC, Czerny C, Brocker EB. Maintenance of clonal anergy by endogenously produced IL-10. *Int Immunol* 1994;6:1605–1612.
75. de Waal Malefyt R, Haanen J, Spits H, et al. Interleukin 10 (IL-10) and viral IL-10 strongly reduce antigen- specific human T cell proliferation by diminishing the antigen- presenting capacity of monocytes via downregulation of class II major histocompatibility complex expression. *J Exp Med* 1991;174:915–924.
76. Maeda H, Kuwahara H, Ichimura Y, Ohtsuki M, Kurakata S, Shiraishi A. TGF-beta enhances macrophage ability to produce IL-10 in normal and tumor-bearing mice. *J Immunol* 1995;155:4926–4932.
77. Guindi M. Role of activated host T cells in the promotion of MALT lymphoma growth. *Semin Cancer Biol* 2000;10:341–344.
78. Hussell T, Isaacson PG, Crabtree JE, Spencer J. Helicobacter pylori-specific tumour-infiltrating T cells provide contact dependent help for the growth of malignant B cells in low-grade gastric lymphoma of mucosa-associated lymphoid tissue. *J Pathol* 1996; 178:122–127.
79. Greiner A, Knorr C, Qin Y, et al. Low-grade B cell lymphomas of mucosa-associated lymphoid tissue (MALT-type) require CD40-mediated signaling and Th2-type cytokines for in vitro growth and differentiation. *Am J Pathol* 1997;150:1583–1593.
80. Tureci O, Sahin U, Pfreundschuh M. Serological analysis of human tumor antigens: molecular definition and implications. *Mol Med Today* 1997;3:342–349.
81. Tsiodras S, Samonis G, Keating MJ, Kontoyiannis DP. Infection and immunity in chronic lymphocytic leukemia. *Mayo Clin Proc* 2000;75:1039–1054.
82. Troy A, Davidson P, Atkinson C, Hart D. Phenotypic characterisation of the dendritic cell infiltrate in prostate cancer. *J Urol* 1998;160:214–219.
83. Troy AJ, Summers KL, Davidson PJ, Atkinson CH, Hart DN. Minimal recruitment and activation of dendritic cells within renal cell carcinoma. *Clin Cancer Res* 1998;4:585–593.

84. Gabrilovich DI, Corak J, Ciernik IF, Kavanaugh D, Carbone DP. Decreased antigen presentation by dendritic cells in patients with breast cancer. *Clin Cancer Res* 1997; 3:483–490.
85. Hart DN, Hill GR. Dendritic cell immunotherapy for cancer: application to low-grade lymphoma and multiple myeloma. *Immunol Cell Biol* 1999;77:451–459.
86. Troy AJ, Hart DN. Dendritic cells and cancer: progress toward a new cellular therapy. *J Hematother* 1997;6:523–533.
87. Allavena P, Piemonti L, Longoni D, et al. IL-10 prevents the differentiation of monocytes to dendritic cells but promotes their maturation to macrophages. *Eur J Immunol* 1998;28:359–369.
88. Steinbrink K, Wolfl M, Jonuleit H, Knop J, Enk AH. Induction of tolerance by IL-10-treated dendritic cells. *J Immunol* 1997;159:4772–4780.
89. Gabrilovich DI, Nadaf S, Corak J, Berzofsky JA, Carbone DP. Dendritic cells in antitumor immune responses. II. Dendritic cells grown from bone marrow precursors, but not mature DC from tumor-bearing mice, are effective antigen carriers in the therapy of established tumors. *Cell Immunol* 1996;170:111–119.
90. Bagdi E, Krenacs L, Krenacs T, Miller K, Isaacson PG. Follicular dendritic cells in reactive and neoplastic lymphoid tissues: a reevaluation of staining patterns of CD21, CD23, and CD35 antibodies in paraffin sections after wet heat-induced epitope retrieval. *Appl Immunohistochem Mol Morphol* 2001;9:117–124.
91. Scoazec JY, Berger F, Magaud JP, Brochier J, Coiffier B, Bryon PA. The dendritic reticulum cell pattern in B cell lymphomas of the small cleaved, mixed, and large cell types: an immunohistochemical study of 48 cases. *Hum Pathol* 1989;20:124–131.
92. Petrasch S, Brittinger G, Wacker HH, Schmitz J, Kosco-Vilbois M. Follicular dendritic cells in non-Hodgkin's lymphomas. *Leuk Lymphoma* 1994;15:33–43.
93. Renard N, Valladeau J, Barthelemy C, et al. Characterization of germinal center dendritic cells in follicular lymphoma. *Exp Hematol* 1999;27:1768–1775.
94. Farag SS, Fehniger TA, Ruggeri L, Velardi A, Caligiuri MA. Natural killer cell receptors: new biology and insights into the graft- versus-leukemia effect. *Blood* 2002;100: 1935–1947.
95. Rosenberg SA. Progress in human tumour immunology and immunotherapy. *Nature* 2001;411:380–384.
96. Ruggeri L, Capanni M, Casucci M, et al. Role of natural killer cell alloreactivity in HLA-mismatched hematopoietic stem cell transplantation. *Blood* 1999;94:333–339.
97. Ruggeri L, Capanni M, Urbani E, et al. Effectiveness of donor natural killer cell alloreactivity in mismatched hematopoietic transplants. *Science* 2002;295:2097–2100.
98. Nadler LM, Stashenko P, Hardy R, et al. Serotherapy of a patient with a monoclonal antibody directed against a human lymphoma-associated antigen. *Cancer Res* 1980;40: 3147–3154.
99. Miller RA, Maloney DG, Warnke R, Levy R. Treatment of B-cell lymphoma with monoclonal anti-idiotype antibody. *N Engl J Med* 1982;306:517–522.
100. White CA, Weaver RL, Grillo-Lopez AJ. Antibody-targeted immunotherapy for treatment of malignancy. *Annu Rev Med* 2001;52:125–145.
101. Keating MJ, Flinn I, Jain V, et al. Therapeutic role of alemtuzumab (Campath-1H) in patients who have failed fludarabine: results of a large international study. *Blood* 2002;99:3554–3561.
102. Leonard JP, Link BK. Immunotherapy of non-Hodgkin's lymphoma with hLL2 (epratuzumab, an anti-CD22 monoclonal antibody) and Hu1D10 (apolizumab). *Semin Oncol* 2002;29:81–86.
103. Press OW, Leonard JP, Coiffier B, Levy R, Timmerman J. Immunotherapy of Non-Hodgkin's lymphomas. *Hematology* (Am Soc Hematol Educ Program) 2001:221–240.

104. McCune SL, Gockerman JP, Rizzieri DA. Monoclonal antibody therapy in the treatment of non-Hodgkin lymphoma. *JAMA* 2001;286:1149–1152.
105. Lewis JP, Denardo GL, Denardo SJ. Radioimmunotherapy of lymphoma: a UC Davis experience. *Hybridoma* 1995;14:115–120.
106. DeNardo GL, DeNardo SJ, Goldstein DS, et al. Maximum-tolerated dose, toxicity, and efficacy of (131)I-Lym-1 antibody for fractionated radioimmunotherapy of non-Hodgkin's lymphoma. *J Clin Oncol* 1998;16:3246–3256.
107. Kaminski MS, Zelenetz AD, Press OW, et al. Pivotal study of iodine I 131 tositumomab for chemotherapy-refractory low-grade or transformed low-grade B-cell non-Hodgkin's lymphomas. *J Clin Oncol* 2001;19:3918–3928.
108. Ostrand-Rosenberg S. Tumor immunotherapy: the tumor cell as an antigen-presenting cell. *Curr Opin Immunol* 1994;6:722–727.
109. Dranoff G, Mulligan RC. Gene transfer as cancer therapy. *Adv Immunol* 1995;58: 417–454.
110. Allison JP, Hurwitz AA, Leach DR. Manipulation of costimulatory signals to enhance antitumor T- cell responses. *Curr Opin Immunol* 1995;7:682–686.
111. Hellstrom KE, Hellstrom I, Chen L. Can co-stimulated tumor immunity be therapeutically efficacious? *Immunol Rev* 1995;145:123–145.
112. Schultze JL. Vaccination as immunotherapy for B cell lymphoma. *Hematol Oncol* 1997; 15:129–139.
113. Liu YJ, Kanzler H, Soumelis V, Gilliet M. Dendritic cell lineage, plasticity and cross-regulation. *Nat Immunol* 2001;2:585–589.
114. Ranheim EA, Kipps TJ. Activated T Cells Induce Expression of B7/BB1 on Normal or Leukemic B Cells through a CD40-dependent Signal. *J Exp Med* 1993;177:925–935.
115. Schultze JL, Michalak S, Seamon MJ, Gribben JG, Nadler LM. CD40 activated follicular lymphoma cells are resistant to and can overcome generalized T cell unresponsiveness induced by IL-10 and TGF beta. *Blood* 1996;88:2534.
116. Cardoso AA, Seamon MJ, Afonso HM, et al. Ex vivo generation of human anti-pre-B leukemia-specific autologous cytolytic T cells. *Blood* 1997;90:549–561.
117. Wierda WG, Cantwell MJ, Woods SJ, Rassenti LZ, Prussak CE, Kipps TJ. CD40-ligand (CD154) gene therapy for chronic lymphocytic leukemia. *Blood* 2000;96:2917–2924.
118. Krolick KA, Isakson PC, Uhr JW, Vitetta ES. BCL1, a murine model for chronic lymphocytic leukemia: use of the surface immunoglobulin idiotype for the detection and treatment of tumor. *Immunol Rev* 1979;48:81–106.
119. Bogen B, Weiss S. Processing and presentation of idiotypes to MHC-restricted T cells. *International Reviews of Immunology* 1993;10:337–355.
120. Weiss S, Bogen B. B-lymphoma cells process and present their endogenous immunoglobulin to major histocompatibility complex-restricted T cells. *Proc Natl Acad Sci USA* 1989; 86:282–286.
121. Chakrabarti D, Ghosh SK. Induction of syngeneic cytotoxic T lymphocytes against a B cell tumor. III. MHC class I-restricted CTL recognizes the processed form(s) of idiotype. *Cell Immunol* 1992;144:455–464.
122. Weiss S, Bogen B. MHC class II-restricted presentation of intracellular antigen. *Cell* 1991;64:767–776.
123. Kwak LW, Young HA, Pennington RW, Weeks SD. Vaccination with syngeneic, lymphoma-derived immunoglobulin idiotype combined with granulocyte/macrophage colony-stimulating factor primes mice for a protective T-cell response. *Proc Natl Acad Sci USA* 1996;93:10,972–10,977.
124. Hsu F, Benike C, Fagnoni F, et al. Vaccination of patients with B-cell lymphoma using autologous antigen pulsed dendritic cells. *Nat Med* 1996;2:52–58.

125. Bendandi M, Gocke CD, Kobrin CB, et al. Complete molecular remissions induced by patient-specific vaccination plus granulocyte-monocyte colony-stimulating factor against lymphoma. *Nat Med* 1999;5:1171–1177.
126. Trojan A, Schultze JL, Witzens M, et al. Immunoglobulin framework-derived peptides function as cytotoxic T-cell epitopes commonly expressed in B-cell malignancies. *Nat Med* 2000;6:667–672.
127. Boon T, Cerottini JC, Van den Eynde B, van der Bruggen P, Van Pel A. Tumor antigens recognized by T lymphocytes. *Annu Rev Immunol* 1994;12:337–365.
128. Gilboa E. The makings of a tumor rejection antigen. *Immunity* 1999;11:263–270.
129. Rosenberg SA. A new era for cancer immunotherapy based on the genes that encode cancer antigens. *Immunity* 1999;10:281–287.
130. Van den Eynde BJ, van der Bruggen P. T cell defined tumor antigens. *Curr Opin Immunol* 1997;9:684–693.
131. Sahin U, Tureci O, Pfreundschuh M. Serological identification of human tumor antigens. *Curr Opin Immunol* 1997;9:709–716.
132. Schultze JL, Vonderheide RH. From cancer genomics to cancer immunotherapy: toward second-generation tumor antigens. *Trends Immunol* 2001;22:516–523.
133. Schultze JL, Maecker B, von Bergwelt-Baildon MS, Anderson KS, Vonderheide RH. Tumor immunotherapy—new tools, new treatment modalities and new T cell antigens. *Vox Sanguinis* 2001;80:81–89.
134. Maecker B, von B-B, Anderson KS, Vonderheide RH, Schultze JL. Linking genomics to immunotherapy by reverse immunology—′immunomics′ in the new millennium. *Curr Mol Med* 2001;1:609–619.
135. Luster AD, Leder P. IP-10, a -C-X-C- chemokine, elicits a potent thymus-dependent antitumor response in vivo. *J Exp Med* 1993;178:1057–1065.
136. Laning J, Kawasaki H, Tanaka E, Luo Y, Dorf ME. Inhibition of in vivo tumor growth by the beta chemokine, TCA3. *J Immunol* 1994;153:4625–4635.
137. Homey B, Muller A, Zlotnik A. Chemokines: agents for the immunotherapy of cancer? *Nat Rev Immunol* 2002;2:175–184.
138. Dilloo D, Bacon K, Holden W, et al. Combined chemokine and cytokine gene transfer enhances antitumor immunity. *Nat Med* 1996;2:1090–1095.
139. Cairns CM, Gordon JR, Li F, Baca-Estrada ME, Moyana T, Xiang J. Lymphotactin expression by engineered myeloma cells drives tumor regression: mediation by CD4+ and CD8+ T cells and neutrophils expressing XCR1 receptor. *J Immunol* 2001;167:57–65.
140. Tatsugami K, Tamada K, Abe K, Harada M, Nomoto K. Local injections of OK432 can help the infiltration of adoptively transferred CD8+ T cells into the tumor sites and synergistically induce the local production of Th1-type cytokines and CXC3 chemokines. *Cancer Immunol Immunother* 2000;49:361–368.
141. Maric M, Chen L, Sherry B, Liu Y. A mechanism for selective recruitment of CD8 T cells into B7-1-transfected plasmacytoma: role of macrophage-inflammatory protein 1alpha. *J Immunol* 1997;159:360–368.
142. Biragyn A, Tani K, Grimm MC, Weeks S, Kwak LW. Genetic fusion of chemokines to a self tumor antigen induces protective, T-cell dependent antitumor immunity. *Nat Biotechnol* 1999;17:253–258.
143. Biragyn A, Surenhu M, Yang D, et al. Mediators of innate immunity that target immature, but not mature, dendritic cells induce antitumor immunity when genetically fused with nonimmunogenic tumor antigens. *J Immunol* 2001;167:6644–6653.
144. King CA, Spellerberg MB, Zhu D, et al. DNA vaccines with single-chain Fv fused to fragment C of tetanus toxin induce protective immunity against lymphoma and myeloma [see comments]. *Nat Med* 1998;4:1281–1286.

145. Armstrong AC, Dermime S, Allinson CG, et al. Immunization with a recombinant adenovirus encoding a lymphoma idiotype: induction of tumor-protective immunity and identification of an idiotype-specific T cell epitope. *J Immunol* 2002;168:3983–3991.
146. Thirdborough SM, Radcliffe JN, Friedmann PS, Stevenson FK. Vaccination with DNA encoding a single-chain TCR fusion protein induces anticlonotypic immunity and protects against T-cell lymphoma. *Cancer Res* 2002;62:1757–1760.
147. Liu Z, Savoldo B, Huls H, et al. Epstein-Barr virus (EBV)-specific cytotoxic T lymphocytes for the prevention and treatment of EBV-associated post-transplant lymphomas. *Recent Results Cancer Res* 2002;159:123–133.
148. Huppi K, Henderson D, Siwarski D, Hochman J, Bergel M, Tuchscherer G. Generation of monospecific peptide antibodies to the DNA binding domain of p53. *Biotechniques* 2000;29:1100–1106.
149. Passoni L, Scardino A, Bertazzoli C, et al. ALK as a novel lymphoma-associated tumor antigen: identification of 2 HLA-A2.1-restricted CD8+ T-cell epitopes. *Blood* 2002;99: 2100–2106.
150. Chiriva-Internati M, Wang Z, Salati E, Bumm K, Barlogie B, Lim SH. Sperm protein 17 (Sp17) is a suitable target for immunotherapy of multiple myeloma. *Blood* 2002; 100:961–965.
151. Davis TA, White CA, Grillo-Lopez AJ, et al. Single-agent monoclonal antibody efficacy in bulky non-Hodgkin's lymphoma: results of a phase II trial of rituximab. *J Clin Oncol* 1999;17:1851–1857.
152. Colombat P, Salles G, Brousse N, et al. Rituximab (anti-CD20 monoclonal antibody) as single first-line therapy for patients with follicular lymphoma with a low tumor burden: clinical and molecular evaluation. *Blood* 2001;97:101–106.
153. Hainsworth JD, Burris HA, 3rd, Morrissey LH, et al. Rituximab monoclonal antibody as initial systemic therapy for patients with low-grade non-Hodgkin lymphoma. *Blood* 2000; 95:3052–3056.
154. Coiffier B, Haioun C, Ketterer N, et al. Rituximab (anti-CD20 monoclonal antibody) for the treatment of patients with relapsing or refractory aggressive lymphoma: a multicenter phase II study. *Blood* 1998;92:1927–1932.
155. Kaminski MS, Zasadny KR, Francis IR, et al. Iodine-131-anti-B1 radioimmunotherapy for B-cell lymphoma. *J Clin Oncol* 1996;14:1974–1981.

17 Immune Dysfunction in Classical Hodgkin's Lymphoma

Arjan Diepstra, MD,
Ewerton M. Maggio, MD, PhD,
Anke van den Berg, PhD,
and Sibrand Poppema, MD, PhD

CONTENTS

1. INTRODUCTION

Immunological mechanisms play a major role in the pathogenesis of Hodgkin's lymphoma (HL), which in terms of the multitude of interactions between different cell types is probably the most complex of all neoplasms. HL is distinct from almost all other malignant tumors because of its unique cellular composition: a minority of neoplastic cells in an abundant inflammatory background. This background consists of varying amounts of T and B lymphocytes, plasma cells, eosinophilic granulocytes, and histiocytes, and usually comprises more than 99% of the tumor mass.

From: *Current Clinical Oncology: Cancer Immunotherapy at the Crossroads: How Tumors Evade Immunity and What Can Be Done*
Edited by: J. H. Finke and R. M. Bukowski © Humana Press Inc., Totowa, NJ

Table 1
World Health Organization Histological Classification of Hodgkin's Lymphoma

Nodular lymphocyte predominant HL
Classical HL
Nodular sclerosis classical HL
Mixed cellularity classical HL
Lymphocyte-rich classical HL
Lymphocyte-depleted classical HL

The formation of this infiltrate is not a simple antitumor-cell response of the immune system. The Hodgkin and Reed-Sternberg (HRS) cells, the neoplastic cells in HL, actively influence their microenvironment through production of cytokines and chemokines (chemoattractant cytokines) and by communication through cell-surface receptors. HRS cells make use of mechanisms to evade the immune response, as do tumor cells in most other neoplasms. However, HRS cells also seem to require the presence of the reactive infiltrate to survive. This chapter explores these seemingly contradictory phenomena and discusses the potential application of immunomodulatory approaches.

2. CHARACTERISTICS OF HRS CELLS

The classical Reed-Sternberg cell is a very large cell with a moderate amount of amphophilic cytoplasm, and it contains two nuclei or nuclear lobes, each with a large nucleolus. This cell type, named after Dorothy Reed and Carl Sternberg, is considered to be the hallmark of HL. Mononuclear variants and so-called lacunar cells are members of the same neoplastic population. The Reed-Sternberg cells, together with the variants, are known as HRS cells. These cells are typical for the classical HL (CHL) subtypes: nodular sclerosis (NS), mixed cellularity (MC), lymphocyte depletion (LD), and lymphocyte rich (LR) *(1)* (Table 1).

There is a non-CHL subtype, the nodular lymphocyte predominant type, which has a strikingly different immunophenotype of the neoplastic cells and lymphocytes in the inflammatory background and a more indolent clinical course as compared to the CHL subtypes. For these reasons, the nodular lymphocyte predominant subtype is considered to be a different entity. This chapter will only address the classical subtypes of HL that account for approx 95% of HL cases worldwide *(2)*.

The cellular origin of HRS cells has long been debated. Immunohistochemical studies showed rare and variable expression of B-cell and/or T-cell antigens with additional expression of markers typical for dendritic cells (DC) or other cell lineages *(3)*. The problem was resolved by single-cell polymerase chain reaction polymerase chain reaction (PCR)-based approaches for immunoglobulin gene-rearrangement analysis using laser-guided micromanipulation of HRS cells from frozen sections of primary CHL biopsies. In the vast majority of cases, the HRS cells were found to have monoclonal immunoglobulin gene rearrangement and a high load of somatic hypermutations, indicating that they are derived from a germinal-center B lymphocyte *(4)*.

Somatic hypermutations in the germinal-center reaction are an important mechanism that results in increased affinity of the B-cell receptor to the antigen presented by follicular dendritic cells (FDC). Since the mutations occur at random, they can also result in lower affinity or truncation of immunoglobulin, and in these instances the B cell undergoes apoptosis within the germinal center. Positively selected high-affinity immunoglobulin-bearing B cells are rescued from apoptosis by induction of bcl-2 expression. The somatic hypermutations found in HRS cells are nonproductive ("crippling") in a proportion of cases, and prevent antibody expression.

Absence of surface immunoglobulin can also be explained by a lack of expression of the immunoglobulin transcription factors Bob-1 and/or Oct-2, both in cases with and without crippling somatic hypermutations. Aside from Bob-1 and Oct-2, low expression or absence of B-cell transcription factors Pax-5 and PU.1 also may account for the loss of the B-cell phenotype of HRS cells *(5–8)*. Because the HRS cell and its precursor do not express immunoglobulin, these cells require an alternative mechanism to escape apoptosis during the germinal-center reaction.

This alternative mechanism is believed to involve the transcription factor NF-κB (RelA/*p50*). In its inactivated state, NF-κB is present in the cytoplasm, and is repressed by IκB that prevents transport of NF-κB into the nucleus. Activation of NF-κB can be initiated by signaling through cell-surface receptors of the tumor necrosis factor (TNF)-receptor family. The signal is transduced by TNF-receptor-associated factor (TRAF) which, together with other proteins in the signaling cascade, recruits and activates IκB kinase complex (IKK). Active IKK phosphorylates IκB and induces ubiquitinization and subsequent degradation of this inhibitor. The activated NF-κB dimer then translocates to the nucleus, where it activates transcription of a variety of genes. These genes encode cytokines, cell-adhesion molecules, acute phase-response proteins, and anti-apoptotic proteins that are involved in survival, proliferation, and inflammation. Nuclear localization of active NF-κB can be detected in the majority of HRS cells in all CHL cases and cell lines, but not in cases of non-Hodgkin's lymphoma (NHL) *(9)*.

A few mechanisms may induce constitutive activation of NF-κB. First, HRS cells express several TNF-receptor family receptors, including CD30. This receptor is present on the HRS cells in virtually all cases of CHL, and the demonstration of CD30 is even used as an immunohistochemical marker to confirm the diagnosis. Other TNF receptors such as CD40, receptor activator of NF-κB (RANK), TNFRI (TNF receptor I), and TNFRII each are expressed in a proportion of cases *(10)*. Moreover, the signal-transducing molecules TRAF1 and TRAF2 are commonly expressed in HRS cells *(11,12)*.

Another mechanism that results in constitutive activation of NF-κB involves inactivation of the IκB gene by somatic mutations, resulting in absence or dysfunction of this inhibitor. IκB mutations have been shown in only a few CHL cases and are usually monoallelic *(13–15)*. A third proposed mechanism involves aberrant and persistent activation of IKK complex, resulting in continuous degradation of IκB *(16)*.

In a considerable proportion of CHL cases, the Epstein-Barr virus (EBV) is involved. The EBV viral genome persists as multiple circular episomes that generally do not integrate into the host genome. The presence of these episomes is representative for latent EBV infection. In EBV-involved cases, each and every HRS cell harbors multiple copies of a monoclonal EBV genome, strongly suggesting that EBV infection of the HRS-cell precursor must have been an early step in transformation. The expression of EBV-latent genes in CHL resembles that of nasopharyngeal carcinoma, but differs from the expression pattern of EBV-related Burkitt lymphoma and lymphomas arising in immune-compromised individuals. Only EBV nuclear antigen 1 (EBNA1), latent membrane protein1 (LMP1), and LMP2 are expressed at the mRNA and protein level. This expression pattern is referred to as latency type II *(17)*. The EBNA1 protein binds to viral DNA and allows the EBV genome to be maintained in the B cell as a circular DNA episome *(18)*. A pathogenetic role for the abundantly expressed EBV-encoded small RNAs (EBERs) 1 and 2 is not apparent.

Cell-surface expression of the LMP1 protein alone can mediate B-lymphocyte growth transformation. This potent oncogene product mimics a constitutively activated CD40 molecule, and can protect B cells from apoptosis by activation of NF-κB *(19)*. The LMP2 gene encodes two distinct proteins: LMP2A and LMP2B. The LMP2A protein contains two immunoreceptor tyrosine-based activation motifs (ITAMs). LMP2B is similar to LMP2A but lacks the ITAMs. LMP2A is essential for blocking B-cell-receptor-mediated signal transduction by negatively regulating protein tyrosine kinase activity *(20)*. The latter prevents reactivation of EBV from latently infected cells *(21)*. However, it has been suggested that in the absence of B-cell-receptor signaling, LMP2A can drive the proliferation and survival of B cells.

Although EBV infection of the HRS precursor cell probably acts as a transforming event, this probably is not the only mechanism of transformation. In the Western world, more than 50% of CHL cases are EBV-negative, and it is possible that transforming events unrelated to viral infection are involved. Alternatively, it has been proposed that in some cases EBV negativity may be caused by a possible "hit and run" behavior of the virus, meaning that it leaves the host cell after it has transformed it. More likely, another viral agent is involved, and this has been the subject of many investigations. However, no alternative viral candidate has consistently been detected to date *(17,22)*.

3. CHARACTERISTICS OF THE INFLAMMATORY INFILTRATE

The cell population surrounding the HRS cells is variable, especially in the most common subtypes, NS and MC. CD4-positive T lymphocytes are invariably present in considerable-to-large numbers. However, irregular nodules of small B lymphocytes are also common. In addition, varying amounts of plasma cells, eosinophilic granulocytes, and histiocytes are typically involved, and in some cases, large numbers of neutrophilic granulocytes are prominent. Macrophages and mast cells can also be found in the infiltrate. The general architecture of CHL-affected lymph nodes is nodular, with sclerotic bands separating individual nodules in the NS subtype, and in MC, the background is diffuse and devoid of sclerotic bands.

Interestingly, the polyclonal CD4-positive T lymphocytes have a peculiar mode of activation. They express early activation markers CD38 and CD69 and are CD45RO+/CD45Rbdim, consistent with a Th2 population. Upon restimulation in vitro, these lymphocytes produce IL-4, IL-5, and IFN-γ but not IL-2. Except for the IFN-γ production, this cytokine profile also suggests a Th2-like phenotype. CD8-positive T lymphocytes and natural killer (NK) cells are scarce in the reactive infiltrate. However, activation marker and costimulatory molecule CD26 is absent in the CD4-positive lymphocytes, and this may be an indication for anergy *(23–25)*.

4. COMMUNICATION BETWEEN HRS CELLS AND OTHER CELL TYPES

The HRS cells consistently produce and express a variety of cytokines, chemokines (cytokines with chemoattracting properties), and cell-surface markers. Expression levels of the cytokines and chemokines are much higher than in reactive lymph nodes and tonsils (Fig. 1). This is presumably a result of the constitutive activation of NF-κB in the HRS cells. The expression of cell-surface molecules is restricted, and many lymphoid markers that are normally expressed on B cells are missing. For several of the molecules that are present on HRS cells, an important role in tumor biology has been proposed (Fig. 2).

4.1. Chemokines

HRS cells produce a multitude of chemokines that are likely to be involved in recruitment of the reactive cells (Table 2). Using serial analysis of gene expression (SAGE) and immunohistochemistry, it has been shown that the CC

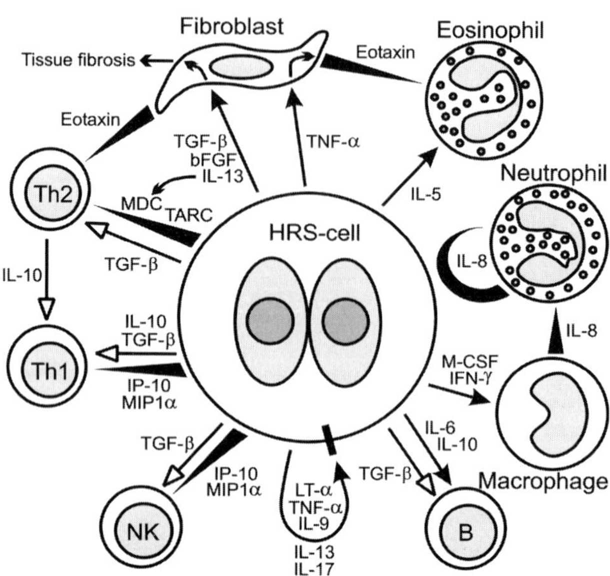

Fig. 1. Chemokines and cytokines in classical HL. Some of the major communications between the HRS cells and cells in the reactive infiltrate are depicted. Chemotaxis is mediated by chemokines (gradient triangles). Cytokines induce proliferation and activation (black arrows) as well as inhibition of activation (white arrows).

chemokine CCL17 or TARC (thymus and activation-related chemokine) is strongly expressed in the neoplastic cells of CHL. It is not detected in NLP HL or NHL *(26)*. TARC binds specifically to the CC chemokine receptor CCR4 that has the highest level of expression in activated Th2 cells. However, activated Th1 cells express CCR5. The influx of lymphocytes with a Th2-like phenotype may thus be explained by the production of TARC by HRS cells *(27)*.

CCL22 or MDC (macrophage-derived chemokine) is a chemokine that maps to the same genomic region as TARC, 16q13. Like TARC, it binds the CCR4 receptor on Th2 lymphocytes; however, unlike TARC, it is also variably expressed in NLP HL and NHL cases. MDC production is stimulated by Th2 cytokines IL-4 and IL-13, and may serve to reinforce the attraction of Th2 lymphocytes initiated by TARC *(28–30)*.

Many chemokines are also produced by HRS cells that can attract Th1 lymphocytes and NK cells—for example, IP-10 (CXCL10), MIP-1α (CCL3), and RANTES (CCL5). These chemokines are expressed more consistently and at higher levels in EBV-positive CHL than in EBV-negative CHL *(28,31)*.

The source of some of the chemokines that may play an important role in CHL is outside the HRS cell. Eotaxin (CCL11) is produced by fibroblasts in the reactive infiltrate in response to TNF-α secreted by HRS cells, and is

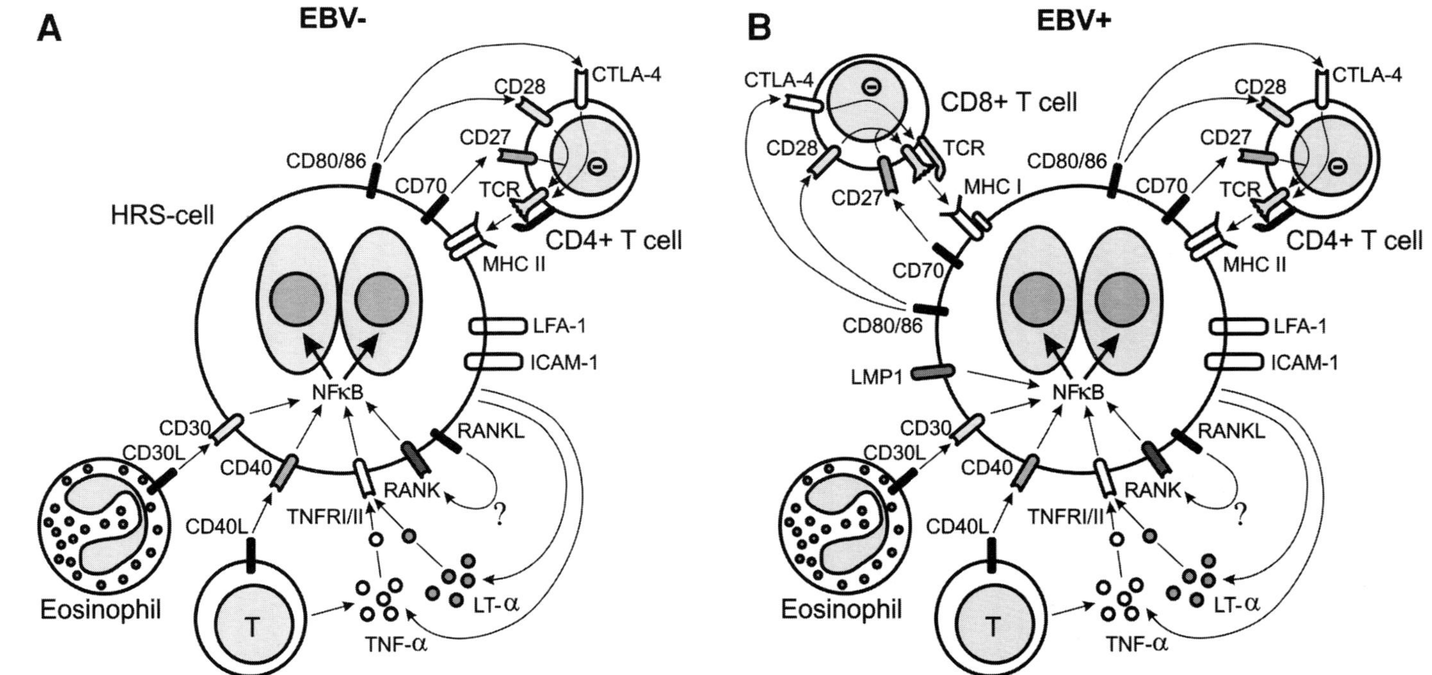

Fig. 2. Cell-surface receptors and ligands in both EBV-negative **(A)** and EBV-positive **(B)** classical HL. TNF receptors CD30, CD40, TNFRI, TNFRII, and RANK as well as the EBV protein LMP1 transduce signals to activate transcription factor NF-κB. Most EBV-positive HRS cells express the MHC class I molecule, yet EBV-negative HRS cells do not. Supposing that MHC molecules present antigens, the HRS cells should be able to trigger CD4 and CD8 T lymphocyte responses. Costimulatory molecules on the T lymphocytes can either reinforce (CD27 and CD28) or dampen (CTLA-4) TCR-transduced signals. LFA-1 and ICAM-1 are major cell-adhesion molecules that mediate contact between the HRS cells and potentially all cell types in the reactive infiltrate. Fas and Fas ligand molecules are not shown.

Table 2
Chemokines Involved in Classical HL

Chemokine	*Source in CHL*	*Receptor(s)*	*Main Target cells*
TARC (CCL17)	HRS cells	CCR4	Th2 cells
MDC (CCL22)	HRS cells	CCR4	Th2, NK, and dendritic cells
IP-10 (CXCL10)	(EBV+) HRS cells	CXCR3	Stimulated T and NK cells
MIP-1α (CCL3)	(EBV+) HRS cells	CCR5	T and NK cells
RANTES (CCL5)	T lymphocytes	CCR1,3,5	Monocytes, T lymphocytes, and eosinophils
Eotaxin (CCL11)	Fibroblasts	CCR3	Eosinophils and Th2 cells
IL-8 (CXCL8)	Monocytes, macrophages, and neutrophils	CXCR1,2	Neutrophils

involved in eosinophil recruitment *(32)*. IL-8 (CXCL8) attracts neutrophils and is produced by macrophages and neutrophils, but not by HRS cells *(33)*.

Several chemokines—including MDC, RANTES, IP-10, and eotaxin—may be natural substrates of CD26. This glycoprotein has intrinsic dipeptidyl-peptidase IV activity and can truncate its substrates, resulting in products with reduced chemotactic activity. Since the T lymphocytes surrounding the HRS cells lack CD26 expression, they are incapable of modulating the chemotaxis exerted by the HRS cells, in contrast to CD26-positive cells, such as Th1 cells and cytotoxic cells that are thus less sensitive to these chemokines *(28)*.

4.2. Cytokines

HRS cells produce a spectrum of cytokines that have a profound effect on the composition and state of activation of surrounding cells in the reactive infiltrate (Table 3). Two major immunosuppressive cytokines involved are IL-10 and transforming growth factor-β (TGF-β). IL-10 is a growth and differentiation factor for B cells, but more importantly, it inhibits Th1 responses by blocking IFN-γ and IL-2 production by Th1 lymphocytes. This cytokine is expressed more frequently and in higher amounts in EBV-positive CHL. The EBV BCRF1 protein shares 70% of its amino acid sequence with human IL-10 and exerts the same effects. However, this viral protein is not expressed in latent EBV infection, and the higher IL-10 level observed in EBV positive CHL is of human origin. Expression of human IL-10 is presumably stimulated by LMP-1 signaling and subsequent NF-κB activation *(34)*. IL-10 expression by the surrounding lymphocytes is also higher in EBV-positive cases *(35)*.

Table 3
Cytokines Involved in Classical HL

Cytokine	*Source in CHL*	*Target Cell*	*Biological Activity*
IL-1	HRS cells and cells in reactive infiltrate	T-lymphocytes Fibroblasts	Activation Proliferation Induction acute-phase proteins
IL-5	HRS cells	Eosinophils	Growth and differentiation
IL-6	(EBV+) HRS cells and surrounding lymphocytes	B lymphocytes	Plasma cell differentiation Production of IL-1, TNF-α, and acute-phase proteins
IL-7	HRS cells	T lymphocytes	Growth and survival
IL-9	HRS cells	HRS cells	Autocrine growth
IL-10	(EBV+) HRS cells and surrounding lymphocytes	Th1 lymphocytes	Blocks IFN-γ and IL-2 production
		B lymphocytes	Growth and differentiation
IL-12	Reactive cells, mainly in EBV+ cases	Th1 lymphocytes	Differentiation
IL-13	HRS cells	HRS cells	Autocrine growth MDC production
		Fibroblasts	Tissue fibrosis
IL-17	HRS cells	HRS cells	Autocrine growth
TGF-β	HRS cells, lymphocytes, and eosinophils	T lymphocytes NK cells B lymphocytes Fibroblasts	Inhibits activation Inhibits cytolytic activity Inhibits proliferation Tissue fibrosis
IFN-γ	Reactive cells and HRS cells; more in EBV+ cases	Macrophages	Activates phagocytosis and production of TNF-α, TGF-β and IL-1
TNF-α	HRS cells and cells in reactive infiltrate	HRS cells Fibroblasts	NF-κB activation Eotaxin production
LT-α	HRS cells	HRS cells	NF-κB activation
bFGF	HRS cells and reactive cells in NS CHL	Fibroblasts	Tissue fibrosis
M-CSF	HRS cells	Macrophages	Growth and differentiation

TGF-β is also a cytokine with strong immunosuppressive potency. It inhibits IL-2-dependent T-cell proliferation and blocks upregulation of the IL-2 receptor (CD25). Moreover, TGF-β inhibits the cytolytic activity of NK cells, and suppresses proliferation and immunoglobulin secretion by B lymphocytes. TGF-β secreted by HRS cells may in turn induce TGF-β production by lymphocytes, resulting in an autocrine-suppressed state of these lymphocytes *(36)*. Eosinophils in the reactive infiltrate are another source of TGF-β *(37)*.

In addition to being strongly immunosuppressive, TGF-β also induces fibroblast proliferation and synthesis of collagen. High TGF-β levels are especially found in NS HL and are believed to be responsible for the formation of the collagen bands in this subtype *(38)*. Other factors that are involved in tissue fibrosis are IL-13 and basic fibroblast growth factor (bFGF). The latter, like TGF-β, is expressed at higher levels in NS HL than in MC HL *(39)*.

HRS cells also secrete a number of cytokines that are not immunosuppressive, but do influence other cell types in the inflammatory infiltrate. IL-5 is essential for the growth and differentiation of eosinophilic granulocytes, and its expression correlates with tissue eosinophilia in CHL *(40)*. IL-5 can also act as a B-cell growth factor for some B cells, in man as well as in mice. IL-6 is produced by HRS cells in EBV-negative cases, and in higher amounts in EBV-positive cases. It is also occasionally expressed by lymphocytes in the reactive infiltrate and induces the maturation of B cells into plasma cells *(41)*. IL-7 may act as a growth factor for T lymphocytes. This cytokine may increase reactivity of surrounding cells to the HRS cells *(42)*.

Finally, HRS cells produce cytokines that act as autocrine growth factors. IL-9, IL-13, IL-17, and their respective receptors are expressed by HRS cells. These cytokines have been shown to stimulate growth in various CHL cell lines. IL-13 has multiple effects, and as already mentioned, also stimulates the synthesis of MDC and tissue fibrosis *(10)*.

Other cytokines that can be produced by cells in the reactive infiltrate are IL-12 and IFN-γ, which are both Th1-type cytokines. IL-12 can promote a Th1-type immune response and induce IFN-γ secretion, but its effects are inhibited by IL-4 and IL-10. IL-12 is especially expressed in EBV-positive CHL with highly variable expression levels *(43)*. IFN-γ enhances the ability of macrophages to phagocytose and kill microorganisms, and stimulates secretion of TNF-α, TGF-β, and IL-1. TNF-α can bind to the TNFRI and TNFRII receptors on HRS cells, and can activate NF-κB.

4.3. Cell-Surface Receptors

HRS cells express a large number of TNF-receptor-family glycoproteins, such as CD30, CD40, RANK, TNFRI, and TNFRII. Cells in the surrounding infiltrate express cell-surface-bound ligands for these receptors; reactive T cells express CD40L, and eosinophils and mast cells express CD30L. RANK-positive HRS cells co-express RANK ligand. The TNFRI and TNFRII ligands TNF-α and lymphotoxin-α (LT-α) both are secreted by HRS cells. TNF-α is also produced by the surrounding lymphocytes and macrophages *(10)* (Table 4). As mentioned previously, EBV-positive cases additionally express LMP1 that mimics a constitutively activated CD40 receptor.

HRS cells show cell-surface expression of the major histocompatibility complex (MHC) class II (HLA-DR) and a number of costimulatory and adhesion molecules—most notably, CD40, CD70, CD80, CD86, ICAM-1 (CD54), and

Table 4
Cell Surface Receptors and Ligands in Classical Hodgkin's Lymphoma

Receptor on HRS Cell	*Ligand*	*Cells in CHL-Expressing Ligand*
TNF Receptor Family		
TNFRI/TNFRII	TNF-α	HRS cells, reactive infiltrate
	LT-α	HRS cells
CD30	CD30L	Eosinophils, mast cells
CD40	CD40L	Surrounding T lymphocytes
RANK	RANKL	HRS cells
Adhesion		
LFA-3 (CD58)	CD2	T lymphocytes
ICAM-1 (CD54)	LFA-1 (CD11a/18)	T lymphocytes, granulocytes, macrophages
	CD43	All cells in reactive infiltrate
Antigen Presentation		
MHC class I	TCR/CD3 complex + CD8	Occasional T lymphocytes
MHC class II	TCR/CD3 complex + CD4	Majority of T lymphocytes
Costimulation		
CD70	CD27	T lymphocytes
CD80/CD86	CD28	T lymphocytes
	CTLA-4	Activated T lymphocytes
Other		
CD95	CD95L	HRS cells, occasional lymphocytes
CD95L	CD95	HRS cells, occasional lymphocytes

LFA-3 (CD58). HRS cells thus have characteristics of professional antigen-presenting cells (APC). It is remarkable that the HRS cells have generally lost the majority of B-cell markers (CD19, CD20, CD22, and CD79a), but consistently express antigen presentation and costimulatory molecules. This suggests that antigen presentation must play an important role in the pathogenesis of CHL. One possibility is that expression of a superantigen results in the attraction of a polyclonal population of lymphocytes. However, there is evidence that endogenously generated antigenic peptides may not be correctly loaded onto the MHC II molecule. Proper loading displaces the CLIP (class II-associated invariant-chain peptide protein) from the MHC II antigen-binding groove, but in fresh CHL lymph node biopsies, a subset of HRS cells express a substantial number of surface MHC II-CLIP complexes *(44)*. It is not clear whether the remaining MHC II dimers express antigenic peptides.

The MHC class I molecule is expressed less frequently than MHC class II. In fact, in most EBV-negative cases, it is entirely absent, and this may help the HRS cells escape cytotoxic T lymphocyte (CTL) responses. However, lack of MHC class I molecules on tumor cells generally leads to recognition and subsequent lysis by NK cells. EBV-positive HRS cells do express MHC class I in more than 75% of cases. LMP1 can induce expression of MHC class I and enhance antigen presentation *(45)*. It has also been shown that EBV antigenic peptides actually are presented, at least in CHL cell lines *(46)*. The antigens presented can evoke EBV-specific CTL responses in CHL patients *(47)*. Therefore, HRS cells need mechanisms to effectively evade these responses.

HRS cells express CD95L (FASL) and can act as veto cells. Thus, any cell that expresses CD95 (FAS) and that is in contact with a HRS cell is threatened to die from FAS-mediated apoptosis. Because activated Th1 cells and CTLs are more sensitive to this mechanism than Th2 cells, FAS-mediated apoptosis is yet another way for the HRS cells to shape the immune response in the reactive infiltrate *(48)*. HRS cells also express CD95 themselves but they appear to be resistant to FAS-mediated apoptosis. This resistance is caused by FAS mutations in a minority of cases. Overexpression of c-FLIP (cellular FLICE inhibitory protein) that can block the downstream FAS signaling pathway is probably the major mechanism *(49,50)*.

HRS cells in a large proportion of cases express CD15, but its pathogenetic relevance is unclear. CD15 is usually present in the non-sialylated form on HRS cells, and in this form has no known ligand. However, when CD15 is sialylated, it is able to bind to selectins. Sialylated CD15 on granulocytes is important in leukocyte rolling and subsequent diapedesis through endothelial cells. Sialylation of CD15 may confer the capacity to metastasize on the HRS cells, most notably to the bone marrow *(51)*.

HRS cells themselves are activated, as shown by the expression of activation markers CD25 (the IL-2 receptor) and CD71 (the transferrin receptor). The latter is necessary for internalizing iron, and its high expression in HRS cells correlates with the high iron demand of proliferating cells.

5. EVASION OF IMMUNE RESPONSES

As in any other malignancy, the HRS cells of CHL need mechanisms to evade immune responses. It should be clear that HRS cells employ a multitude of strategies to achieve this. First, HRS cells influence their microenvironment in order to shield themselves from CTLs and NK cells. They establish a Th2-like reactive infiltrate through secretion of the Th2 lymphocyte-attracting chemokines TARC and MDC. This Th2-like infiltrate suppresses Th1 responses and hinders interactions of Th1 lymphocytes, CTLs, and NK cells with the HRS cells.

In addition, the HRS cells also suppress Th1 activation directly by producing IL-10, especially in EBV-positive cases. Moreover, when an activated Th1 lymphocyte or CTL reaches a HRS cell, it can be killed by FAS-mediated apoptosis. In EBV-positive CHL, EBV specific CTL responses are largely evaded by not presenting the immunodominant EBNA3 antigenic peptide or, in a smaller number of cases, through the absence of or abnormal expression of the MHC class I molecule. LMP1 and LMP2, however, are subdominant targets for EBV-specific CTL responses, and are restricted to common MHC haplotypes *(52,53)*. Thus, less common MHC haplotypes in CHL patients may contribute to ineffectiveness of recognizing HRS cells.

Finally, the T lymphocytes in the reactive infiltrate are influenced in such a way that they cannot become fully activated. Attenuation of activation is caused by TGF-β, and there may be another contributing mechanism. This other mechanism requires that HRS cells do present a still unidentified MHC class II restricted antigen. Signals that are transduced through the T-cell receptor need a costimulatory signal to induce full activation. This costimulation can be provided through the CD80 and CD86 that are present on HRS cells. Usually, T cells are positively costimulated through CD28. However, when the T cell expresses CTLA-4 instead of CD28, costimulation leads to inhibition of the T-cell-receptor signal cascade. CTLA-4 is indeed expressed on CD4-positive lymphocytes in the reactive infiltrate in CHL *(54, 55)*. It has also been shown that lymphocytes from peripheral blood in CHL express more CTLA-4 upon stimulation than controls *(56)*.

6. REVERSE IMMUNE SURVEILLANCE

Although evasion of immune responses is clearly important for the survival of HRS cells, a trophic effect of the immune response is probably even more critical in the pathogenesis of CHL. The concept of reverse immune surveillance implies that recognition of tumor-cell antigens and a response by the host immune system constitute a requirement for tumor growth *(57)*.

One very important characteristic of HRS cells is the constitutive activation of NF-κB. TNF receptor signaling is likely to be responsible for this activation in the majority of cases. Assuming that constitutive activation of NF-κB is crucial for the survival of the HRS cells, constitutive TNF-receptor engagement is then a prerequisite. Cells in the reactive infiltrate (e.g., CD40L on lymphocytes) provide cell-surface-bound ligands for the TNF receptor as well as soluble ligands (TNF-α by lymphocytes and macrophages). Although HRS cells also produce TNF-receptor ligands themselves, this is often insufficient for continuous stimulation. Consequently, HRS cells really are critically dependent on the reactive infiltrate.

A practical observation underscoring the importance of reverse immune surveillance in CHL is the difficulty to establish HRS cell lines. When trying to culture a primary CHL affected lymph-node cell suspension, we will find that cells can be maintained for only a limited number of weeks. As soon as the lymphocyte numbers in the culture drop to a critical level, the HRS cells die. Many attempts in the past only resulted in establishment of lymphoblastoid cell lines from EBV transformed bystander B lymphocytes that are unrelated to the HRS cells. Indeed, the 15 CHL cell lines that have been established to date, all originated from advanced stage and vigorously treated CHL cases, mostly from pleural effusions or from peripheral blood *(58)*. The HRS cells obtained from these sites are likely to have progressed to grow independent of reactive cells. A major criticism on the use of HL cell lines as an in vitro model for the disease is that these cell lines may not be fully representative of HRS cells.

7. IMMUNOTHERAPEUTIC APPROACHES

HL was the first malignant lymphoma for which effective radiation and chemotherapy treatment was available. Advances in radiation therapy and a later combination with polychemotherapy have improved survival rates in HL dramatically. Today, the cure rate approaches 80%, and HL is the lymphoma with the best prognosis. Nevertheless, there is still room for improvement. Conventional treatment regimens have high rates of late adverse effects, such as occurrence of second malignancies and cardiovascular disease. Also, for patients with a relapse of CHL the long-term prognosis is poor *(59)*. Clinical trials with various immunotherapeutic approaches have demonstrated some clinical response in patients with advanced-stage (Ann Arbor stages III and IV in which multiple lymph nodes on both sides of the diaphragm or extranodal sites respectively are affected) and relapsed CHL. In most trials, complete remissions are rare and partial remission rates usually lie within the range of 5–20%. It is conceivable that the clinical efficacy in these trials is reduced by high tumor load. Immunotherapeutic approaches may be more effective in eradicating residual HRS cells after primary conventional treatment of bulky disease *(60)*.

Most immunotherapeutic strategies that have been explored focus on targeting the HRS cells. Antibodies that are specific for markers on HRS cells have been fused to toxins such as Pseudomonas exotoxin A, ricin A, angiogenin, and ribosome-inactivating proteins. In most approaches, these so-called immunotoxins are directed at CD30, because this molecule has a high expression on HRS cells in virtually all CHL cases. Moreover, only a minority of non-neoplastic cells expresses CD30, most notably a small number of activated T or B lymphocytes. Other molecules that have been occasionally targeted are CD25 and CD80 *(61)*.

Also epitopes outside the HRS cells have been targeted. Ferritin is a tumor marker associated with CHL and is present in the tumor interstitium, especially when tumor size exceeds 1 cm. Application of radiolabeled anti-ferritin antibodies reduces lymphomatous mass by radiation-induced damage and not by immunologic effects, as unlabeled antibodies do not reduce tumor size *(62)*. Another approach has been used in mice that bear a CHL cell line tumor and has been directed at the vasculature of the tumor. The target antigen vascular cell adhesion molecule (VCAM-1) is expressed on endothelium and is upregulated by TNF-α and IL-1. A murine VCAM-1 antibody covalently linked to human tissue factor was found to specifically target to a CHL cell line tumor in mice. The human tissue-factor component of this so-called coaguligand induces thrombosis and subsequent infarction of the tumor, resulting in retarded tumor growth *(63)*.

These immunotherapeutic approaches use specific targets to deliver locally damaging agents. However, given the role of the reactive infiltrate in CHL, the immune system itself can also be used to damage the HRS cells *(64)*.

7.1. Potentiation of the Immune Response

Bispecific monoclonal antibodies (MAbs) for example with specificity for both CD30 and CD16, can specifically potentiate immune responses. CD16 is the Fcγ receptor IIIA, and is present on NK cells, macrophages, and activated monocytes. Application of the CD30/CD16 bispecific antibodies recruits these cells to the HRS cells, and CD16 engagement induces the direct release of cytotoxic molecules by these cells *(65)*. A similar approach utilizes a combination of CD30/CD3 and CD30/CD28-bispecific antibodies. When administered simultaneously, these antibodies can activate and properly costimulate lymphocytes in the direct environment of the HRS cells, resulting in proliferation, increased IL-2 production, and antigen-specific cytotoxicity *(66,67)*.

In EBV-positive CHL, EBV-specific CTLs can be applied *(68)*. Autologous EBV-specific CTLs are activated in vitro to recognize LMP1- and/or LMP2-derived antigenic peptides. This can be achieved by stimulating these CTLs in the presence of autologous EBV-infected lymphoblastoid cell lines or in the presence of antigen presenting DC *(69–72)*. Results with this approach have been suboptimal, and this has been ascribed to the evasion strategies observed in CHL. Therefore, attempts have been made to equip the EBV-specific CTLs with additional mechanisms to escape from the immunomodulating influences of the HRS cells. For example, EBV-specific CTLs have been transduced to express the dominant-negative TGF-β type II receptor, thus escaping the suppressing effect of TGF-β *(73)*.

7.2. Attenuation of the Immune Response

To date, no attempts have been made to specifically attenuate the immune response in CHL. However, a portion of the effect of classical radiotherapy and chemotherapy may involve disruption of the inflammatory background, since activated T cells are extremely sensitive to low doses of irradiation and steroids. The relative importance of this effect is impossible to measure.

Although attenuation of the immune response theoretically may be as efficient as potentiation of the immune response, it is difficult to determine which targets are most appropriate for immunotherapy. One possibility is to neutralize the effects of the chemokines TARC and MDC by neutralizing antibodies or antibodies directed at the CCR4 receptor. Alternatively, the immunosuppressive cytokines TGF-β and IL-10 may be blocked with antibodies or anti-sense probes. Yet another approach might involve blocking of the supposed antigen presentation by HRS cells. Finally, interfering with TNF receptor and TNF-receptor ligand interactions may break the cycle of constitutive NF-κB activation.

8. SUMMARY

CHL is a hematological malignancy in which an intricate network of immunological interactions appears to be crucially involved. The neoplastic HRS cells use a variety of strategies to evade immune reactions, but also shape the immune response to their own benefit. Immunotherapeutic approaches can be used to potentiate the immune response and direct this response to the HRS cells. Theoretically, attenuation of immune responses should also be effective. It is difficult to predict which of both immunotherapeutic approaches will be most effective in the end. Immunotherapy in CHL is indeed at the crossroads, and the paths have only partially been explored. Many potential immunotherapeutic strategies have not been investigated properly or are not yet developed. Improved knowledge about the pathogenesis of CHL is needed to set the horizon. The development of reliable models of human HL in severe combined immunodeficiency (SCID) mice is an important prerequisite to test such strategies.

REFERENCES

1. Stein H, Delsol G, Pileri S, Said J, Mann R, Poppema S, et al. (2001) Classical Hodgkin lymphoma. In: World Health *Organization Classification of Tumours. Pathology and Genetics of Tumours of Haematopoietic and Lymphoid Tissues* (Jaffe ES, Harris NL, Stein H, Vardiman JW, eds.), IARCPress, Lyon, France, pp. 244–253.
2. Stein H, Delsol G, Pileri S, Said J, Mann R, Poppema S, et al. (2001) Nodular lymphocyte predominant Hodgkin Lymphoma. In: *World Health Organization Classification of Tumours. Pathology and Genetics of Tumours of Haematopoietic and Lymphoid Tissues* (Jaffe ES, Harris NL, Stein H, Vardiman JW, eds.), IARCPress, Lyon, France, pp. 240–243.
3. Drexler HG. Recent results on the biology of Hodgkin and Reed-Sternberg cells. I. Biopsy material. Leuk *Lymphoma* 1992;8(4–5):283–313.
4. Kanzler H, Kuppers R, Hansmann ML, Rajewsky K. Hodgkin and Reed-Sternberg cells in Hodgkin's disease represent the outgrowth of a dominant tumor clone derived from (crippled) germinal center B cells. *J Exp Med* 1996;184(4):1495–1505.

5. Hertel CB, Zhou XG, Hamilton-Dutoit SJ, Junker S. Loss of B cell identity correlates with loss of B cell-specific transcription factors in Hodgkin/Reed-Sternberg cells of classical Hodgkin lymphoma. *Oncogene* 2002;21(32):4908–4920.
6. Theil J, Laumen H, Marafioti T, Hummel M, Lenz G, Wirth T, et al. Defective octamer-dependent transcription is responsible for silenced immunoglobulin transcription in Reed-Sternberg cells. *Blood* 2001;97(10):3191–3196.
7. Re D, Muschen M, Ahmadi T, Wickenhauser C, Staratschek-Jox A, Holtick U, et al. Oct-2 and Bob-1 deficiency in Hodgkin and Reed Sternberg cells. *Cancer Res* 2001;61(5): 2080–2084.
8. Stein H, Marafioti T, Foss HD, Laumen H, Hummel M, Anagnostopoulos I, et al. Down-regulation of BOB.1/OBF.1 and Oct2 in classical Hodgkin disease but not in lymphocyte predominant Hodgkin disease correlates with immunoglobulin transcription. *Blood* 2001;97(2):496–501.
9. Bargou RC, Emmerich F, Krappmann D, Bommert K, Mapara MY, Arnold W, et al. Constitutive nuclear factor-kappaB-RelA activation is required for proliferation and survival of Hodgkin's disease tumor cells. *J Clin Investig* 1997;100(12):2961–2969.
10. Skinnider BF, Mak TW. The role of cytokines in classical Hodgkin lymphoma. *Blood* 2002;99(12):4283–4297.
11. Izban KF, Ergin M, Martinez RL, Alkan S. Expression of the tumor necrosis factor receptor-associated factors (TRAFs) 1 and 2 is a characteristic feature of Hodgkin and Reed-Sternberg cells. *Mod Pathol* 2000;13(12):1324–1331.
12. Murray PG, Flavell JR, Baumforth KR, Toomey SM, Lowe D, Crocker J, et al. Expression of the tumour necrosis factor receptor-associated factors 1 and 2 in Hodgkin's disease. *J Pathol* 2001;194(2):158–164.
13. Jungnickel B, Staratschek-Jox A, Auninger A, Spieker T, Wolf J, Diehl V, et al. Clonal deleterious mutations in the IkappaBalpha gene in the malignant cells in Hodgkin's lymphoma. *J Exp Med* 2000;191(2):395–402.
14. Cabannes E, Khan G, Aillet F, Jarrett RF, Hay RT. Mutations in the IkBa gene in Hodgkin's disease suggest a tumour suppressor role for IkappaBalpha. *Oncogene* 1999;18(20): 3063–3070.
15. Emmerich F, Meiser M, Hummel M, Demel G, Foss HD, Jundt F, et al. Overexpression of I kappa B alpha without inhibition of NF-kappaB activity and mutations in the I kappa B alpha gene in Reed-Sternberg cells. *Blood* 1999;94(9):3129–3134.
16. Krappmann D, Emmerich F, Kordes U, Scharschmidt E, Dorken B, Scheidereit C. Molecular mechanisms of constitutive NF-kappaB/Rel activation in Hodgkin/Reed-Sternberg cells. *Oncogene* 1999;18(4):943–953.
17. Jarrett RF, MacKenzie J. Epstein-Barr virus and other candidate viruses in the pathogenesis of Hodgkin's disease. *Semin Hematol* 1999;36(3):260–269.
18. Caldwell RG, Wilson JB, Anderson SJ, Longnecker R. Epstein-Barr virus LMP2A drives B cell development and survival in the absence of normal B cell receptor signals. *Immunity* 1998;9(3):405–411.
19. Izumi KM, Kieff ED. The Epstein-Barr virus oncogene product latent membrane protein 1 engages the tumor necrosis factor receptor-associated death domain protein to mediate B lymphocyte growth transformation and activate NF-kappaB. *Proc Natl Acad Sci USA* 1997; 94(23):12,592–12,597.
20. Fruehling S, Longnecker R. The immunoreceptor tyrosine-based activation motif of Epstein-Barr virus LMP2A is essential for blocking BCR-mediated signal transduction. *Virology* 1997;235(2):241–251.
21. Miller CL, Burkhardt AL, Lee JH, Stealey B, Longnecker R, Bolen JB, et al. Integral membrane protein 2 of Epstein-Barr virus regulates reactivation from latency through dominant negative effects on protein- tyrosine kinases. *Immunity* 1995;2(2):155–166.

22. Weiss LM. Epstein-Barr virus and Hodgkin's disease. *Curr Oncol Rep* 2000;2(2):199–204.
23. Poppema S. Immunology of Hodgkin's disease. *Baillieres Clin Haematol* 1996;9(3): 447–457.
24. Poppema S, Potters M, Visser L, van den Berg AM. Immune escape mechanisms in Hodgkin's disease. *Ann Oncol* 1998;9(Suppl 5):S21–S24.
25. Poppema S. The nature of the lymphocytes surrounding Reed-Sternberg cells in nodular lymphocyte predominance and in other types of Hodgkin's disease. *Am J Pathol* 1989;135(2): 351–357.
26. van den Berg A, Visser L, Poppema S. High expression of the CC chemokine TARC in Reed-Sternberg cells. A possible explanation for the characteristic T-cell infiltrate in Hodgkin's lymphoma. *Am J Pathol* 1999;154(6):1685–1691.
27. Ohshima K, Tutiya T, Yamaguchi T, Suzuki K, Suzumiya J, Kawasaki C, et al. Infiltration of Th1 and Th2 lymphocytes around Hodgkin and Reed-Sternberg (H&RS) cells in Hodgkin disease: Relation with expression of CXC and CC chemokines on H&RS cells. *Int J Cancer* 2002;98(4):567–572.
28. Maggio EM, van den BA, Visser L, Diepstra A, Kluiver J, Emmens R, et al. Common and differential chemokine expression patterns in rs cells of NLP, EBV positive and negative classical hodgkin lymphomas. *Int J Cancer* 2002;99(5):665–672.
29. Imai T, Chantry D, Raport CJ, Wood CL, Nishimura M, Godiska R, et al. Macrophage-derived chemokine is a functional ligand for the CC chemokine receptor 4. *J Biol Chem* 1998;273(3):1764–1768.
30. Andrew DP, Chang MS, McNinch J, Wathen ST, Rihanek M, Tseng J, et al. STCP-1 (MDC) CC chemokine acts specifically on chronically activated Th2 lymphocytes and is produced by monocytes on stimulation with Th2 cytokines IL-4 and IL-13. *J Immunol* 1998; 161(9):5027–5038.
31. Teruya-Feldstein J, Jaffe ES, Burd PR, Kingma DW, Setsuda JE, Tosato G. Differential chemokine expression in tissues involved by Hodgkin's disease: direct correlation of eotaxin expression and tissue eosinophilia. *Blood* 1999;93(8):2463–2470.
32. Jundt F, Anagnostopoulos I, Bommert K, Emmerich F, Muller G, Foss HD, et al. Hodgkin/Reed-Sternberg cells induce fibroblasts to secrete eotaxin, a potent chemoattractant for T cells and eosinophils. *Blood* 1999;94(6):2065–2071.
33. Foss HD, Herbst H, Gottstein S, Demel G, Araujo I, Stein H. Interleukin-8 in Hodgkin's disease. Preferential expression by reactive cells and association with neutrophil density. *Am J Pathol* 1996;148(4):1229–1236.
34. Herbst H, Foss HD, Samol J, Araujo I, Klotzbach H, Krause H, et al. Frequent expression of interleukin-10 by Epstein-Barr virus-harboring tumor cells of Hodgkin's disease. *Blood* 1996;87(7):2918–2929.
35. Dukers DF, Jaspars LH, Vos W, Oudejans JJ, Hayes D, Cillessen S, et al. Quantitative immunohistochemical analysis of cytokine profiles in Epstein-Barr virus-positive and -negative cases of Hodgkin's disease. *J Pathol* 2000;190(2):143–149.
36. Obberghen-Schilling E, Roche NS, Flanders KC, Sporn MB, Roberts AB. Transforming growth factor beta 1 positively regulates its own expression in normal and transformed cells. *J Biol Chem* 1988;263(16):7741–7746.
37. Kadin M, Butmarc J, Elovic A, Wong D. Eosinophils are the major source of transforming growth factor-beta 1 in nodular sclerosing Hodgkin's disease. *Am J Pathol* 1993; 142(1):11–16.
38. Kadin ME, Agnarsson BA, Ellingsworth LR, Newcom SR. Immunohistochemical evidence of a role for transforming growth factor beta in the pathogenesis of nodular sclerosing Hodgkin's disease. *Am J Pathol* 1990;136(6):1209–1214.
39. Ohshima K, Sugihara M, Suzumiya J, Haraoka S, Kanda M, Shimazaki K, et al. Basic fibroblast growth factor and fibrosis in Hodgkin's disease. *Pathol Res Pract* 1999;195(3):149–155.

40. Samoszuk M, Nansen L. Detection of interleukin-5 messenger RNA in Reed-Sternberg cells of Hodgkin's disease with eosinophilia. *Blood* 1990;75(1):13–16.
41. Herbst H, Samol J, Foss HD, Raff T, Niedobitek G. Modulation of interleukin-6 expression in Hodgkin and Reed-Sternberg cells by Epstein-Barr virus. *J Pathol* 1997; 182(3):299–306.
42. Foss HD, Hummel M, Gottstein S, Ziemann K, Falini B, Herbst H, et al. Frequent expression of IL-7 gene transcripts in tumor cells of classical Hodgkin's disease. *Am J Pathol* 1995;146(1):33–39.
43. Schwaller J, Tobler A, Niklaus G, Hurwitz N, Hennig I, Fey MF, et al. Interleukin-12 expression in human lymphomas and nonneoplastic lymphoid disorders. *Blood* 1995; 85(8):2182–2188.
44. Bosshart H, Jarrett RF. Deficient major histocompatibility complex class II antigen presentation in a subset of Hodgkin's disease tumor cells. *Blood* 1998;92(7):2252–2259.
45. Rowe M, Khanna R, Jacob CA, Argaet V, Kelly A, Powis S, et al. Restoration of endogenous antigen processing in Burkitt's lymphoma cells by Epstein-Barr virus latent membrane protein-1: coordinate up-regulation of peptide transporters and HLA-class I antigen expression. *Eur J Immunol* 1995;25(5):1374–1384.
46. Lee SP, Constandinou CM, Thomas WA, Croom-Carter D, Blake NW, Murray PG, et al. Antigen presenting phenotype of Hodgkin Reed-Sternberg cells: analysis of the HLA class I processing pathway and the effects of interleukin-10 on epstein-barr virus-specific cytotoxic T-cell recognition. *Blood* 1998;92(3):1020–1030.
47. Chapman AL, Rickinson AB, Thomas WA, Jarrett RF, Crocker J, Lee SP. Epstein-Barr virus-specific cytotoxic T lymphocyte responses in the blood and tumor site of Hodgkin's disease patients: implications for a T-cell-based therapy. *Cancer Res* 2001;61(16):6219–6226.
48. Poppema S, Potters M, Emmens R, Visser L, van den Berg A. Immune reactions in classical Hodgkin's lymphoma. *Semin Hematol* 1999;36(3):253–259.
49. Thomas RK, Kallenborn A, Wickenhauser C, Schultze JL, Draube A, Vockerodt M, et al. Constitutive expression of c-FLIP in Hodgkin and Reed-Sternberg cells. *Am J Pathol* 2002;160(4):1521–1528.
50. Maggio E, van den Berg A, de Jong D, Diepstra A, Poppema S. Low frequency of FAS mutations in Reed-Sternberg cells of Hodgkin Lymphoma. *Am J Pathol* 2003;162(1):29–35.
51. Benharroch D, Dima E, Levy A, Ohana-Malka O, Ariad S, Prinsloo I, et al. Differential expression of sialyl and non-sialyl-CD15 antigens on Hodgkin-Reed-Sternberg cells: significance in Hodgkin's disease. *Leuk Lymphoma* 2000;39(1-2):185–194.
52. Lee SP, Thomas WA, Murray RJ, Khanim F, Kaur S, Young LS, et al. HLA A2.1-restricted cytotoxic T cells recognizing a range of Epstein-Barr virus isolates through a defined epitope in latent membrane protein LMP2. *J Virol* 1993;67(12):7428–7435.
53. Lee SP, Tierney RJ, Thomas WA, Brooks JM, Rickinson AB. Conserved CTL epitopes within EBV latent membrane protein 2: a potential target for CTL-based tumor therapy. *J Immunol* 1997;158(7):3325–3334.
54. Vandenborre K, Van Gool SW, Kasran A, Ceuppens JL, Boogaerts MA, Vandenberghe P. Interaction of CTLA-4 (CD152) with CD80 or CD86 inhibits human T-cell activation. *Immunology* 1999; 98(3):413–421.
55. Vandenborre K, Delabie J, Boogaerts MA, De Vos R, Lorre K, Wolf-Peeters C, et al. Human CTLA-4 is expressed in situ on T lymphocytes in germinal centers, in cutaneous graft-versus-host disease, and in Hodgkin's disease. *Am J Pathol* 1998;152(4):963–973.
56. Kosmaczewska A, Frydecka I, Bocko D, Ciszak L, Teodorowska R. Correlation of blood lymphocyte CTLA-4 (CD152) induction in Hodgkin's disease with proliferative activity, interleukin 2 and interferon-gamma production. *Br J Haematol* 2002;118(1):202–209.
57. Ponzio NM, Thorbecke GJ. Requirement for reverse immune surveillance for the growth of germinal center-derived murine lymphomas. *Semin Cancer Biol* 2000;10(5):331–340.

58. Drexler HG. Recent results on the biology of Hodgkin and Reed-Sternberg cells. II. Continuous cell lines. *Leuk Lymphoma* 1993;9(1-2):1–25.
59. Fung HC, Nademanee AP. Approach to Hodgkin's lymphoma in the new millennium. *Hematol Oncol* 2002;20(1):1–15.
60. Schnell R, Borchmann P, Schulz H, Engert A. Current strategies of antibody-based treatment in Hodgkin's disease. *Ann Oncol* 2002;13(Suppl 1):57–66.
61. Barth S, Huhn M, Matthey B, Tawadros S, Schnell R, Schinkothe T, et al. Ki-4(scFv)-ETA′, a new recombinant anti-CD30 immunotoxin with highly specific cytotoxic activity against disseminated Hodgkin tumors in SCID mice. *Blood* 2000;95(12):3909–3914.
62. Vriesendorp HM, Quadri SM. Radiolabeled immunoglobulin therapy in patients with Hodgkin's disease. *Cancer Biother Radiopharm* 2000;15(5):431–445.
63. Ran S, Gao B, Duffy S, Watkins L, Rote N, Thorpe PE. Infarction of solid Hodgkin's tumors in mice by antibody-directed targeting of tissue factor to tumor vasculature. *Cancer Res* 1998;58(20):4646–4653.
64. Huhn M, Sasse S, Tur MK, Matthey B, Schinkothe T, Rybak SM, et al. Human angiogenin fused to human CD30 ligand (ang-CD30L) exhibits specific cytotoxicity against CD30-positive lymphoma. *Cancer Res* 2001;61(24):8737–8742.
65. Hartmann F, Renner C, Jung W, Pfreundschuh M. Anti-CD16/CD30 bispecific antibodies as possible treatment for refractory Hodgkin's disease. *Leuk Lymphoma* 1998; 31(3–4):385–392.
66. Renner C, Jung W, Sahin U, Denfeld R, Pohl C, Trumper L, et al. Cure of xenografted human tumors by bispecific monoclonal antibodies and human T cells. *Science* 1994; 264(5160):833–835.
67. da Costa L, Renner C, Hartmann F, Pfreundschuh M. Immune recruitment by bispecific antibodies for the treatment of Hodgkin disease. *Cancer Chemother Pharmacol* 2000; 46(Suppl):S33–S36.
68. Finberg RW. Epstein-Barr virus-specific T cells for the management of Epstein-Barr virus lymphomas. *Curr Opin Oncol* 2001;13(5):349–353.
69. Gahn B, Siller-Lopez F, Pirooz AD, Yvon E, Gottschalk S, Longnecker R, et al. Adenoviral gene transfer into dendritic cells efficiently amplifies the immune response to LMP2A antigen: A potential treatment strategy for Epstein-Barr virus-positive Hodgkin's lymphoma. *Int J Cancer* 2001;93(5):706–713.
70. Su Z, Peluso MV, Raffegerst SH, Schendel DJ, Roskrow MA. The generation of LMP2a-specific cytotoxic T lymphocytes for the treatment of patients with Epstein-Barr virus-positive Hodgkin disease. *Eur J Immunol* 2001;31(3):947–958.
71. Sing AP, Ambinder RF, Hong DJ, Jensen M, Batten W, Petersdorf E, et al. Isolation of Epstein-Barr virus (EBV)-specific cytotoxic T lymphocytes that lyse Reed-Sternberg cells: implications for immune-mediated therapy of EBV+ Hodgkin's disease. *Blood* 1997; 89(6):1978–1986.
72. Roskrow MA, Suzuki N, Gan Y, Sixbey JW, Ng CY, Kimbrough S, et al. Epstein-Barr virus (EBV)-specific cytotoxic T lymphocytes for the treatment of patients with EBV-positive relapsed Hodgkin's disease. *Blood* 1998;91(8):2925–2934.
73. Bollard CM, Rossig C, Calonge MJ, Huls MH, Wagner HJ, Massague J, et al. Adapting a transforming growth factor beta-related tumor protection strategy to enhance antitumor immunity. *Blood* 2002;99(9):3179–3187.

18 Lung Cancer and Immune Dysfunction

Steven M. Dubinett, MD,
Sherven Sharma, PhD, *Min Huang,* MD,
Jenny T. Mao, MD, *and Raj K. Batra,* MD

CONTENTS

1. THE PROBLEM OF LUNG CANCER

Lung cancer accounts for more than 28% of all cancer deaths each year, and is the leading cause of cancer-related mortality in the United States *(1)*. Despite focused research in conventional therapies, the 5-year survival rate remains at 14%, and has improved only minimally in the past 25 years. Newly discovered molecular mechanisms in the pathogenesis of lung cancer provide novel opportunities for targeted therapies of non-small-cell lung cancer (NSCLC) *(2,3)*. Immune-based targeted therapies have focused on the elicitation of specific

From: *Current Clinical Oncology: Cancer Immunotherapy at the Crossroads: How Tumors Evade Immunity and What Can Be Done*
Edited by: J. H. Finke and R. M. Bukowski © Humana Press Inc., Totowa, NJ

tumor antigen-directed responses. Although various methods of immune stimulation have been attempted for the treatment of lung cancer, none have proven to be reliably effective *(4)*. In contrast, immune-based therapies have proven more successful in melanoma and renal cell carcinoma (RCC) *(5,6)*, leading to the misconception that thoracic malignancies are nonimmunogenic and are not amenable to immunologic interventions. However, protective immunity is now known to be generated against non-immunogenic murine tumors *(7,8)*. These studies suggest that a tumor's apparent lack of immunogenicity indicates a failure to elicit an effective host response rather than a lack of tumor antigen (TA) expression *(9,10)*. Accordingly, a new paradigm has emerged that focuses on generating antitumor responses by therapeutic vaccination *(11,12)*. In this setting, vaccination refers to an intervention that unmasks TAs, leading to generation of specific host-immune responses against the tumor.

Despite the identification of a repertoire of TAs, hurdles persist in the pathway to finding successful immune-based therapies. First, an immune response to a malignancy may not develop as a result of tolerance *(13)*. It has been suggested that the single most important determinant of tumor rejection antigen potency is the avidity of the cognate cytotoxic T lymphocyte (CTL) *(14)*. The tolerogenic response appears to eliminate high-avidity T cells, but spares the low-avidity CTL effector populations *(15)*. Thus, the most effective cancer immunotherapies may be those interventions that significantly activate the low-avidity T-cell populations. A second major problem, well-documented in thoracic and other malignancies, is the active immune suppression induced by the tumor itself *(13)*. Here, we review tumor-induced immune dysfunction in lung cancer.

2. CYTOKINE NETWORKS IN IMMUNE DYSFUNCTION IN LUNG CANCER

The effective elicitation of specific immune responses requires the regulated balance of cytokine production that serves to direct both antigen presentation and effector responses. Lung-cancer cells elaborate immunosuppressive mediators, including type 2 cytokines, PGE2 and transforming growth factor β (TGF-β) that may interfere directly with cell-mediated antitumor immune responses *(16–19)*. In addition to producing their own suppressive factors, tumor cells may also direct surrounding inflammatory cells to release suppressive cytokines in the tumor milieu *(17,20)*. It has previously been demonstrated that NSCLC cells express a Th2 cytokine pattern *(18)*. In particular, interleukin (IL)-10 is the predominant Th2 cytokine expressed by the tumor cells. Effective cell-mediated immune responses depend on IL-12 and IFN-γ to mediate a range of biological effects that facilitate anticancer immunity. In contrast, Type 2 cytokines inhibit Type 1 cytokines, and can suppress cell-mediated antitumor immune responses *(21)*. In both patients and murine tumor models, progressive tumor growth has often been associated with a marked limitation in Type 1 cytokine production, along with upregulated IL-10 and other Type 2 cytokines *(22–26)*. IL-10 inhibits a broad array of immune parameters in vitro, including pro-inflammatory cytokine production by macrophages *(27)*, antigen (Ag) presentation *(28)*, Ag-specific T-cell proliferation *(29,30)*, and type 1 cytokine production by T cells *(31,32)*. Therefore, elevated IL-10 production at the tumor site in vivo may potently suppress Ag presentation, enabling the tumor to escape immune detection *(18,33)*. In addition to secreting their own suppressive mediators, tumor cells may also signal surrounding inflammatory cells to release suppressive cytokines, such as IL-10 *(34)*. To evaluate the impact of enhanced T cell-derived IL-10 on antitumor immunity in vivo, Sharma et al. *(21)* and Hagenbaugh et al. *(35)* utilized a novel transgenic mouse model in which IL-10 is expressed under the control of the IL-2 promoter. Lewis lung carcinoma cells (3LL) grew more rapidly in IL-10 transgenic mice compared with their control littermates *(35)*. Transfer of T cells from IL-10 transgenic mice to control littermates transferred the IL-10 immunosuppressive effect and led to enhanced 3LL tumor growth. In addition to changes in T cell-mediated immunity, professional APC from IL-10 transgenic mice were found to have significantly suppressed capacity to induce major histocompatibility complex (MHC) alloreactivity, CTL responses, and IL-12 production. Tumor Ag-pulsed dendritic cells (DC) from IL-10 transgenic mice also failed to generate antitumor reactivity. These results suggest that increased levels of T-cell-derived IL-10 severely impair antitumor immunity in vivo because of defects in both T cell and APC function *(21)*. These preclinical investigations are consistent with findings from clinical studies. For example, Hidalgo et al. found increased PGE2 levels and enhanced monocyte derived IL-10 in NSCLC patients *(36)*. Studies suggest that IL-10 may be a poor prognostic factor in human NSCLC *(37–39)*. This has been postulated to be the result of immune suppression *(16,17,40)* or promotion of angiogenesis *(41)*. Therapeutic immunosuppression has long been known to cause a marked increase in non-melanoma skin cancer *(42)*. More recently, increased incidence of several epithelial tumors, including lung cancer has also been linked to immunosuppression *(43)*.

3. TUMOR COX-2-DEPENDENT REGULATION OF IMMUNE SUPPRESSION IN LUNG CANCER

Cyclooxygenase (also referred to as prostaglandin endoperoxidase or prostaglandin G/H synthase) is the rate-limiting enzyme for the production of prostaglandins (PGs) and thromboxanes from free arachidonic acid *(44)*. The enzyme is bifunctional, with fatty acid cyclooxygenase (producing PGG2 from arachidonic acid) and PG hydroperoxidase activities (converting PGG2 to PGH2). Two forms of cyclooxygenase (COX) have now been described: a constitutively expressed enzyme, COX-1, that is present in most cells and tissues, and an inducible isoenzyme, COX-2 (also known as PGS-2), expressed in response to cytokines, growth factors, and other stimuli *(44–47)*. COX-2 has been reported to be constitutively overexpressed in a variety of malignancies *(47–53)*; our studies and others have reported that COX-2 is often constitutively elevated in human NSCLC *(16,54–57)*. Mounting evidence from several studies indicates that tumor COX-2 activity has a multifaceted role in conferring the malignant and metastatic phenotypes. Multiple genetic alterations are necessary for lung-cancer invasion and metastasis, COX-2 may be a central element in orchestrating this process *(16,55–58)*. Studies indicate that overexpression of COX-2 is associated with resistance to apoptosis *(59–62)*, angiogenesis *(50,63–65)*, decreased host immunity *(16,40)*, and enhanced invasion and metastasis *(66)*. In the first report of COX-2 overexpression in human lung cancer, it was observed that the tumor-derived, high-level PGE2 production mediated dysregulation of host immunity by altering the balance of interleukins 10 and 12 *(16)*. Indeed, specific inhibition of COX-2 led to significant in vivo tumor reduction in murine lung-cancer models *(40,64)*. Tumor-cell overexpression of COX-2 strongly upregulates lymphocyte and macrophage IL-10 in a PGE2-dependent manner *(16,17)* (Fig. 1). Recently, other studies have corroborated and expanded on these initial findings documenting the importance of COX-2 expression in lung cancer *(54–57,67,68)*. COX-2 activity can be detected throughout the progression of a pre-malignant lesion to the metastatic phenotype *(55)*. Markedly higher COX-2 expression was observed in lung-cancer lymph-node metastasis and compared to primary adenocarcinoma *(55)*. In addition to these direct effects on immune function, it was recently reported that stable overexpression of COX-2 in NSCLC results in upregulation of CD44, the cell-surface receptor for hyaluronate *(69)*. A CD44-dependent increase in invasion in Matrigel matrix assays was also documented. In contrast, abrogation of tumor-COX-2 expression results in decreased PGE2 production, diminished CD44 expression, and decreased invasion *(69)*. Khuri et al. recently reported that COX-2 overexpression appears to portend a shorter survival among patients with early-stage NSCLC *(70)*. COX-2 expression in specimens from 160 patients with stage I NSCLC was evaluated. The strength of COX-2 expression was associated with a decreased overall survival rate (p = 0.001) and a diminished disease-free survival rate (p = 0.022). These reports, together with studies documenting an increase in COX-2 expression in precursor lesions *(56,57)*, suggest the involvement of COX-2 overexpression in the pathogenesis of lung cancer. Epidemiological studies showing a decreased incidence of lung cancer in subjects who regularly use aspirin also support this hypothesis *(71–73)*. In human lung-cancer cell lines, tumor COX-2 strongly dysregulates host cell-mediated antitumor immunity by creating an imbalance in interleukins 10 and 12 (Fig. 1). Inhibition of tumor COX-2 or inhi-

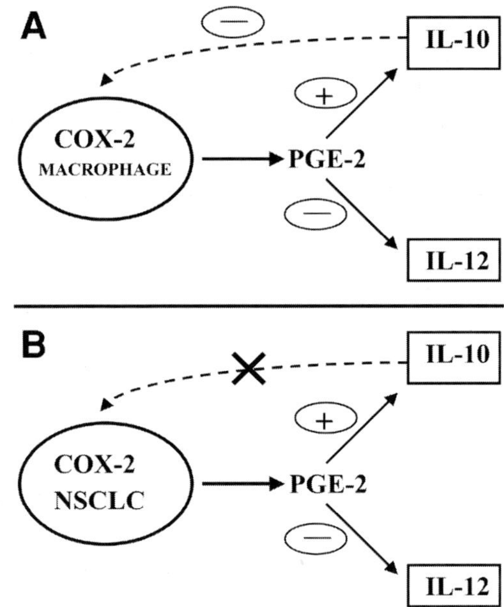

Fig. 1. (A) PGE2 serves as an important regulator of the Th1/Th2 cytokine balance in normal host cells by inhibiting the production of IL-12 by antigen-presenting cells (APC) while potently inducing IL-10 production by lymphocytes and macrophages. IL-10 in turn is known to potently suppress COX-2 in normal cells such as macrophages. Thus, the capacity of IL-10 to down regulate COX-2 expression and PGE2 production in normal host cells constitutes an important homeostatic regulatory loop in the maintenance of normal cytokine balance. **(B)** In contrast, IL-10 does not have the capacity to downregulate COX-2 in NSCLC cells. This appears to be caused by the lack of lung cancer-cell-surface expression of the IL-10 receptor α. Deficiency of the IL-10-mediated COX-2 regulatory feedback loop in NSCLC cells may contribute to COX-2 overexpression and maintenance of high-level PGE_2 in the lung cancer microenvironment. In addition to suppression of immune responses, the persistent elevation of tumor COX-2 may cause enhanced angiogenesis, tumor-cell apoptosis resistance, and invasion, leading to the promotion of tumorigenesis.

bition of the COX-2 metabolite PGE_2 restored the normal balance *(16)*. In murine models of established lung cancer, specific genetic or pharmacological inhibition of COX-2 in vivo led to significant tumor regression. COX-2 inhibition was accompanied by a significant decrement in the immunosuppressive cytokine IL-10 and a concomitant restoration of IL-12 production in vivo *(40)*. Subsequent studies in which COX-2-knockout mice were challenged with 3LL tumor were consistent with these findings: tumor growth was markedly attenuated in COX-2-knockout mice *(46)*. Thus, tumors as well as host-derived COX-2 expression could contribute to COX-2-dependent suppression of immunity. These intriguing preclinical and clinical studies have led to the initiation of chemoprevention trials utilizing COX-2 inhibitors in patients at high risk for lung cancer, as well as several trials for early and advanced-stage disease in which COX-2 inhibitors are combined with surgery, chemotherapy, or radiation.

4. ANTIGEN-PRESENTING CELL AND LYMPHOCYTE DYSFUNCTION

Antitumor immune responses require the coordinated activities of lymphocyte effectors and professional antigen-presenting cells (APC) *(74)*. Dendritic cells (DCs) are professional APC that are pivotal participants in the initiation of T-cell responses *(75)*. DCs acquire Ag in the periphery and subsequently transport it to lymphoid organs, where they prime specific immune responses *(75)*. The tumor microenvironment can adversely affect DC maturation and function *(76)*. Tumor-derived cytokines that have been shown to mediate DC dysfunction include IL-10, vascular endothelial growth factor (VEGF), macrophage colony-stimulating factor (M-CSF), IL-6 *(77–79)* and PGE2 *(80)*. Recent studies indicate that murine bone marrow-derived DC reveal altered maturation when exposed to tumor supernatants during their in vitro differentiation with GM-CSF and IL-4 *(81)*. Functional analyses indicated that tumor supernatant caused a decrease in DC capacity to i) process and present antigens, ii) induce alloreactivity, and iii) secrete IL-12. These limitations in DC activity were prevented when DC were cultured in tumor supernatant from COX-2 inhibited tumors. Whereas tumor supernatant-exposed DC showed a significant reduction in cell-surface expression of CD11c, DEC205, MHC class I, MHC class II, CD80, and CD86 as well as a reduction in the transporter-associated proteins, TAP1 and TAP2, these changes were not evident when DCs were cultured in supernatant from COX-2-inhibited tumors. Antibody-mediated depletion of PGE2 also abrogated the deleterious effects of the tumor supernatant. Although pulsed with tumor-specific peptides, the tumor supernatant-exposed DCs were incapable of generating antitumor immune responses in vivo. When injected into established murine lung cancer, DCs generated in tumor supernatant caused immunosuppressive effects that correlated with enhanced tumor growth *(81)*. These findings support the studies of Almand et al. *(82)*, who found that immature myeloid cells generated in large numbers in cancer patients can directly inhibit Ag-specific T-cell responses.

Tumor-derived factors can subvert effective antitumor immunity *(16,21, 40,83)* and incapacitate cytotoxic T-cell mediators of cell death through induced apoptosis or signaling defects *(84)*. Inhibition of effector-cell NF-κB-activation has been described as a pathway that leads to impairment of T-cell survival in the tumor milieu *(85–87)*. The renal cell cancer-induced alterations in T-cell NF-κB-activation also appear to be mediated by soluble factors, and have provided a rationale to investigate whether similar alterations were present in lung cancer *(85–87)*. The role of NF-κB as a survival factor has been extensively described *(88,89)*, and this ubiquitous factor has been implicated in the transcriptional regulation of many inhibitors of apoptosis *(90,91)*. Batra et al. found that NSCLC tumor supernatant significantly enhanced apoptosis in PMA/ionomycin and anti-CD3-stimulated lymphocytes *(92)*. Enhanced lymphocyte apoptosis was associated with an impairment of NF-κB nuclear translocation and diminished IκBα degradation. In lymphocytes that were stimulated following exposure to tumor supernatant, cytoplasmic IκBα persisted as a result of alterations in IκB-kinase (IKK)-activity. Accordingly, although there were no apparent differences in the amount of IKK-component concentrations, lymphocytes that were pre-exposed to tumor supernatant exhibited markedly reduced IKK activity. It was concluded that NSCLC-derived soluble factor(s) promote apoptosis in activated lymphocytes through an IKK-dependent pathway *(92)*.

5. REGULATORY T CELLS IN LUNG CANCER

Regulatory T cells have been shown to function as suppressor cells, and may play a role in the progression of cancer *(93,94)*. A variety of T-regulatory subsets have been identified *(95)*. Failure of tumor immunosurveillance or enhanced tumor growth could be caused by an increase of these regulatory T cells, which produce inhibitory cytokines such as TGF-β and IL-10, or directly inhibiting immunity via specific cellular interactions at the tumor site *(96)*. In mice, CD4+CD25+ regulatory cells have been shown to inhibit T-cell proliferation *(97)*. The Carl June laboratory recently documented an increase in the CD4+CD25+ regulatory T-cell population at the tumor site in NSCLC *(94,98)*. These studies clearly demonstrated that greater than one third of the CD4+ TIL from NSCLC consisted of CD4+CD25+ regulatory cells, and these cells were capable of exerting inhibition of autologous T-cell proliferation *(94,98)*. These findings are consistent with recent studies in murine models, which demonstrate that the depletion of CD4+CD25+ T cells can significantly augment the efficacy of cancer vaccination *(99)*. Together, these studies assist in the understanding of T regulatory cells in the lung-cancer environment. These findings also provide a basis for the development of clinical strategies to address the suppressive effects of regulatory T cells in lung cancer.

6. NONCLASSICAL HUMAN LEUKOCYTE ANTIGEN (HLA) EXPRESSION IN LUNG CANCER

In addition to inducing limitation in effector-cell survival, lung-tumor cells may specifically interfere with lymphocyte and natural killer (NK)-cell functions. It has previously been demonstrated that lung-tumor cells have limited

MHC class I and II expression *(100)*. Coupled with the paucity of classical MHC expression is the concomitant overexpression of nonclassical MHC molecules such as HLA-G that have been implicated as inhibitors of cellular immune responses. The HLA-G gene has been observed to have a limited polymorphism, and the alternative transcription of spliced mRNAs encode at least seven different isoforms *(101)*. Three of these isoforms are membrane-bound, and the remainder are soluble. HLA-G cell-surface expression may limit cytotoxicity and antigen presentation by binding inhibitory receptors *(101–104)*. Soluble HLA-G molecules can suppress alloreactivity *(105)*, limit peripheral-blood NK activity *(102)*, and induce CD95 ligand-mediated apoptosis in CD8+ T cells *(106)*. Moreau found that IL-10 selectively induces HLA-G expression in human trophoblasts and monocytes *(107)*. Although IL-10 selectively upregulates HLA-G in these cells, it also downregulates classical MHC class I expression. In keeping with these findings, Urosevic found that upregulation of HLA-G expression in lung cancer is associated with high-grade histology and loss of HLA class I and IL-10 production *(108)*. Pengault et al. noted that HLA-G expression in pulmonary macrophages and DC infiltrating lung cancers. It was therefore suggested that in addition to tumor-cell expression, host-cell expression of HLA-G could also limit immune responsiveness, and thus favor tumor progression *(109)*.

7. CAN IMMUNE-BASED THERAPIES REVERSE TUMOR-DEPENDENT IMMUNE SUPPRESSION IN LUNG CANCER?

Several clinical strategies are being developed to specifically address the defined immune deficits in lung cancer. One example of this is the therapeutic use of professional APC to augment tumor-specific responses. Lung-cancer cells have defects in antigen processing and diminished MHC expression *(110,111)*, rendering them ineffective as APC. Thus, as defined in elegant studies by Huang and colleagues *(74)*, professional APC play a major role in the immune response against cancer. This has led to the recent emphasis on the use of professional APC as the major source of tumor antigen presentation in vivo in genetic immunotherapies. DCs are highly specialized, professional APCs with a strong capacity to capture, process, and present antigen to T cells *(75)*. Unfortunately, tumor cells interfere with host DC maturation and function *(77,112)*. To circumvent the in vivo inhibition of DC maturation and function, protocols have been developed that enable DC to undergo cytokine-stimulated maturation ex vivo. These cells can then be used to generate antigen-specific CTL responses in a variety of models, as well as in clinical trials *(113,114)*. In this context, delivery of tumor antigens by ex vivo-stimulated DC may be superior to purified peptides in avoiding CTL tolerization *(115)*, and vaccination with multiple tumor antigens may be superior to the use of a single epitope *(115,116)*. Thus, another method of exposing the DC to a wide range of tumor antigens is the administration of DC intratumorally after ex vivo maturation. The introduction of immune-potentiating cytokine genes into these DC further enhances the antitumor response. For example, intratumorally administered, cytokine gene-modified DC were found to take up antigen at the tumor site, traffick to regional and systemic lymph nodes, and generate systemic antitumor responses and long-term immunity *(117)*. Intratumoral therapy with cytokine gene-modified DC yielded systemic antitumor effects that were comparable to those achieved with specific tumor-antigen-pulsed DC. This finding may have important implications in human lung cancer, for which specific tumor antigen-based therapies are difficult to achieve at this time *(12)*. Although additional specific tumor antigens may be identified, immunization with individual peptides may contribute to tolerance *(115)*. Peptide-induced tolerization of CTL has resulted in the inability of animals to reject antigen-expressing tumors *(115)*, and strong evidence has been presented to support immunoselection of antigen-loss variants in human cancer *(6,118)*. These limitations may be circumvented by the use of intratumoral DC-based genetic immunotherapies in which the tumor provides an array of immunogenic epitopes *in situ*. The effective use of activated DC administered intratumorally without antigen pulsing ex vivo implies that cross-presentation—the MHC class I-restricted presentation of exogenous antigens leading to CD8+ T-cell responses *(119)*—is operative. In fact, DC have been implicated as the APC predominantly effective in cross-presentation *(120)*. In agreement with these findings, novel tumor antigen-delivery systems using cytokine gene-transduced tumor cells and DC *(114,121)*, or fusion of tumor cells with DC, have resulted in the induction of antitumor immunity *(122,123)*.

Other approaches for the use of DC in lung cancer have been suggested *(124)*. NKT lymphocytes have been implicated in host resistance to tumor formation *(125,126)*. Numerous NKT-cell subsets have been described but important regulatory properties have been ascribed to those that express a conserved T-cell (TCR), receptor encoded by the Vα24–JαQ gene segments in human cells and Vα14–Jα281 segments in murine cells *(127)*. Vα24 NKT cells are activated by α-galactosylceramide (αGalCer) in a CD1-dependent manner *(128–130)*. αGalCer is a synthetic glycolipid derived from mollusks, originally identified as having potent antitumor properties in murine models *(131)*. αGalCer presented to NKT cells results in significant activation and cytokine release. αGalCer-loaded DC can induce prolonged IFN-γ production by NKT cells. Toura et al. have documented inhibition of experimental metastasis by DC pulsed with αGalCer *(11)*. Motahashi et al. found that although reduced in number, the function of Vα24 NKT cells were preserved *(124)*. The capacity for αGalCer presentation by lung-cancer patients' DC was also preserved.

These findings suggest that αGalCer-pulsed DC could be applicable in immunotherapy of human lung cancer *(124)*.

Despite the recent advances in identification of tumor antigens and the technical advances in genetic immunotherapy, our understanding of the host's failure to respond to these antigens is in its infancy. The pathway to successful clinical application of immunotherapy for lung cancer will require further studies that contribute to a more complete picture of the complex tumor–host interactions that foster progressive tumor growth.

ACKNOWLEDGMENTS

Supported by the UCLA SPORE in Lung Cancer (National Institutes of Health Grant P50 CA90388)

REFERENCES

1. Greenlee RT, Murray T, Bolden S, Wingo PA. Cancer statistics, 2000. *CA Cancer J Clin* 2000;50:7–33.
2. Dy GK, Adjei AA. Novel targets for lung cancer therapy: part I. *J Clin Oncol* 2002; 20:2881–2894.
3. Dy GK, Adjei AA. Novel targets for lung cancer therapy: part II. *J Clin Oncol* 2002; 20:3016–3028.
4. O'Reilly EM, Ilson DH, Saltz LB, Heelan R, Martin L, Kelsen DP. A phase II trial of interferon alpha-2a and carboplatin in patients with advanced malignant mesothelioma. *Cancer Investig* 1999;17:195–200.
5. Kugler A, Stuhler G, Walden P, et al. Regression of human metastatic renal cell carcinoma after vaccination with tumor cell-dendritic cell hybrids. *Nat Med* 2000;6:332–336.
6. Thurner B, Haendle I, Roder C, et al. Vaccination with mage-3A1 peptide-pulsed mature, monocyte-derived dendritic cells expands specific cytotoxic T cells and induces regression of some metastases in advanced stage IV melanoma. *J Exp Med* 1999;190:1669–1678.
7. Van Pel A, Boon T. Protection against a nonimmunogenic mouse leukemia by an immunogenic variant obtained by mutagenesis. *Proc Natl Acad Sci USA* 1982;79:4718–4722.
8. Boon T, Old L. Cancer tumor antigens. *Curr Opin Immunol* 1997;9:681–683.
9. Boon T, Gajewski TF, Coulie PG. From defined human tumor antigens to effective immunization? *Immunol Today* 1995;16:334–336.
10. Boon T, van der Bruggen P. Human tumor antigens recognized by T lymphocytes. *J Exp Med* 1996;183:725–729.
11. Pardoll D. Cancer vaccines. *Nat Med* 1998;4(5 Suppl):525–531.
12. Dubinett SM, Miller PW, Sharma S, Batra RK. Gene therapy for lung cancer. *Hematol Oncol Clin N Am* 1998;12:569–594.
13. Sogn JA. Tumor immunology: the glass is half full. *Immunity* 1998;9:757–763.
14. Zeh HJ, 3rd, Perry-Lalley D, Dudley ME, Rosenberg SA, Yang JC. High avidity CTLs for two self-antigens demonstrate superior in vitro and in vivo antitumor efficacy. *J Immunol* 1999;162:989–994.
15. Poplonski L, Vukusic B, Pawling J, et al. Tolerance is overcome in beef insulin-transgenic mice by activation of low-affinity autoreactive T cells. *Eur J Immunol* 1996;26:601–609.
16. Huang M, Stolina M, Sharma S, et al. Non-small cell lung cancer cyclooxygenase-2-dependent regulation of cytokine balance in lymphocytes and macrophages: up-regulation

of interleukin 10 and down-regulation of interleukin 12 production. *Cancer Res* 1998; 58:1208–1216.
17. Huang M, Sharma S, Mao JT, Dubinett SM. Non-small cell lung cancer-derived soluble mediators and prostaglandin E_2 enhance peripheral blood lymphocyte IL-10 transcription and protein production. *J Immunol* 1996;157:5512–5520.
18. Huang M, Wang J, Lee P, et al. Human non-small cell lung cancer cells express a type 2 cytokine pattern. *Cancer Res* 1995;55:3847–3853.
19. Neuner A, Schindel M, Wildenberg U, Muley T, Lahm H, Fischer JR. Cytokine secretion: clinical relevance of immunosuppression in non-small cell lung cancer. *Lung Cancer* 2001;34:S79–S82.
20. Alleva DG, Burger CJ, Elgert KD. Tumor-induced regulation of suppressor macrophage nitric oxide and TNF-alpha production: role of tumor-derived IL-10, TGF-beta and prostaglandin E2. *J Immunol* 1994;153:1674–1686.
21. Sharma S, Stolina M, Lin Y, et al. T cell-derived IL-10 promotes lung cancer growth by suppressing both T cell and APC function. *J Immunol* 1999;163:5020–5028.
22. Rohrer JW, Coggin JH, Jr. CD8 T cell clones inhibit antitumor T cell function by secreting IL-10. *J Immunol* 1995;155:5719–5727.
23. O'Hara RJ, Greenman J, McDonald AW, et al. Advanced colorectal cancer is associated with impaired interleukin 12 and enhanced interleukin 10 production. *Clin Cancer Res* 1998; 4:1943–1948.
24. O'Hara RJ, Greenman J, Drew PJ, et al. Impaired interleukin-12 production is associated with a defective anti-tumor response in colorectal cancer. *Dis Colon Rectum* 1998;41: 460–463.
25. Asselin-Paturel C, Echchakir H, Carayol G, et al. Quantitative analysis of Th1, Th2 and TGF-b1 cytokine expression in tumor, TIL and PBL of non-small cell lung cancer patients. *Int J Cancer* 1998;77:7–12.
26. Yamamura M, Modlin RL, Ohmen JD, Moy RL. Local expression of anti-inflammatory cytokines in cancer. *J Clin Investig* 1993;91:1005–1010.
27. Fiorentino DF, Zlotnik A, Mosmann TR, Howard M, Ogarra A. IL-10 inhibits cytokine production by activated macrophages. *J Immunol* 1991;147:3815–3822.
28. Mitra RS, Judge TA, Nestle FO, Turka LA, Nickoloff BJ. Psoriatic skin-derived dendritic cell function is inhibited by exogenous IL-10. *J Immunol* 1995;154:2668–2677.
29. Taga K, Tosato G. IL-10 inhibits human T cell proliferation and IL-2 production. *J Immunol* 1992;148:1143–1148.
30. de Waal-Malefyt R, Haanen J, Spits H, et al. Interleukin-10 (IL-10) and viral IL-10 strongly reduce antigen-specific human T-cell proliferation by diminishing the antigen-presenting capacity of monocytes via down-regulation of class-II major histocompatibility complex expression. *J Exp Med* 1991;174:915–924.
31. Mosmann T, Moore KW. The role of IL-10 in cross-regulation of TH1 and TH2 responses. *Immunol Today* 1991;12:A49–A53.
32. Fiorentino DF, Zlotnik A, Vieira P, et al. IL-10 acts on the antigen-presenting cell to inhibit cytokine production by Th1 cells. *J Immunol* 1991;146:3444–3451.
33. Kim J, Modlin RL, Moy RL, et al. IL-10 production in cutaneous basal and squamous cell carcinomas: A mechanism for evading the local T cell immune response. *J Immunol* 1995;155:2240–2247.
34. Halak BK, Maguire HC, Jr., Lattime EC. Tumor-induced interleukin-10 inhibits type 1 immune responses directed at a tumor antigen as well as a non-tumor antigen present at the tumor site. *Cancer Res* 1999;59:911–917.
35. Hagenbaugh A, Sharma S, Dubinett S, et al. Altered immune responses in IL-10 transgenic mice. *J Exp Med* 1997;185:2101–2110.

36. Hidalgo GE, Zhong L, Doherty DE, Hirschowitz EA. Plasma PGE-2 levels and altered cytokine profiles in adherent peripheral blood mononuclear cells in non-small cell lung cancer (NSCLC). *Mol Cancer* 2002;1:5–11.
37. Hatanaka H, Abe Y, Kamiya T, et al. Clinical implications of interleukin (IL)-10 induced by non-small-cell lung cancer. *Ann Oncol* 2000;11:815–819.
38. De Vita F, Orditura M, Galizia G, et al. Serum interleukin-10 levels as a prognostic factor in advanced non-small cell lung cancer patients. *Chest* 2000;117:365–373.
39. Neuner A, Schindel M, Wildenberg U, Muley T, Lahm H, Fischer JR. Prognostic significance of cytokine modulation in non-small cell lung cancer. *Int J Cancer* 2002;101:287–292.
40. Stolina M, Sharma S, Lin Y, et al. Specific inhibition of cyclooxygenase 2 restores antitumor reactivity by altering the balance of IL-10 and IL-12 synthesis. *J Immunol* 2000; 164:361–370.
41. Hatanaka H, Abe Y, Naruke M, et al. Significant correlation between interleukin 10 expression and vascularization through angiopoietin/TIE2 networks in non-small cell lung cancer. *Clin Cancer Res* 2001;7:1287–1292.
42. Birkeland SA, Storm HH, Lamm LU, et al. Cancer risk after renal transplantation in the Nordic countries, 1964–1986. *Int J Cancer* 1995;60:183–189.
43. Hecht SS. Chemoprevention by isothiocyanates. *J Cell Biochem Suppl* 1995:195–209.
44. Herschman H. Review: Prostaglandin synthase 2. *Biochim Biophys Acta* 1996; 1299:125–140.
45. Herschman HR. Regulation of prostaglandin synthase-I and prostaglandin synthase-2. *Cancer Metastasis Rev* 1994;13:241–256.
46. Williams CS, Tsujii M, Reese J, Dey SK, DuBois RN. Host cyclooxygenase-2 modulates carcinoma growth. *J Clin Investig* 2000;105:1589–1594.
47. Soslow RA, Dannenberg AJ, Rush D, et al. COX-2 is expressed in human pulmonary, colonic, and mammary tumors. *Cancer* 2000;89:2637–2645.
48. Yip-Schneider M, Miao W, Lin A, Barnard D, Tzivion G, Marshall M. Regulation of the Raf-1 kinase domain by phosphorylation and 14-3-3 association. *Biochem J* 2000; 351:151–159.
49. Sheng H, Shao J, Dixon DA, et al. Transforming growth factor-beta1 enhances Ha-ras-induced expression of cyclooxygenase-2 in intestinal epithelial cells via stabilization of mRNA. *J Biol Chem* 2000;275:6628–6635.
50. Liu XH, Kirschenbaum A, Yao S, Lee R, Holland JF, Levine AC. Inhibition of cyclooxygenase-2 suppresses angiogenesis and the growth of prostate cancer in vivo. *J Urol* 2000;164:820–825.
51. Shamma A, Yamamoto H, Doki Y, et al. Up-regulation of cyclooxygenase-2 in squamous carcinogenesis of the esophagus. *Clin Cancer Res* 2000;6:1229–1238.
52. Chan G, Boyle JO, Yang EK, et al. Cyclooxygenase-2 expression is up-regulated in squamous cell carcinoma of the head and neck. *Cancer Res* 1999;59:991–994.
53. Dannenberg AJ, Zakim D. Chemoprevention of colorectal cancer through inhibition of cyclooxygenase-2. *Semin Oncol* 1999;26:499–504.
54. Hida T, Kozaki K, Muramatsu H, et al. Cyclooxygenase-2 inhibitor induces apoptosis and enhances cytotoxicity of various anticancer agents in non-small cell lung cancer cell lines. *Clin Cancer Res* 2000;6:2006–2011.
55. Hida T, Yatabe Y, Achiwa H, et al. Increased expression of cycloxygenase 2 occurs frequently in human lung cancers, specifically in adenocarcinomas. *Cancer Res* 1998;58:3761–3764.
56. Wolff H, Saukkonen K, Anttila S, Karjalainen A, Vainio H, Ristimaki A. Expression of cyclooxygenase-2 in human lung carcinoma. *Cancer Res* 1998;58:4997–5001.
57. Hosomi Y, Yokose T, Hirose Y, et al. Increased cyclooxygenase 2 (COX-2) expression occurs frequently in precursor lesions of human adenocarcinoma of the lung [In Process Citation]. *Lung Cancer* 2000;30:73–81.

58. Achiwa H, Yatabe Y, Hida T, et al. Prognostic significance of elevated cyclooxygenase 2 expression in primary, resected lung adenocarcinomas. *Clin Cancer Res* 1999;5:1001–1005.
59. De Flora S, Cesarone CF, Balansky RM, Albini A, D'Agostini F, Bennicelli C, et al. Chemopreventive properties and mechanisms of N-Acetylcysteine. The experimental background. *J Cell Biochem Suppl* 1995;22:33–41.
60. Van Zandwijk N, Dalesio O, Pastorino U, et al. EUROSCAN, a randomized trial of vitamin A and N-acetylcysteine in patients with head and neck cancer or lung cancer. *J Natl Cancer Inst* 2000;95:977–986.
61. Goodman G. Prevention of lung cancer. *Critical Reviews in Oncology/Hematology* 2000; 33:187–197.
62. Li X, Liu J, Park J-K, et al. T cells from renal cell carcinoma patients exhibit an abnormal pattern of kB-specific DNA-binding activity: a preliminary report. *Cancer Res* 1994; 54:5424–5429.
63. Leahy K, Koki A, Masferrer J. Role of cyclooxygenases in angiogenesis. *Curr Med Chem* 2000;7:1163–1170.
64. Masferrer JL, Leahy KM, Koki AT, et al. Antiangiogenic and antitumor activities of cyclooxygenase-2 inhibitors. *Cancer Res* 2000;60:1306–1311.
65. Uefuji K, Ichikura T, Mochizuki H. Cyclooxygenase-2 expression is related to prostaglandin biosynthesis and angiogenesis in human gastric cancer. *Clin Cancer Res* 2000;6: 135–138.
66. Tsujii M, Kawano S, DuBois R. Cyclooxygenase-2 expression in human colon cancer cells increases metastatic potential. *Proc Natl Acad Sci USA* 1997;94:3336–3340.
67. Watkins DN, Lenzo JC, Segal A, Garlepp MJ, Thompson PJ. Expression and localization of cyclo-oxygenase isoforms in non-small cell lung cancer. *Eur Respir J* 1999;14: 412–418.
68. Ochiai M, Oguri T, Isobe T, Ishioka S, Yamakido M. Cyclooxygenase-2 (COX-2) mRNA expression levels in normal lung tissues and non-small cell lung cancers. *Jpn J Cancer Res* 1999;90:1338–1343.
69. Dohadwala M, Luo J, Zhu L, et al. Non small cell lung cancer cylooxygenase-2-dependent invasion is mediated by CD44. *J Biol Chem* 2001;276:20,809–20,812.
70. Khuri F, Wu H, Lee J, et al. Cyclooxygenase-2 overexpression is a marker of poor prognosis in stage I non-small cell lung cancer. *Clin Cancer Res* 2001;7:861–867.
71. Schreinemachers DM, Everson RB. Aspirin use and lung, colon, and breast cancer incidence in a prospective study. *Epidemiology* 1994;5:138–146.
72. Harris RE, Beebe-Donk J, Schuller HM. Chemoprevention of lung cancer by non-steroidal anti-inflammatory drugs among cigarette smokers. *Oncol Rep* 2002;9:693–695.
73. Akhmedkhanov A, Toniolo P, Zeleniuch-Jacquotte A, Koenig KL, Shore RE. Aspirin and lung cancer in women. *Br J Cancer* 2002;87:49–53.
74. Huang AYC, Golumbek P, Ahmadzadeh M, Jaffee E, Pardoll D, Levitsky H. Role of bone marrow-derived cells in presenting MHC class I-restricted tumor antigens. *Science* 1994;264:961–965.
75. Banchereau J, Steinman RM. Dendritic cells and the control of immunity. *Nature* 1998;392:245–252.
76. Almand B, Resser JR, Lindman B, et al. Clinical significance of defective dendritic cell differentiation in cancer. *Clin Cancer Res* 2000;6:1755–1766.
77. Gabrilovich DI, Chen HL, Girgis KR, et al. Production of vascular endothelial growth factor by human tumors inhibits the functional maturation of dendritic cells [published erratum appears in *Nat Med* 1996 Nov;2(11):1267]. *Nat Med* 1996;2:1096–1103.
78. Alavena P, Piemonti L, Longoni D, et al. IL-10 prevents the differentiation of monocytes to dendritic cells but promotes their maturation to macrophages. *Eur J Immunology*1998;28:359–363.

79. Caux M, Montmain CG, Dieu MC, et al. Inhibition of the differentiation of dendritic cells from CD34 + progenitors by tumor cells: role of interleukin 6 and macrophage colony stimulating factor. *Blood* 1998;92:4778–4791.
80. Sombroek CC, Stam AG, Masterson AJ, et al. Prostanoids play a major role in the primary tumor-induced inhibition of dendritic cell differentiation. *J Immunol* 2002;168: 4333–4343.
81. Sharma S, Stolina M, Yang SC, et al. Tumor cyclooxygenase 2-dependent suppression of dendritic cell function. [In Press]. *Clin Cancer Res* 2003;9:961–968.
82. Almand B, Clark JI, Nikitina E, et al. Increased production of immature myeloid cells in cancer patients: a mechanism of immunosuppression in cancer. *J Immunol* 2001; 166:678–689.
83. Sulitzeanu D. Immunosuppressive factors in human cancer. *Adv Cancer Res* 1993; 60:247–267.
84. Bladergroen BA, Meijer CJ, ten Berge RL, et al. Expression of the granzyme B inhibitor, protease inhibitor 9, by tumor cells in patients with non-Hodgkin and Hodgkin lymphoma: a novel protective mechanism for tumor cells to circumvent the immune system? *Blood* 2002;99:232–237.
85. Ng CS, Novick AC, Tannenbaum CS, Bukowski RM, Finke JH. Mechanisms of immune evasion by renal cell carcinoma: tumor-induced T-lymphocyte apoptosis and NFkappaB suppression. *Urology* 2002;59:9–14.
86. Uzzo RG, Kolenko V, Froelich CJ, et al. The T cell death knell: immune-mediated tumor death in renal cell carcinoma. *Clin Cancer Res* 2001;7:3276–3281.
87. Uzzo RG, Clark PE, Rayman P, et al. Alterations in NFkappaB activation in T lymphocytes of patients with renal cell carcinoma. *J Natl Cancer Inst* 1999; 91:718–721.
88. Van Antwerp DJ, Martin SJ, Kafri T, Green DR, Verma IM. Suppression of TNF-α-induced apoptosis by NF-κB. *Science* 1996;274:787–789.
89. Liu ZG, Hsu H, Goeddel DV, Karin M. Dissection of TNF receptor 1 effector functions: JNK activation is not linked to apoptosis while NF-kappaB activation prevents cell death. *Cell* 1996;87:565–576.
90. Goyal L. Cell death inhibition: keeping caspases in check. *Cell* 2001;104:805–808.
91. Deveraux QL, Reed JC. IAP family proteins—suppressors of apoptosis. *Genes Dev* 1999;13:239–252.
92. Batra RK, Lin Y, Sharma S, et al. Non small cell lung cancer derived soluble mediators enhance apoptosis in activated T lymphocytes through an IκB-Kinase dependent mechanism. *Cancer Res* 2003;63:642–646.
93. Dye ES, North RJ. T cell-mediated immunosuppression as an obstacle to adoptive immunotherapy of the P815 mastocytoma and its metastases. *J Exp Med* 1981;154: 1033–1042.
94. Woo EY, Yeh H, Chu CS, et al. Regulatory T cells from lung cancer patients directly inhibit autologous T cell proliferation. *J Immunol* 2002;168:4272–4276.
95. Shevach EM. Regulatory T cells in autoimmunity. *Annu Rev Immunol* 2000;18: 423–449.
96. Maloy KJ, Powrie F. Regulatory T cells in the control of immune pathology. *Nat Immunol* 2001;2:816–822.
97. Thornton AM, Shevach EM. CD4+CD25+ immunoregulatory T cells suppress polyclonal T cell activation in vitro by inhibiting interleukin 2 production. *J Exp Med* 1998;188: 287–296.
98. Woo EY, Chu CS, Goletz TJ, et al. Regulatory CD4(+)CD25(+) T cells in tumors from patients with early-stage non-small cell lung cancer and late-stage ovarian cancer. *Cancer Res* 2001;61:4766–4772.

99. Sutmuller RP, van Duivenvoorde LM, van Elsas A, et al. Synergism of cytotoxic T lymphocyte-associated antigen 4 blockade and depletion of CD25(+) regulatory T cells in antitumor therapy reveals alternative pathways for suppression of autoreactive cytotoxic T lymphocyte responses. *J Exp Med* 2001;194:823–832.
100. Redondo M, Concha A, Oldiviela R, et al. Expression of HLA class I and II antigens in bronchogenic carcinomas: its relationship to cellular DNA content and clinical-pathological parameters. *Cancer Res* 1991;51:4948–4954.
101. Rouas-Freiss N, Khalil-Daher I, Riteau B, et al. The immunotolerance role of HLA-G. *Semin Cancer Biol* 1999;9:3–12.
102. Carosella ED, Rouas-Freiss N, Paul P, Dausset J. HLA-G: a tolerance molecule from the major histocompatibility complex. *Immunol Today* 1999;20:60–62.
103. Le Gal FA, Riteau B, Sedlik C, et al. HLA-G-mediated inhibition of antigen-specific cytotoxic T lymphocytes. *Int Immunol* 1999;11:1351–1356.
104. Allan DS, Colonna M, Lanier LL, et al. Tetrameric complexes of human histocompatibility leukocyte antigen (HLA)-G bind to peripheral blood myelomonocytic cells. *J Exp Med* 1999;189:1149–1156.
105. Mitsuishi Y, Miyazawa K, Sonoda A, Terasaki PI. Cellular function of soluble HLA-G., Twelfth Interantional Histocompatibility Worshop and Conference, Paris, 1997. Vol. 2. Medical and Scientific International Publishers.
106. Fournel S, Aguerre-Girr M, Huc X, et al. Cutting edge: soluble HLA-G1 triggers CD95/CD95 ligand-mediated apoptosis in activated CD8+ cells by interacting with CD8. *J Immunol* 2000;164:6100–6104.
107. Moreau P, Adrian-Cabestre F, Menier C, et al. IL-10 selectively induces HLA-G expression in human trophoblasts and monocytes. *Int Immunol* 1999;11:803–811.
108. Urosevic M, Kurrer MO, Kamarashev J, et al. Human leukocyte antigen G up-regulation in lung cancer associates with high-grade histology, human leukocyte antigen class I loss and interleukin-10 production. *Am J Pathol* 2001;159:817–824.
109. Pangault C, Le Friec G, Caulet-Maugendre S, et al. Lung macrophages and dendritic cells express HLA-G molecules in pulmonary diseases. *Hum Immunol* 2002;63: 83–90.
110. Restifo NP, Esquivel F, Kawakami Y, et al. Identification of human cancers deficient in antigen processing. *J Exp Med* 1993;177:265–272.
111. Hiraki A, Kaneshige T, Kiura K, et al. Loss of HLA haplotype in lung cancer cell lines: implications for immunosurveillance of altered HLA class I/II phenotypes in lung cancer. *Clin Cancer Res* 1999;5:933–936.
112. Kiertscher SM, Luo J, Dubinett SM, Roth MD. Tumors promote altered maturation and early apoptosis of monocyte-derived dendritic cells. *J Immunol* 2000;164: 1269–1276.
113. Mayordomo JI, Zorina T, Storkus WJ, et al. Bone marrow-derived dendritic cells pulsed with synthetic tumor peptides elicit protective and therapeutic antitumor immunity. *Nat Med* 1995;1:1297–1302.
114. Miller PW, Sharma S, Stolina M, et al. Dendritic cells augment granulocyte-macrophage colony-stimulating factor (GM-CSF)/herpes simplex virus thymidine kinase-mediated gene therapy of lung cancer. *Cancer Gene Ther* 1998;5:380–389.
115. Toes R, van der Voort E, Schoenberger S, et al. Enhancement of tumor outgrowth through CTL tolerization after peptide vaccination is avoided by peptide presentation on dendritic cells. *J Immunol* 1998;160:4449–4456.
116. Fields RC, Shimizu K, Mule JJ. Murine dendritic cells pulsed with whole tumor lysates mediate potent antitumor immune responses in vitro and in vivo. *Proc Natl Acad Sci USA* 1998;95:9482–9487.

117. Miller PW, Sharma S, Stolina M, et al. Intratumoral administration of adenoviral interleukin 7 gene-modified dendritic cells augments specific antitumor immunity and achieves tumor eradication. *Hum Gene Ther* 2000;11:53–65.
118. Jager E, Ringhoffer M, Karbach J, Arand M, Oesch F, Knuth A. Inverse relationship of melanocyte differentiation antigen expression in melanoma tissues and CD8+ cytotoxic-T-cell responses: evidence for immunoselection of antigen-loss variants in vivo. *Int J Cancer* 1996;66:470–476.
119. Bevan MJ. Antigen presentation to cytotoxic T lymphocytes in vivo. *J Exp Med* 1995; 182:639–641.
120. Waldrop S, Pitcher C, Peterson D, Maino V, Picker L. Determination of antigen-specific memory/effector CD4+ T cell frequencies by flow cytometry. *J Clin Investig* 1997; 99:1739–1750.
121. Sharma S, Miller P, Stolina M, et al. Multi-component gene therapy vaccines for lung cancer: effective eradication of established murine tumors in vivo with interleukin 7/Herpes Simplex Thymidine Kinase-transduced autologous tumor and ex vivo-activated dendritic cells. *Gene Therapy* 1997;4:1361–1370.
122. Gong J, Chen D, Kashiwaba M, Kufe D. Induction of antitumor activity by immunization with fusions of dendritic and carcinoma cells. *Nat Med* 1997;3:558–561.
123. Celluzzi C, Falo LJ. Cutting edge: physical interaction between dendritic cells and tumor cells result in an immunogen that induces protective and therapeutic tumor rejection. *J Immunol* 1998;160:3081–3085.
124. Motohashi S, Kobayashi S, Ito T, et al. Preserved IFN-alpha production of circulating Valpha24 NKT cells in primary lung cancer patients. *Int J Cancer* 2002;102:159–165.
125. Kawano T, Cui J, Koezuka Y, et al. Natural killer-like nonspecific tumor cell lysis mediated by specific ligand-activated Valpha14 NKT cells. *Proc Natl Acad Sci USA* 1998; 95:5690–5693.
126. Cui J, Shin T, Kawano T, et al. Requirement for Vα14 NKT cells in IL-12-mediated rejection of tumors. *Science* 1997;278:1623–1626.
127. Grant EP, Degano M, Rosat JP, et al. Molecular recognition of lipid antigens by T cell receptors. *J Exp Med* 1999;189:195–205.
128. Brossay L, Chioda M, Burdin N, et al. CD1d-mediated recognition of an alpha-galactosylceramide by natural killer T cells is highly conserved through mammalian evolution. *J Exp Med* 1998;188:1521–1528.
129. Kawano T, Tanaka Y, Shimizu E, et al. A novel recognition motif of human NKT antigen receptor for a glycolipid ligand. *Int Immunol* 1999;11:881–887.
130. Spada FM, Koezuka Y, Porcelli SA. CD1d-restricted recognition of synthetic glycolipid antigens by human natural killer T cells. *J Exp Med* 1998;188:1529–1534.
131. Morita M, Motoki K, Akimoto K, et al. Structure-activity relationship of alpha-galactosylceramides against B16-bearing mice. *J Med Chem* 1995;38:2176–2187.

19 Primary Malignant Brain Tumors

Immune Defects and Immune Evasion

Lucinda H. Elliott, PhD,
Lorri A. Morford, PhD,
William H. Brooks, MD,
and Thomas L. Roszman, PhD

CONTENTS

1. INTRODUCTION

Although primary malignant brain tumors are rare among the general population, accounting for less than 2.4% of all cancer deaths, they are the second leading cause of cancer deaths among individuals under 34 yr of age, and rank fourth among cancer deaths for men between 35 and 55 yr of age. Glioblastoma multiforme represent 30% of all primary malignant tumors and 50% of all astrocytomas, and are the most common primary malignant tumor in middle-aged men. Despite significant advancements in therapy over the past 30 yr, the outcome for most patients who harbor these tumors remains poor, with an average mean survival of approx 62 wk after diagnosis and treatment. Several factors play a significant role in the poor prognosis for patients who harbor these tumors. One factor can be attributed to the aggressive growth characteristics and the highly invasive nature of gliomas. Although gliomas rarely metastasize outside of the brain, they often migrate along nerve tracks across the corpus

From: *Current Clinical Oncology: Cancer Immunotherapy at the Crossroads: How Tumors Evade Immunity and What Can Be Done*
Edited by: J. H. Finke and R. M. Bukowski © Humana Press Inc., Totowa, NJ

callosum to seed secondary/tertiary sites in the brain, which frequently result in recurrences. Another factor involves the sequestration of gliomas away from aggressive immune attack in an immunologically privileged site. Finally, many studies suggest that glioma-derived soluble factors suppress immune-effector cells at the tumor site and systemically contribute to the broad-based immunocompromised state that has been observed in patients with gliomas. Thus, this tumor model offers an excellent opportunity to define mechanisms that are involved in immune modulation by soluble tumor-derived products. Furthermore, the model may provide insight into the mechanisms that contribute to immune privilege in the brain. This chapter reviews significant studies that have contributed to the characterization of the impaired immune status of patients with gliomas and the role of glioma-derived factors in the modulation of immune function in these patients.

2. IMMUNE DEFECTS IN PATIENTS WHO HARBOR GLIOMAS

2.1. Quantitative and Qualitative Defects in Peripheral-Blood Lymphocytes Obtained From Patients

Impaired immune responsiveness has been extensively documented in patients with primary central nervous system (CNS) neoplasia since the 1970s. These early studies demonstrated that patients with gliomas exhibit profound T-lymphopenia and suppressed in vivo responsiveness to common recall and neoantigens when compared to normal healthy age-matched controls, head trauma patients, and patients with other types of brain tumors *(1–6)*. In the 1970s and 1980s, a series of in vitro studies further elucidated the mechanisms that contributed to the immunocompromised status of patients with brain tumors. These studies demonstrated that peripheral-blood lymphocytes (PBL) obtained from patients exhibit decreased responsiveness to a number of T-cell mitogens and antigens *(7)*, which could not be attributed to decreased binding of the mitogens *(8–10)* or increased suppressor-cell activity *(8)*. The decreased proliferative response is the result of both quantitative and qualitative defects in PBL obtained from patients *(8,11,12)*. This is evidenced by reduced percentages of CD3+, and CD4+ T-lymphocyte populations in PBL isolated from patients when compared to normal values *(12)*. Moreover, limiting dilution analysis demonstrated that PBL from patients contain sixfold fewer phytohemagglutinin (PHA)-responsive cells when compared to similar numbers of cells obtained from normal healthy individuals. In the same study, cytokinetic analysis using colchicine synchronized cells suggested that the decreased responsiveness of PBL obtained from patients results from a block in G1 to S cell-cycle progression and the subsequent failure of these cells to expand into a pool of proliferating cells. However, the diminished proliferative response to mitogens observed in these cells cannot be attributed solely to T-cell lymphopenia, as mitogen responsiveness is equally diminished in purified populations of T cells *(7,11)*. Although PBL from patients who exhibit decreased in vitro antibody production in response to the T-cell-dependent B-cell mitogen, pokeweed mitogen (PWM), further evidence suggested that the diminished humoral response observed in these patients could be attributed to deficient T-helper-cell activity *(12)*. This was supported by the observation that PBL from patients contained normal levels of B cells *(4)* and that T cells obtained from patients could not provide helper activity in allogenic PWM cultures *(12)*. In addition, the PBL obtained from patients displayed normal levels of responsiveness to the T-independent B-cell mitogens, *Staphylococcus aureus* Cowen strain (SAC) as well as phorbol-12, 13-dibutyrate (PDBu) plus anti-IgM *(13)*. As a whole, these data suggest that the immunocompromised state of patients who harbor gliomas is confined primarily to the T-cell compartment, and deficiencies in humoral immunity can be attributed to insufficient T-cell help. In contrast, this broad T-cell deficiency was not observed in patients with head trauma or other types of brain tumors *(1,8,13)*.

2.2. Intrinsic Defects in T-Helper Cells Obtained from Patients

With the discovery that immune dysfunction in patients with brain tumors was confined primarily to T-helper-cell populations, studies were initiated to determine the mechanisms involved. The data from these studies indicated that PHA-activated PBL obtained from brain-tumor patients secreted significantly reduced amounts of interleukin 2 (IL-2) when compared to similarly stimulated PBL from normal individuals *(11)*. Moreover, the depressed PHA responsiveness of PBL from patients was not restored to normal levels with the addition of exogenous recombinant IL-2 (rIL-2). Together with the observation that PHA activated PBL obtained from patients contain significantly fewer numbers of CD25 (alpha chain of the IL-2R)-positive cells *(10)*, these data suggest that the reduced proliferative capacity of stimulated T cells from patients is linked to the inability of these cells to secrete and respond appropriately to IL-2. RNase protection assays demonstrated that IL-2 mRNA peaks early after stimulation with anti-CD3 monoclonal antibodies (MAbs) in T cells obtained from patients, but is completely absent by 8 h after stimulation, as opposed to normal T cells, which maintain IL-2 mRNA synthesis throughout (L. Morford, unpublished observation). Subsequent binding assays with radiolabeled rIL-2 confirmed that purified T cells from patients that were stimulated for 48 h with PHA express fivefold fewer high-affinity (K_d 8.3 pM) IL-2R than normal T cells treated similarly *(14)*. Expression of intermediate-affinity IL-2Rs (K_d 83 pM) is within the normal range. Fluorescence-activated cell sorting (FACS) analysis revealed that the relative density of CD25 is significantly decreased on PHA-activated PBL from patients. In contrast, Northern analysis demonstrated normal steady-state levels of mRNA for the IL-2R alpha chain in purified PHA-activated T cells from patients. Because the appropriate translation and post-translational modification of the alpha chain appear to occur normally, decreased expression of *p55* on the cell surface was believed to reside in events that involved insertion of the alpha protein into the cell membrane and its subsequent association with components of the intermediate IL-2R. Alternatively, reduced expression of CD25 on the surface of T cells could result from rapid shedding of the alpha chain from the T-cell surface after stimulation *(13)*. These studies were completed before the complete elucidation of the structure of the functional high-affinity IL-2R, which exists as a heterotrimeric complex containing an alpha chain (CD25), beta chain (CD122), and gamma chain (CD132) *(15)*. The intermediate-affinity IL-2R, which consists of the beta and gamma chain, is constitutively expressed on resting T cells. Activation of T cells by mitogens or via the T-cell receptor (TCR)/CD3 complex stimulates the expression of the IL-2 alpha chain and the subsequent production of high levels of CD25, which then associate with intermediate IL-2R to form high-affinity IL-2R that is functional at physiological concentrations of IL-2 *(16)*. The IL-2R binding studies performed with T cells obtained from patients *(14)* were completed before the discovery of the gamma chain, and thus, the role played by this important subunit in assembly of functional high-affinity receptors on patient T cells has not been addressed.

Because expression of the IL-2 gene is dependent upon the generation of appropriate TCR/CD3-coupled biochemical activation signals, studies were initiated to determine whether decreased IL-2 synthesis was associated with anomalies in TCR/CD3-induced signaling events. Perturbation of the TCR/CD3 complex by antigens or mitogens results in the activation of at least two interrelated second-messenger systems; one mediated by the activation of protein tyrosine kinases (PTK) and the other initiated by phospholipase Cγ1 (PLCγ1)-catalyzed hydrolysis of membrane polyphosphoinositides *(17–20)*. Activation of the PTK pathway results in tyrosine phosphorylation of a number of protein substrates, including the zeta chain of CD3, PLCγ, and several PTKs—namely, $p56^{lck}$, and $p59^{fyn}$—that are involved in the initiation of downstream signaling events such as the Ras activation pathway *(21–24)*. Phosphorylation of PLCγ results in the activation of this membrane-associated hydrolase and the subsequent cleavage of membrane phosphoinositol-4, 5-bisphosphate (PIP_2) to diacylglycerol (DAG) and inositol-1,4,5-trisphosphate (IP_3) *(18,24)*. These products act as second messengers with DAG, directly activating protein kinase C (PKC) and IP_3 mediating the release of calcium into the cytosol from intracellular stores *(25,26)*.

Anomalies in early transmembrane signaling events were discovered in peripheral-blood T cells obtained from patients, as evidenced by reduced tyrosine phosphorylation of a number of substrate proteins after stimulation with PHA or anti-CD3 MAbs when compared to T cells from control individuals *(27)*. In particular, phosphorylation of pp100 and PLCγ are markedly decreased in anti-CD3-stimulated T cells from patients. Although the function of pp100 has not been identified, its phosphorylation has been well-documented in activated T cells, and it does not appear to be vav *(18,28,29)*. Reduced tyrosine phosphorylation of PLCγ and pp100 in patient T cells is correlated with reduced protein levels of $p56^{lck}$ *(27)*, while $p59^{fyn}$ protein levels are not reduced. Association of $p56^{lck}$ with the zeta chain of CD3 is a key requirement for the induction of activation signals in stimulated T cells *(20,22,30)*, and there are reports that link the induction of anergic signals to the association of $p59^{fyn}$ with the zeta chain *(31)*. Further evidence for a signaling defect in T cells obtained from patients comes from the observation that calcium mobilization is impaired, as revealed both by spectrophotometric and FACS analysis *(27)*. Although the temporal increase in intracellular calcium is not altered in mitogen- or ionomycin (IONO)-stimulated T cells obtained from patients when compared to normal T cells, the magnitude is significantly reduced. Reduced calcium mobilization may be attributed to decreased PLCγ activity. However, stimulation of glioma patient T cells with PMA and IONO, which should bypass the requirement for PLCγ activation and directly activate the $p21^{Ras}$ signaling pathway, does not restore the proliferative capacity of these T cells *(27)*. These findings support the theory that additional defects exist in more distal biochemical events after PKC activation or in the $p21^{Ras}$ activation pathway. Together, these studies suggest that the decreased responsiveness of T cells from patients with gliomas is associated with multiple defects in TCR/CD3-coupled signaling events, which result in the induction of an anergic state in these T cells. This T-cell anergy shares many characteristic features with other models of anergy, namely altered substrate tyrosine phosphorylation patterns after stimulation *(31–34)*, reductions in PTK levels *(35)*, decreased calcium mobilization *(33)*, inability to secrete and respond to IL-2, and altered IL-2R expression *(36,37)*. Unlike other models of T-cell anergy, T cells from patients cannot be rescued from their unresponsive state with the addition of exogenous IL-2 alone or together with appropriate costimulation via CD2 or CD28 (A.R. Dix and L. Morford, unpublished observation).

2.3. Apoptosis of T Cells in Brain-Tumor Patients

T-cell lymphopenia, most notably in the T-helper-cell subpopulation, is a prominent hallmark of patients with gliomas *(3,4,12)*. One probable explanation for this deficiency can be attributed to increased apoptosis in the CD4+

T-cell populations associated with the generation of anergic signals. Engagement of the antigen receptor on normal quiescent T cells initiates a cascade of activation signals that induce the cell to enter Gap 1 (G1) of the cell cycle *(38, 39,40)*. However, additional costimulatory signals via the engagement of CD28 with B71/B72 on professional antigen-presenting cells (APC) as well as the interaction IL-2 with high-affinity IL-2R are required to drive the T cell into S and subsequently through the cell cycle *(41)*. The absence of appropriate costimulatory signals via CD28 and the IL-2R is associated with the induction of an anergic state and increased sensitivity to apoptosis *(41)*. In fact, the induction of apoptosis in antigen-activated T cells serves as an important homeostatic mechanism to remove activated T cells late in the immune response when they are no longer needed, and as a mechanism to guard against the generation of autoimmune responses *(42–44)*. Activation-induced apoptosis has also been implicated as an important mechanism for the prevention of potentially detrimental inflammatory responses in immunoprivileged sites such as the interior chamber of the eye and the brain *(44)*.

Apoptotic elimination of antigen-stimulated T cells is generally mediated by specific surface receptors that, upon appropriate engagement, generate "death signals" into the cell *(44)*. Prominent among these receptors is Fas/APO-1, which is a 43-kDa transmembrane glycoprotein that is a member of the tumor necrosis factor (TNF)-receptor family of proteins *(45)*. The natural ligand for Fas (FasL or CD95L), is a 40-kDa transmembrane protein that is a member of the TNF family *(46)*. There is increasing evidence that Fas-mediated apoptosis of tumor-specific T cells is a potential mechanism used by tumors to escape the immune system. In fact, gliomas have been demonstrated to express both Fas and FasL *(47,48)*, and CD95-dependent killing of Fas-positive T-cells by gliomas has been implicated as an important mechanism for immune evasion *(48)*. In support of this hypothesis, cultured FasL-positive glioma-cell lines kill murine Fas-transfected P815 targets and human Jurkat T-cells via Fas/FasL interactions *(48,49)*.

In our studies, we found that the level of Fas/APO-1-positive T cells is normal or slightly elevated when compared to control T cells (AR Dix, unpublished observation), but there is a significant increase in the percentage of apoptotic peripheral blood T cells obtained from patients with gliomas *(50)*. Stimulation of peripheral T cells from patients in vitro with anti-CD3 MAb further elevates the level of apoptotic cells when compared to similarly treated T cells from normal individuals. Also, CD28 expression is significantly decreased in T-cell populations from patients, and FasL/APO-1 expression appears to be selectively elevated on the CD28-negative T-cells (AR Dix, unpublished observation), which is not surprising, as the absence of CD28-coupled costimulated signaling is associated with an increase in apoptosis of T cells.

Further analysis using freshly isolated peripheral T cells from patients indicated that resting T cells or T cells in the early stages of activation after stimulation with anti-CD3 are targeted for apoptosis *(50)*. The observation that peripheral T cells from patients exhibit increased levels of Fas/Apo-1-associated apoptosis suggests that direct contact with FasL-expressing glioma cells is not required for the induction of apoptosis in T cells obtained from patients. In fact, there is evidence to suggest that glioma-derived factors play a major modulatory role in the induction of T-cell anergy and apoptosis in patients by shifting the pattern of immune cytokine secretion from a Th-1 to Th-2 profile *(50,51)*. The data indicate that although Th-1 cytokines, particularly IL-2 and interferon γ (IFN-γ) rescue T cells from programmed cell death *(52)*, Th-2 cytokines—namely IL-4 and IL-10—promote apoptosis of T cells in a number of tumor models *(53)*. Thus a glioma-induced cytokine shift to a Th-2 environment would promote loss of T cells and, in turn, promote tumor growth and survival.

2.4. Cytokine Dysregulation in Patients With Gliomas

Induction of the appropriate cytokine network, Th-1 or Th-2, is a critical component for the production of a protective immune response to pathogens and tumors. It is becoming more apparent that one mechanism used by pathogens and tumors to evade the immune response is to shift the cytokine profile in their environment from one that inhibits the induction of a protective immune response to one that favors growth and survival of the pathogen or tumor. In fact, the induction of an inappropriate immune response as the result of cytokine dysregulation has been shown to play a major role in a variety of diseases including, cancer, acquired immunodeficiency syndrome (AIDS), leshmaniasis, leprosy, and lupus *(51,53–59)*. There is increasing evidence to suggest that gliomas escape immune destruction by inducing a shift from a protective Th-1 cytokine environment (IL-2, IL-12, IFN-γ) to a Th-2 cytokine profile (IL-10, IL-4), which alters macrophage and T-cell function to promote tumor growth (refs. *27,51*; A.R. Dix, unpublished observation). This theory is supported by several observations. First, mitogen- or antigen-stimulated PBL obtained from patients secrete significantly reduced levels of the Th1 cytokines, IL-2 *(10,11)* and IFN-γ *(60,61)*. Second, PBL obtained from patients when stimulated in vitro with the SAC 1 produced significantly more IL-10 and decreased amounts of IL-12 and IFN-γ when compared to similarly treated PBL from healthy controls (ref. *51*; A.R. Dix, unpublished observation). Third, tumor-infiltrating leukocytes isolated from gliomas secrete predominantly Th-2 cytokines *(62)*. Finally, glioma-cell lines secrete Th-2 cytokines, including TGF-β, IL-6, and IL-10, and other factors such as PGE_2, which favor a shift to a Th-2 cytokine environment that is favorable to tumor growth *(51,58,63–65)*. There is significant evidence to suggest that tumor-derived moieties alter macrophage function to promote tumor growth *(58)*, and that the cytokine shift observed in PBL obtained from patients is mediated by glioma-derived factors via alterations in monocyte activity (ref. *51*; AR Dix, unpublished observations).

2.5. Alterations in Monocyte/Macrophage Function in Patients With Gliomas

Macrophages represent a critical component of host immunity to tumors, both directly and indirectly. In addition to presenting tumor antigens to T cells and providing the necessary costimulatory signals for T-cell activation, macrophages secrete a variety of soluble factors that are directly cytotoxic to tumors and can modulate immune function of T helper cells, cytotoxic T-cells, and natural killer (NK) cells. However, in addition to their positive roles, it is well-established that macrophages can also exert negative regulatory influences on the immune system *(58)*. Furthermore, there is increasing evidence that macrophage function can be redirected by tumors to alter the immune response and promote tumor growth *(51,58)*. Although our data indicate that immune defects in patients with gliomas are confined primarily to the T-cell compartment *(7,10,50)*, recent observations suggest that glioma-induced altered monocyte/macrophage function plays a significant role in the induction of the intrinsic defects observed in patients with gliomas. For example, CD14+ monocytes isolated from patients express reduced levels of HLA-DR class II molecules and secrete decreased amounts of IL-1β upon stimulation with lipopolysaccharide (LPS) when compared to normal controls and patients with low-grade astrocytomas *(65)*. The percentage of human leukocyte antigen (HLA)-DR positive cells, but not the density of expression and secretion of IL-1β by LPS-stimulated monocytes is partially restored when the tumor mass is debulked *(65)*. These observations, together with the evidence that partially purified culture supernatant from glioma cell lines downmodulate expression of MHC Class II molecules as well as B71/B72 (CD80/86) *(51)*, suggests that gliomas directly alter macrophage activity and reduce their capacity to function as professional APC, which in turn would contribute to the induction of T-cell anergy and promotion of apoptosis. In fact, purified monocytes from patients can facilitate apoptosis of unstimulated normal autologous T-cells in vitro (A.R. Dix, unpublished observation). This is further supported by studies showing that macrophages kill target cells by multiple mechanisms that result in the induction of apoptosis *(66)*.

Further evidence that gliomas can redirect monocyte/macrophage function to promote tumor growth is supported by several observations. For example, the shift from a Th-1 to Th-2 cytokine profile by gliomas is modulated by alterations in the secretion patterns of monokines *(51)*. Thus, stimulation of monocytes isolated from patients with *Staphylococcus aureus* Cowan strain 1 (SAC) induces a prolonged shift from Th-1 to Th-2 profiles over 96 h in culture when compared to similarly treated cells from normal individuals (ref. *51*; A.R. Dix, unpublished observation). Moreover, supernatants collected from SAC-stimulated patient PBL inhibit the proliferative response of T cells obtained from normal individuals to immobilized anti-CD3 MAb (A.R. Dix, unpublished observation), suggesting that monocyte-derived factors may be directly involved in the induction of T-cell anergy. Finally, some monokine-derived growth factors may theoretically augment tumor growth. For example, tumor-infiltrating monocytes secrete epidermal growth factor (EGF) *(67,68)* and IL-1β *(69,70)*. Since gliomas express receptors for both of these growth factors, these monokines could further support growth of the tumor.

3. IMMUNE MODULATION BY GLIOMA-DERIVED SOLUBLE FACTORS

3.1. Evidence for Immune Modulation by Glioma-Derived Factors

Because gliomas rarely metastasize outside of the brain, the systemic immunosuppression observed in these patients suggests that the release of glioma-derived soluble factors into the periphery may play a significant role in modulating the immune response of the host (reviewed in ref. *71*). This is supported by the following observations. First, T-cell anergy is directly correlated with the size, but not the location, of the tumor *(27)*. Second, mitogen responsiveness of peripheral T cells obtained from patients returns to near normal levels after surgical resection of the tumor, but diminishes again upon tumor recurrence *(72)*. Third, autologous and homologous lymphocyte reactivity in vitro is suppressed by sera, cerebral spinal fluid, and tumor cyst fluid *(1,73–76)*. Fourth, partially purified culture supernatants (GCS) from cloned glioma-cell lines, when added to normal T-cells, reproduce many of the immunologic anomalies noted in patients *(51,77,78)*. Finally, gliomas secrete growth factors, cytokines, and other soluble factors that are known immune modulators *(50,51)*.

3.2. Survey of Soluble Immunomodulatory Factors Secreted by Gliomas

Gliomas are known to secrete several growth factors and cytokines, including IL-1, IL-6, Il-10, TGF-β1, and CGRP, as well as other immunomodulatory compounds such as prostaglandin E_2 (PGE_2) and gangliosides *(51,69,77–79)*. Although the secretion of soluble factors that are capable of immune modulation is well-documented in gliomas, the role these factors play in vivo in redirecting the immune response and promoting tumor growth in patients has not been completely defined.

PGE_2 is a product of the cyclooxygenase pathway of arachidonic acid metabolism that is primarily produced by activated monocytes/macrophages, endothelial cells, platelets, and mast cells. As a potent inflammatory mediator, many of the cardinal signs of inflammation—including fever, pain, and increased vascular permeability—can be attributed to the direct action of prostaglandins on endothelial cells *(80–82)*. However, PGE_2 also has inhibitory effects on T-cell activation, presumably by promoting a shift from Th-1 to Th-2 cytokine profiles. Thus, PGE_2 inhibits the synthesis of IL-12 and enhances the production of IL-10 by monocytes *(83)*. Studies using naïve T-cell precursor cells isolated from cord blood demonstrate that PGE_2 inhibits the differentiation of IL-2-producing Th-1 cells, but promotes the development of Th-2 cells *(84)*. PGE_2 selectively inhibits the synthesis of IL-2 and IFN-γ by Th-1 effector cells, but has no effect, or even slightly enhances, the production of IL-4 and IL-5 by Th-2-effector cells *(85)*. Although increased levels of PGE_2 production by gliomas has been noted and proposed to contribute to the T-cell dysfunction in patients *(86,87)*, some studies suggest that there is not a prominent role for PGE_2 in the T-cell anomalies noted in these patients. Thus, the concentration of PGE_2 observed in glioma-cell supernatants does not correlate with the concentration required to inhibit T-cell activation or alter cytokine profiles *(51,88)*. Moreover, the addition of naproxin and indomethacin—potent inhibitors of PGE_2 synthesis—to glioma cell lines does not abrogate the production of glioma-derived suppressor factors by these cells *(77)*.

TGF-β was one of the first growth factors to be isolated and cloned from glioma-cell lines known to possess immunomodulatory capabilities *(79,89)*. The modulatory effects of TGF-β can both augment and suppress the immune response, by regulating downstream activation signals involved in progression through the cell cycle *(89)*. Some of the reported inhibitory effects of TGF-β on the immune response are: i) inhibition of the proliferative responses of thymocytes, T cells, and B cells to mitogens and specific antigens; ii) blockage of the generation of cytotoxic T cells and LAK activity; iii) suppression of cytokine release by monocytes/macrophages; iv) downregulation of surface MHC Class II expression on monocytes/macrophages; and v) induction of apoptosis in T cells (reviewed in ref. *89*). Despite the plethora of immunomodulatory effects of TGF-β on the immune response, the role this cytokine plays in contributing to the immune defects observed in patients with gliomas is unclear. In fact, recent evidence suggests that TBF-β plays only a marginal role in this tumor model. For example, the concentration of TGF-β measured in culture supernatants from glioma-cell lines does not correlate with the concentration of this cytokine required to inhibit T-cell function in vitro *(65,88)*. Moreover, neutralizing antibodies to TGF-β do not reverse the inhibitory effects of glioma-derived factors on T-cell function (refs. *64,90*, L. Morford, unpublished observation). Likewise, the glioma-induced cytokine shift from Th-1 to Th-2 profiles cannot be attributed to TGF-β, as evidenced by the fact that addition of TGF-β to PBMC, either alone or in combination with IL-6, does not induce such a shift; nor does neutralization or removal of TGF-β from glioma-culture supernatants abrogate the ability of the supernatant to stimulate a TH-1-to-Th-2 cytokine shift in normal PBL *(51)*. Together, these studies suggest that although TGF-β possesses potent immunomodulatory capacities and is secreted at high levels by some gliomas, other glioma-derived moieties in addition to TGF-β play substantial roles in the generation of the immune anomalies noted in patients who harbor gliomas.

IL-10 is a 17-kDa type II Th-2 cytokine produced primarily by activated monocytes, T cells, and B cells (reviewed in ref. *91*). It is an immunomodulatory cytokine that plays a significant role in regulating the balance between Th-1 and Th-2 profiles. IL-10 inhibits the production of a number of Th-1 cytokines, including IL-2, IL-12, TNF, and IFN-γ and thus is a major inhibitor of the generation of Th-1-mediated responses. Suppression of T-cell activation and IL-2 production by IL-10 has been attributed to the direct inhibition of macrophage-mediated antigen presentation. Thus, IL-10 directly inhibits macrophage activation as well as the subsequent upregulation of MHC class II expression and secretion of proinflammatory mediators by specific subsets of macrophages *(91)*. The expression of IL-10 by gliomas appears to be directly related to the grade of the tumor as 88% of grade III-IV astrocytomas (gliomas) express significant levels of steady-state IL-10 mRNA, and only 4% of Grade II astrocytomas are positive for IL-10 mRNA *(65)*. Moreover, highly invasive gliomas express greater levels of IL-10 than localized tumors *(63)*. However, not all glioma-cell lines secrete detectable levels of IL-10, but partially purified GCS from these negative cell lines can induce the expression and secretion of IL-10 by SAC-stimulated monocytes from normal donors *(51)*. Moreover, SAC-stimulated monocytes from patients secrete higher levels of IL-10. Interestingly, SAC-stimulated monocytes from patients secrete decreased levels of IL-12, and supernatant from glioma-cell lines mimic these observations by inhibiting the expression of IL-12 by SAC-stimulated monocytes. Together, these observations suggest that monocytes play an intermediary role in the observed glioma-induced cytokine shift from Th-1 to Th-2 profiles. The studies also indicated that the inhibitory effect of glioma-derived factors on IL-12 secretion occurs partly by an IL-10-independent mechanism, as neutralizing antibodies to IL-10 do not restore IL-12 secretion levels of GCS-treated SAC-stimulated monocytes to normal levels. This is supported by the observation that addition of IL-10-neutralizing antibodies does not alleviate the direct inhibitory effect of GCS on T-cell responsiveness to anti-CD3 MAb (L. Morford, unpublished observation). Thus, although some of the immune anomalies observed in patients with glioma can be attributed to increased production of IL-10 by monocytes or the glioma tumor itself, other IL-10-independent mechanisms are also operant.

Gangliosides are glycosphingolipids that are primarily anchored in the outer leaflet of cell membranes, but can be shed into the extracellular environment at especially high levels by malignant cells *(92)*. These have been detected in culture supernatants of cloned tumor-cell lines, including gliomas, as well as in the serum of cancer patients *(92,93)*. Gangliosides that are shed into extracellular fluids can bind to lipids and proteins *(94)*, but can also be picked up by adjacent cells and inserted into their membranes *(92)*. As ubiquitous membrane components, gangliosides function primarily in cellular adhesion, recognition, signaling, and growth regulation *(92)*, but have also been demonstrated to possess potent immunosuppressive activities that affect APC and T-cell function *(92,95–100)*. These observations, together with the fact that they are expressed at high levels in the CNS *(101–103)*, make gangliosides potential candidates for the maintenance of immunoprivilege in the brain, as well as likely mediators of immune evasion by tumors. This is supported by studies that demonstrate that brain-derived gangliosides inhibit murine T-cell function in vitro, as evidenced by impaired dose-dependent proliferative responses to mitogens and decreased gene expression of IL-2 and IFN-γ *(92)*. Interestingly, expression of the Th-2 cytokines IL-4 and IL-10 are not suppressed by gangliosides. The inhibition of T-cell proliferation is associated with a block in T-cell signaling downsteam of early transmembrane signaling events that are required for the activation of NF-κB transcription factor. Furthermore, the proliferative response cannot be restored with the addition of exogenous IL-2, and persists because the entry into the cell cycle is blocked. Gangliosides inhibit expression of CD4 on human and murine T-cells and block the generation of both cytotoxic T lymphocytes (CTL) and NK cell activity *(95,98,104)*.

3.3. In Vitro Correlates of Glioma-Induced Immune Suppression

Studies from our laboratory suggest that the immunocompromised state of patients with gliomas—which is correlated with a Th-1-to-Th-2 cytokine profile shift and intrinsic T-cell defects—results from direct and/or indirect effects of tumor-derived immunosuppressive factors (reviewed in revs. *71* and *105*). In these studies, we demonstrate that glioma-culture supernatant (GCS) from freshly explanted gliomas as well as the cloned glioma-cell lines, SNB-19, SNB-56 *(106)*, and U251 *(107)* when added to T cells isolated from normal donors, reproduce many of the T-cell anomalies that we have previously observed in patients with gliomas *(50,77,78)*. These studies, which used GCS-treated normal T cells as an in vitro correlate to our tumor model, have provided us with the opportunity to better define the inherent cellular and molecular defects mediated by glioma-derived immunosuppressive factors, and to develop a model for the glioma induced T-cell anergy and increased sensitivity to apoptosis observed in patients with gliomas (Fig. 1).

The results of these in vitro studies demonstrated that GCS collected from freshly explanted gliomas obtained from patients and cloned glioma-cell lines inhibit mitogen responsiveness of both CD4- and CD8-positive T cells in a dose-

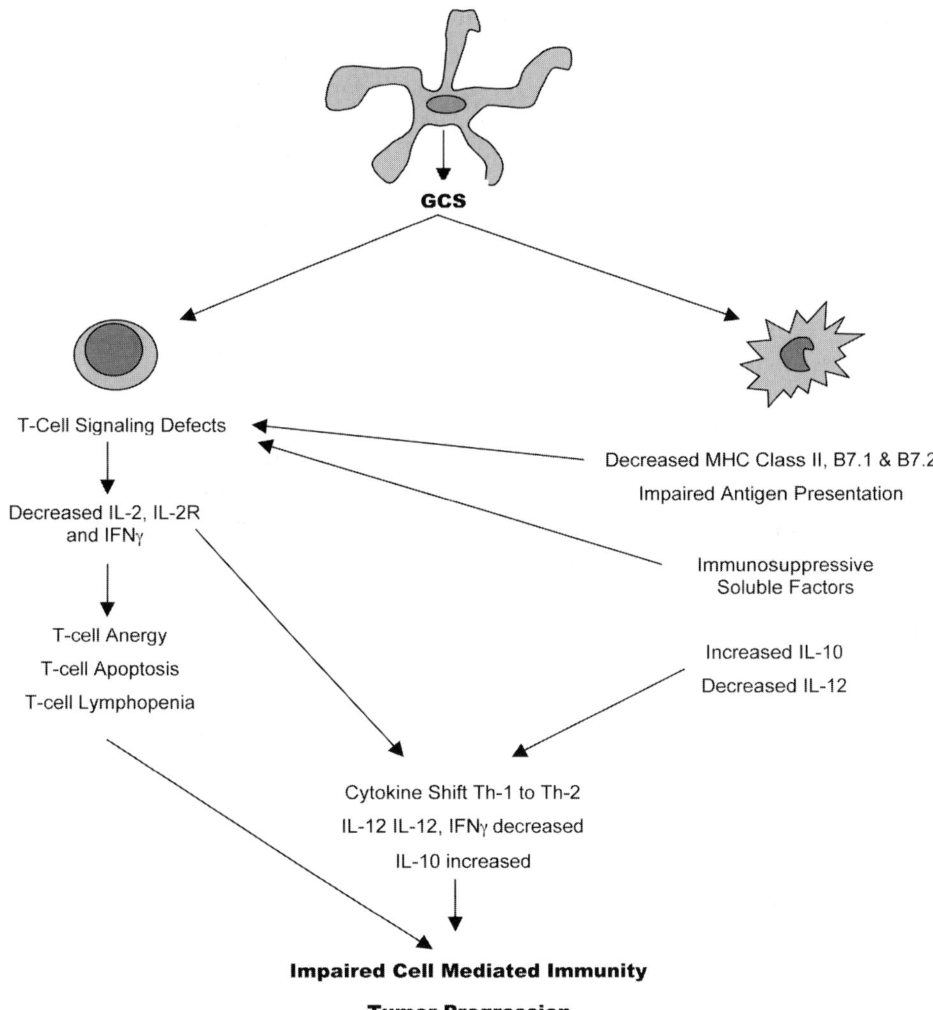

Fig. 1. Immune modulation by gliomas. Immunomodulatory factors secreted by gliomas (GCS) directly or indirectly, via monocyte actions, suppress T-cell function in patients. Suppression of immune function of monocytes and/or T cells by GCS results in alterations in the cytokine profile from a protective Th-1 response to a nonprotective Th-2 response that ultimately contributes to tumor progression.

dependent manner, as evidenced by decreased DNA *(77)* and RNA (L. Morford, unpublished observation) synthesis, and induce apoptosis of mitogen activated T cells 72–96 h post-exposure to GCS *(50)*. The block in T-cell activation appears to occur in early activation events, as GCS must be added within the first 24 h of culture in order to cause maximal inhibition *(77)*. The studies also indicated that GCS-induced T-cell anergy is correlated with suppression of IL-2 secretion as well as a block in the expression of high-affinity IL-2 receptors *(78)*. GCS-induced T-cell anergy cannot be rescued with the addition of an exogenous source of rIL-2 alone *(78)*, or in the presence of additional costimulation via CD2 or CD28 accessory molecules (AR Dix, unpublished observation).

Although GCS appears to have some direct effects on T-cell function of purified T cells, recent data suggest that monocytes also play a definitive role in mediating the immunoregulatory effects of GCS *(51)*. As previously discussed, these data indicate that GCS induces a shift in cytokine production of SAC-stimulated monocytes, inhibiting IL-12 and stimulating IL-10. GCS also reduces the antigen-presenting capabilities of monocytes by decreasing the expression of MHC class II molecules as well as B7.1 and B7.2. The intermediary role of monocytes and monocyte-derived factors in this tumor model (Fig. 1) is further supported by data collected from recent experiments using purified monocytes from normal donors as well as the monocyte cell lines, THP-1 and U947. In these studies, the GCS pretreated monocytes were placed in the upper chamber of a transwell culture system, and T-cells obtained from normal donors were stimulated with immobilized anti-CD3 MAb in the lower chamber. The studies indicate that GCS pretreated monocytes secrete soluble factors, which block the proliferative response of normal T cells to anti-CD3 mAb (AR Dix, unpublished observation).

In an attempt to identify potential immunoregulatory moieties in the GCS, enzyme-linked immunosorbent assays (ELISAs) were used to screen six different lots of supernatants collected from SNB-19 for the presence of known immunomodulatory cytokines and growth factors *(51)*. These studies indicated that GCS collected from SNB-19 contain significant amounts of IL-6, transforming growth factor (TGF)-β1, calcitonin gene-related peptide (CGRP) and very low levels of PGE_2 (<7 pg/mL). The culture supernatant does not contain detectable levels of IL-10, IL-12, TNF-α, or IFN-γ. However, IL-6, TGF-β, CGRP, or PGE_2 do not appear to play significant roles in the immunomodulatory activity of GCS obtained from SNB-19. PGE_2 is not a likely candidate, because the concentration found in SNB-19 is less than that reported to modulate cytokine production by PBL *(51)*, and the addition of naproxin or indomethacin to the cell lines does not block secretion of factors, which block the mitogen responsiveness of normal T cells *(77)*. A potential role for IL-6, TGF-β, and (CGRP) in GCS modulation of cytokine production was ruled out when neutralizing antibodies to these cytokines or removal by immunoprecipitation did not alter the immunomodulatory capacity of SNB-19 GCS *(51)*. These data suggest that other unknown glioma-derived moieties are involved in the GCS induced immune modulation of T cells and monocytes.

Attempts to purify the unknown suppressor factor(s) contained in the GCS from the cloned glioma-cell lines studied in our laboratory have been unsuccessful thus far, but the moieties that mediate the immunomodulatory activities of GCS have been partially characterized *(51,77,78)*. Thus, GCS was exposed to a variety of physical and chemical treatments before assaying its activity in two biological assays: i) inhibition T-cell proliferation to PHA; ii) modulation of cytokine production by SAC-stimulated monocytes. The data suggest that multiple factors or complexes of factors are involved in the modulation of T cells and monocytes. For example, GCS-mediated inhibition of T-cell proliferation is sensitive to heating at 56°C and 100°C for 30 min and treatment with immobilized trypsin for 15 min, but stable to both alkaline (to pH 11.0) and acidic (to pH 2.0) exposure. On the other hand, GCS modulation of monokine secretion is resistant to heating at 56°C as well as acid and alkali exposure, but sensitive to heating at 100°C. Both biological activities are retained by anion-exchange columns (Q and DEAE Sepharose) but not cation-exchange columns (SP and CM Sepharose), and have a minimum molecular mass of 45 kDa. However, both activities are eluted at higher molecular masses (68 kDa and 150 kDa), suggesting that the factors form large aggregates with other proteins or lipids (L Morford, unpublished observation).

Together, these data support a model of immunosuppression by glioma-derived factors, which involves numerous pathways and targets (Fig. 1). Thus, GCS can act directly on T helper cells, inducing anergy and increasing sensitivity to apoptosis. T-cell anergy is coupled to defects in early transmembrane signaling that block the expression of IL-2, and high-affinity receptors. As a result, clonal expansion of stimulated T cells does not occur, and the concurrent induction of apoptotic signals contributes to the T-cell lymphopenia observed in these patients. However, the data also suggest an intermediary role for monocytes in this tumor model. Thus, GCS downmodulates the expression of Class II MHC and B7 accessory molecules on monocytes, severely blocking their antigen-presenting capability, which could in turn contribute to the induction of T-cell anergy and apoptosis. Furthermore, soluble mediators elicited by GCS-treated monocytes can also impair T-cell function and induce apoptosis of T cells. Finally, GCS can redirect monocyte cytokine production to modulate the shift in cytokine profiles from Th-1 to Th-2, as evidenced by increased secretion of IL-10 and decreased expression of IL-12 by monocytes, which in turn contributes to the decreased production of IFN-γ by T cells.

REFERENCES

1. Brooks W, Netsky M, Normansell D, Horwitz D. Depressed cell-mediated immunity in patients with primary intracranial tumors. Characterization of a humoral immunosuppressive factor. *N Engl J Med* 1972;136:1631–1647.
2. Brooks W, Caldwell H, Mortara R. Immune responses in patients with gliomas. *Surg Neurol* 1974;2:419–423.

3. Brooks, W, Roszman T, Rogers A. Impairment of rosette-forming T-lymphocytes in patients with primary intracranial tumors. *Cancer* 1976;37:1869–1873
4. Brooks W, Roszman T, Mahaley M, Woosley R. Immunobiology of primary intracranial tumors: II Analysis of lymphocytes subpopulations in patients with primary brain tumors. *Clin Exp Immunol* 1977;29:61–66.
5. Young H, Kaplan A. Cellular immune deficiency in patients with glioblastoma. *Surg Forum* 1976;27:476–478.
6. Mahaley M, Brooks W, Roszman T, Bigner D, Dudka L, Richardson S. Immunobiology of primary intracranial tumors: Part 1: studies of the cellular and humoral general immune competence of brain-tumor patients. *J Neurosurg* 1977;46:467–476.
7. Elliott L, Brooks W, Roszman T. Activation of immunoregulatory lymphocytes obtained from patients with malignant glomas. *J Neurosurg* 1987;67:231–236.
8. Roszman T, Brooks W. Immunobiology of primary intracranial tumors: III. Demonstration of a qualitative lymphocyte abnormality in patients with primary brain tumors. *Clin Exp Immunol* 1980;39:395–402.
9. Roszman T, Brooks W, Elliott L. Immunobiology of primary intracranial tumors: VI. Suppressor cell function and lectin-binding lymphocyte subpopulations in patients with cerebral tumors. *Cancer* 1982;50:1273–1279.
10. Elliott L, Brooks W, Roszman T. Role of interleukin-2 (IL-2) and IL-2 receptor expression in the proliferative defect observed in mitogen-stimulated lymphocytes from patients with gliomas. *J Natl Cancer Inst* 1987;78:919–922.
11. Elliott L, Brooks W, Roszman T. Cytokinetic basis for the impaired activation of lymphocytes from patients with primary intracranial tumors. *J Immunol* 1984;132:1208–1215.
12. Roszman T, Brooks W, Steele C, Elliott L. Pokeweed mitogen-induced immunoglobulin secretion by peripheral blood lymphocytes from patients with primary intracranial tumors. Characterization of T helper and B cell function. *J Immunol* 1985; 134:1545–1550.
13. Ashkenazi E, Deutsch M, Tirosh R, Weinreb A, Tsukerman A, Brodie C. A selective impairment of the IL-2 system in lymphocytes of patients with glioblastomas: increased level of soluble IL-2R and reduced protein tyrosine phosphorylation. *Neuroimmunomodulation* 1997; 4:49–56.
14. Elliott L, Brooks W, Roszman, T. Inability of mitogen-activated lymphocytes obtained from patients with malignant primary intracranial tumors to express high affinity interleukin 2 receptors. *J Clin Investig* 1990;86:80–86.
15. Kamio M, Arima N, Tsudo M, Imada K, Ohkuma M, Uchiyama T. The third molecule associated with interleukin 2 receptor α and β chain. *Biochem Biophys Res Comm* 1992; 184:1288–1292.
16. Taniguchi T, Minami Y. The IL-2 receptor system: a current overview. *Cell* 1993;73:5–8.
17. Imboden J, Stobo J. Transmembrane signaling by the T cell antigen receptor. Perturbation of the T3-antigen receptor complex generates inositol phosphates and releases calcium ions from intracellular stores. *J Exp Med* 1985;262:446–456.
18. June C, Fletcher M, Ledbetter J, Samelson L. Increases in tyrosine phosphorylation are detectable before phospholipase C activation after T cell receptor stimulation. *J Immunol* 1990;144:1591–1599.
19. Chan A, Irving B, Fraser J, Weiss A. The zeta chain is associated with a tyrosine kinase and upon T-cell antigen receptor stimulation associates with ZAP-70, a 70-kDa tyrosine phosphoprotein. *Proc Natl Acad Sci USA* 1991;88:9166–9170.
20. Straus D, Weiss A. Genetic evidence for the involvement of the lck tyrosine kinase in signal transduction through the T cell antigen receptor. *Cell* 1992;70:585–593.
21. His E, Siegel J, Minami Y, Luong E., Klausner R, Samelson L. T cell activation induces rapid tyrosine phosphorylation of a limited number of cellular substrates. *J Biol Chem* 1989; 264:10,836–10,842.

22. Veillette A, Brookman M, Horak E, Samelson L, Bolen J. Signal transduction through the CD4 receptor involves the activation of the internal membrane tyrosine-protein kinase p56[lck]. *Nature* 1989;338:257–259.
23. Secrist J, Karnitz L, Abraham R. T-cell antigen receptor ligation induces tyrosine phosphorylation of phospholipase C-γ1. *J Biol Chem* 1991:12,135–12,139.
24. Weiss A, Koretzky G, Schatzman R, Kadlecek T. Functional activation of the T-cell antigen receptor induces tyrosine phosphorylation of phospholipase C-γ1. *Proc Natl Acad Sci USA* 1991;88:5484–5488.
25. Imboden J, Weiss A. The T-cell antigen receptor regulates sustained increases in cytoplasmic free Ca^{2+} influx and ongoing intracellular Ca^{2+} mobilization. *Biochem J* 1987;247:695–700.
26. Isakov N, Mally M, Schotz W, Atlman A. T-lymphocyte activation: The role of protein kinase C and the bifurcating inositol phospholipid signal transduction pathway. *Immunol Rev* 1987;95:89–111.
27. Morford L, Elliott L, Carlson S, Brooks W, Roszman. T cell receptor-mediated signaling is defective in T cells obtained from patients with primary intracranial tumors. *J Immunol* 1997;159:4415–4425.
28. Anel A, Kleinfeld A. Tyrosine phosphorylation of a 100kDa protein is correlated with cytotoxic T-lymphocyte function. Evidence from cis unsaturated fatty acid and phenylarsineoxide inhibition *J Biol Chem* 1993;268:17,578–17,587.
29. Skalhegg B, Rasmussen A, Tasken K, Hansson V, Jahnsen T, Lea T. Cyclic AMP sensitive signaling by the CD28 marker requires concomitant stimulation by the T-cell antigen receptor (TCR/CD3) complex. *Scand J Immunol* 1994;40:202–208.
30. Abraham N, Miceli M, Parnes J, Veillette A. Enhancement of T-cell receptor responsiveness by the lymphocyte specific tyrosine protein kinase p56. *Nature* 1991;350:62–66.
31. Cho E, Riley M, Sillman A, Quill H. Altered protein tyrosine phosphorylation in anergy Th1 cells. *J Immunol* 1993;151:20–28.
32. Bhandoola A, Cho E, Yui K, Saragovi H, Greene M, Quill H. Reduced CD3-mediated protein tyrosine phosphorylation in anergic CD4+ and CD8+ T cells. *J Immunol* 1993;151:2355–2367.
33. Gajewski T, Qian D, Fields P, Fitch F. Anergic T-lymphocyte clones have altered inositol phosphate, calcium and tyrosine kinase signaling pathways. *Proc Natl Acad Sci USA* 1994;91:38–42.
34. Migita K, Eguchi K, KawabeY Y, Tsukada T, Ichinose Y, Nagataki S, Ochi A. Defective TCR-mediated signalin in anergic T cells *J Immunol* 1995;155:5083–5087, published erratum appears in *J Immunol* 1996;156;8:following 3088.
35. Quill H, Riley M, Cho E, Casnellie J, Reed J, Torigoe T. Anergic Th1 cells express altered levels of the protein tyrosine kinases p56[lck] and p59[fyn]. *J Immunol* 1992;149:2887–2839.
36. Schwartz RH. A cell culture model for T lymphocyte clonal anergy. *Science* 1990;248:1349–1356.
37. Schwartz RH. Models of T cell anergy: is there a common molecular mechanism? *J Exp Med* 1996;184:1–8.
38. Clevers H, Alarcon B, Willeman T, Terhorst C. The T cell receptor/CD3 complex: a dynamic protein ensemble. *Annu Rev Immunol* 1988;6:629–662.
39. Weiss A. Molecular and genetic insights into T cell antigen receptor structure and function. *Annu Rev Genet* 1991;8:139–168.
40. Crabtree G, Clipstone N. Signal transmission between the plasma membrane and nucleus of T lymphocytes *Annu Rev Biochem* 1994;63:1045–1083.
41. Schwartz RH. Costimulation of T lymphocytes: the role of CD28, CTLA-4, and B7/BB1 in interleukin-2 production and immunotherapy. *Cell* 1992;71:1065–1068.

42. Boise LH, Minn AT, Noel PJ, June CH, Accavitti MA, Landsten T. CD28 costimulation can promote T cell survival by enhancing the expression of Bcl-x_L. *Immunity* 1995;3:87–98.
43. Vella AT, Mitchell T, Groth B, Linsley PS, Green JM, Thompson CB. CD28 engagement and proinflammatory cytokines contribute to T cell expansion and long-term survival in vivo. *J Immunol* 1997:158:4714–4720.
44. Thompson C. (1999) Apoptosis. In: *Fundamental Immunology*, 4th ed. (Paul WE, ed.), Lippincott-Raven, Philadelphia, PA, pp. 813–829.
45. Itoh N, Yonehara S, Ishii A, Yonehara M, Mizushima S, Sameshima M, et al. The polypeptide encoded by the cDNA for human cell surface antigen FAS can mediate apoptosis. *Cell* 1991;66:233–243.
46. Suda T, Nagata S. Purification and characterization of the Fas-ligand that induces apoptosis. *J Exp Med* 1994;179:873–879.
47. Tachibana O, Nakazawa H, Lampe J, Watanabe K, Kleihues P, Ohgaki H. Expression of Fas/APO-1 during the progression of astrocytomas. *Cancer Res* 1995;55:5528–5530.
48. Weller M, Kleihues P, Dichgans J, Ohgaki H. CD95 ligand: lethal weapon against malignant glioma? *Brain Pathol* 1998;8:285–293.
49. Saas P, et al. Fas ligand expression by astrocytoma in vivo; maintaining immune privilege in the brain?. *J Clin Investig* 1997;99:1173–1178.
50. Morford L, Dix A, Brooks W, Roszman T. Apoptotic elimination of peripheral T-lymphocytes in patients with primary intracranial tumors. *J Neurosurg* 1999;6:935–946.
51. Zou J-P, Morford L, Chougnet C, Dix A, Brooks A, Torres N, et al. Human glioma-induced immunosuppression involves soluble factor(s) that alter monocyte cytokine profile and surface markers. *J Immunol* 1999;162:4882–4892.
52. Adachi Y, Oyaizu N, Than S, McCloskey T, Pahwa S. IL-2 rescues in vitro lymphocyte apoptosis in patients with HIV infection: correlation with its ability to block culture-induced downmodulation of Bcl-2. *J Immunol* 1996;157:4184–4193.
53. Clerici M, Shearer G, Clerici E. Cytokine dysregulation in invasive cervical carcinoma and other human neoplasias: time to consider the Th1/Th2 paradigm. *J Natl Cancer Inst* 1998;18:261–263.
54. Clerici m, Shearer G. A TH1 to TH2 switch is a critical step in the etiology of HIV infection. *Immunol Today* 1993;15:575–581.
55. Kaufmann S. Immunity to intracellular microbial pathogens. *Immunol Today* 1995;215: 221–238.
56. Daugelat S, Kaufmann S. (1996) Role of Th1 and Th2 cells in bacterial infections. In: *Th1 and Th2 Cells in Health and Disease* (Romagnani S, ed.), Switzerland, Karger, Basel, pp. 66–97.
57. Yang B-C, Wang Y, Lin L-C, Lui M. Induction of apoptosis and cytokine gene expression in T-cell lines by sera of patients with systemic lupus erythematosis. *Scand J Immunol* 1997;46:96–102.
58. Elgert K, Alleva D, Mullins D. Tumor-induced immune dysfunction: the macrophage connection. *J Leukoc Biol* 1998;64:275–290.
59. Das G, Vohra H, Rao K, Saha B, Mishra G. *Leshmania donovani* infection of a susceptible host results in CD4+ T-cell apoptosis and decreased Th1 cytokine production. *Scand J Immunol* 1999;49:307–310.
60. Ausiello C, Maleci A, Cassone A. Modulation of immune function by glioma. *Immunol Today* 1992;13(4):148.
61. Urbani F, Maleci A, La Sala A, Lande R, Ausiello C. Defective expression of interferon-gamma, granulocyte-macrophage colony-stimulating factor, tumor necrosis factor alpha and interleukin-6 in activated peripheral blood lymphocytes from glioma patients. *J Interferon Cytokine Res* 1995;15:421–429.

62. Roussel E, Gingras M, Grimm E, Bruner J, Moser R. Predominance of a type 2 intratumoural immune response in fresh tumour-infiltrating lymphocytes from human gliomas. *Clin Exp Immunol* 1996;105:344–352.
63. Nitta T, Hishii M, Sato K, Okumura K. Selective expression of interleukin-10 within glioblastoma multiforme. *Brain Res* 1994;649:122–128.
64. Hishii M, Nitta T, Ishida H, Ebato M, Kurosu A, Yagita H, et al. Human glioma-drived interleukin-10 inhibits antitumor immune response in vitro. *Neurosurgery* 1995;37: 1160–1166.
65. Huettner C, Czub S, Kerkau S, Roggendorf W, Tonn J. Interleukin 10 is expressed in human gliomas in vivo and increases glioma cell proliferation and motility in vitro. *Anticancer Res* 1997;17:3217–3224.
66. Woiciechowsky C, Asadullah K, Nestler D, Schoning B, Glockner F, Docke W, Volk H. Diminished monocytic HLA-DR expression and ex vivo cytokine secretion capacity in patients with glioblastoma: effect of tumor extirpation. *J Neuroimmunol* 1998;84:164–171.
67. Aliprantis A, Diez-Roux G, Mulder L, Zychlinsky A, Lang R. Do macrophages kill through apoptosis? *Immunol Today* 1996;17:573–576.
68. Fries G, Perneczky A, Kempski O. Glioblastoma-associated circulating monocytes and the release of epidermal growth factor. *Neurosurgery* 1996;85:642–647.
69. Giometto B, Bozza F, Faresin F, Alessio L, Mingrino S, Tavolato B. Immune infiltrates and cytokines in gliomas. *Acta Neurochir* 1996;138:50–56.
70. Fries G, Perneczky A, Kempski O. Enhanced interleukin-1 beta release and longevity of glioma-associated peripheral blood monocytes in vitro. *Neurosurgery* 1994;35:264–270.
71. Roszman T, Elliott L, Brooks W. Modulation of T-cell function by gliomas. *Immunol Today* 1991;12:370–374.
72. Brooks W, Latta R, Mahaley M, Roszman T, Dudka L, Skaggs C. Immunobiology of primary intracranial tumors: Part 5: correlation of a lymphocyte index and clinical status. *J Neurosurg* 1981;54:331–337.
73. Young H, Sakalas R, Kaplan A. Inhibition of cell-mediated immunity in patients with brain tumors. *Surg Neurol* 1976;5:19–20.
74. Levy N. Cell-mediated cytotoxicity and serum-mediated blocking: evidence that their associated determinants on human tumor cells are different. *J Immunol* 1978;121:916–922.
75. Kikuchi K, Neuwelt E. Presence of immunosuppressive factors in brain-tumor cyst fluid. *J Neurosurg* 1983;59:790–799.
76. Tada T, Yabu K, Kobayashi S. Detection of active form of transforming growth factor-beta in cerebrospinal fluid of patients with glioma. *Jpn J Cancer Res* 1993;84:544–548.
77. Roszman T, Brooks W, Elliott L. Inhibition of lymphocyte responsiveness by a glial tumor cell-derived suppressor factor. *J Neurosurg* 1987;67:874–879.
78. Elliott L, Brooks W, Roszman T. Suppression of high affinity IL-2 receptors on mitogen activated lymphocytes by glioma-derived suppressor factor. *J Neurooncol* 1992;14:1–7.
79. Wrann M, Bodmer S, de Martin R, Siepl C, Hofer-Warbinek R, Frei K, et al. T cell suppressor factor from human glioblastoma cells is a 12.5-kd protein closely related to transforming growth factor-beta. *EMBO J* 1987;6:1633–1636.
80. Davies P, MacIntyre DE. (1992) Prostaglandins and inflammation. In: *Inflammation*, 2nd ed. (Gallin JL, Goldstein IM, Snyderman R, eds.), Raven Press, New York, NY, pp. 123–138.
81. Goetzl EJ, An S, Smith WL. Specificity of expression and effects of eicosanoid mediators in normal physiology and human disease. *FASEB J* 1995;44:1–10.
82. Seibert K, Masferrer J, Zhang Y et al. Mediation of inflammation by cyclooxygenase-2. *Agents Actions Suppl* 1995;46:41–50.
83. van der Pouw, Kraan TC, Boeije LC, Smeenk RJ, Wijdenes J, Aarden LA. Prostaglandin-E2 is a potent inhibitor of human interleukin 12 production. *J Exp Med* 1995;181 :775–779.

84. Katamura K, Shintaku N, Yamauchi Y, et al. Prostglandin E2 at priming of naïve CD4+ T cells inhibits acquisition of ability to produce IFN-gamma and IL-2, but not IL-4 and IL-5. *J Immunol* 1995;146:4406–4612.
85. Hilkens CM, Vermeulen H, van Neervens RJ, Snijdewint FG, Wierenga EA, Kapsenberg ML. Differential modulation of T helper type 1 (Th1) and T helper type 2 (Th2) cytokine secretion by prostaglandin E2 critically depends on interleukin-2. *Eur J Immunol* 1995;25:59–63.
86. Castelli MG, Chiabrando C, Fanelli R, Martelli L, Butti B, Gaetani P, et al. Prostaglandin and thromboxane synthesis by human intracranial tumor. *Cancer Res* 1989;49:1504–1508
87. Black KL, Chen K, Becker DP, Merrill JE. Inflammatory leukocytes associated with increased immunosuppression by glioblastoma. *J Neurosurg* 1992;77:120–126.
88. Couldwell WT, Dore-Duffy P, Apuzzo ML, Antel JP. Malignant glioma modulation of immune function: relative contribution of different soluble factors. *J Neuroimmunol* 1991;33:89–96.
89. Weller M, Fontana A. The failure of current immunotherapy for malignant glioma. Tumor-derived TGF-beta, T-cell apoptosis and the immune privilege of the brain. *Brain Res Rev* 1995;21:128–151.
90. Munz C, Naumann U, Grimmel C, Rammensee HG, Weller M. TGF-beta-independent induction of immunogenicity by decorin gene transfer in human malignant glioma cells. *Eur J Immunol* 1999;29:1032–1040.
91. Moore KW, O'Garra A, de Waal Malefyt R, Vieira P, Mosmann TR. Interleukin 10. *Annu Rev Immunol* 1993;11:165–190.
92. Irani DN, Lin Kuo-I, Griffin DE. Brain-derived gangliosides regulate the cytokine production and proliferation of activated T cells. *J Immunol* 1996;157:4333–4340.
93. Ladisch S, Wu Z-L. Detection of a tumor-associated ganglioside in plasma of patients with neuroblastoma. *Lancet J* 1985;1:136–138.
94. Valentino LA, Ladisch S. Localization of shed human tumor gangliosides: association with serum lipoproteins. *Cancer Res* 1992;52:810–814.
95. Ikeda T, Nakakuma H, Shionoya H, Kawaguchi T, Yamatsu K, Takatsuki K. Ganglioside-induced inhibition of in vivo immune response in mice. *Life Sci* 1992;51;847–851.
96. Whisler RL, Yates AJ. Regulation of lymphocyte responses by human gangliosides: I. Characteristics of inhibitory effects and the induction of impaired activation. *J Immunol* 1980;125:2106–2111.
97. Landisch S, Ulsh L, Gillard B, et al. Modulation of the immune response by gangliosides: inhibition of human adherent accessory cell function. *J Clin Investig* 1984;74:2074–2081.
98. Merrit WD, Bailey JM, Pluznik DH, Inhibition of interleukin-2-dependent cytotoxic T-lymphocyte growth by gangliosides. *Cell Immunol* 1984;89:1–10.
99. Landisch L, Becker H, Ulsh L. Immunosuppression by human gangliosides: I. Relationship of carbohydrate structure to the inhibition of T cell responses. *Biochem Biophys Acta* 1992;1125:180–188.
100. Li R, Villacreses N, Ladisch S. Human tumor gangliosides inhibit murine immune responses in vivo. *Cancer Res* 1995;55:211–214.
101. Fredman P, von Holst H, Collins VP, Granholm L, Svennerholm L. Sialyllactotetraosylceramide, a ganglioside marker for human malignant gliomas. *J Neurochem* 1988;50: 912–919.
102. Fredman P, Mansson J-E, Delheden B, Bostrom K, von Holst H. Expression of the GM1-species, [NeuN]-GM1, in a case of human glioma. *Neurochem Res* 1999;24; 275–279.
103. Kawai K, Takahashi H, Watarai S, Ishizu H, Fukai K, Tanabe Y, et al. Occurrence of ganglioside GD3 in neoplastic astrocytes. An immunocytochemical sutudy in humans *Virchows Arch* 1999;434:201–205.

104. Offner H, Thieme T, Vandernbark AA. Gangliosides induce selective modulation of CD4 helper T lymphocytes. *J Immunol* 1987;139:3295–3305.
105. Dix AR, Brooks WH, Roszman TL, Morford LA. Immune defects observed in patients with primary malignant brain tumors. *J Neuroimmunol* 1999;100:216–232.
106. Welch WC, Morrison RS, Gross JL, Gollin SM, Kitson RB, Golfarb RH, et al. Morphologic, immunologic, biochemical and cytogenetic characteristics of the human glioblastoma-derived cell line, SNB-19. *In Vitro Cell Dev Biol Anim* 1995;31;610–616.
107. Bigner DD, Bigner SH, Ponten J, Westermark B, Mahaley MS, Ruoslahti E, et al. Heterogeneity of genotypic and phenotypic characteristics of fifteen permanent cell lines derived from human gliomas. *J Neuropathol Exp Neurol* 1981;40:201–229.

Index

f: figure
t: table

B

C

I

M

N

U

V

W

Z